QUALITY MANAGEMENT
IN THE IMAGING SCIENCES

Seventh Edition

QUALITY MANAGEMENT

IN THE **IMAGING SCIENCES**

Jeffrey Papp, PhD, RT(R)(QM)

Emeritus Professor of Physics and Diagnostic Imaging
College of DuPage
Glen Ellyn, IL

ELSEVIER

Elsevier
3251 Riverport Lane
St. Louis, Missouri 63043

QUALITY MANAGEMENT IN THE IMAGING SCIENCES, SEVENTH EDITION   ISBN: 978-0-323-83292-2

Notices

Knowledge and best practice in this field are constantly changing. As new research and experience broaden our understanding, changes in research methods, professional practices, or medical treatment may become necessary.

Practitioners and researchers must always rely on their own experience and knowledge in evaluating and using any information, methods, compounds, or experiments described herein. In using such information or methods they should be mindful of their own safety and the safety of others, including parties for whom they have a professional responsibility.

With respect to any drug or pharmaceutical products identified, readers are advised to check the most current information provided (i) on procedures featured or (ii) by the manufacturer of each product to be administered, to verify the recommended dose or formula, the method and duration of administration, and contraindications. It is the responsibility of practitioners, relying on their own experience and knowledge of their patients, to make diagnoses, to determine dosages and the best treatment for each individual patient, and to take all appropriate safety precautions.

To the fullest extent of the law, neither the Publisher nor the authors, contributors, or editors, assume any liability for any injury and/or damage to persons or property as a matter of products liability, negligence or otherwise, or from any use or operation of any methods, products, instructions, or ideas contained in the material herein.

Previous editions copyrighted 2019, 2015, 2011, 2006, 2002, 1998.

Content Strategist: Meg Benson
Content Development Manager: Ranjana Sharma
Senior Content Development Specialist: Vaishali Singh
Senior Project Manager: Manchu Mohan
Designer: Ryan Cook

Printed in India.

Last digit is the print number: 9 8 7 6 5 4 3 2 1

To my wonderful family and all of my
students, past, present, and future.

The author and publisher wish to acknowledge the following previous edition contributors.

Lorrie Kelley, MS, RT(R)(MR)(CT)
Associate Professor and Director
CT/MRI Programs
Boise State University
Boise, Idaho

James M. Kofler Jr., PhD
Assistant Professor of Radiologic Physics
Department of Diagnostic Radiology, Mayo College of Medicine
Mayo Clinic
Rochester, Minnesota

Joanne M. Metler, MS, CNMT
Assistant Professor Emeritus
Nuclear Medicine Technology Program
College of DuPage
Glen Ellyn, Illinois

James A. Zagzebski, PhD
Professor Emeritus
Departments of Medical Physics, Human Oncology, and Radiology
University of Wisconsin
Madison, Wisconsin

Quality Management in the Imaging Sciences includes the most up-to-date information available on the quality control aspects of digital imaging systems, image processing, radiographic equipment and accessories, fluoroscopic and advanced imaging equipment, radiographic image artifacts, repeat analysis, mammographic quality standards, computed tomography, magnetic resonance imaging, diagnostic ultrasound, and nuclear medicine. Quality assurance organizations and their websites are listed in Appendix A, and full-page documentation forms are available in Evolve Resources.

The following special features are included, as in the first six editions:

- Federal regulations are set in boldface type in the text and the symbol appears beside them.
- Procedures are highlighted as separate elements with step-by-step guidelines.
- Key terms are identified at the beginnings of chapters, set in boldface type, and explained within chapters.
- Learning objectives, chapter outlines, and chapter review questions (with answers) are provided as study tools.
- Key term definitions are collected in a glossary.

NEW TO THE SEVENTH EDITION

Additional updates continue to benefit the reader:

1. Revisions to the mammography chapter correspond with new digital mammographic systems that have received Food and Drug Administration approval.
2. The material on Evolve Resources that accompanies the text offers these features:
   a. Full-size sample documentation forms that can be used "as is" or modified to meet the needs of a particular department.
   b. Student experiments and analyses of them to correspond with appropriate chapters that have been modified for digital-only departments.
   c. Questions for analysis and critical thinking that challenge the reader to prepare for real-life situations.
3. An updated chapter on image quality that is common to all imaging modalities.
4. Additional material on dose levels, dose reporting, and workflow.
5. Expanded material for digital imaging and quality control procedures for electronic image monitors and picture archiving and communication systems.
6. The latest changes in technology and current regulations have been updated throughout.

Quality Management in the Imaging Sciences continues to provide the wealth of information needed for instructors to guide students through quality management issues, and for students and for technologists to succeed in the delivery of high-quality services.

INSTRUCTOR RESOURCES

Instructor ancillaries, including a test bank of more than 400 questions; an electronic image collection of the images in the text; an instructor's manual of chapter outlines, teaching tips, and teaching strategies; and a new PowerPoint lecture presentation are all available at http://evolve.elsevier.com.

Jeffrey Papp, PhD, RT(R)(QM)

ACKNOWLEDGMENTS

Just as with the first six editions of this text, the production of this seventh edition has required the help and input of many people. I must start with my now former associates in the Diagnostic Medical Imaging program at the College of DuPage, namely Shelli Thacker and Sue Dumford, for all of their support and understanding while I was preoccupied with writing this text. I also thank Patty Holvey of Advocate Good Samaritan Hospital in Downers Grove, Illinois; Janet Petersen of Elmhurst Memorial Hospital, Elmhurst, Illinois; and Pam Verkuilen of Ascension Saint Alexius Medical Center in Hoffman Estates, Illinois, for all of their help in gathering information on digital imaging.

I am deeply indebted to my contributing authors: Lorrie Kelley, program director for CT/MRI at Boise State University; James M. Kofler, assistant professor, Department of Diagnostic Radiology, Mayo Clinic; Joanne M. Metler, emeritus coordinator for Nuclear Medicine at the College of DuPage; and James A. Zagzebski, professor of medical physics at the University of Wisconsin, Madison.

I would also like to thank Meg Benson, Sonya Seigafuse, Vaishali Singh, Charu Bali, and everyone at Elsevier for their help, support, and patience in the production of this text and the accompanying material found in the Evolve Resources.

Finally, I must thank Professor Gerard Lietz of DePaul University for giving me the knowledge, inspiration, and love of medical physics that allowed me to be successful in this profession.

Jeffrey Papp, PhD, RT(R)(QM)

CONTENTS

QUALITY MANAGEMENT
IN THE IMAGING SCIENCES

Introduction to Quality Management

OBJECTIVES

At the completion of this chapter, the reader should be able to do the following:

- Identify the need for quality management in diagnostic imaging
- Discuss the impact of government regulation and The Joint Commission accreditation on quality management
- Explain the differences between QA, quality control, and quality management
- Identify the five steps of a process
- List the basic administrative responsibilities of a quality management program
- Describe the various components of a risk management program
- Describe the radiation safety protocols for patients and radiation personnel

KEY TERMS

Action
Accreditation
Achievable dose
American Recovery and
  Reinvestment Act
As low as reasonably achievable
Cost of quality
Consolidated Appropriations Act of
  2016
Customer
Deficit Reduction Act
Det Norske Veritas
Diagnostic reference levels
Dose area product
Dose creep

Error
Health Information Technology for
  Economic and Clinical Health Act
The Health Insurance Portability
  and Accountability Act (HIPAA)
Image Gently
Image Wisely
Incident
Input
Kerma area product (KAP)
Key input variables
Key output variable
Loss potential
Mammography Quality Standards
  Reauthorization Act

Meaningful use rules
Medicare Access and Children's
  Health Insurance Program (CHIP)
  Reauthorization Act of 2015
Medicare Improvements for Patients
  and Providers Act
Metrics
Output
Patient Protection and Affordable
  Care Act
Process
Protecting Access to Medicare Act
  of 2014
Quality assessment
Quality assurance

Quality care
Quality control
Regulation
Risk

Risk management
Safety
Standard
Supplier

System
Tax Cuts and Jobs Act of 2017
Workflow

Diagnostic imaging is a multistep process by which information concerning patient anatomy and physiology is gathered and displayed with the use of modern technology. Unfortunately, numerous sources of variability, in both human factors and equipment factors, can produce subquality images if not properly controlled. This can result in repeat exposures that increase both patient dose and department cost and possibly decrease the accuracy of image interpretation. This in turn can result in decreased customer satisfaction (customers being providers, vendors, insurance companies, employees, and patients) that ultimately costs the healthcare provider lost business and revenue. The purpose of a quality management program is to control or minimize these variables as much as possible. In a diagnostic imaging department, these variables include equipment; image receptor system; quality of image processing; viewing or display conditions; and competency of the technologist, support staff, and the observer or interpreter. By reducing these variables, the quality of imaging services should increase, inefficiencies that increase the cost of these services should decrease, and the satisfaction of the customer should increase.

In healthcare environments, quality care is should be the main focus, because it will lead to higher customer satisfaction and continued success for the healthcare organization. The National Academy of Medicine (NAM) defines quality care as providing patients with appropriate service in a technically competent manner, with good communication, shared decision-making, and cultural sensitivity. With diagnostic imaging departments, the quality of patient care and the diagnostic images that are produced are the main outcome. When discussing the *quality* of particular goods or services, one must keep in mind the three levels on which quality is determined:

1. *Expected quality*. This is the level of quality of the product or service that is expected by the customer and may be influenced by outside factors such as prior word of mouth from friends and relatives. A diagnostic imaging professional would likely have the least amount of impact on this level of quality because it is present before the patient comes into the imaging department.
2. *Perceived quality*. This is the customer's perception of the product or service. It is based on the customer's perception of the product or service and is highly subjective and more difficult to measure quantitatively. For patients undergoing diagnostic imaging, their experience (such as how long they had to wait or how they were treated) during the procedures greatly influences their perception of quality. Therefore how well an imaging professional performs his or her respective responsibilities will

have the greatest impact on this level of quality. Because perceived quality is often what brings patients back to a hospital or imaging center, it can be more important than the actual quality.
3. *Actual quality*. This level of quality uses statistical data to measure outcomes and considers all factors that can influence the final outcome (e.g., the quality of the image, accuracy of diagnosis, timeliness of report to primary provider). It also can compare the quality of the product or service with that of a competitor. This type of quality is most useful in quality management programs because it allows for data-driven decision-making that can be used by management to revise or replace business processes as well as other management decisions. The success of the data-driven approach is reliant upon the quality of the data gathered and the effectiveness of its analysis and interpretation.

In diagnostic imaging departments, we can ultimately define quality as the extent to which the right procedure is done in the right way at the right time, and the correct interpretation is accurately and quickly communicated to the patient and referring provider. Measuring and improving quality is essential not only to ensure optimum effectiveness of care and comply with increasing regulatory requirements but also to combat current trends leading to commoditization of radiology services.

Since the early 1980s, healthcare delivery in the United States has undergone dramatic changes that have affected diagnostic imaging departments and their ability to provide quality care. These changes include the following:

- *Advances in technology, equipment, and procedures.* The digitization of radiography, along with expensive technologies such as magnetic resonance imaging (MRI), spiral computed tomography (CT), electron beam tomography, positron emission tomography (PET), digital radiography (DR) and fluoroscopy, and single photon emission computed tomography (SPECT), have increased the cost of equipment acquisition, installation, and maintenance.
- *Legislation and government regulations.* Legislation such as the Safe Medical Devices Act (SMDA) of 1990, the Mammography Quality Standards Act (MQSA) of 1992, Mammography Quality Standards Reauthorization Act (MQSRA) of 1998, and the Medicare Improvements for Patients and Providers Act of 2008 has increased the responsibility of diagnostic imaging department managers and staff to document proper equipment operation and procedures. This is in addition to requirements from the Occupational Safety and Health Administration (OSHA), the Environmental Protection Agency (EPA), and the Food and Drug Administration (FDA) that affect matters

ranging from blood-borne pathogens to disposal of processing chemicals.

- *Accreditation Procedures.* The accreditation procedures of The Joint Commission (TJC) and others have gone from the philosophy of quality assurance (QA) to one of total quality management (TQM) (explained in more detail later in this chapter).
- *Corporate buyouts and mergers.* In the United States, over 30% of all hospitals that were open and functioning in 1980 have closed (especially in rural areas), while a relatively few number of new hospitals have opened to replace them. Many others have been purchased by "for-profit" healthcare organizations or have merged to condense costs or reduce competition, or both.
- *Methods of reimbursement for services rendered.* The previous method of "fee for service" reimbursement of healthcare expenses is rapidly being replaced by managed care plans such as health maintenance organizations (HMOs) and point of service plans such as preferred provider organizations (PPOs). The lower rate of reimbursement from these plans has reduced the operating budgets of many diagnostic imaging departments. In addition, many insurers are now employing radiology benefits management companies to determine the necessity of various diagnostic imaging orders. Federal legislation such as the Deficit Reduction Act (DRA) of 2005, Medicare Improvements for Patients and Providers Act of 2008, and the Patient Protection and Affordable Care Act of 2010 all attempt to cap reimbursements for medical exams and procedures. The Patient Protection and Affordable Care Act contains a provision whereby reimbursement will change from a "fee for service" to a "bundled payment." This would result in a single payment to a hospital or provider group for a defined episode of care (such as a fractured hip) rather than individual payments for itemized fees and services. On December 18, 2015, President Obama signed into law the Consolidated Appropriations Act of 2016, bipartisan legislation that provided funding for the federal government for the 2016 fiscal year (October 1, 2015–September 30, 2016). Within this extensive legislation were radiology provisions related to the reimbursement for analog radiography (film), computed radiography (CR), and DR imaging services. The law is implemented by the Centers for Medicare and Medicaid Services (CMS) and took effect on January 1, 2017. The rule follows the same framework that CMS used to implement the CT reimbursement scheme codified in the Protecting Access to Medicare Act of 2014 designed around NEMA XR 29.

Medicare reimbursements of the technical component under the Provider Fee Schedule and the Hospital Outpatient Prospective Payment System were reduced by 20% for radiologic exams conducted using a film/screen system. On January 1, 2018, a reduction of 7% occurred for images obtained with CR systems, which was further reduced to 10% on January 1, 2022. Only radiographs performed with DR receive 100% reimbursement.

These changes have made a quality management program essential to the operation and survival of a diagnostic imaging department. The cost of such a program in the form of personnel time and test equipment is more than offset by the savings from lower repeat rates, less equipment downtime, film and chemical savings in analog departments, greater department efficiency, and increased customer satisfaction because waiting time can be reduced. When assessing the effectiveness of a quality management program, one must consider the cost of quality. This is defined as the expense of not doing things right the first time. In diagnostic imaging departments, this could be considerable because the result could lead to lost business at the very least or the injury or death of a patient at the very worst.

STANDARDS, REGULATIONS, AND QUALITY MANAGEMENT

A quality management program has to incorporate standards and regulations that must be met for the healthcare organizations to remain in business. A standard is a statement that is defined and promoted by a professional body or organization by which the quality of practice or service can be evaluated. Standards are to be viewed as the minimum, rather than the maximum expectation of care. Standards are important because all healthcare professions have standards that guide practice. Healthcare organizations also establish standards that apply to their staff and work processes within the organization. Accrediting agencies (such as TJC and DNV-GL that are discussed later in this chapter) have standards that must be applied to all healthcare organizations to maintain accreditation. Accreditation is a method that is used to assess organizations and determine if they meet minimum established standards. Technologists also must commit to their profession's scope of practice standards (such as those established by the American Society of Radiologic Technologists [ASRT] and American Registry of Radiologic Technologists [ARRT] for imaging technologists) to meet certification and licensure requirements.

Standards that have been written into local, state, or federal law that are employed in controlling, directing, or managing an activity, organization, or system are known as regulations. Regulations are usually enforced by a regulatory agency (such as the Center for Devices and Radiological Health, which is a part of the FDA). Quality management programs can ensure compliance with standards and regulations as well as provide data for revision or replacement of standards when they become obsolete or when new technology is developed.

HISTORY OF QUALITY MANAGEMENT IN DIAGNOSTIC IMAGING

One of the earliest known methods of evaluating the quality of clinical healthcare by assessing patient outcomes was carried out by Florence Nightingale in the 1860s. She was one of the first to use a systematic approach to collecting and analyzing mortality rates and other data in hospitals and recommending changes based on these data. In 1910, Ernest Codman, MD (who helped found the American College of Surgeons), proposed the "end result system of hospital standardization." With this system, a hospital would track patients to determine whether the treatment given was effective. If the treatment was not effective, the hospital would then attempt to determine why, so a more successful treatment could be used in future patients.

The origins of modern quality management can be traced back to the early 1900s in the work of an industrial engineer named Frederick Winslow Taylor. Taylor was a mechanical engineer who sought to improve industrial efficiency. He is considered the "Father of Scientific Management" because of his philosophy that the planning function and the execution stage of production be separate and that numerous individuals be assigned specific tasks within the production process to minimize the complexity of the task. With complexity minimized, the hope was to maximize efficiency because, theoretically, fewer mistakes would occur. Job tasks were broken down into simple, separate steps that could be performed over and over again (i.e., assembly lines). Only specific persons were assigned the task of quality control inspection.

Taylor's scientific management consisted of four principles:

- Replace rule-of-thumb work methods with methods based on a scientific study of the tasks.
- Scientifically select, train, and develop each employee rather than passively leaving them to train themselves.
- Provide "detailed instruction and supervision of each worker in the performance of that worker's discrete task."
- Divide work nearly equally between managers and workers, so that the managers apply scientific management principles to planning the work and the workers actually perform the tasks.
- This philosophy was common practice, both in American industry and in healthcare settings (including diagnostic imaging), until the 1980s.

During the 1980s, the concept of quality improvement began to gradually replace the concept of scientific management. This concept is credited to W. Edwards Deming and Joseph Juran (working separately), who used the quality improvement philosophy to revitalize the economy of Japan after World War II. This concept combines quality control with an overall management philosophy that gives input to all persons involved in the process of creating the specific good(s) or service(s) (Deming). It also emphasizes that top management must be quality minded or else little quality will occur at lower levels (Juran). Many diagnostic imaging departments have been systematically monitoring their equipment and procedures (quality control) since the 1930s, independent of any government regulation or accreditation agency. The main motivations were to save money and increase efficiency and quality of care. Since then, governmental action and policies mandated by accreditation agencies have all but required that an extensive quality management program be implemented by diagnostic imaging departments. In 1992, the Accreditation Manual for Hospitals, published by TJC, began a multiyear transition to standards that emphasize performance improvement concepts inspired by the work of Deming and Juran.

Beginning in the late 1990s, the National Academy of Sciences Institute of Medicine began researching how healthcare is delivered in the United States. In March 2016, this group changed its name to National Academy of Sciences-Health and Medicine Division (NAS/HMD). This nonprofit agency that is based in Washington, DC, is not connected to the government but serves as an advisory group to the government, businesses, educators and healthcare professionals. This group published two key reports, the first of which was *To Err Is Human* (1999), which recognized that there was a need to know more about the healthcare delivery system and its quality. The second publication, *Crossing the Quality Chasm* (2001) concluded that the US healthcare delivery system was dysfunctional, with great variety in performance, fragmented and poorly organized, confusing, and complex. It also noted a need for systematic monitoring of healthcare quality to better improve care. This led to the creation of the *National Healthcare Quality Report,* which is published annually by the Agency for Healthcare Research and Quality. The Agency for Healthcare Research and Quality is an agency in the Department of Health and Human Services and distributes the *National Healthcare Quality Report* on its website (www.ahrq.gov). The conclusions of these publications made quality improvement (a key component in quality management programs) a professional responsibility of all healthcare providers and personnel as well as a quality of care issue rather than a managerial tactic.

Governmental Action

The federal government's first step toward requiring that diagnostic imaging departments implement quality management programs came in 1968 with the Radiation Control for Health and Safety Act (Public Law 90-602). This law required the US Department of Health, Education, and Welfare (now called Health and Human Services) to develop and administer standards that would reduce human exposure to radiation from electronic products. The Bureau of Radiological Health (BRH) (now called the National Center for Devices and Radiological Health) was given the responsibility for implementing this act. The BRH set forth regulatory action, beginning in 1974, with several amendments to control the manufacture and installation of medical and dental diagnostic equipment to reduce the production of useless radiation. These regulations are contained in the document Title 21 of the Code of Federal Regulations Part 1020 (21 CFR 1020). Title 21 refers to the FDA. In 1978, the BRH published the "Recommendations for Quality Assurance Programs in Diagnostic Radiology Facilities." Accrediting agencies, along with most state public health agencies, have adopted these recommendations into their various policies governing diagnostic imaging departments.

In 1981, the Consumer-Patient Radiation Health and Safety Act (Public Law 112-90) addressed issues such as unnecessary repeat examinations, QA techniques, referral criteria, radiation exposure, and unnecessary mass screening programs. It also established minimum standards for accreditation of educational programs in the radiologic sciences and for the certification of radiographic equipment operators. This law motivated many states to enact licensure laws for radiologic technologists. However, there is no legal penalty for noncompliance contained within the law, and eight states, plus the District of Columbia, currently have no minimum educational or certification criteria for healthcare workers who perform radiologic procedures. As of the writing of this edition, the eight states are Alabama, Alaska, Georgia, Idaho, Missouri, North Carolina, Oklahoma, and South Dakota. The states of Michigan and Nevada license mammographers but not radiographers, and Wisconsin does not license radiographers but does require American Registry of Radiologic Technologists certification. In September 2000, the Consumer Assurance of Radiologic Excellence (CARE) Act was first introduced in Congress by Representative Rick Lazio (R-NY) as H.R. 5624. In 2006, the CARE bill was retitled the Consistency, Accuracy, Responsibility and Excellence in Medical Imaging and Radiation Therapy Bill because many of the imaging disciplines included in the CARE legislation are not directly related to radiology. The CARE Act mandated educational and training requirements for all technologists performing imaging procedures (thereby mandating the standards contained in the Consumer-Patient Radiation Health and Safety Act of 1981). In addition to improving the quality of care nationwide, enacting the CARE Act would have saved considerable money each year. According to the Radiologic Society of North America journal, *Radiology*, approximately 130 million diagnostic radiology procedures are performed on 36 million Medicare enrollees per year. Over $10 billion is spent by Medicare on medical imaging procedures each year (according to the Medicare Payment Advisory Commission MedPAC). If the national repeat examination rate is between 4% and 7% (averaging 5.5%) and the CARE bill would have lowered repeat rates from 5.5% to 4.5%, enacting education and credentialing standards could save Medicare over $100 million a year. Unfortunately, the bill was never passed and there are currently no plans to reintroduce the bill.

In July 2008, Congress passed the Medicare Improvements for Patients and Providers Act of 2008, which mandates that any nonhospital institution performing advanced diagnostic services (such as nuclear medicine and PET) had to be accredited as of January 1, 2012, to receive federal funding (Medicare reimbursement). Accreditation must be by one of three US CMS-approved agencies. These are (1) American College of Radiology (ACR), (2) TJC, and (3) Intersocietal Accreditation Commission (IAC). Basic areas of CMS requirements are: (1) personnel qualifications for nonprovider medical staff, medical directors, and supervising providers; (2) image quality standards; (3) equipment performance standards; (4) safety standards for staff and patients; and (5) QA and quality control standards must be established.

In the mid-1980s, OSHA, in response to the outbreak of human immunodeficiency virus and hepatitis B virus, amended the existing federal regulations concerning infection control in the workplace and mandated a policy on blood-borne pathogens. All workplaces had to implement these new regulations by the spring of 1992. This policy states that an exposure control plan must be in place for all industries in which workers may come in contact with blood and other infectious materials. Included in this policy are standard precaution procedures (also known as *Tier 1 procedures*), education programs for employees, free hepatitis B immunization for staff who might be exposed to blood or body substances, followup care to any staff member accidentally exposed to blood or bodily fluids through needlesticks and so on, personal protective equipment supplied by the employer (including gloves, gowns, laboratory coats, face shields, eye protection, pocket masks, and ventilation devices), and disposal procedures. These infection control procedures also must include transmission-based precautions (also known as *Tier 2* or *category-specific precautions*) that are used in addition to Tier 1 or standard precautions. They are used when a specific communicable disease is suspected or confirmed and are designed to place a barrier between the patient with the disease and everyone else. They are specifically geared toward preventing infection by minimizing the three specific modes of disease transmission: air, droplet, and contact. The complete OSHA policy on infection control blood-borne pathogens can be found in the Federal Register under Title 29 of the Code of Federal Regulations Part 1910 (29 CFR 1910). OSHA also is responsible for monitoring the workplace environment, including the requirements for occupational exposure to radiation and to chemicals found in processing solutions. OSHA also has proposed an Ergonomics Standard with the objective of reducing the rising incidence of work-related injury and workers' compensation claims.

The SMDA of 1990 (Public Law 101-629) was enacted to increase the amount of information the FDA and device manufacturers receive about problems with medical devices. Under the act, medical facilities must report to the FDA and the manufacturer, if known, any medical devices (e.g., malfunctioning bed, nonworking defibrillator, nonworking pacemaker, malfunctioning radiation therapy unit, or excessive radiation dose during diagnostic procedures such as interventional fluoroscopy) that have caused the death or serious injury of a patient or employee. Facilities also must report device-related serious injuries to the device manufacturer or to the FDA if the manufacturer is not known. In addition, the SMDA requires that device user facilities must submit to the FDA, on a semiannual basis, a summary of all facility records submitted during that time period. It also authorizes civil penalties to healthcare workers or facilities that do not report defects and failures in medical devices. When any incidents of unsafe medical devices are reported to the FDA, Form 3500 should be used for voluntary reporting, and Form 3500 A should be used for mandatory reporting. Mandatory reporting requirements for user facilities are shown in Fig. 1.1). A full listing of requirements of the SMDA can be found in the Code of Federal Regulations, 21 CFR 803.

In 1992, the MQSA or Public Law 102-539 mandated QA programs for all facilities that want to perform mammographic procedures to obtain FDA approval. Specific requirements were designed for dedicated equipment, providers

Reset Form

U.S. Department of Health and Human Services
Food and Drug Administration

MEDWATCH

FORM FDA 3500 (2/19)
The FDA Safety Information and
Adverse Event Reporting Program

For VOLUNTARY reporting of
adverse events, product problems
and product use/medication errors

Page 1 of _2

Form Approved: OMB No. 0910-0291, Expires: 11-30-2021
See PRA statement on reverse.

FDA USE ONLY
Triage unit sequence #
FDA Rec. Date

Note: For date prompts of "dd-mmm-yyyy" please use 2-digit day, 3-letter month abbreviation, and 4-digit year; for example, 01-Jul-2018.

A. PATIENT INFORMATION

1. **Patient Identifier**

In Confidence

2. **Age**
☐ Year(s) ☐ Month(s)
☐ Week(s) ☐ Day(s)

or Date of Birth (e.g., 08 Feb 1925)

3. **Gender** (check one)
☐ Female
☐ Male
☐ Intersex
☐ Transgender
☐ Prefer not to disclose

4. **Weight**
☐ lb
☐ kg

5. **Ethnicity** (check one)
☐ Hispanic/Latino
☐ Not Hispanic/Latino

6. **Race** (check all that apply)
☐ Asian   ☐ American Indian or Alaskan Native
☐ Black or African American   ☐ White
☐ Native Hawaiian or Other Pacific Islander

B. ADVERSE EVENT, PRODUCT PROBLEM

1. **Type of Report** (check all that apply)
☐ Adverse Event   ☐ Product Problem (e.g., defects/malfunctions)
☐ Product Use/ Medication Error   ☐ Problem with Different Manufacturer of Same Medicine

2. **Outcome Attributed to Adverse Event** (check all that apply)
☐ Death   Date of death (dd-mmm-yyyy):
☐ Life-threatening   ☐ Disability or Permanent Damage
☐ Hospitalization (initial or prolonged)   ☐ Congenital Anomaly/Birth Defects
☐ Other Serious or Important Medical Events
☐ Required Intervention to Prevent Permanent Impairment/Damage

3. **Date of Event** (dd-mmm-yyyy)

4. **Date of this Report** (dd-mmm-yyyy)

5. **Describe Event, Problem or Product Use/Medication Error**

(Continue on page 2)

6. **Relevant Tests/Laboratory Data**   **Date** (dd-mmm-yyyy)

(Continue on page 2)

7. **Other Relevant History, Including Preexisting Medical Conditions** (e.g., allergies, pregnancy, smoking and alcohol use, liver/kidney problems, etc.)

(Continue on page 2)

C. PRODUCT AVAILABILITY

1. **Product Available for Evaluation?** (Do not send product to FDA)
☐ Yes ☐ No ☐ Returned to Manufacturer on (dd-mmm-yyyy)

2. **Do you have a picture of the product?** (check yes if you are including a picture) ☐ Yes

D. SUSPECT PRODUCTS

1. **Name, Strength, Manufacturer/Compounder** (from product label).   #1 ☐ Yes
Does this report involve cosmetic, dietary supplement or food/medical food? #2 ☐ Yes

#1 – Name and Strength	#1 – NDC # or Unique ID
#1 – Manufacturer/Compounder	#1 – Lot #
#2 – Name and Strength	#2 – NDC # or Unique ID
#2 – Manufacturer/Compounder	#2 – Lot #

2. **Dose or Amount**   **Frequency**   **Route**

#1
#2

3. **Treatment Dates/Therapy Dates** (give best estimate of length of treatment (start/stop) or duration.)
#1 Start
#1 Stop
Is therapy still on-going? ☐ Yes ☐ No
#2 Start
#2 Stop
Is therapy still on-going? ☐ Yes ☐ No

4. **Diagnosis for Use** (Indication)
#1

#2

5. **Product Type** (check all that apply)
#1 ☐ OTC   #2 ☐ OTC
☐ Compounded   ☐ Compounded
☐ Generic   ☐ Generic
☐ Biosimilar   ☐ Biosimilar

6. **Expiration Date** (dd-mmm-yyyy)
#1

#2

7. **Event Abated After Use Stopped or Dose Reduced?**
#1 ☐ Yes ☐ No ☐ Doesn't apply
#2 ☐ Yes ☐ No ☐ Doesn't apply

8. **Event Reappeared After Reintroduction?**
#1 ☐ Yes ☐ No ☐ Doesn't apply
#2 ☐ Yes ☐ No ☐ Doesn't apply

E. SUSPECT MEDICAL DEVICE

1. **Brand Name**

2a. **Common Device Name**   2b. **Procode**

3. **Manufacturer Name, City and State**

4. **Model #**   **Lot #**   5. **Operator of Device**
Catalog #   **Expiration Date** (dd-mmm-yyyy)   ☐ Health Professional
Serial #   **Unique Identifier** (UDI) #   ☐ Patient/Consumer
☐ Other

6a. **If Implanted, Give Date** (dd-mmm-yyyy)   6b. **If Explanted, Give Date** (dd-mmm-yyyy)

7a. **Is this a single-use device that was reprocessed and reused on a patient?** ☐ Yes ☐ No
7b. **If Yes to Item 7a, Enter Name and Address of Reprocessor**

8. **Was this device serviced by a third party servicer?**
☐ Yes ☐ No ☐ Unknown

F. OTHER (CONCOMITANT) MEDICAL PRODUCTS

1. **Product names and therapy dates** (Exclude treatment of event)

(Continue on page 2)

G. REPORTER (See confidentiality section on back)

1. **Name and Address**

Last Name:	First Name:
Address:	
City:	State/Province/Region:
ZIP/Postal Code:	Country:
Phone #:	Email:

2. **Health Professional?** ☐ Yes ☐ No
3. **Occupation**
4. **Also Reported to:**
☐ Manufacturer/Compounder
☐ User Facility
☐ Distributor/Importer

5. **If you do NOT want your identity disclosed to the manufacturer, please mark this box:** ☐

FORM FDA 3500 (2/19)   Submission of a report does not constitute an admission that medical personnel or the product caused or contributed to the event.
* Please see instructions

Fig. 1.1 FDA Form 3500.

Reset Form

U.S. Department of Health and Human Services
Food and Drug Administration

MEDWATCH

FORM FDA 3500 (2/19) *(continued)*
The FDA Safety Information and
Adverse Event Reporting Program

(CONTINUATION PAGE)
For VOLUNTARY reporting of
adverse events, product problems
and product use/medication errors

Page 2 of 2

B.5. **Describe Event or Problem** *(continued)*

Back to Item B.5

B.6. **Relevant Tests/Laboratory Data** *(continued)*

Date *(dd-mmm-yyyy)*   **Relevant Tests/Laboratory Data**   **Date** *(dd-mmm-yyyy)*

Additional comments

Back to Item B.6

B.7. **Other Relevant History** *(continued)*

Back to Item B.7

F.1. **Concomitant Medical Products and Therapy Dates** *(Exclude treatment of event) (continued)*

Back to Item F.1

Fig. 1.1, cont'd.

Continued

ADVICE ABOUT VOLUNTARY REPORTING
Detailed instructions available at: http://www.fda.gov/medwatch/report/consumer/instruct.htm

Report adverse events, product problems or product use errors with:

- Medications (drugs or biologics)
- Medical devices (including diabetes glucose-test kit, hearing aids, breast pumps, and many more)
- Combination products (medication & medical devices)
- Blood transfusions, gene therapies, and human cells and tissue transplants (for example, tendons, bone, and corneas)
- Special nutritional products (dietary supplements, medical foods, infant formulas)
- Cosmetics (such as moisturizers, makeup, shampoos and conditioners, face and body washes, deodorants, nail care products, hair dyes and relaxers, and tattoos)
- Food (including beverages and ingredients added to foods)

Report product problems – quality, performance or safety concerns such as:

- Suspected counterfeit product
- Suspected contamination
- Questionable stability
- Defective components
- Poor packaging or labeling
- Therapeutic failures (product didn't work)

Report SERIOUS adverse events. An event is serious when the patient outcome is:

- Death
- Life-threatening
- Hospitalization (initial or prolonged)
- Disability or permanent damage
- Congenital anomaly/birth defect
- Required intervention to prevent permanent impairment or damage
- Other serious (important medical events)

Report even if:

- You're not certain the product caused the event
- You don't have all the details
- Just fill in the sections that apply to your report

How to report:

- Use section D for all products except medical devices
- Attach additional pages if needed
- Use a separate form for each patient
- Report either to FDA or the manufacturer (or both)

How to submit report:

- To report by phone, call toll-free: 1-800-FDA (332)-1088
- To fax report: 1-800-FDA(332)-0178
- To report online: www.fda.gov/medwatch/report.htm

If your report involves a serious adverse event with a device and it occurred in a facility outside a doctor's office, that facility may be legally required to report to FDA and/or the manufacturer. Please notify the person in that facility who would handle such reporting.

If your report involves an adverse event with a vaccine, go to http://vaers.hhs.gov to report or call 1-800-822-7967.

Confidentiality:

The patient's identity is held in strict confidence by FDA and protected to the fullest extent of the law. The reporter's identity, including the identity of a self-reporter, may be shared with the manufacturer unless requested otherwise.

The information in this box applies only to requirements of the Paperwork Reduction Act of 1995.

The burden time for this collection of information has been estimated to average 40 minutes per response, including the time to review instructions, search existing data sources, gather and maintain the data needed, and complete and review the collection of information. Send comments regarding this burden estimate or any other aspect of this collection of information, including suggestions for reducing this burden to:

Department of Health and Human Services
Food and Drug Administration
Office of Chief Information Officer
Office of Chief Information Officer
Paperwork Reduction Act (PRA) Staff
PRAStaff@fda.hhs.gov

Please DO NOT RETURN this form to the PRA Staff e-mail above.

OMB statement:

"An agency may not conduct or sponsor, and a person is not required to respond to, a collection of information unless it displays a currently valid OMB control number."

U.S. DEPARTMENT OF HEALTH AND HUMAN SERVICES
Food and Drug Administration

Fig. 1.1, cont'd.

interpreting the images, medical physicists, and technologists. Most of these standards were formulated by or in conjunction with the ACR and were in use by many facilities before enactment of the MQSA. This law became effective October 1, 1994. The MQSA was replaced by the MQSRA of 1998, also known as Public Law 105-248. As part of the new law, final FDA regulations concerning mammographic procedures became effective April 28, 1999, replacing interim regulations that were used during the original law. The final regulations emphasize performance objectives rather than specify the behavior and manner of compliance. More specific information on the MQSA and MQSRA can be found in Chapter 11.

The Health Insurance Portability and Accountability Act (HIPAA) of 1996 (also known as the Kennedy-Kassebaum Act or Public Law 104-191) was enacted to simplify healthcare standards and save money for healthcare businesses by encouraging electronic transactions, but it also required new safeguards to protect patient security and confidentiality. HIPAA established national standards for healthcare e-commerce that include the following:

1. Electronic patient record system security requirements (security standard): This created a new national standard for the administrative, technical, and physical safety of protected health information.
2. Standard electronic formats for insurance transactions such as enrollment, encounters, and claims (transaction standard): This standard requires the implementation of a uniform set of codes and forms, such as the American National Standards Institute ASC X12N format for electronic healthcare transactions or professional and institutional claims.
3. Standard identifiers and codes for institutions, personnel, diagnoses, and treatments (national identifier standard): This created national numbers to identify employers, health plans, and healthcare providers (National Provider Identifiers). It also contains a set of codes that are used to encode all healthcare data. The four categories of these codes are (1) diseases International Classification of Diseases (ICD-9); (2) injuries (ICD-10); (3) actions taken to prevent, diagnose, treat, or manage diseases (Current Procedural Terminology [CPT]-4); and (4) substances, equipment, and supplies.
4. Patient information, confidentiality, and privacy rules (privacy standard): This created a new national standard for privacy of protected health information.

The Department of Health and Human Services first issued proposed regulations for these standards in November 1999, with final rules approved in December 2000. They took effect April 14, 2001, and all healthcare organizations had to comply with and implement them by April 14, 2005. All medical records and patient information, whether electronic, on paper, or oral, are covered by these final rules.

Failure to comply with these standards resulted in significant penalties ranging from as little as $10 to $250,000 and 10 years in prison. The American Recovery and Reinvestment Act (ARRA) of 2009 included the Health Information Technology for Economic and Clinical Health Act that amended HIPAA's enforcement regulations by adding several categories of violations and established ranges of penalty amounts for each category of violation. These regulations took effect on February 18, 2009, and include the following categories of violations and their respective penalty amounts available:

Violation Category— Section 1176 (a)(1)	Each Violation	All Such Violations of an Identical Provision in a Calendar Year
(A) Did not know	$100–$50,000	$1,500,000
(B) Reasonable cause	$1000–$50,000	$1,500,000
(C) (i) Willful neglect— corrected	$10,000–$50,000	$1,500,000
(C) (ii) Willful neglect—not corrected	$50,000	$1,500,000

Further information can be found in the *Federal Register*, Vol. 74, No. 209, Friday, October 30, 2009: Rules and Regulations 56127, and complete HIPAA guidelines can be found in the *Federal Register* under Title 45 of the Code of Federal Regulations Parts 160–164 (45 CFR 160–164).

This means that healthcare administrators must have policies and procedures including establishing a system of security and confidentiality, training all personnel in these policies, and appointing a staff member to act as a security officer to monitor compliance with these policies. This is discussed further in Chapter 2. The ARRA of 2009 also requires certain criteria (known as meaningful use rules) that health information technology departments must meet to receive payment for services from the CMS. Since picture archiving and communication systems (PACS) are a part of electronic health records (EHR), these rules impact diagnostic imaging departments.

The current CMS-EHR objectives and measures that eligible hospitals must meet are:

1. Protect electronic protected health information created or maintained by the certified electronic health record technology (CEHRT) through the implementation of appropriate technical capabilities.
2. Use clinical decision support to improve performance on high-priority health conditions.
3. Use computerized provider order entry for medication, laboratory, and radiology orders directly entered by any licensed healthcare professional who can enter orders into the medical record per state, local, and professional guidelines.
4. Generate and transmit permissible discharge prescriptions electronically.
5. Health Information Exchange—The eligible hospital that transitions their patient to another setting of care or provider of care or refers their patient to another provider of care provides a summary care record for each transition of care or referral.
6. Use of clinically relevant information from the CEHRT to identify patient-specific education resources and provide those resources to the patient.
7. The eligible hospital that receives a patient from another setting of care or provider of care or believes an encounter is relevant performs medication reconciliation.
8. Patient Electronic Access—Provides patients the ability to view online, download, and transmit their health information within 36 hours of hospital discharge.
9. Public Health Reporting—The eligible hospital is in active engagement with a public health agency to submit electronic health data from the CEHRT except where prohibited and in accordance with appropriate law and practice.

Hospitals must apply these criteria to their health information technology departments and connect them to their quality improvement programs.

The Deficit Reduction Act of 2005 (DRA), also known as Public Law 109-362, was enacted to help make $11 billion in cuts from 2007 (when the DRA went into effect) to 2015 in Medicare and Medicaid programs. One aspect of the program is to reduce payments for freestanding diagnostic imaging centers by capping some CPT codes that were higher than hospital outpatient rates and freezing CPT codes already lower than hospital outpatient rates. Current procedural terminology codes were developed by the American Medical Association and adopted by the federal government and private insurance providers to classify medical, surgical, and diagnostic services. The DRA also requires imaging centers to have quality control standards in place to receive reimbursement.

Having an effective quality management program also has become necessary as a condition of receiving reimbursement for services by the federal government. The US Department of Health and Human Services, through its subbranch the CMS, emphasizes effective quality management procedures be documented for healthcare facilities to receive reimbursement for any healthcare service, and many private insurance companies have followed this practice.

The Patient Protection and Affordable Care Act of 2010, commonly known as "Obamacare" or Public Law 111-148, was enacted to increase health insurance coverage for Americans as well as reducing the overall cost of healthcare. There are far too many provisions of this bill to cover in a chapter of a book, so I will only mention the ones that should have a direct impact on diagnostic imaging departments. One provision (discussed earlier in this chapter) would change Medicare reimbursement from "fee for service" to a bundled payment for a "defined episode of care," which could lower the reimbursement rate to healthcare providers. Another provision adds a 2.3% excise tax on all medical devices (such as diagnostic imaging equipment) that is collected at the time of purchase. This could lead to more equipment being leased rather than purchased. It is also thought that having more people insured will increase the demand for healthcare services, thereby increasing the demand for imaging professionals in the workplace. Since many provisions were scheduled to become effective gradually between 2014 and 2020, it will take time to evaluate the impact of the law. The Patient Protection and Affordable Care Act also introduced penalties for providers who do not submit qualifying data to the Provider Quality Reporting System (PQRS). The PQRS system is a healthcare quality improvement incentive program initiated by the CMS. In 2015, the program began applying a negative payment adjustment to individual EPs and PQRS group practices that did not satisfactorily report data on quality measures for Medicare Part B Provider Fee Schedule covered professional services in 2013. Those who report satisfactorily for a program year will avoid the PQRS negative payment adjustment two years later. The Tax Cuts and Jobs Act of 2017 canceled the penalty enforcing individual mandate of the Affordable Care Act.

To ensure Medicare provider reimbursement rates (and therefore Medicare patient's access to their providers), the Protecting Access to Medicare Act of 2014 or Public Law 113-93 (also known as the sustainable growth rate or sustainable growth rate patch) was enacted. Some of the provisions in this law that affect diagnostic imaging departments include requiring ordering providers of advanced imaging procedures to provide support using appropriate use criteria; improved and stricter patient radiation dose safety controls and levels (such as CT dose index and dose length product); and that all CT equipment must meet NEMA standards.

In April of 2015, the Medicare Access and Children's Health Insurance Program (CHIP) Reauthorization Act of 2015 or Public Law 114-10, was enacted to modify the Protecting Access to Medicare Act of 2014. The law:

- Repeals the sustainable growth rate methodology for determining updates to the Medicare Provider Fee Schedule
- Establishes annual positive or flat fee updates for 10 years and institutes a two-track fee update beginning in 2019
- Establishes the Merit-Based Incentive Payment System that consolidates existing Medicare quality programs
- Establishes a pathway for providers to participate in an Alternative Payment Model

This law focuses on quality—both a set of evidence-based, specialty-specific standards as well as practice-based improvement activities; cost; and use of CEHRT to support interoperability and advanced quality objectives in a single, cohesive program that avoids redundancies.

In December 2016, Congress passed the Consolidated Appropriations Act of 2016, or Public Law 114-113 (also known as the 2016 omnibus spending bill). This bill provided funding to the federal government through September 30, 2016. The most important aspect of this bill for diagnostic imaging departments was the incentives for healthcare institutions to convert to DR. The act accomplished this by reducing reimbursement for plain film X-rays by "20 percent in 2017 and all subsequent years," and also reducing CR reimbursement by 7 percent from 2018 to 2022 and 10 percent thereafter.

The Joint Commission

TJC, formerly known as the Joint Commission for the Accreditation of Healthcare Organizations or JCAHO, was founded in 1951, and is an independent, not-for-profit organization that accredits and certifies more than 20,000 healthcare organizations and programs in the United States. In the 1970s, TJC began requiring hospitals and other healthcare providers to perform and document specific QA procedures for these facilities to obtain accreditation. Accreditation is voluntary, but hospitals and medical centers that do not have it may not possess Medicaid certification, hold certain licenses, have a residency program for training providers, obtain reimbursements from insurance companies, or receive malpractice insurance. However, some hospitals may choose not to be accredited by TJC and instead have inspections by their state public health departments or other organizations such as DNV-GL Healthcare (discussed later in this chapter). These hospitals include many rural hospitals that may be critical access hospitals and would still receive Medicaid and Medicare reimbursements. TJC accredits not only hospitals but also facilities for long-term care, ambulatory care, mental health, and chemical dependency. TJC standards are based on the Medicare Conditions of Participation (CoPs) that must be met for institutions to receive Medicare and

Medicaid reimbursement. TJC puts the CoPs in context for hospital leaders through a larger set of standards that define how high-quality/safe patient care should be delivered. The standards have evolved over time through the work of healthcare leaders and subject matter experts, along with input from accredited organizations. There are also leadership standards that focus on aligning the organization around a set of improvement priorities. TJC standards also mandate a quality management system be in place as well as consistent process execution. The TJC quality management procedures are extensive and specific in nature. For example, any equipment that is inspected daily (Monday through Friday) also must be inspected on Saturday and Sunday if the opportunity exists that a patient would need that piece of equipment on the weekend. Second, refrigerators that contain medical supplies must have a thermometer, and a log of the daily recorded temperature (including weekends) must be kept. TJC also requires accredited institutions to have a process in place for correcting customer complaints (a process known as *service recovery*). This means that proper performance and documentation of quality management procedures are essential to pass TJC inspections. Standards set by TJC to receive accreditation require that healthcare organizations have a planned, systematic, and organization-wide approach for monitoring, evaluating, and improving the quality of care, as well as those of management, governance, and support activities. TJC standards also require that healthcare organizations must perform routine inspections of all equipment, devices, and supplies.

The main tenets of TJC are:
- Performance Standards
- Measurement of Actual Quality
- Documentation
- Service Recovery

Before 1991, TJC used the concepts of QA and quality control requiring systematic monitoring and evaluation, with the responsibility left to the medical director or department head. Because these concepts now have been incorporated into the newer quality management philosophy, an understanding of QA and quality control is still important and is discussed later in this chapter.

Det Norske Veritas Healthcare

DNV Healthcare, Inc. is part of Det Norske Veritas, a global foundation that was established in Oslo, Norway, in 1864 and has been operating in the United States since 1898. Their stated purpose is to safeguard life, property, and the environment. On September 26, 2008, DNV Healthcare was granted authority by the CMS to accredit hospitals, and is therefore an alternative to TJC for hospitals to receive accreditation. DNV Healthcare merged with Germanischer Lloyd, a nonprofit association based in Hamburg, Germany, to become DNV-GL. The newly formed DNV-GL Group became operational on September 12, 2013. DNV-GL accreditation standards combine the standards created by the National Integrated Accreditation for Healthcare Organizations with those created by the International Organization for Standardization (ISO) based in Geneva, Switzerland

(www.iso.org). These standards are based on very similar quality management principles as TJC standards, namely:
1. Customer focus
2. Leadership
3. Involvement of people
4. Process approach
5. System approach to management
6. Continual improvement
7. Factual approach to decision-making
8. Mutually beneficial supplier relationships

DNV-GL accreditation requires that institutions achieve ISO 9001 certification, or at least ISO 9001 compliance, within the first 3 years. Within the ISO 9001 standards is a major focus on alignment with strategy, a clear and effective quality management system, as well as consistent process execution. DNV-GL accreditation does not supplement the CoPs with any additional patient care standards or patient safety goals that TJC requires. How care is provided is left up to the individual healthcare organization, and the framework for deciding which processes to focus on, how to design/improve them, and how to manage their performance lies within the ISO 9001 requirements that the organization must learn and be in compliance with by their third year of accreditation under DNV-GL.

Imaging-Specific Accrediting Bodies

In addition to accrediting the entire healthcare facility, accreditation is available for specific imaging modalities. The main agencies for diagnostic imaging are the ACR and the IAC. The ACR began accrediting radiation therapy departments in 1986, followed by mammography accreditation in 1987. Over the years, they have added several other modalities, including:
- MRI
- Breast MRI
- Ultrasound
- Breast ultrasound
- Computed tomography
- Nuclear medicine
- Positron emission tomography
- Stereotactic breast biopsy

The goals of ACR accreditation are:
- Set quality standards for imaging practices
- Provide recommendations for improvement
- Help sites improve quality of patient care
- Recognize quality imaging practice

The IAC began accrediting in healthcare more than 30 years ago with the inception of the first of the IAC accreditation divisions, the IAC Vascular Testing (formerly the Intersocietal Commission for the Accreditation of Vascular Laboratories), in 1991. From this first accrediting body, the IAC has continued its path of developing standards and methods for the evaluation of the quality of care delivered. Holding true to its original mission, the IAC's scope has expanded to provide similar peer review processes for multiple imaging modalities within the medical community. The modalities accredited by the IAC include:

- Vascular testing
- Echocardiography
- Nuclear/PET
- MRI
- Diagnostic CT
- Dental CT
- Carotid stenting
- Vein treatment and management
- Cardiac electrophysiology
- Cardiovascular catheterization

Quality Assurance

Quality assurance (QA) is an all-encompassing management program used to ensure excellence in healthcare through the systematic collection and evaluation of data. The primary objective of a QA program is the enhancement of patient care; this includes patient selection parameters and scheduling, management techniques, departmental policies and procedures, technical effectiveness and efficiency, in-service education, and image interpretation with timeliness of reports. The main emphasis of the program is on the human factors that can lead to variations in quality care. QA should not be confused with quality assessment, which is the measurement of the level of quality at some point in time with no effort to change or improve the level of care.

Quality Control

Quality control (QC) is the part of the QA program that deals with techniques used in monitoring and maintaining the technical elements of the systems that affect the quality of the image. Therefore quality control is the part of the QA program that deals with instrumentation and equipment. A quality control program includes the following three levels of testing:

Level I: Noninvasive and Simple. Noninvasive and simple evaluations can be performed by any technologist and include tests such as the wire mesh test for screen contact and the spinning top test for timer accuracy.

Level II: Noninvasive and Complex. Noninvasive and complex evaluations should be performed by a technologist who has been specifically trained in quality control procedures. This is because more sophisticated equipment, such as special test tools, meters, or the noninvasive evaluation of a radiation output computerized multiple function unit, is used. Many educational programs now include this level of competency for graduation, so the number of technologists with these skills is increasing. The ASRT includes quality control and QA duties in its practice standards for radiographers, sonographers, nuclear medicine technologists, CT technologists, MRI technologists, mammographers, interventional radiographers, and bone densitometry technologists. The ARRT offers an advanced level certification examination for technologists wishing to document their knowledge of QA and quality control procedures and protocols. This can be used to verify qualification for a quality management technologist position.

Level III: Invasive and Complex. Invasive and complex evaluations involve some disassembly of the equipment and are normally performed by engineers or physicists. This textbook focuses on levels I and II of quality control testing. The following are the three types of quality control tests on various levels:

1. Acceptance testing is performed on new equipment or equipment that has undergone major repair to demonstrate that it is performing within the manufacturer's specifications and criteria. It also can detect any defects that may exist in the equipment. The results obtained during acceptance testing are also used to establish the baseline performance of the equipment that is used as a reference point in future quality control testing.

2. Routine performance evaluations are specific tests performed on the equipment in use after a certain amount of time has elapsed. These evaluations can verify that the equipment is performing within previously accepted standards and can be used to diagnose any changes in performance before becoming radiographically apparent.

3. Error correction tests evaluate equipment that is malfunctioning or not performing to the manufacturer's specifications and are also used to verify the correct cause of the malfunction so that the proper repair can be made.

Continuous Quality Improvement

The older QA/QC program ensured that a certain level of quality was met; it required monitoring only periodically for maintenance. It was segmented in approach because each department in a facility monitored and evaluated its own structural outcomes, creating a tendency to view individual performances rather than the process or system in which that individual was functioning. In turn, the program was externally motivated because its emphasis was on demonstrating compliance with externally developed standards. As long as the standards were met, no further work was required to improve the system.

In 1991, TJC began incorporating the concepts of continuous quality improvement (CQI), which is defined as a structured organizational process for involving personnel in planning and executing a continuous flow of improvements to provide quality healthcare that meets or exceeds expectations, to replace the older QA/QC philosophy into their program of accreditation of healthcare organizations. CQI evolved from *total quality management* concept in the manufacturing industry, also referred to as *total quality control*, *total quality leadership*, *total quality improvement*, and *statistical quality control*. This concept is based on the "14 Points for Management" developed by W. Edwards Deming (Box 1.1) and the Japanese management style.

The CQI concept does not replace the concept of QA/quality control but incorporates it at a higher conceptual level. Instead of just ensuring and maintaining quality, it continually improves quality by focusing on improving the system or process in which individual workers function rather than on the individuals themselves. For these processes to improve, it

BOX 1.1 Deming's 14 Points of Management

1. Create constancy of purpose.
2. Adopt a new philosophy.
3. Cease dependence on mass inspection.
4. End the practice of awarding business on the basis of price alone.
5. Continually seek out problems to improve.
6. Institute on-the-job training.
7. Institute leadership to help people do the job better.
8. Drive out fear.
9. Break down barriers between departments.
10. Eliminate slogans and exhortations.
11. Eliminate targets and quotas.
12. Permit pride of workmanship.
13. Institute education.
14. The transformation to total quality improvement is everyone's job.

is essential to focus on the organization as a whole rather than on individual departments. It is important that each healthcare organization have a clear mission, values, and objectives that performance improvement processes are designed and implemented to support. It also promotes the need for objective data involving statistics to analyze and improve processes (known as data-driven or evidence-based analysis). Every employee should be actively involved in CQI (rather than just management or the quality control technologist) for the program to be successful. In this way, CQI can be internally motivating because employees will see that their involvement is tied to the success of the hospital, creating an atmosphere in which employees are motivated to do better because they are participating actively. Management must take the responsibility to promote this atmosphere, effectively allocate resources needed for improvement, treat employees as assets and not expenses, and work together toward shared goals. Managers/leaders should establish unity of purpose and direction of the organization. They should create and maintain the internal environment in which people can become fully involved in achieving the organization's objectives. For healthcare institutions, this should allow the ultimate focus to be on improving patient care, which should build a satisfied customer base and benefit the institution in the long term.

PROCESS IMPROVEMENT THROUGH CONTINUOUS QUALITY IMPROVEMENT

As mentioned earlier, CQI focuses on the process in which employees operate rather than on the employees themselves. The rationale is that problems and variability with the process are the main cause of poor quality. The concept of process improvement through CQI is based on the following premises:

- 85/15 Rule—the process or system in place is the cause of problems 85% of the time, and the people or personnel within the process are the cause of problems 15% of the time.
- 80/20 Rule—80% of the problems are the result of 20% of the causes.

- Workers who are closest to the problem probably know what is wrong with the process and are better able to fix it.
- Structured problem-solving processes that use statistical means to verify performance produce better long-term solutions than processes that are not structured.
- Improving quality is the responsibility of everyone within an organization because all are a part of the process. People at all levels are the essence of an organization, and their involvement enables their abilities to be used for the organization's benefit.

For healthcare organizations, most of the processes should be oriented toward the deliverance of high-quality care and the achievement of customer satisfaction. A process is an ordered series of steps that help achieve a desired outcome or all the tasks directed at accomplishing one particular outcome grouped in a sequence. A system is a group of related processes. Identifying, understanding, and managing interrelated processes contributes to the healthcare organization's effectiveness and efficiency in achieving its objectives. The parts of any process include a supplier, input, action, output, and the customer.

- A supplier is an individual or entity that furnishes input to a process (e.g., person, department, organization) or one who provides the institution with goods or services. For diagnostic imaging departments, examples may include imaging equipment vendors and referring providers. An organization and its suppliers are interdependent, and a mutually beneficial relationship enhances the ability of both to create value for both parties.
- Input is information or knowledge necessary to achieve the desired outcome or everything that is used (mostly as variables) to produce one or more outputs from a process. For diagnostic imaging departments, examples may include patient information, examination requested, technologists' knowledge of procedures, and workload.
- Action is the means or activity used to achieve the desired outcome or the steps or activities carried out to convert inputs to one or more outputs. Examples for diagnostic imaging departments may include computer entry and form completion and assignment of patients to appropriate rooms. The action steps are sometimes referred to as the workflow. A more technical definition of workflow is the sequence of physical and mental tasks performed by various people within and between work environments.

These first three steps are variable factors that influence the next portion of the process called the *output*.

- Output refers to the desired outcome, result, product, or characteristics that satisfy the customer, or one or more outcomes or physical products emerging from a process. In diagnostic imaging departments, examples may include completed paperwork, completed diagnostic examination, and an accurate radiologist report. A desired result is achieved more efficiently when activities and related resources are managed as a process.
- Customer refers to a person, department, or organization that needs, uses or wants the desired outcome or a process. In diagnostic imaging, customers can be the patient,

referring provider, or even other departments in the healthcare organization.

According to Deming, the customer determines what constitutes quality. This can be broken down into the following groups:

- **Internal customers:** Generally, these are individuals or groups from within the organization such as referring providers, hospital employees, departments, and department employees.
- **External customers:** These are individuals or groups from outside the organization, such as patients and their families, third-party payers, and the community.

The satisfaction of the customer, both internal and external, is the driving force behind CQI because it focuses on the needs and expectations of customers and the continuous improvement of the product or service. By continually meeting or exceeding customer satisfaction, the process is considered to be successful. Both customer satisfaction and health outcomes should be used as performance measures to evaluate the success of a process in a healthcare environment. Organizations depend on their customers, and therefore should understand current and future customer needs, meet customer requirements, and strive to exceed customer expectations.

Improvement projects can be taken up on output or input metrics whenever a performance issue is found and variations seen in the process. The improvement efforts should not only be directed internally to improve process capabilities but also externally to the suppliers who provide critical inputs. The organization can now establish clear control plans for managing the suppliers, inputs, and processes effectively to ensure control over the outputs and to satisfy the customers. These plans will typically include actions to be taken, the frequency of the actions, responsibility, status check, and governance on the entire plan by the quality and internal audit functions. A comprehensive control plan should include at least the following:

- Data collection trackers such as patient waiting time and repeat analysis
- Control charts or other information display tools (covered in the next chapter) for display and analysis of critical metrics
- Action plan trackers with responsibility and timelines to address out-of-control situations
- Review mechanism (internal with management and external with customer)

Key Quality Characteristics

Key quality characteristics are those qualities or aspects that have been identified as being most important to the customer, and are sometimes referred to as healthcare metrics. These characteristics must be constantly measured and improved for customer satisfaction to increase. At an organizational level, healthcare metrics can be classified into the following basic types:

- Financial—track the financial performance of the healthcare system from a business perspective (usually standard financial/accounting data)

- Utilization—characterize the number and type of basic services rendered, the resources that are used, and the availability of care (e.g., MRI, PET)
- Cost/productivity—used to reduce supply/labor costs and increase productivity
- Clinical performance—also known as patient outcome data; these measure the quality of patient care, such as mortality rates and accuracy of diagnosis
- Patient safety—metrics that characterize preventable medical mistakes that are made
- Patient satisfaction—measure satisfaction from a patient's perspective

In diagnostic imaging departments, the important metrics can be found in the imaging process sequence listed in the following table:

Event	Metrics
Referring provider orders examination	Appropriateness guidelines, intended examination (ordering error)
Appointment scheduled	Access time
Initial imaging department encounter	Patient wait time, patient education (preparation)
Protocol selection	Standardized protocol: best practice
Patient examination	Environment of care, safety, and comfort; protocol complications
Interpretation (peer-reviewed credentials)	Correct subspecialty interpretation, accuracy, structured report; report answers clinical question
Finalization errors	Timelines, succinctness
Communication of final report	Referring provider satisfaction; query answered or addressed
Measuring and monitoring performance improvement in quality, safety, and efficiency	Turnaround time in examinations and reporting, patient complications, and patient satisfaction

Key Process Variables

Key process variables are the components of any process that may affect the final output of the process. Variability can have a negative impact on the quality of the final output, and systems must be developed to properly manage any variability that may arise. Unfortunately, patients, providers, and diagnostic categories found in healthcare are highly variable. There are major categories of key process variables: manpower, machines, materials, environment, and policies.

- **Manpower** refers to the personnel involved in the process.
- **Machines** refers to the equipment used in the process.
- **Materials** refers to the type and quality of materials used in the process.
- **Environment** refers to the physical and psychological aspects on people involved in the process.
- **Policies** refers to the steps in the procedure or policy manual that have been used in the process.

Key process variables can be divided into two groups—key input variables (KIVs) and key output variables (KOVs). KIVs are process inputs that have a significant impact on the variation found in a key process output variable and are the most important input(s) to a process. That is, if the key process input variables were controlled (e.g., held constant), the process would produce predictable and consistent outputs. KIVs are the components of a process that we can directly control to deliver a quality product or service. KIVs are quick glimpses of the only real process controls at our disposal. Examples would include entry of the correct examination requested by the ordering provider, or the proper patient identification before they are brought into the examination room. KOVs are measurable on, within, or about the product or service itself, and are the attributes seen by the customer. They are the process outputs that are affected by KIVs and are known collectively as quality. The quality of the diagnostic image and the accuracy of the radiologist's report would be examples of KOVs. In short, they are characteristics that have a big impact on efficiency and/or customer satisfaction. Variation in key process output variables leads to lower levels of quality and reliability and, ultimately, higher costs.

COMPONENTS OF A QUALITY MANAGEMENT PROGRAM IN DIAGNOSTIC IMAGING

A comprehensive quality management program consists of many different components, depending on the size and complexity of the healthcare organization. Programs for diagnostic imaging departments, regardless of the size, should contain at least the following components:

1. *Equipment quality control.* This aspect of a quality management program involves evaluation of equipment performance to ensure proper image quality, as well as patient and operator safety. These procedures are covered extensively in Chapters 3–13.
2. *Administrative responsibilities.* This aspect of the quality management program involves the establishment of various processes to accomplish the specific departmental tasks that are required, such as departmental procedure manuals for performing diagnostic examinations or procedures for scheduling and routing of patients. It also involves data collection and analysis to continuously improve these processes. Other responsibilities include cost control, management of personnel, education of personnel (education for newly hired personnel and continuing education for existing workers), equipment acquisition, communication with various vendors, communication with other departments within the healthcare organization, and various other activities.
3. *Risk management.* The ability to identify potential risks to patients, employees, and visitors at the healthcare institution and establish processes that would minimize these risks is extremely important to healthcare organizations. Civil litigation and workers' compensation judgments can severely deplete the financial resources of even the largest healthcare organization.

4. *Regulatory and standards compliance.* Diagnostic imaging departments must be in compliance with state, federal, and local regulatory agencies, as well as accrediting bodies to continue to be in business.
5. *Radiation safety program.* This is to ensure that patient exposure is kept as low as reasonably achievable (ALARA) and that department personnel, medical staff, and members of the general public are protected from overexposure to ionizing radiation.

ADMINISTRATIVE RESPONSIBILITIES

Earlier in Chapter 1, a distinction between QA (which deals with human factors) and QC (which deals with equipment factors) is made. Merging these entities in a TQM program requires certain administrative procedures (Box 1.2) to be implemented by radiologists, department administrators, quality management technologists (Box 1.3), quality improvement committees, and imaging professionals (since they have direct patient contact and are therefore on the front line in demonstrating quality of care). Some of the more important administrative procedures follow.

Threshold of Acceptability

The threshold of acceptability includes levels of accuracy, sensitivity, and specificity of diagnosis (see Chapter 3). It also should include such items as the number of radiographs per examination, the amount of radiation per examination, and the performance thresholds of the equipment. These should be established according to both external factors (such as federal and state guidelines or professional and accrediting agencies) and internal factors, which are based on the needs and resources of the individual department.

Communication Network

Proper communication among all members of a diagnostic imaging department is essential for a successful quality management program. Items such as the proper examination ordered for a particular patient must be supplied to the technologist from the ordering provider and office support staff. The technologist also must communicate the appropriate patient history to the radiologist and ensure proper film identification and marking. Administrative personnel and radiologists must then communicate with technologists about proper procedures and guidelines for patient care and image parameters. Diagnostic imaging departments also should have proper communication with other departments within

---

BOX 1.2   Administrative Procedures

Establish thresholds of acceptability
Establish an effective communication network
Provide for patient comfort
Ensure accepted performance of diagnostic imaging personnel
Develop a record-keeping system
Establish corrective action procedures

BOX 1.3 Quality Management Technologist Duties

The scope of practice of the medical imaging and radiation therapy professional includes:

- Providing optimal patient care
- Receiving, relaying, and documenting verbal, written, and electronic orders in the patient's medical record
- Corroborating a patient's clinical history with procedure and ensuring information is documented and available for use by a licensed independent practitioner
- Verifying informed consent for applicable procedures
- Assuming responsibility for patient needs during procedures
- Preparing patients for procedures
- Applying principles of ALARA to minimize exposure to patient, self, and others
- Performing venipuncture as prescribed by a licensed independent practitioner
- Starting, maintaining, and/or removing intravenous access as prescribed by a licensed independent practitioner
- Identifying, preparing, and/or administering medications as prescribed by a licensed independent practitioner
- Evaluating images for technical quality, ensuring proper identification is recorded
- Identifying and responding to emergency situations
- Providing education
- Educating and monitoring students and other healthcare providers
- Performing ongoing QA activities
- Applying the principles of patient safety during all aspects of patient care

The scope of practice of the quality management technologist also includes:

1. Coordinating, performing, and monitoring quality control procedures for all types of equipment
2. Creating policies and procedures to meet regulatory, accreditation, and fiscal requirements
3. Determining and monitoring exposure factors and/or procedural protocols in accordance with ALARA principles and age-specific considerations
4. Ensuring adherence to federal, state, and local regulatory requirements
5. Facilitating change through appropriate management processes
6. Facilitating performance improvement processes
7. Facilitating the department's quality assessment and improvement plan
8. Performing physics surveys independently on general radiographic and fluoroscopic equipment, with medical physicist oversight
9. Providing assistance to staff for image optimization, including patient positioning, proper equipment use, and image critique
10. Providing input for equipment and software purchase and supply decisions when appropriate or requested
11. Providing practical information regarding quality management topics
12. Serving as a resource regarding regulatory, accreditation, and fiscal requirements
13. Supporting and assisting a medical physicist with modality physics surveys

Data from American Society of Radiologic Technologists: *Practice Standards for Medical Imaging and Radiation Therapy*, Albuquerque, 2019, ASRT.

---

the healthcare setting such as the emergency department staff or floor nurses so the patient can be cared for properly. Proper communication also includes report dictation, transcription, and distribution to the ordering provider and other interested parties. Modern imaging departments rely on electronic reporting and electronic record keeping (i.e., Hospital Information Systems and Radiology Information Systems), so a major administrative responsibility is making sure that all personnel have competency in computer usage and knowledge of HIPAA requirements.

Patient Comfort

Patient comfort, convenience, and privacy should be provided within reasonable limits in diagnostic imaging departments. Factors such as patient scheduling, preparation, waiting time, ambient room temperature, and politeness and consideration of personnel should be monitored regularly. This is best accomplished by a patient survey or questionnaire, which should be sent to patients 3–7 days after the procedure for maximum reliability. These can be administered in various formats including comment cards, mail surveys, web-based or social network surveys (using tools such as SurveyMonkey, etc.), or telephone interviews (personal interviews with patients via telephone by trained interviewers). Some healthcare organizations may also utilize point-of-service interviews, which are either self-administered or interviewer-administered

questionnaires that are usually completed following service delivery at the clinical site. The method of delivery of patient satisfaction surveys is usually determined by which method will yield the greatest response rate. As discussed in Chapter 2, respect and caring, and timeliness of care, are key clinical performance indicators that require measurement by accrediting agencies. Acute care hospitals subject to the Inpatient Prospective Payment System must survey recently discharged patients on their hospital experience using the Hospital Care Quality Information from the Consumer Perspective survey. This survey was developed by the CMS and the Agency for Healthcare Research and Quality in 2002. The core of the survey consists of 21 items that ask whether patients experienced a critical aspect of hospital care, rather than whether they were "satisfied" with their care. Also included in the survey are four screener items that direct patients to relevant questions, five items to adjust for the mix of patients across hospitals, and two items that support congressionally mandated reports. Hospitals may include additional questions after the core Hospital Care Quality Information from the Consumer Perspective items. Further information can be found at www. hcahpsonline.org.

Personnel Performance

Policies should be developed to ensure that diagnostic personnel are performing their duties within accepted professional standards for areas such as proper equipment operation, critical thinking, and interaction with patients and other personnel. Information obtained from repeat analysis studies and patient surveys can be useful in assessing performance. Documentation of data, periodic review of these data, and any corrective actions that have been taken also should be included. Personnel education programs also should be offered and documented to improve performance and maintain staff competency. In addition to continuing education in topics that are specific to each modality (i.e., new equipment operation, radiation safety), departments should also try to educate their personnel in quality management topics such as working in interdisciplinary teams, applying quality improvement activities, and using informatics.

Record-Keeping System

A record-keeping system is necessary to document that quality management and quality control procedures are being implemented and that they are in compliance with accepted norms. Items that should be included are processor control charts (film/screen departments only), phantom image results, equipment checklists, examination requisitions, equipment service records, incident reports, personnel dosimetry reports of radiation exposure, and image interpretation reports.

Corrective Action

If equipment or personnel are not performing to accepted standards, corrective action must be taken and documented. Equipment downtime and failure should be documented using established forms and procedures. In-service education or other corrective action procedures may be necessary for department personnel. A flowchart is a useful tool in demonstrating corrective actions for possible problems.

RISK MANAGEMENT

An important aspect of a quality management program for diagnostic imaging departments is risk management. This is the system or process for the identification, analysis, and evaluation of risks and the selection of the most advantageous method for minimizing them. Other names for risk management include *safety and loss prevention, total loss control*, or *loss control management*. Risk can be defined as the chance of an event or incident happening that may threaten or damage an organization. Measuring risk can take place in the form of either the likelihood of something happening or the consequences should something actually happen. The purpose of a risk management program is to maintain quality patient care and a safe environment for employees and visitors, while conserving the healthcare institution's financial resources. When studying risk management, it is important to note two important terms, safety and error. Safety is defined as the freedom from accidental injury or death and is a key dimension of healthcare quality. Error is defined as the failure of a planned action to be completed as intended or the use of a wrong plan to achieve an outcome. Preventing errors in the first

place or resolving errors that do occur is a key objective of a risk management program. In quality management, blaming individual staff for errors rather than the processes and system in place should be avoided. Therefore processes need to be in place to reduce the likelihood of an event occurring (risk reduction) as well as to minimize the consequences of an event should one occur. The overall responsibility for risk management may lie with a risk management coordinator, a risk management team, the individual department manager, or the department quality management person, depending on the size and structure of the institution. However, all employees must be made aware of their role in the risk management process. This includes proper education in both departmental and institutional policies and procedures, awareness of safety issues, and the immediate reporting of incidents and hazardous conditions to the appropriate person.

Risk Analysis

The first step in developing risk management policies and procedures for diagnostic imaging departments is to perform a risk analysis. This means identifying the potential risks to patients, employees, students, and visitors to the diagnostic imaging department.

- *Risks to patients*. The potential risks to patients in diagnostic imaging departments are considerable. For example, patients may slip and fall, be hit by equipment, have a reaction to contrast media, have entered the department with a traumatic injury and be improperly manipulated, or receive the wrong diagnostic procedure (all are considered to be sentinel events). Other more subtle risks can include excess radiation exposure (due to additional radiation from repeat images), exposure to infectious disease (due to failure of the technologist to maintain room cleanliness), and breach of confidentiality (due to technologists discussing patient information near waiting areas or other unauthorized persons). These potential risks can be reduced by having the appropriate policies and procedures in place and making sure that employees have knowledge of and follow these procedures. Accrediting agencies such as TJC and DNV-GL publish extensive safety guidelines for patients for various types of healthcare institutions on their websites. Documentation of adherence to these guidelines is essential in obtaining and maintaining accreditation.
- *Risks to employees and medical staff*. Risks to employees and professional staff include injuries from falls, back injury from lifting patients or heavy equipment, repetitive stress injuries, needlesticks, exposure to infectious diseases, exposure to ionizing radiation, and exposure to toxic chemicals such as processing solutions. Most of the risks to employees and medical staff (like those to the patient) also can be reduced by implementing appropriate policies and procedures. Information to better ensure safe labor practices and workplace safety is available from two federal agencies, namely the National Institute for Occupational Safety and Health and OSHA. The National Institute for Occupational Safety and Health is

a part of the Health and Human Services Center for Disease Control and Prevention. Their goals are to (1) conduct research to reduce worker illness and injury and to advance worker well-being; (2) promote safe and healthy workers through intervention, recommendations, and capacity building; and (3) enhance international worker safety and health through global collaborations. OSHA is a part of the US Department of Labor. The function of this agency is to ensure safe and healthful working conditions for employees by setting and enforcing standards and by providing training, outreach, education, and assistance. Information concerning work-related employee injuries and illness is available in the OSHA 2000 Log. This report must be posted at the work site each year during the month of February. These reports may be maintained by the human resources department, risk manager, or employee health department, depending on the institution. Potential workplace concerns for employees in diagnostic imaging departments may include infections, blood-borne pathogen exposure, injuries from lifting or moving patients, radiation exposure, chemical exposure, and magnetic field dangers for MRI technologists. Good policies and procedures in place, along with proper training and supervision, should reduce the likelihood of these dangers.

- *Risk to others.* This category includes such persons as students, visitors, and volunteers, and is probably the most difficult category to assess. This is due to the potential size of this group and the variety of persons that can be included. Another potential difficulty is that the individuals within this group probably have little or no knowledge of the policies and procedures of the healthcare institution. The greatest potential risks to members of this group are injuries from falling, exposure to infectious disease, and HIPAA violations (such as they may not have knowledge of privacy concerns). It is imperative to have appropriate policies and procedures in place to address these risks and to encourage employees (because they should have been educated in risk management) to report any hazardous conditions (e.g., liquid spills) immediately.
- Once a risk analysis is performed and policies and procedures have been created to reduce any potential risks, the next step in a risk management program is to create an investigation procedure for any incidents that may occur. An **incident** is any occurrence that is not consistent with the routine care of a patient or the normal course of events at a particular facility. Facilities should have some type of "incident report" form that is to be completed as soon as possible after an incident. The completed reports should be reviewed immediately by the department manager and then forwarded to the risk manager for additional review. The risk manager should then determine whether any followup action is necessary. This can include additional investigation, notification of government agencies (e.g., the FDA, OSHA, the Nuclear Regulatory Commission [NRC], the EPA), or the obtainment of legal counsel.

A risk management program also should include policies and procedures addressing claims prevention and loss potential. **Loss potential** refers to any activity that costs a facility either money or its reputation. Educating employees on safety policies and procedures, emphasizing quality patient care, and communicating effectively within the healthcare facility can greatly reduce the occurrence of incidents and therefore the cost of defending any claims that may result from these incidents. With these policies in place and documentation that they are being implemented, loss potential can be reduced, first by minimizing the chance of an incident and second, by showing that the healthcare facility did all that it could to minimize risk, which should cast a more favorable opinion if litigation becomes necessary.

Policies and Procedures

Finally, if an incident does occur, a risk management program should have policies and procedures in place that address responsibility of the healthcare institution for the outcome of the incident, for example, paying the medical bills for a patient or employee who is injured in a diagnostic imaging department. Having effective policies and procedures addressing this type of responsibility and loss can often prevent the filing of a claim or reduce the amount of a claim after litigation. As with all quality management components, keeping proper records of all incidents, documents, reports, and policies is imperative for the process to be successful. The following list summarizes the key concepts of an effective risk management program:

- *Risk analysis*—to identify all potential hazards and risks that can occur
- *Written policies and procedures*—to reduce all risks and deal with incidents as they occur
- *Employee education*—to inform employees of all policies and procedures, as well as seek input from employees (such as a brainstorming session) to identify and reduce further risks
- *Periodic inspection*—to make sure that all policies and procedures are being implemented
- *Record keeping*—to document that all policies and procedures have been implemented

REGULATORY AND STANDARDS COMPLIANCE

Policies and procedures must be in place to ensure adherence to accreditation, federal, state, and local regulatory requirements. Institutional and/or image specific accrediting agencies were discussed earlier in this chapter, as well as noncompliance (i.e., loss of accreditation and therefore inability to receive reimbursement for fees). Failure to comply with federal, state, and local requirements generally results in significant fines, which can increase the expenses for the department as well as result in the loss of a business license. Therefore adherence to these standards is a key job responsibility for a quality management technologist.

RADIATION SAFETY PROGRAM

Diagnostic imaging procedures (with the exception of MRI and sonography) contribute the largest single exposure to artificial radiation (more than 90%) in the United States. The average effective dose equivalent for diagnostic radiographs is 39 millirem (mrem) (0.39 millisievert [mSv]) and 14 mrem (0.14 mSv) for nuclear medicine procedures. This is in addition to the 360 mrem (3.6 mSv) per year that is received from natural sources such as cosmic radiation (from outer space), terrestrial radiation (from the earth, air, and drinking water), and internal radiation (from our own body tissues). The 360 mrem (3.6 mSv) per year is an average for the United States and can vary considerably from one location to the next. Persons who live in areas where the altitude is high or where exposure to radon-222 is common may experience considerably more than 360 mrem per year. It is therefore imperative that patients, visitors, hospital staff, and radiographers themselves receive as little radiation exposure as possible. It is the primary responsibility of each radiographer to ensure that this indeed occurs. A quality management program should have radiation safety policies and procedures in place to make sure that all employees who administer ionizing radiation to patients are aware of this responsibility. The NRC (or state radiation governing body) and TJC require a radiation safety committee, administered by a radiation safety officer, to implement these policies. Additional responsibilities of this committee would include creating policies and procedures for the safe handling and disposal of radioactive materials, radiation accidents, and care of patients exposed to radiation.

Implementation of proper radiation safety protocols is mandated by the federal government and most state governments. The more important federal laws are described in this chapter. The enactment of the laws mentioned earlier in Chapter 1 means that diagnostic imaging professionals may have to interact with one or more regulatory agencies that oversee compliance. These federal agencies include the following:

- *The FDA*. As mentioned previously, the FDA, through the Center for Devices and Radiological Health, regulates the design and manufacture of X-ray equipment. These regulations are contained in the document Title 21 of the Code of Federal Regulations Part 1020 (21 CFR 1020). Title 21 refers to the FDA. The FDA also must certify the administrative, professional, and technical aspects of mammographic services to obtain Medicare and most private insurance reimbursement. The FDA uses three classifications of all medical devices:
  - *Class I—general controls.* Class I devices are subject to the least regulatory control and present minimal potential for harm to the user. Examples would include image receptors, grids, and lead aprons.
  - *Class II—special controls.* Class II devices are those for which general controls alone are insufficient to assure safety and effectiveness. In addition to complying with general controls, class II devices also are subject to special

controls. Examples would include collimators, pressure injectors for contrast media, and barium enema tips.
  - *Class III—premarket approval.* Class III is the most stringent regulatory category for devices. Class III devices are those for which insufficient information exists to ensure safety and effectiveness solely through general or special controls. Class III devices are usually those that support or sustain human life; are of substantial importance in preventing impairment of human health; or present a potential, unreasonable risk of illness or injury. Examples include angioplasty catheters and cardiovascular stents.
- *The NRC.* This agency is responsible for enforcing both equipment standards and radiation safety practices. This information is published in Title 10 of the Code of Federal Regulations Part 20 (10 CFR 20). Title 10 refers to the Department of Energy, which contains the NRC. In some states called *agreement states*, the NRC allows the state to have the responsibility to enforce equipment standards and radiation safety practices. As of the writing of this edition, there are currently 37 agreement states. The nonagreement states are Montana, Idaho, South Dakota, Missouri, Indiana, Michigan, West Virginia, Connecticut, Delaware, Alaska, and Hawaii, as well as Washington, DC. The states of Vermont and Wyoming have signed letters of intent to become agreement states.
- *OSHA.* This agency is responsible for establishing standards for safety and monitoring the workplace environment, including the requirements for occupational exposure to radiation, handling and disposal of hazardous materials, universal precautions (Tier 1) for protection of employees from infectious diseases, and personal protective equipment. This information is contained in Title 29 of the Code of Federal Regulations Part 1910 (29 CFR 1910). Title 29 refers to OSHA.

Patient Radiation Protection

Radiographic Examinations

The federal government recommends that the ALARA concept be used during all diagnostic X-ray procedures. ALARA is covered in detail in the National Council on Radiation Protection (NCRP) Report #107. Some of the main recommendations of the ALARA program for radiographic examinations include the following:

- *Use of high kilovolt (peak) (kVp) and low milliampere-second (mAs) exposure factors.* This is the most effective method of reducing patient exposure because milliampere-second selection is the primary control of the quantity of radiation emitted by the X-ray source. This is even more critical with CR systems and DR systems. With these systems, the computer can compensate for overexposure to radiation when it displays the final image on the monitor. This can lead technologists to become careless in their milliampere-second selection; they can overexpose the patient, resulting in dose creep. This is an increase in patient radiation exposure that occurs in CR and DR imaging, since these systems can compensate for overexposure up to 500% above the ideal amount but only compensate for underexposure of about 60% below the ideal value. It is extremely important to adhere to your system's recommended exposure indicator values (e.g., dose index (DI) numbers, S-numbers) to avoid overexposure to your patient. The radiographer must keep in mind that the kilovolt (peak) that is used must be kept in an optimum range for the particular part of the body that is being radiographed, because excessive kilovolt (peak) can produce images that may be of poor diagnostic quality (especially with film/screen image receptors).

- *Use of high-speed image receptor systems.* This is the second most effective method of reducing patient exposure because a faster speed system requires a lower milliampere-second value to obtain a diagnostic image. With conventional film/screen imaging systems, most departments use rare earth phosphors that are high speed and demonstrate acceptable recorded detail. When deciding which image receptor to use, one must consider that faster speed film/screen systems can demonstrate poorer resolution than slower speed systems. Most current CR and DR systems possess a system speed that is comparable to a 200- to 300-speed film/screen system.

- *Use of proper filtration.* Filtration removes lower-energy X-rays from the primary beam before contact with the patient. This can reduce the patient's entrance skin dose by as much as 90%. There is usually a certain amount of inherent filtration (filtering performed by the window of the X-ray tube, as well as any cooling oil) present and added aluminum or copper between the X-ray tube window and the top of the collimating device.

- *Use of the smallest field size possible, along with proper collimation.* This reduces the amount of the patient's body that is exposed to radiation, thereby reducing the total dose. The effect of field size can be seen by calculating a value known as the **dose area product** (DAP) or **kerma area product (KAP)**. These values incorporate the total dose of radiation or air kerma value along with the area of field that is being used. The units that can be used to measure DAP can be roentgen (R) × square centimeter (R × cm²), coulomb per kilogram (C/kg) × square centimeter (C/kg × cm²), or Rad × square centimeter (R × cm²). For KAP measurement, the milliGray × square centimeter (mGy × cm²) or microGray × square centimeter (μGy × cm²) may be used. For example, a field size of 5 × 5 cm (25 cm²) can receive a dosage of 4 R, yielding a DAP of 100 R × square centimeter. A field size of 20 × 20 cm (400 cm²) can receive a much lower dose of only 0.25 R but still yield the same DAP of 100 R × square centimeter because of the increase in the size of the X-ray field.

- *Use of optimum processing conditions.* Regardless of whether one is using film/screen radiography or a digital radiographic imaging system, proper image processing must exist to obtain consistent image quality. Automatic film processor quality control is extremely important in lowering the patient dose in conventional film/screen radiography. For example, if the developer temperature were too low, the resulting radiographs would appear to lack optical density. This can lead to a repeat image (increasing the dose for that particular patient) or to an increase in technical factors for subsequent images (increasing patient dose for all subsequent patients). For CR and DR systems, proper manipulation of both preprocessing and postprocessing software factors by the radiographer is necessary to obtain proper image quality.

- *Avoidance of repeat examinations.* The ideal overall repeat rate for diagnostic imaging departments is no greater than 4%–6% (2% for mammographic procedures). This figure can vary depending on the patient population and acceptance standards of a particular imaging department but should never exceed 10%–12%. Proper patient instructions, along with correct positioning and technique selection by the radiographer, should help reduce the need for repeat examinations. Digital radiographic systems can reduce the repeat rate due to technique error because postprocessing software can yield some correction of image brightness (optical density in film/screen imaging) and image gray scale (contrast in film/screen imaging). Proper positioning is extremely important when automatic exposure control devices are used with both film/screen imaging (to be sure the correct portion of the anatomy is over the cell that has been selected) and with CR and DR systems (because the computer must compare the image obtained with its preprogrammed ideal image to obtain the correct image).

- Use of a posteroanterior (PA) projection instead of an anteroposterior (AP) projection for scoliosis series on young female patients. Normally, radiographic views of the spine are performed with an AP projection to place the spine as close to the image receptor as possible. However, the breast tissue in female adolescents is extremely sensitive to the development of radiation-induced breast cancer (with a latent period of 5–15 years). When the examination is performed with the PA projection instead of the AP projection, the breast tissue receives the exit dose instead of the entrance dose of radiation. This can reduce the mean glandular dose to the breast tissue by as much as 98%. Shielding of the breast areas with specialized devices also should be used to reduce the dose even further.

- *Use of gonadal shielding.* The FDA recommends that gonadal shielding with at least 0.5-mm lead equivalence should be used whenever the gonads lie within 5 cm of the collimation line and do not interfere with the anatomy of interest (21CFR1000.50). This can reduce the dose to the reproductive organs by as much as 90%. Gonadal shielding may be a flat contact, a shaped contact, or a shadow type of shield. In April of 2019, the American Association of Physicists in Medicine (AAPM) issued a position statement that "[p]atient gonadal and fetal shielding during X-ray based diagnostic imaging should be discontinued as routine practice. Because of these risks and the minimal to nonexistent benefit associated with fetal and gonadal shielding, AAPM recommends that the use of such shielding should be discontinued." In January 2021, the NCRP concurred, stating, "NCRP now recommends that gonadal shielding (GS) not be used routinely during abdominal and pelvic radiography, and that federal, state, and local regulations and guidance should be revised to remove any actual or implied requirement for routine GS. GS use may remain appropriate in some limited circumstances. The recommendations in this Statement are limited to patient GS during abdominal and pelvic radiography. NCRP recognizes that adoption of these new recommendations requires addressing the impact of this substantial change on ingrained medical practice." As of the writing of this edition, the FDA has not changed its requirement on gonadal shielding, so each department should discuss and develop policies on gonadal shielding.

Fluoroscopic Examinations

Fluoroscopic examinations have the potential to deliver a considerable dose of radiation to the patient. Therefore ALARA protocols, including the following, should be in place for these examinations:

Make sure that the fluoroscopic system does not exceed maximum entrance exposure or air kerma rates. Fluoroscopic systems that are provided with automatic exposure rate control (AERC) shall not be operable at any combination of tube potential and current that will result in an exposure rate (air kerma rate) in excess of 2.58×10^{-3} coulomb per kilogram per minute (C/kg per minute), 10 roentgens per minute (10 R/min or 100 mGy/min) at the point where the center of the useful beam enters the patient. AERC, also known as automatic brightness control (or automatic brightness stabilization) is a system that adjusts X-ray output parameters when moving from various regions of the body to maintain uniform image brightness. Fluoroscopic systems that are not provided with AERC shall not be operable at any combination of tube potential and current that will result in an exposure rate (air kerma rate) in excess of 1.29×10^{-3} C/kg per minute (5 R/min or 50 mGy/min) at the point where the center of the useful beam enters the patient. For systems equipped with high-level control, the fluoroscopic system shall not be operable at any combination of tube potential and current that will result in an exposure rate (air kerma rate) in excess of 5.16×10^{-3} C/kg per minute (20 R/min or 200 mGy/min) at the point where the center of the useful beam enters the patient. Special means of activation of high-level controls shall be required. The high-level control shall only be operable when continuous manual activation is provided by the operator. A continuous signal audible to the fluoroscopist shall indicate that the high-level control is being employed.

- *Keep fluoroscopic milliampere (mA) and time as low as possible when performing fluoroscopy.* The mA is usually kept in a relatively narrow range (0.5–3 mA), so reducing the fluoroscopic time is one of the most effective means of reducing patient dose during fluoroscopic procedures.
- *Use high kilovolt (peak) if possible.* Fluoroscopic examinations should be performed in the 85- to 125-kVp range (depending on the contrast media being used). The use of a higher kVp reduces the fluoroscopic mA required to obtain adequate image brightness, thereby reducing the patient's dose.

- *Limit field size as much as possible.* This is done with the fluoroscopic collimation shutters and with a smaller size image intensifier. This has the same effect as collimation, which was previously discussed.
- *Use intermittent fluoroscopy (periodic activation of the fluoroscopic X-ray tube rather than continuous activation).* This can reduce patient dose by as much as 90%. Many departments have incorporated a procedure of recording the total fluoroscopic exposure time of a patient in their medical records or in a department log sheet. This information also should include the name of the radiologist/provider who performed the fluoroscopy, along with the patient case number.
- *Use the last-image-hold feature.* This feature holds the last image obtained in digital storage and displays it on the monitor. This can reduce total fluoroscopic time by 50% to 80%.
- *Avoid the magnification mode.* The magnification mode found with multifield tube-type image intensifiers can increase patient dose 2–10 times that of the standard mode. This is because the magnification mode reduces the brightness gain of the image intensifier tube, requiring an increase in fluoroscopic milliampere to compensate.
- Keep the patient-to-image intensifier distance as short as possible during mobile fluoroscopic studies with a C-arm. This reduces the source-to-skin distance to the patient.
- *Reduce the number of spot images and reduce the spot image size.* Patient dose increases as the number of spot images increases. In addition, larger spot size formats require more radiation; therefore, patient dose is increased.

One program to help reduce patient exposure during radiographic, CT, and fluoroscopic procedures in adults is called Image Wisely. This was developed by the ACR, Radiologic Society of North America, ASRT, and AAPM to raise public and professional awareness about the risks and benefits of the use of ionizing radiation used in medically necessary diagnostic imaging studies and eliminating unnecessary procedures. For pediatric patients, a program known as Image Gently was created by Society of Pediatric Radiology, ACR, ASRT, and AAPM in 2007. The goal of this program is to provide safe, high-quality pediatric imaging through raising awareness of the need to adjust radiation dose when imaging children.

Diagnostic reference levels. In addition to these ALARA concepts, radiology departments should be aware of diagnostic reference levels (DRLs). According to the ACR and the American Association of Physicists in Medicine, a DRL is an investigational level used to identify unusually high radiation doses for common diagnostic medical X-ray imaging procedures. DRLs are suggested action levels above which a facility should review its methods and determine if acceptable image quality can be achieved at lower doses. DRLs are based on standard phantom or patient measurements under specific conditions at a number of representative clinical facilities. DRLs have been set at approximately the 75th percentile of measured patient or phantom data. This means that procedures performed at 75% of the institutions surveyed have exposure levels at or below the DRL. Achievable dose (AD) can be used with DRLs to assist in optimizing image

TABLE 1.1 DRL and AD for Radiography		
Examination	DRL (mGy)	AD (mGy)
Adult PA chest (23 cm) with grid	0.15	0.11
Pediatric PA chest (12.5 cm), without grid	0.06	0.04
Pediatric PA chest (12.5 cm), with grid	0.12	0.07
Adult AP Abdomen (22 cm)	3.4	2.4
Adult AP lumbosacral spine (22 cm)	4.2	2.8

AD, Achievable dose; *AP*, anteroposterior; *DRL*, diagnostic reference level; *mGy*, milliGray; *PA*, posteroanterior.

TABLE 1.2 DRL and AD for Fluoroscopy		
Phantom: Adult PA Abdomen with Grid	DRL	AD
Upper GI fluoroscopy without oral contrast media	54 mGy min^{-1}	40 mGy min^{-1}
Upper GI fluoroscopy with oral contrast media	80 mGy min^{-1}	72 mGy min^{-1}
Fluorographic image without contrast		
Film	3.9 mGy	2.5 mGy
Digital	1.5 mGy	0.9 mGy
Fluorographic image with contrast		
Film	27.5 mGy	18.7 mGy
Digital	9.9 mGy	5.3 mGy

AD, Achievable dose; *DRL*, diagnostic reference level; *GI*, gastrointestinal; *mGy*, milliGray; *PA*, posteroanterior.

quality and dose. ADs are set at approximately the median (50th percentile) of the study dose distribution (i.e., half of the facilities are producing images at lower doses and half are using higher doses). The DRL and AD values from these two groups are as follows.

Radiography. For radiography, including screen-film and digital imaging, this practice parameter bases DRLs and ADs on a measurement of air kerma in milliGray at the skin plane (without backscatter) to a standard phantom using the X-ray technique factors the facility would typically select for an average size adult or pediatric patient (see Table 1.1).

Fluoroscopy. For fluoroscopy, the DRLs and ADs are based on a measurement of air kerma in milliGray at the skin plane (with some backscatter due to the geometry) to a standard phantom using the X-ray technique factors the facility would typically select for an average-size adult patient. Published reference levels are currently not available for pediatric patients (see Table 1.2).

Computed tomography. The DRLs and ADs for CT are based on the volume CT dose index (CTDIvol) in milliGray. For the values reported herein, the 16-cm diameter phantom was used for all head and pediatric abdomen CT examinations, and the 32-cm diameter phantom was used for all adult body CT examinations (see Table 1.3).

Patient dose tracking. Diagnostic medical imaging performs over 4 billion studies worldwide each year, which means that populations are being exposed to increasing doses of ionizing radiation. The majority of this exposure is justified, with medical benefits for patients, but reports in a variety of clinical settings have identified a number of

radiological examinations that may not meet appropriateness criteria. The International Atomic Energy Agency initiated the Smart Card project in 2006 with the objective of developing a flexible template for tracking cumulative radiation exposure (number and type of radiological procedures) and wherever possible, dose for individual procedure. This program was subsequently named as SmartCard/SmartRadTrack. This was to dispel the myth that the purpose is to develop a card that contains patient dose history and to indicate a mechanism to track procedures and doses. Since that time, efforts worldwide have begun to require patient dose tracking for diagnostic imaging examinations and have this information become part of the patient's EHR. Examples include:

1. Veterans Health Administration—The Veterans Health Administration Handbook dated July 6, 2012, states: "A record must be kept of each fluoroscopic procedure. The record must list the fluoroscopy unit, date of the procedure, type of procedure, information identifying the patient, and the name of the provider operating or directing the operation of the device. The record must also list the cumulative fluoroscopy time, number of static images, total time of dynamic cinefluorography series, the cumulative air kerma or skin dose from both fluoroscopy and from static image recording, if available, and the dose-area-product, if available. Dose can be stored as a Digital Imaging and

TABLE 1.3 DRL and AD for CT				
	Patient Lateral (LAT) Dimension	CTDI Phantom Diameter (cm)	DRL (mGy)	AD (mGy)
Adult head	16	16	75	57
Adult abdomen-pelvis	38	32	25	17
Adult chest	35	32	21	14
Pediatric 5-year-old head	15	16	40	31
Pediatric 5-year-old abdomen-pelvis	20	16	20	14

AD, Achievable dose; *CTDI*, computed tomography dose index; *DRL*, diagnostic reference level; *GI*, gastrointestinal; *mGy*, milliGray; *PA*, posteroanterior.

Communications in Medicine Radiation Dose Structured Report."

2. TJC—revised TJC requirements also specify that the radiation dose of every CT examination must be recorded, and that high radiation dose incidents must be evaluated against industry benchmarks (found under the Provision of Care, Treatment, and Services PC.0102.15):

- The [critical access] hospital documents in the patient's medical history record the radiation dose index (CTDIvol, DLP [dose length product], or size-specific dose estimate [SSDE]) on every study produced during a diagnostic CT examination. The radiation dose index must be exam specific, summarized by series or anatomic area, and documented in a retrievable format.

- The [critical access] hospital reviews and analyzes incidents where the radiation dose index (CTDIvol, DLP, or size-specific dose estimate [SSDE]) from diagnostic CT examinations exceeded expected dose index ranges identified in imaging protocols. These incidents are then compared to external benchmarks.

3. The ACR—The ACR hosts a Dose Index Registry (DIR) that allows facilities to compare their CT dose indices to regional and national values. The information collected is masked, transmitted to the ACR, and stored in a database. Facilities receive quarterly feedback reports comparing their results to aggregate results by body part and examination type. According to TJC, the ACR DIR provides benchmark data. The intent of Performance Improvement Standard PI.02.01.01 is to ensure that the organization is committed to dose optimization and stays current with standard of practice. Since the frequency of data collection and analysis is under the organization's purview, participation in the ACR DIR would meet compliance with PI.02.01.01.

4. Individual State Requirements—As of the writing of this edition, the states of California and Texas have enacted legislation to require patient dose tracking in certain radiologic procedures. The state of Ohio has proposed dose tracking of cumulative air kerma or dose area product/kerma area product for fluoroscopic procedures involving interventional procedures and cardiac catheterization of pediatric or pregnant patients.

- California—Senate Bill 1237 took effect in January of 2011, and requires the reporting to the State of California Health and Human Services Agency all CT scans that are repeated or occurred to the wrong body part that exceeded an effective dose equivalent of 0.05 Sievert (5 rem), 0.5 Sievert (50 rem) to a specific organ or tissue, and 0.5 Sievert (50 rem) shallow dose to the skin. The CTDIvol or DLP are required to calculate the effective dose equivalent. It also requires that CT departments must be accredited in CT by an organization that is approved by the CMS.

- Texas—Texas Administrative Code 25 TAC 289.227 took effect in May of 2013. One provision of the law is for departments to establish radiation protocol committees (RPCs) for CT systems and fluoroscopically guided interventional procedures. These committees

are responsible for establishing DRLs for these procedures, specify methods that are to be used to monitor radiation output for these procedures, and specify actions that are to be taken when reference levels are exceeded. For fluoroscopy, the RPC must make and maintain a record of radiation output information so the radiation dose to the skin may be estimated, and must include cumulative air kerma or dose area product (if available on system) and fluoro mode, cumulative exposure time, and number of recorded exposures. The RPC for CT systems must make and maintain a record of radiation output information so the radiation dose to the skin may be estimated using CTDIvol and DLP (if system capable of calculating and displaying) or an index described by the AAPM Task Group 111.

It is expected that more states and the federal government will expand patient dose tracking or dose monitoring requirements in the near future. Luckily, commercial dose tracking software packages are available to accomplish this task (see Table 1.4 for a listing of leading dose management software). Features of these systems include transmission of dose information from imaging device or PACS, advanced analysis and reporting capabilities, and can integrate with PACS, radiology information system (RIS), and electronic health record (EHR) systems. Problems that have been encountered with patient dose tracking software include no uniform dose metrics across all systems and difficulty working on older equipment.

Visitor Protection

"Visitors" to diagnostic imaging departments are persons other than patients or radiology department staff. They may include relatives or friends of patients, hospital volunteers, security personnel, or other hospital employees who do not normally work in radiation areas (e.g., nurses, patient care technicians, respiratory therapists). Although these persons are in the diagnostic imaging department or near mobile X-ray equipment in use (e.g., the emergency department or surgical suite), they are entitled to a safe environment with no unnecessary exposure to ionizing radiation. The NCRP lists maximum effective dose equivalent limits for members of the general population in its report, number 116. For members of the general population who may be exposed to frequent or continuous exposure from artificial sources other than medical irradiation (this includes radiography students younger than the age of 18), the NCRP recommends a maximum effective dose equivalent limit of 0.1 rad equivalent, man (rem) (1 mSv) per year. For those who may receive infrequent exposure (e.g., a parent who may be asked to hold a child for an X-ray procedure), a maximum of 0.5 rem (5 mSv) per year is recommended. To help minimize exposure to department visitors, radiographers can make sure that all examination room doors remain closed during radiographic procedures.

During mobile radiographic procedures, visitors should leave the area if possible or move at least 8 ft away from the source of radiation. Visitors who want to accompany patients or observe a radiographic examination (such as a prospective radiography student or a radiology resident) should remain

TABLE 1.4 Various Dose Management/Patient Dose Tracking Software Vendors and Products

Company	Product	URL
Agfa Healthcare	Dose Monitor	https://www.dosemonitor.com
Bayer Healthcare LLC	Radimetrics Enterprise Platform	https://www.radimetrics.com
Canon Medical	Dose Tracking System	https://global.medical.canon
Canon Medical	SPOT Fluoroscopy	https://global.medical.canon
Fujifilm Medical Systems U.S.A., Inc.	FDX console (common acquisition workstation for all Fujifilm DR portable and room solutions)	http://www.fujimed.com
Fujifilm Medical Systems U.S.A., Inc.	Aspire AWS Console (common acquisition workstation for all Fujifilm mammography solutions)	http://www.fujimed.com
GE HealthCare	DoseWatch	https://www3.gehealthcare.com
GE HealthCare	DoseWatch Explore	https://www3.gehealthcare.com
Guerbet LLC	Dose&Care	https://www.guerbet.com
Imalogix	ImalogixT	https://imalogix.com
Infinitt Healthcare	DoseM	https://www.infinittna.com
Medic Vision Imaging Solutions Ltd.	SafeCT-29	http://www.medicvision.com/usa/
Medic Vision Imaging Solutions Ltd.	SafeCT Dose Report	http://www.medicvision.com/usa/
Medic Vision Imaging Solutions Ltd.	SafeCT Dose Report	http://www.medicvision.com/usa/
Medsquare	Radiation Dose Monitor (RDM)	https://www.medsquarehealth.com
MyXrayDose Ltd.	MyXrayDose	https://myxraydose.com
Novarad	Novadose	https://www.novarad.net/
Numa, Inc.	Numa (for nuclear medicine and PET)	https://www.ec2software.com
PACSHealth, LLC/PHS Technologies Group, LLC	DoseMonitor, NexoDose (Bracco), NovaDose (Novarad), Agfa Healthcare Dose Management (Agfa), Radiation Dose Monitor by NTT (Dell)	https://pacshealth.com
Primordial Design	Primordial	https://www.nuance.com/healthcare/diagnostics-solutions/workflow-radiology-reporting/powerscribe-one.html
Philips Healthcare	DoseWise Portal	http://www.usa.philips.com/health-care/clinical-solutions/dosewise
ScImage, Inc.	PICOM365	https://scimage.com
Sectra	Sectra Dosetrak	https://medical.sectra.com
Siemens Healthineers	Right Dose	https://www.siemens-healthineers.com/en-us/products-services
Qaelum	DOSE	https://qaelum.com
Volpara Solutions, Inc.	VolparaDoseRT	http://www.volparasolutions.com/
Volpara Solutions, Inc.	Volpara Analytics	http://www.volparasolutions.com/

behind a protective barrier or wear protective apparel, or both. In some cases (e.g., pediatric patients), a visitor (nurse, patient care technician, parent, or other relative) may be asked to help hold a patient during a radiographic procedure. These persons should be provided with protective apparel (such as lead aprons and gloves) to prevent overexposure to radiation that can occur during the procedure. Avoiding repeat exposure is also important in these instances because repeat exposure increases the patient's and visitor's dose.

Personnel Protection

Personnel who perform diagnostic procedures using ionizing radiation can potentially receive significant amounts of radiation and must therefore follow proper radiation practices.

According to NCRP report number 116, maximum total effective dose equivalent for occupational personnel are as follows:

Whole body exposure	5 rem (50 mSv) per year
Eye lens	15 rem (150 mSv) per year
All other body parts (such as hands)	50 rem (500 mSv) per year

Examinations in which mobile equipment, fluoroscopy, cardiac catheterization, and interventional procedures are used pose a greater risk of higher dosages to radiographers and radiologists' assistants than traditional radiographic procedures. Occupational radiation dosage should be monitored with a dosimeter obtained from a licensed provider. The most common of these are film badges, optically stimulated luminescent dosimeters, and thermoluminescent dosimeters. These are checked at either 1- or 3-month intervals, with a report sent back to the institution indicating the dosage measured. For whole body measurement, these dosimeters are worn at either the waist or collar area. Finger dosimeters can also be issued in cases where the hands may receive relatively high dosages (i.e., nuclear medicine technologists and interventional technologists).

The embryonic/fetal dose of occupational workers should not exceed 0.0025 mrem (0.025 mSv) per day, 0.05 rem (0.5 mSv) in any 1 month of the 9-month gestation period and 0.5 rem (5 mSv) for the entire gestation period. When a radiographer, radiologist, or radiologist assistant has confirmation that they are pregnant, they must first declare their pregnancy to their employer or many institutions will not accept liability for proper precautions to protect a pregnant worker from radiation. Once the declaration is on file, the fetus is treated like a member of the general population. Most institutions will also issue a second dosimeter to act as a fetal dose monitor. This should be worn at the waist level under a lead apron. The institution should also provide the pregnant employee a full explanation of the potential risks of fetal radiation exposure, dose limits, as well as any state, local, or institutional policies. Technologists who become pregnant should not work with patients who have been treated with radionuclides since these materials could deliver a dose that would exceed acceptable limits.

Medical facilities must have an orientation program on radiation safety for newly employed technologists and a continuing education program to update the skills of all department personnel. Personnel who work in proximity to radiographic and fluoroscopic procedures (e.g., emergency department, operating room, intensive care unit) also should have the same in-service training.

Periodic surveys with properly calibrated instruments such as Geiger–Müller counters and ionization chambers should be performed to assess that radiation in the workplace does not exceed accepted standards. Warning signs marked "Caution: Radiation Area" should be posted for any areas where dosage can exceed 5 milliroentgen (mR)/h or 0.05 milligray (mGy)/h. The cardinal principles of radiation protection (time, distance, and shielding) should be followed by all radiologic technologists to minimize their occupational exposure.

Time

Radiographers should keep the time of exposure to radiation as short as possible because the amount of exposure is directly proportional to the time of exposure, as indicated by the following equation:

$$\text{Total exposure} = \text{exposure rate} \times \text{time}$$

The exposure rate is the output of radiation from the source per unit time. For example, if a radiation source creates an exposure rate of 225 mR/h at a position occupied by an occupational worker, and the worker remains at that position for 36 min, what is the total exposure?

$$\text{Total exposure} = \frac{(225\,\text{mR/h})}{(36/60\,\text{h})} = 135\,\text{mR}$$

The factor of time is especially important during fluoroscopic, angiographic, and interventional procedures.

Distance

Radiographers should always maintain as large a distance as possible between the source of radiation and themselves. The reason is that radiation continually diverges from its source, so as distance is increased, less radiation exists per unit area. Reduction in radiation intensity follows an inverse square relationship and can be determined from the following equation:

$$\frac{\text{New intensity}}{\text{Old intensity}} = \frac{\text{Old distance}^2}{\text{New distance}^2}$$

For example, if the radiation intensity at 90 cm from a radiation source is 1.3 mGy/min, at 270 cm (three times the distance as 90 cm), the radiation intensity is reduced to only 0.14 mGy/min (nine times less than the amount received at 90 cm). Therefore a small increase in the distance from the source causes a large decrease in the amount of radiation exposure that is received. This factor is especially important in fluoroscopy because it may require the operator of the X-ray equipment to remain in the examination room. As a rule of thumb, the occupational radiation exposure during tableside fluoroscopy is about 1 mrem/min. Moving back away from the side of the examination table (if possible) can significantly reduce this amount, according to the inverse square law. Standing on the image receptor side of a C-arm fluoroscopic unit rather than the X-ray tube side will also minimize radiation dose.

Shielding

Any material that can be placed between you and a source of radiation is considered shielding. Materials with a high atomic number (such as lead) that are not naturally radioactive are best for shielding because the greatest amount of photoelectric absorption occurs in these materials. Shielded booths are required for protecting the area around the control panel of radiographic units. The walls of the examination room are designed to protect personnel, other hospital employees, and the general public from unnecessary exposure. Lead aprons and gloves must be provided to employees when the possibility of exposure rate could exceed 5 mR/h (i.e., technologists who must be outside of the control booth during fluoroscopic or mobile procedures). Lead aprons must have a minimum lead equivalent thickness of at least 0.25 mm and cover 75%–80% of the active bone marrow of the person wearing it. Protective gloves require a minimum lead equivalent thickness of 0.25 mm, with 0.5 mm preferred. Thyroid shields are available for general fluoroscopic, angiographic, and interventional procedures, and must have a minimum lead equivalent thickness of 0.5 mm. Protective eyeglasses with a minimum lead equivalence of 0.35 mm or 0.5 mm are also available. Fluoroscopic and cardiovascular/interventional suites can also be equipped with leaded shields made of either radiation-absorbing acrylic or glass panels that are mounted on wheels for portability or are suspended from the ceiling.

SUMMARY

In modern diagnostic imaging departments, the radiologists, department administrators and supervisors, technologists, and support staff should work together to ensure that adequate processes are in place to properly care for the patient, achieve the highest-quality image possible, and obtain the correct diagnosis from that image. These processes also are necessary to meet accreditation standards or government requirements, or both. The processes also should be reviewed continuously by all parties and modified as the need arises. Any quality management plan should have specific objectives (what the program is intending to achieve), an outline of the chain of command and responsibilities within the organization, the scope of the program, a mechanism for monitoring various aspects of patient management, evaluation of the program's effectiveness in meeting the objectives, and the efficacy of the program. Having an effective quality management program also has become necessary as a condition of receiving reimbursement for services by the federal government and many private insurance companies.

Implementing a quality management program requires considerably more than just equipment monitoring and maintenance. A basic knowledge of administrative responsibilities, risk management, and radiation safety practices is essential for a quality management technologist to implement a successful quality management program.

Refer to the Evolve website at https://evolve.elsevier.com for Student Experiment 1.1: Attenuation or Transmission of Radiation.

REVIEW QUESTIONS

1. Which levels of quality control testing can usually be performed by a QA/quality management technologist: level I, level II, or level III?
   a. I and II
   b. I and III
   c. II and III
   d. I, II, and III
2. Which government agency mandates a policy on exposure to blood-borne pathogens?
   a. FDA
   b. EPA
   c. OSHA
   d. Center for Devices and Radiological Health
3. Which of the following terms best describes information or knowledge necessary to achieve a desired outcome?
   a. Supplier
   b. Input
   c. Action
   d. Output
4. Which of the following terms best describes a person, department, or organization that needs or wants a desired outcome?
   a. Supplier
   b. Input
   c. Action
   d. Customer
5. Who is considered to be the "Father of Scientific Management"?
   a. W. Edwards Deming
   b. Joseph Juran
   c. Raymond Smith
   d. Frederick Winslow Taylor

6. The unit of measure used to express the dose equivalent to occupational workers is which of the following?
   a. Coulomb per kilogram of air
   b. Gray
   c. Sievert
   d. Relative biological effectiveness
7. Which of the following does not affect patient dose during diagnostic radiography?
   a. Inherent filtration
   b. Added filtration
   c. Focal spot size
   d. Source-to-image distance
8. The current US regulatory dose limit to the fetus of a radiation worker is:
   a. mSv/month
   b. mSv/month
   c. 0.5 mSv/month
   d. mSv/month
9. The current US regulatory dose limit for the annual whole body effective dose to radiation workers is:
   a. mSv
   b. 5 mSv
   c. 20 mSv
   d. 50 mSv
10. Who regulates the use of radioactive materials in the United States?
    a. NAS-BEIR
    b. NRC
    c. NCRP
    d. FDA

Quality Improvement Tools and Procedures

OBJECTIVES

At the completion of this chapter, the reader should be able to do the following:
- List and define the basic terms used in statistical analysis
- Discuss the seven types of graphs and charts used to organize and present data in total quality management
- List the various tools of group dynamics
- Explain TJC 10-step monitoring and evaluation process and cycle for improving performance
- Describe the components of a quality improvement plan
- Describe the various quality management/quality improvement models

KEY TERMS

Accuracy
Aggregate data indicator
Appropriateness of care
Assess
Benchmarking
Brainstorming
Cause-and-effect diagram
Central tendency
Concurrent data
Continuous variables
Control chart
Critical path
Dashboards
Data
Database
Dataset
Dependent variable
Design
Dichotomous variables
Effectiveness of care
Efficacy of care

Efficiency of care
Enterprise data warehouse
Expectation
Failure mode and effects analysis (FMEA)
Flowchart
Focus group
FOCUS-PDCA
Frequency
Gaussian distribution
Histogram
Improve
Independent variable
Indicators
Key performance indicators
Lean process improvement
Mean
Median
Measure
Mode
Pareto chart
Poisson distribution

Population
Precision
Prejudice
Problem
Qualitative data
Quantitative data
Quality improvement team
Root cause analysis (RCA)
Range
Reliability
Sample
Scatterplot
Sentinel event indicator
Six Sigma
Standard deviation
SWOT analysis
Trend chart
Trending
Validity
Variance
Variation

INFORMATION ANALYSIS

To implement the various components of a quality management program, a considerable amount of data must be collected and analyzed, which requires the use of statistics. Statistics is the mathematical science pertaining to the collection, analysis, interpretation, and presentation of data. These data then can be used to verify the success of organizational processes or provide justification for changing and improving these processes. Data can be defined as discrete entities described objectively without interpretation and can be classified as either quantitative data or qualitative data. Quantitative data are measurable data that focus on numbers and frequencies, such as repeat analysis data or patient waiting time. Qualitative data provide information about descriptive characteristics and are based on observation rather than measurable data. A method that can be used to organize data so that they are easy to store, manage, and access is known as a database. A collection of databases that can be accessed and analyzed in known as an enterprise data warehouse. Examples of enterprise data warehouses include the Agency for Healthcare Research and Quality (AHRQ) and the National Quality Forum. To assist in the implementation of a quality management program, diagnostic imaging personnel need a basic knowledge of the terminology and data presentation tools used in statistical analysis.

Terminology Used in Statistical Analysis

Population

A population comprises the entire set or group of items being measured. Identifying the population to be measured is one of the first steps in performing a statistical analysis. For example, if you perform a statistical analysis of the number of repeat chest radiographs during a particular month, you focus on just the patients receiving chest examinations (that particular population) rather than each patient receiving each type of radiographic procedure.

Sample

A sample is the number of items actually measured from a population. Some populations may be extremely large and therefore difficult to study. Sampling involves choosing a portion or evaluating a subset of the population that makes data collection more practical, timely, and efficient. An example of sampling is the nationwide measurement of persons watching particular television programs. Only certain persons have their television viewing patterns actually monitored by the ratings services, and the results are extrapolated to be indicative of the entire population. This is known as *statistical inference*. Sampling must be performed carefully to ensure that the sample chosen is representative of the entire population.

Dataset

A dataset is the information or measurements acquired by evaluating the particular sample.

Frequency

The frequency is the number of times a particular value of a variable occurs or the number of observations of an event. For example, during a repeat study of chest examinations, 37 chest views had to be repeated during a particular month. Therefore the frequency of repeated chest views for that month was 37.

Dependent Variables

Dependent variables are those variables that are observed in statistical studies to change in response to independent variables and are not controlled during the study. Dependent variables also can be referred to as response variables, measured variables, or output variables. For example, if one were to study how different brands of contrast media cause allergic reactions in diagnostic imaging patients, a researcher could compare the frequency and intensity of a reaction to the different brands of contrast media. In this study, the frequency and cause of allergic reactions would be the dependent variables.

Independent Variables

Independent variables are those that are deliberately manipulated to invoke a change on the dependent variables. Independent variables also may be referred to as predictor variables or input variables. In the example presented under dependent variables comparing how different brands of contrast media cause allergic reactions in diagnostic imaging patients, the different brands of contrast media given to diagnostic imaging patients would be the independent variable.

Continuous Variables

Continuous variables are those variables being studied that have an infinite range of possible mathematical values. Examples might include the age of patients, weight of patients, height of patients, and time of a particular event.

Dichotomous Variables

Dichotomous variables are those variables being studied that have only two opposing choices, such as on or off, black or white, etc.

Central Tendency

The central tendency is the central position of a sample frequency. In statistical analysis, there are several possible measures of central tendency, three of which are the mean, the median, and the mode.

- *Mean*. The mean is the calculated average set of observations and can be denoted by either μ, $\overline{X}$, or M. The mean provides the greatest reliability of the three measures of central tendency.

$$\text{Mean} = \frac{\text{Sum of observed values}\,(\Sigma)}{\text{Total number of values}\,(N)}$$

For example, if the values 7, 3, 6, and 4 are observed, the mean is determined by taking 20 (the sum of the observed values) divided by 4 (the total number of values observed), which yields a mean of 5.

- The median is a point in a data distribution above which are exactly one-half of the values and below which are the other half. In other words, it is the numeric middle or halfway point in the observed dataset. For example, if the values 4, 6, 8, 10, and 12 are observed, the median is 8.

- The mode is the one value that occurs with the greatest frequency in the dataset. For example, if the values 2, 3, 4, 4, 4, 5, and 5 are observed, the mode is 4. The mode provides information about the most typical occurrence, but this is usually just a rough estimate of central value. In a histogram graph (discussed later in this chapter), the mode is the highest point.

Reliability

Reliability refers to the consistency of repeated measurements of the same thing or the reproducibility or variation of a result, and is sometimes known as precision. Many factors, such as the sample size (larger samples are usually more reliable), the design of the data collection process (e.g., are the questions on a survey worded in a "biased" way?), and the collection and interpretation of the data (e.g., is the person collecting the data including all of the information given?), can affect the reliability of statistical information. In diagnostic imaging, the quality of the equipment and the skill of the quality management technologist can also affect reliability or precision. The most common result of low reliability in diagnostic imaging equipment and image assessment evaluations is higher levels of noise. This can be compensated for by collecting more photons during the testing or more signal measurements (i.e., larger sample size). A new quality management program may have unreliable data at first because of the "startup effect." This effect can cause an unusually high or low data result because the human tendency is to be hyperaware when new studies are begun. To counteract the startup effect, a sufficient period of time needs to elapse to allow the data to change and stabilize before reliable data analysis is obtained. Reliability or precision does not imply accuracy.

Accuracy

Accuracy refers to the ability to measure what is purported to be measured and is sometimes referred to as validity. In other words, do the data collected reflect the reality of the situation being studied (i.e., the truth)? One also can think of accuracy as how well a value that has been studied and measured agrees with the true value. The differences between accuracy and reliability (precision) is demonstrated in Fig. 2.1. In the figure, imagine throwing darts at a dart board. Accuracy would refer to how close you got to the bull's-eye or at least

hitting the target. Reliability or precision would refer to the amount of variation or scattering that occurs.

Bias

Bias is a systematic or nonrandom difference between the true value of a property and individual measurements of that property or the presence of a systematic error. Sometimes bias in a statistical context is thought of as being synonymous with the term prejudice. This is an incorrect assumption because prejudice refers to an individual's state of mind that would create a desire for a particular outcome.

Error

Measurement error refers to the difference between the measured value and the true value of the variable being measured. Errors of measurement can be divided into two categories, systematic errors and random errors. Systematic errors, also known as determinate errors, result from factors such as malfunctioning equipment, not correcting all outside influences, and poor design of the data collection process. Examples in imaging would include equipment not calibrated properly or incorrect exposure factors selected by a technologist. Random errors, also known as indeterminate errors, are caused by statistical fluctuations or uncertainties such as quantum mottle.

Range

Range refers to the difference between the highest and lowest values or the width of the distribution of values and is a measure of the dispersion of the data distribution.

Standard Deviation

The standard deviation is the range of variation or dispersion of a set of values surrounding the mean, or the spread or distribution of a dataset. It can apply to a random variable, a population, a probability distribution, or a multiset. This can be symbolized by the capital letters SD or the small Greek letter sigma (σ). It is defined as the root-mean-square deviation of the values from their mean. Since standard deviation is a measure of statistical dispersion, it measures how widely spread the values in a dataset are from the mean. If many data points are close to the mean, then the standard deviation is small; if many data points are far from the mean, then the standard deviation is large. If all data values are equal, then the standard deviation is zero.

$$\sqrt{SD = \frac{\sum x^2}{M}}$$

The small letter x is the amount of deviation of a value X from the mean (M). $x = X - M$. For example, with the values 7, 3, 6, and 4, the mean is 5. The standard deviation is determined with the following equation:

$$SD = \sqrt{\frac{(7-5)^2 + (3-5)^2 + (6-5)^2 + (4-5)^2}{5}}$$

The standard deviation is 1.41.

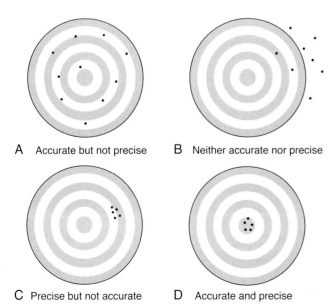

A Accurate but not precise   B Neither accurate nor precise

C Precise but not accurate   D Accurate and precise

Fig. 2.1 Concept of accuracy versus reliability (precision). Parts A-D demonstrate the difference between accuracy and reliability (precision).

When a large standard deviation is obtained (i.e., a large variation has occurred from the mean), it is important to analyze why this has occurred. Possibilities to consider include that this may be a normal occurrence and that the data are valid. It is also possible that the ways in which the measurements were obtained, calculated, or determined were not correctly performed. The validity of the standard deviation value must be determined before the results of the study being performed can be considered valid.

Variance

Variance is the square of the standard deviation in Poisson statistics (discussed later) and is used to determine if the separate means of several different groups differ significantly from each other (e.g., between male and female patients, different age groups). Like standard deviation, it is used as a measure of the dispersion or spread of a set of values. As the mean increases, the variance will increase as well.

Gaussian Distribution

A Gaussian distribution, named after German mathematician Carl Friedrich Gauss, is also known as a *normal distribution* and creates a bell-shaped curve that is continuous, with both tails extending to infinity (Fig. 2.2). The distribution is symmetric about the mean value of the measurement set, with the spread of the measurements characterized by the standard deviation of the measurements. With this distribution, 68% of all values will fall within one standard deviation on either side of the mean, 95% will fall within two standard deviations, and 99% will fall within three standard deviations. (This is the basis of Six Sigma, discussed later in this chapter, whereby 99% of all variables are covered.) The Gaussian distribution is the most commonly used statistical distribution in medical imaging and quality management studies.

Poisson Distribution

A Poisson distribution, named after French mathematician Simeon Poisson, is a discrete probability distribution that is used to determine whether events occur randomly or not (such as the number of particles emitted by a radioactive source in a given period of time). The shape of a Poisson distribution is determined by only one parameter, whereas the shape of a Gaussian distribution is governed by two parameters. In this Poisson distribution, the variance is equal to the mean. This distribution is generally asymmetrical (the opposite of Gaussian distribution) for low mean values (<10). In Poisson statistics, the standard deviation can be estimated by taking the square root of the mean. For example, if a sample has a mean of 144, the standard deviation is 12. Both X-ray and gamma ray counting statistics obey the Poisson distribution, so it is relevant to radiography, mammography, fluoroscopy, computed tomography, and nuclear medicine.

Variation

Variation refers to anything that would cause a process to deviate from acceptable standards (or the norm). It is related to the statistical concepts of variance and standard deviation, since it describes the range of output around the central measure of a process. For example, a chest X-ray examination on a patient in a hospital radiology department may average 16 min to complete. However, the examination may take as few as 11 min or as long as 25 min. This range would indicate the extent of variation of the process. Sources of variation in diagnostic imaging might include materials and supplies, equipment, procedures and methods, personnel, and management. Two basic types of variation are encountered in diagnostic imaging: special cause variation and common cause variation. Common cause variation is generally due to the process or system in place, as well as the people within the system (i.e., personnel or patient population). Special cause variation is assignable to a specific cause or causes and arises because of special circumstances.

Validity

As mentioned previously, validity is sometimes referred to as *accuracy*. In survey measurement, there are three main types

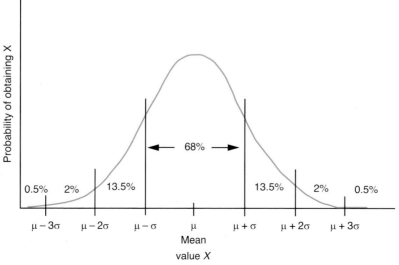

Fig. 2.2 Gaussian probability (normal) distribution

of validity: construct validity, content validity, and criterion validity. Construct validity is the extent to which a measure would agree with other survey instruments that have been used to measure the same parameters and have a proven accuracy. Content validity is the extent to which a survey will cover all of the content area. Criterion validity compares the results obtained in a survey to an established criterion measure or benchmark.

Information Analysis Tools

As mentioned previously, total quality management is devoted to process improvement so that goods and services can be delivered more efficiently to increase customer satisfaction. This means that data must be collected about how well the various processes are being implemented, identify sources of variation, conduct in-depth analysis to clarify knowledge and present results, measure improvements, and monitor progress. Customer satisfaction surveys and repeat analysis of radiographic images are examples of data collection. Once these data are collected, they then must be organized and presented in a format that is easy to analyze. Seven basic statistical tools can be used to display data for interpretation and analysis: flowcharts, cause-and-effect diagrams, histograms, Pareto charts, scatterplots, trend charts, and control charts.

Flowchart

A flowchart is a pictorial representation of the individual steps that can be contained in a process. It is designed to present the sequence of events in the process from its beginning point to its end point. When correctly constructed, it can demonstrate potential problem areas, inconsistencies, or redundancies that can produce variations in the output of the process, which may result in system failure. It also can help document current processes, redesign current processes,

> ### BOX 2.1   The Flowchart
> - The terminal symbol is a rounded rectangle or oval that identifies the beginning or end of a process.
> - The activity symbol in a flowchart is a rectangle.
> - The decision symbol is a diamond.

and design new processes. Flowcharts are relatively easy to construct but are best developed by persons who are directly involved in or have knowledge of the particular process to be presented.

Before constructing a flowchart, one must identify all of the inputs, outputs, and actions within the process, as well as the sequence in which they occur. Then the appropriate symbol must be chosen to characterize each step within the process. For an explanation of the symbols used in a flowchart, see Box 2.1. Computer software programs are available for help in constructing a satisfactory flowchart. With all of the steps in a process accurately diagrammed, it should be easier to communicate the process and its outcomes to all staff (especially new hires). It should also allow a project improvement team to examine the process in order to be able to improve it. An example of a flowchart is shown in Fig. 2.3.

Cause-and-Effect Diagram

A cause-and-effect diagram is a causal analysis tool (also called a *fishbone chart* or *Ishikawa diagram*). This tool was developed by Kaoru Ishikawa of the University of Tokyo in 1943. It is used to demonstrate graphically the causes and effects of different variables or conditions on a key quality characteristic and, thereby, potential areas for improvement. It is most useful in identifying sources of variation within a process. It is especially useful in identifying multiple causes of problems during root cause analysis (RCA) studies.

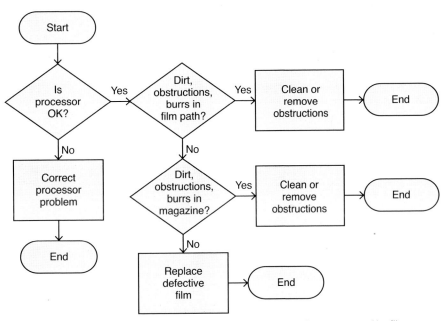

Fig. 2.3 A flowchart diagrams the process of eliminating scratches on images caused by film processors.

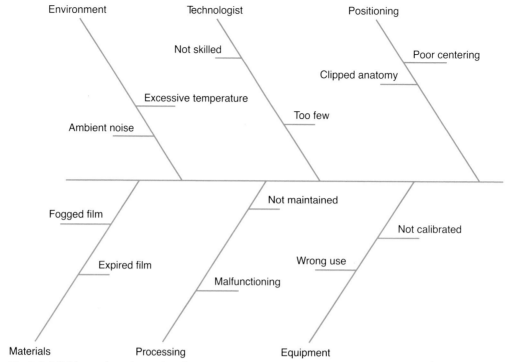

Fig. 2.4 A fishbone chart shows the effect of various parameters on key quality characteristics or outcomes of proper image quality.

To construct a cause-and-effect diagram, you must first determine the key quality characteristic to be improved. Then potential causes of the effect must be identified so they are included in the chart. Brainstorming by a quality improvement team or similar group may be helpful in this identification. The main ideas are listed on branches flowing toward the main branch of the diagram and grouped according to categories. All possible problems or causes for each of these main ideas must then be listed as subcauses within each branch. An example of a cause-and-effect diagram is shown in Fig. 2.4.

Histogram

A histogram is a data display tool in the form of a bar graph that often plots the most frequent occurrence of a quantity in the center. After a cause-and-effect diagram has been created, data are usually collected to see how often different causes of process variation are occurring. A histogram differs from a bar graph in that it is the area of the bar(s) that denotes the value and not the height of the bars. The distribution of continuous data is often best accomplished with a histogram. It also can help demonstrate the amount of variation within an individual process. Histograms often are used in diagnostic imaging to depict such continuous variables as the monthly repeat rate of a department or the number of examinations performed monthly. They also are programmed into digital radiography systems to create satisfactory images (see Chapter 8). Software programs such as Microsoft Excel can generate histograms from information contained in a spreadsheet. Fig. 2.5 shows an example of a histogram. Histograms can also be adapted in a "scorecard display" in which the bars are color coded to indicate whether certain goals or benchmarks have been achieved. Green is used if the goal or

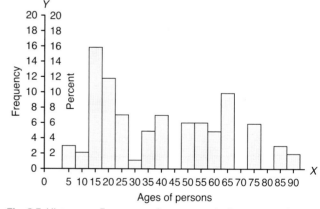

Fig. 2.5 Histogram. Frequency of occurrence is demonstrated on the y-axis, and category or class interval is demonstrated on the x-axis. This example plots percentage of patients undergoing diagnostic procedures versus ages of patients.

benchmark has been met or exceeded, yellow is used if it is within a certain percentage of the goal, and red would indicate that the goal or benchmark has not been met. Histograms can also be designed so that the bars in the graph run vertically rather than horizontally. The most common of these used in quality management is the Gantt chart. This was devised by Henry Gantt in the 1910s and is used to illustrate a project's schedule, including start date, progress status, and projected completion date(s) (Fig. 2.6).

Pareto Chart

A Pareto chart is a causal analysis tool that is named after Wilfredo Pareto, a seventeenth-century Italian political

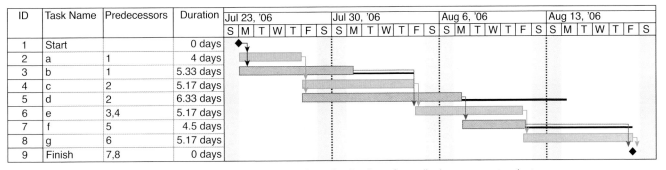

ID	Task Name	Predecessors	Duration	Jul 23, '06							Jul 30, '06							Aug 6, '06							Aug 13, '06						
				S	M	T	W	T	F	S	S	M	T	W	T	F	S	S	M	T	W	T	F	S	S	M	T	W	T	F	S
1	Start		0 days																												
2	a	1	4 days																												
3	b	1	5.33 days																												
4	c	2	5.17 days																												
5	d	2	6.33 days																												
6	e	3,4	5.17 days																												
7	f	5	4.5 days																												
8	g	6	5.17 days																												
9	Finish	7,8	0 days																												

Fig. 2.6 A Gantt chart can be used to show the timeline of a quality improvement project.

economist. The Pareto chart is a variation of the histogram or bar graph, which prioritizes the most frequent problems at the y-axis (far left) of the graph and the other problems in decreasing order to the right. The Pareto chart was developed to illustrate the 80/20 Rule (that 80% of the problems stem from 20% of the causes). The horizontal axis, or x-axis, indicates the factors or problems to be evaluated, whereas the vertical axis, or y-axis, demonstrates the frequency of occurrence. Pareto charts also may include a horizontal reference, or norm (normal occurrence). The Pareto chart is useful in identifying the main causes (i.e., those that occur with the greatest frequency) of problems and in demonstrating the results of improvement strategies that have been implemented. It is important to note that Pareto charts document the frequency of causes and not necessarily the severity of a cause. An example of a Pareto chart is shown in Fig. 2.7.

Scatterplot

A scatterplot (also called a *scatter diagram*) is a traditional two-axis graph (x-axis and y-axis), with several data points that have been plotted throughout. It is designed to determine whether a relationship exists between two different variables in a process. When looking for ideas for improvement or the causes of problems, it can be important to determine whether or not one event or variable is related to another. Once the data points are plotted, the scatterplot then is examined to see if these points are scattered in any particular pattern. If

so, a correlation may exist between the two variables. A positive correlation is indicated when both the x and y values increase in relation to each other. A negative correlation is demonstrated when there is an increase in the x variable in relation to a decrease in the y variable. Scatterplots are often used in regression analysis studies, which are statistical forecasting models based on data demonstrated in scatterplots. An example of a scatterplot is shown in Fig. 2.8.

Trend Chart

A trend chart (also called a *run chart* or *run-sequence plot*) pictorially demonstrates whether key indicators are moving up or down over a given period of time on an ongoing basis. Trending refers to the evaluation of data collected over a period of time for the purpose of identifying patterns or changes. The variable being measured is placed on the vertical axis, or y-axis, and the time factor is placed on the horizontal axis, or x-axis. Often, some measure of central tendency (mean or median) of the data is indicated by a horizontal reference line. The trend chart can display the performance of, and any variation in, a process over a given period of time. For a trend chart to be constructed, the measurement or indicator to be measured must first be identified, then all relevant data must be collected and analyzed. Next, all data points are plotted and connected with a linear line.

Once the chart has been constructed, the plotted points and lines must be analyzed to determine the degree of variation within the indicator. If there are no large spikes (upward or downward) and the line is relatively flat, then the process is considered to be under control. If unusual trends are observed, then the potential causes must be investigated and corrected. Trend charts cannot determine the source of any problem within a process, only if and when they have occurred. An example of a trend chart is shown in Fig. 2.9.

Control Chart

A control chart is a modification of the trend chart in which statistically determined upper and lower control limits are placed with a central line that indicates an accepted norm. If the plotted data points fall above or below these control limits, then the process is considered unstable. The control chart was invented by Walter A. Shewhart while working at Bell Labs in the 1920s, so it is sometimes referred to as the Shewhart chart or process/behavior chart. Like the trend chart, the control

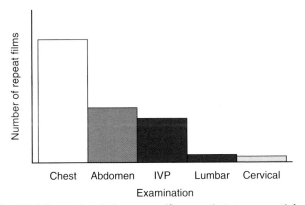

Fig. 2.7 A Pareto chart indicates specific areas that cause unsatisfactory outcomes so improvement actions can be appropriately directed. *IVP*, Intravenous pyelography.

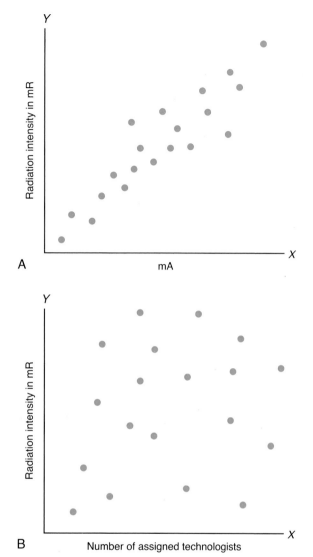

Fig. 2.8 A scatterplot graph shows the relationship between a key outcome or characteristic (y-axis) and a key process variable (x-axis). Graph (A) indicates a positive correlation between two values, and graph (B) indicates that no correlation exists. *mA,* Milliampere; *mR,* milliroentgen.

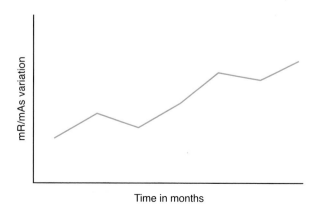

Fig. 2.9 A trend graph displays amount of variation of indicator (radiation emitted from an X-ray generator) as a function of time. *mAs,* Milliampere-second; *mR,* milliroentgen.

chart cannot identify a specific cause of a problem, but rather if and when it has occurred. The control chart is often used for demonstrating phantom image analysis in mammographic units over time (see Chapter 9). An example of a control chart is shown in Fig. 2.10.

QUALITY IMPROVEMENT PLANNING

All quality management programs will incorporate quality improvement planning. A quality improvement plan (also known as a strategic plan) is an organizational plan that describes the goals and proposed activities of a particular quality improvement program. It must incorporate current standards and benchmarks, performance appraisal, professional assessment and improvement, and specific program needs. The purpose of the plan is to provide a formal ongoing process by which an organization utilizes objective measures to monitor and evaluate the quality of services, both clinical and operational, provided to patients. In other words, the quality improvement plan should serve as a road map for all other quality improvement program activities, and will require a structure to support its function (most often provided by a quality improvement team, discussed later in this chapter). According to the Department of Health and Human Services, a quality improvement plan should include the following:

- A systematic process with identified leadership, accountability, and dedicated resources
- Use of data and measurable outcomes to determine progress toward relevant, evidence-based benchmarks
- Focus on linkages, efficiencies, and provider and patient expectations in addressing outcome improvement
- A continuous process that is adaptive to change and fits within the framework of other programmatic quality and quality improvement activities (such as The Joint Commission [TJC], DNV-GL, or American College of Radiology accreditation)
- Assurance that goals are accomplished and are concurrent with improved outcomes based on the data that are collected

Quality improvement plans should address performance measures, performance measurement, and performance management, focusing on core areas of clinical care, operations, and finance.

- **Performance measures** are designed to measure systems of care and are derived from clinical or practice guidelines. Data from these measures are sorted into specific measurable elements that provide the healthcare organization with a meter to measure the quality of its care.
- **Performance measurement** is a process by which a healthcare organization monitors important aspects of its programs, systems, and processes. This includes the operational processes that are used to collect the data necessary to assess performance measures.
- **Performance management** is a forward-looking process that is used to set goals and regularly check progress toward achieving those goals. Healthcare organizations set

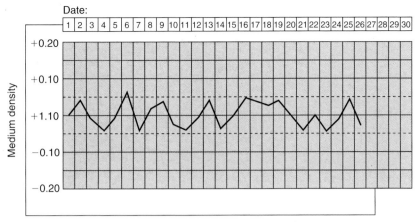

Fig. 2.10 A control graph displays amount of variation of indicator (speed or medium density value from a sensitometry film) as a function of time, with upper and lower control limits indicated.

goals and evaluate their success in achieving those goals by reviewing actual data of their performance.

A key challenge to implementing quality improvement programs is to develop methods to collect knowledge related to quality care and to deliver that knowledge to practitioners at the point of care. There are many dimensions to quality in diagnostic imaging that need to be measured:

- Examination appropriateness—radiologists and referring providers must be knowledgeable about which imaging procedure is appropriate for each clinical indication.
- Procedure protocol or workflow—the technologist who will perform the study must have knowledge of the correct procedure protocol and workflow process. Diagnostic imaging modalities are complex, requiring that many different parameters be specified to customize the imaging procedure to the patient and clinical indication. These parameters may include use of contrast material, section thickness, acquisition protocols, and a variety of postprocessing steps.
- Accuracy of interpretation—the interpreting physician must have good-quality images and technical skill to achieve an accurate diagnosis.
- Communication of imaging result—optimal communication of clinical information between the radiologist and referring provider is critical to patient care.
- Measuring and monitoring performance improvement in quality, safety, and efficiency—institutions must measure and monitor indicators of quality, safety, and efficiency in their services to prove that imaging and their interventions are of high quality.

To measure and monitor performance improvement, key performance indicators need to be developed. **Key performance indicators** (KPIs) are the critical indicators of progress toward an intended result. KPIs provide a focus for strategic and operational improvement, create an analytical basis for decision making, and help focus attention on what matters most. There are three basic types of KPIs in radiology:

- Financial—a measurable value that indicates how well an organization or department is doing regarding generating revenue and profits. Examples include actual expenses and total revenue.

- Operational—measures how busy the department is as well as how efficient it is in handling the work volume. Examples include total examination volume and examination volume by modality.
- Quality—measure the desired outcome of the department. Examples include accuracy of interpretation, correct examination performed, communication of critical tests and critical results, and report turnaround time.

To manage the data measured from KPIs, many radiology departments utilize digital **dashboards** to display the data in real time. A dashboard is a concise, context-specific display of KPIs for quick evaluation of multiple subsystems. It can consist of control charts, fishbone diagrams, and other display tools discussed earlier in this chapter (Fig. 2.11).

Problem Identification and Analysis

Group Dynamics

For the continual improvement of the processes involved in customer satisfaction, several tools must be used to identify and analyze the data obtained. Groups or teams of individuals who are familiar with or are using the processes are generally the most successful in helping with problem identification in continuous quality improvement (CQI). This is because a single individual may not have enough knowledge or experience, or both, with all of the aspects of a process. A team consists of at least two persons. For healthcare organizations, the ideal number for most teams or groups is 6–12 persons. To be effective, these teams should be goal oriented, share equal responsibility, and be empowered by management. By working together, team members not only can improve older processes and develop new and better ones but also develop a sense of ownership within the organization (and therefore be more productive workers). Group dynamic tools that can be used in quality management include brainstorming, focus groups, quality improvement teams, quality circles, multivoting, consensus, work teams, and problem-solving teams.

Brainstorming. **Brainstorming** is a group process used to develop a large collection of ideas without regard to their merit or validity. For example, a department meeting of all

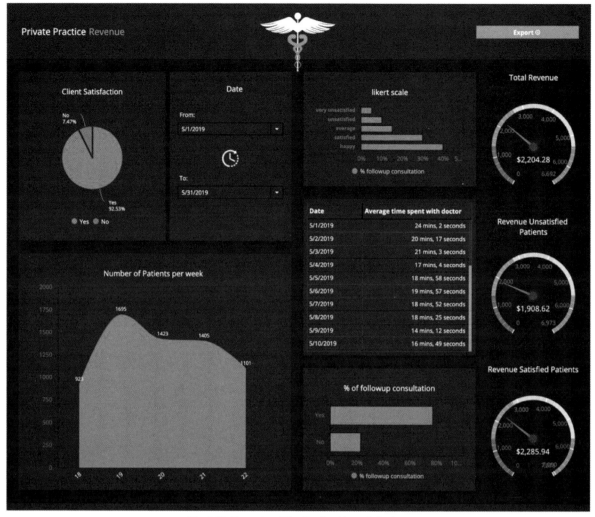

Fig. 2.11 Example of Quality Dashboard display.

staff could be used to solicit ideas or suggestions for a particular topic. The leader of this session should encourage participation by everyone, not criticize any contribution made, and record all ideas for future assessment. It is also important to announce the topic to be discussed to all team members before the session. It also may be more effective for the leader to review the particular subject at the beginning of the session and then phrase the topic that will be discussed in the form of a question. However, the discussion should be relevant to the topic being discussed, and the leader must direct members to adhere to this topic.

Focus groups. A focus group is a small group that focuses on a particular problem and then hopefully derives a solution. Generally, the applicable ideas on a particular problem obtained from brainstorming are considered in this smaller group, which can come to a consensus. Focus groups also may be responsible for obtaining additional data such as the interviewing of customers and patient surveys. This may add to a higher implementation cost for focus groups as compared with other group dynamic tools. A focus group must have a skilled facilitator to be successful.

Quality improvement team. A quality improvement team is a group of individuals who implement the solutions that were derived by the focus group. This may or may not include members of the focus group. Ideally, quality improvement teams should have six or seven members who are key customers or suppliers, or both, of the steps in the process (i.e., the people who actually do the steps in the process). It is best to avoid teams of managers only because they usually do not have detailed knowledge of the process. Input from other customers and suppliers should be sought by the team.

Quality circles. This type of group dynamic tool is normally composed of supervisors and workers who are from the same department or who may have the same function in a similar department. Quality circles should be scheduled to meet regularly and have the specific function of identifying potential problems with departmental processes and then formulate solutions. Levels of productivity and quality of images produced within a department are possible issues that may be discussed by quality circles.

Multivoting. This method is normally used after a brainstorming session to dismiss nonessential or nonrealistic ideas and then concentrate on those that can realistically solve the problem. All members of the brainstorming session are given a list of all of the ideas that were formulated and then asked to vote on which one they consider the most important. The ideas with the fewest votes are discarded and the process repeated (thus the name, *multivoting*) until just one key idea remains. This method reduces a large number of ideas or options to a manageable few judged important by the participants.

Consensus. This is another method that can follow a successful brainstorming session. After the initial ideas are formulated during the brainstorming session, the group members, through discussion and teamwork, come to an agreement on the most important idea to be addressed. Total agreement within the group is unnecessary, but any decision should at least be acceptable to all group members.

Work teams. These teams focus on solving a complete problem or completing an entire task rather than focusing on any one particular step in a process. Some work teams, known as *self-managed teams*, are composed of 6–18 persons and are empowered by management to take any corrective action necessary to solve the assigned problem or task. The self-managed team members should be highly trained in the particular area in which they are working. The teamwork created by these teams is highly successful in facilitating CQI and solving potential problems.

Problem-solving teams. These teams work on specific tasks and meet to solve particular problems, as well as root cause analysis (RCA), which tries to identify the root causes of faults or problems within the process. A problem is defined as a gap between the current condition (what is actually happening) and the target condition (what should be happening or what is needed). These teams normally function to identify, analyze, and then solve both quality and productivity issues. Problem-solving teams must have a knowledgeable facilitator who is responsible for teaching team members the appropriate problem-solving tools for guiding them through the process. According to the AHRQ, the RCA should include the following steps:

1. Select the team to complete the RCA.
2. Create a flowchart to visualize the steps in a process and identify possible and potential cases of problems.
3. Examine the flowchart for areas of failure.
4. Use the team methods (such as brainstorming) to assist in discussing and identifying underlying causes.
5. Analyze the data collected to specify possible root causes. Focus should be on the system and not individual staff.
6. Redesign the process for improvement (if required) based on the analysis results.
7. Implement the changes first through a pilot, and then spread to other areas as appropriate for the improvement strategy.

Three common RCA tools are *5 Whys*, the *Thought Process Map (TPM)*, and the *Analysis Question Matrix*.

5 Whys. This is a question-asking method developed by the Toyota Corporation that is used to explore the cause-and-effect relationships that may underlie a particular problem. Its ultimate goal is to determine the root cause of a problem. For example:

The department waiting time is excessive (the problem).
1. Why?—One of the five X-ray rooms in the department is always malfunctioning.
2. Why?—The unit in the room is used 24 h/day, 7 days/week.
3. Why?—The unit is 10 years old.
4. Why?—It is beyond its useful service life and has never been replaced.
5. Why?—Administration will not approve the purchase of a new unit.

Once the root cause is identified, a solution can then be devised to solve it. A fishbone diagram (discussed earlier in this chapter) is most helpful in identifying multiple causes of problems during RCA.

Thought process map. The TPM is one of the first tools that should be employed for a process improvement project. It presents thoughts, ideas, and questions at the beginning of a project to help a team or person identify all information and progress. There are five basic steps to create a TPM:

• Define the project's goal(s). The project improvement team needs to clearly define what needs to be accomplished or what problem needs to be solved. Brainstorming among the group is a good way to define the goal.
• List the knowns and unknowns. The team leader should use a large poster board or easel pad and make two columns—one for what the team knows and one for what the team does not know. This can help identify the amount and type of data necessary to complete the project.
• Ask grouped questions or questions that define, measure, analyze, improve, or control (DMAIC). Focusing on the unknowns from step 2, create questions from the categorical perspectives of DMAIC. These perspectives are discussed in more detail later in this chapter.
• Sequence and link the questions. The questions in step 4 are now linked together using a flowchart, described earlier in this chapter.
• Identify possible tools to be used. This step involves identifying potential tools that can be used to answer the questions posed in step 3. The most effective way to accomplish this step is to create a four-column matrix that assigns a column for the question, the tool or method, who is responsible, and the due date.

Analysis questions matrix. This matrix lists a series of analysis questions that seek to find the root cause of a particular issue and to uncover why parts of the process occurred or didn't occur when they should have (see Fig. 2.12). This should then be followed up by an action plan that can be used to reduce or alleviate the problem (see Fig. 2.13).

#	Question	Prompts	Organization Response	Root cause	Plan of Action
1	What was the intended process flow?	List the relevant process steps as defined by the policy, procedure, protocol, or guidelines in effect at the time of the event. You may need to include multiple processes. **Note:** The process steps *as they occurred in the event* will be entered in the next question. Examples of defined process steps may include, but are not limited to: • Site verification protocol • Instrument, sponge, sharps count procedures • Patient identification protocol • Assessment (pain, suicide risk, physical, and psychological) procedures • Fall risk/fall prevention guidelines			
2	Were there any steps in the process that did not occur as intended?	Explain in detail any deviation from the intended processes listed in Analysis Item #1 above.			
3	What human factors were relevant to the outcome?	Discuss staff-related human performance factors that contributed to the event. Examples may include, but are not limited to: • Boredom • Failure to follow established policies/procedures • Fatigue • Inability to focus on task • Inattentional blindness/ confirmation bias • Personal problems • Lack of complex critical thinking skills • Rushing to complete task • Substance abuse • Trust			

Fig. 2.12 Analysis question matrix used in root cause analysis.

Specific Quality Management Quality Improvement Processes

TJC 10-Step Process

In 1985, TJC introduced the 10-step monitoring and evaluation process as the mechanism for satisfaction of accreditation. Although it is still in use today, the emphasis of some of its steps has changed from quality assurance (QA) to CQI.

Step 1: Assign responsibility for the department's monitoring and evaluation activities. In QA, the medical director is ultimately responsible, but the task is usually delegated to a supervisor or QA technologist. With CQI, both intradepartmental and interdepartmental committees work together with hospital management participation. A separate quality management department is found in many healthcare facilities, and others use a unit or section within the diagnostic imaging area for QM responsibilities. Regardless, each department or committee is responsible for creating its quality management program structure and functions, documenting the effectiveness of its quality management activities and for reporting such activities to the organization-wide program. Staff members who perform quality management responsibilities also should make sure that the overall organizational program is functional and effective.

Step 2: Delineate the scope of care and service provided by the department. With the QA model, the major services of a particular department are listed (e.g., imaging modalities offered, types of patients served, credentials of staff), whereas under CQI, the scope of care or service for the hospital as a whole is defined.

Step 3: Identify important aspects of care and service. Under QA, specific departmental tasks or functions are identified, with emphasis on high volume (chest radiography), high risk (mammography interpretations and angiography), and high risk/problem prone (diagnostic imaging procedures requiring intravenous contrast media). With CQI, the entire hospital determines the key functions to be monitored. This should include important functions relating to patients, care of patients, leadership, use of medications, use of blood and blood components, and determination of the appropriateness of admissions and continued hospitalization.

Step 4: Identify indicators or performance measures. A **measure** is a standard used as a basis for comparison or reference point against which other things can be evaluated. Measures are specific measurements of variables that affect quality, such as patient waiting time. TJC defines an indicator as a valid and reliable quantitative process or outcome measure related to one or more dimensions of performance. An indicator is an aggregate of measures for a specific operation. The most common type of performance indicator is an aggregate data indicator. An aggregate data indicator quantifies a

Action Plan	Risk Reduction Strategies	Measures of Effectiveness
For each of the findings identified in the analysis as needing an action, indicate the planned action expected, implementation date and associated measure of effectiveness. OR. …	Action Item #1:	
If after consideration of such a finding, a decision is made not to implement an associated risk reduction strategy, indicate the rationale for not taking action at this time.	Action Item #2:	
Check to be sure that the selected measure will provide data that will permit assessment of the effectiveness of the action.	Action Item #3:	
Consider whether pilot testing of a planned improvement should be conducted.	Action Item #4:	
Improvements to reduce risk should ultimately be implemented in all areas where applicable, not just where the event occurred. Identify where the improvements will be implemented.	Action Item #5:	
	Action Item #6:	
	Action Item #7:	
	Action Item #8:	

Fig. 2.13 Action plan used in root cause analysis.

process or outcome related to many cases. It may occur frequently and may be desirable or undesirable. Examples include the number of cesarean sections, interventional procedures, and reported medication errors. Quality indicators and performance measures applicable to healthcare organizations have been developed by organizations such as the AHRQ, Centers for Medicare and Medicaid Services, the National Quality Forum, the National Committee for Quality Assurance, TJC, DNV-GL, and the American College of Radiology. These indicators/measures can be accessed on the websites of each of the above organizations.

Using QA, each department identifies indicators, whereas under CQI, an interdisciplinary team identifies indicators that focus more on the process of care. The performance indicators that are most relevant to healthcare organizations would include the following:

- Appropriateness of care is whether the type of care (i.e., specific test, procedure, or service) that has been requested is necessary. In other words, is it relevant to the patient's clinical needs, given the current state of knowledge (are you doing the right thing?)?

- Continuity of care is the degree to which the care/intervention for the patient is coordinated among practitioners or organizations, or both, over time.
- Effectiveness of care is the level of benefit when services are rendered under ordinary circumstances by average practitioners for typical patients, as defined by K.N. Lohr. It also may be defined as the degree to which the care/intervention is provided in the correct manner, given the current state of knowledge, to achieve the desired/projected outcome for the patient.
- Efficacy of care is the level of benefit expected when healthcare services are applied under ideal conditions and the best possible circumstances or the degree to which the care/intervention has been shown to accomplish the desired outcome (i.e., are you doing the right thing well?). Most healthcare systems deliver care that is somewhere between effectiveness and efficacy. QA attempts to bring effectiveness to efficacy, whereas CQI goes a step further in allowing for continued improvement once effectiveness has been reached.
- Efficiency of care refers to the outcome obtained when the highest quality of care is delivered in the shortest amount of time, with the least amount of expense, and with a positive outcome for the patient's condition.

An aggregate data indicator involves the relationship between the outcomes (results of care) and the resources used to deliver patient care.

- **Respect and caring** is defined as the degree to which the patient or a designee is involved in his or her own care decisions and to which those providing services do so with sensitivity and respect for the patient's needs, expectations, and individual differences. Respect and caring refers to how well patients are treated during the delivery of healthcare service, what the patient's level of satisfaction is, and how well a patient's complaints are handled by staff and management.
- **Safety in the care environment**. This is the degree to which the risk of an intervention and the risk in the care environment are reduced for the patient and others, including the healthcare provider. Safety in the care environment includes equipment functioning and operation, application of universal precautions, and competency of staff. There are two important types of indicators based on patient safety events (a patient safety event is an event, incident, or condition that could have resulted or did result in harm to a patient): adverse event indicator and sentinel event indicator.

Adverse event indicator. An adverse event (or complication) is a patient safety event that resulted in harm to a patient. It is an untoward, undesirable, and usually unanticipated event that is caused by medical management rather than by the underlying disease or condition of the patient. In general, adverse events prolong the hospitalization, produce a disability at the time of discharge, or both. Examples might include perforation of a vessel during an angiographic or interventional procedure. Incidents such as patient falls or improper administration of medications are also considered adverse events, even if there is no permanent effect on the patient.

Sentinel event indicator. A subcategory of adverse events, a sentinel event is a patient safety event (not primarily related to the natural course of the patient's illness or underlying condition) that reaches a patient and results in any of the following: death, permanent harm, or severe temporary harm. A sentinel event is an unexpected occurrence involving death or serious physical or psychological injury, or the risk thereof. Serious injury specifically includes loss of limb or function. The phrase "or the risk thereof" includes any process variation for which a recurrence would carry a significant chance of a serious adverse outcome. The events are called "sentinel" because they signal the need for immediate investigation and response. A sentinel event indicator identifies an individual event or phenomenon that is significant enough to trigger further review each time it occurs. These events are undesirable and occur infrequently, such as the death of a patient during a diagnostic examination as a result of contrast media reaction, erythema of a patient's skin occurring during a fluoroscopic procedure, suicide of a patient in a setting where the patient receives around-the-clock care, unanticipated death of a full-term infant, infant abduction or discharge to the wrong family, sexual assault of a patient, hemolytic transfusion reaction involving administration of blood or blood products having major blood group incompatibilities, and surgery on the wrong patient or wrong body part.

- **Timeliness of care**. This is defined as the degree to which the care/intervention is provided to the patient at the most beneficial or necessary time. Timeliness of care refers to the delivery of healthcare within a reasonable amount of time, with minimal waiting time.
- **Cost of care**. Cost of care refers to the delivery of healthcare that is reasonable for the current marketplace.
- **Availability of care**. This is defined as the degree to which appropriate care/intervention is available to meet the patient's needs. Availability of care refers to the availability at the clinical facility of the type of care or procedure required by the patient. A good example would be how early a patient who has a breast lump would be able to have a mammogram.

According to a survey of the members of the Society of Chairmen of Academic Radiology Departments in the United States, the three main categories of quality management performance indicators used are:

1. Customer satisfaction—in diagnostic imaging, customers are not only patients but are also referring providers and employees of the department, and their satisfaction is based on impressions formed at all points of contact with the institution
2. Patient access to appointments—addresses availability of care
3. Reporting time—addresses timeliness of care

Step 5: Establish a means to trigger evaluation. Under QA, a level of expectation is to be identified for each indicator. TJC identifies a level of expectation (formerly known as a *threshold*) as a preestablished level of performance applied to a specific indicator. The levels can be determined internally (on the basis of past performance of the facility) or externally (on the basis of federal and state regulations or professional guidelines such as those of TJC). As long as the indicator is below the expectation level in a negative event or condition, no further action or evaluation is required. For a highly desirable condition or event, the level of expectation is set at 100%. Under CQI, interdisciplinary teams use statistical methods to determine levels or patterns that trigger evaluation.

Step 6: Collect and organize data. Under QA, the department determines the protocol for data collection. First, the method of collection is determined. These data must be collected systematically and on important processes and outcomes that are related to the care of the patient or the functions of the healthcare organization. Options for collection include the following:

- *Patient surveys and questionnaires.* These should be sent to patients 3–7 days after discharge or on service dates for outpatients. These are the simplest mechanisms for obtaining customer/patient information. These should be brief (completed in 15 min or less to generate a high response rate), have responses that can be measured quantitatively (such as multiple choice or Likert scale—a response that ranges from strongly disagree to strongly agree), and be clearly worded so that patients understand what is being asked of them.
- *Patient records.* Information such as sentinel events or other data are easily obtained.
- *Staff reports.* These include patient care logs, diaries, drug reaction reports, medication variance reports, and so on.

- *Focus groups.* As previously discussed, these small groups collect data that focus on finding a solution to a specific problem.
- *Computer database.* Considerable patient information and relevant data from across the country may be available in some computer databases. However, privacy concerns such as those addressed in the Health Insurance Portability and Accountability Act (previously discussed) may limit access to database information.

Next, the size of the sample is determined (e.g., how many patients, cases). Then the frequency of collection is determined (e.g., concurrently, daily, weekly, monthly). Concurrent data are any data collected during the time of care. Data that should be collected and processed on a continuous basis include patient deaths (dependent on the patient mix and regional factors) and serious complications to treatment. The frequency at which data are collected for a specific indicator is reviewed annually to indicate whether the data are adequately capturing the desired information. The final task is to analyze the data and determine how they are manipulated for comparison with the level of expectation or with preestablished criteria. Under CQI, an interdisciplinary team determines the protocol for data collection from various areas of the hospital.

Step 7: Initiate evaluation. With QA, the staff evaluates the level of performance for an indicator by comparing it with the expectation level. With CQI, the leaders identify areas for evaluation according to the data collected.

Step 8: Take actions to improve care and service. With QA, individuals are evaluated as to whether expectation levels were achieved and corrective action taken accordingly. The CQI method looks at the process used in providing the care or service rather than at the individual.

Step 9: Assess effectiveness of actions and maintain improvements. The QA method examines whether the actions taken in step 8 are effective in ensuring quality, whereas the CQI method shows that improvement is continually being sustained. Documentation of these methods is important.

Step 10: Communicate results to affected individuals and groups. With the QA method, all results are given to a QA committee and then shared with the department staff and hospital QA committee, whereas with CQI, all results are reported to the leaders and other affected individuals. All data collected must be consolidated for distribution in a final report. A common method of presenting such results is with a storyboard (Fig. 2.14). A storyboard can summarize a whole report or process with photographs and graphs and a minimum of text. The final report should include a description of a process identified for improvement and the method used to identify that process; the department involved; the source of all data collected; any cause of variation that is identified; any corrective action that was taken; the person or persons who implemented this action; the timetable for implementation; whether or not the process was actually improved; future plans to monitor the process; and any plans to restudy, if applicable.

TJC Cycle for Improving Performance

TJC 10-step monitoring and evaluation process is still valid and is the basis of their "cycle for improving performance," which identifies the steps design, measure, assess, and improve.

Design. Systematic planning and implementation are key to the design of any function or process. When new functions and processes are being designed and planned, the following factors should be considered:

- The organization's overriding purpose (mission), view of its future (vision), and strategies for carrying out its mission and fulfilling its vision (strategic plan)
- Needs and expectations of patients, staff, accrediting agencies, and payers (customers and suppliers)

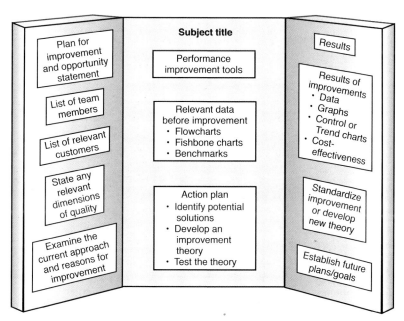

Fig. 2.14 Model for a storyboard.

- Current knowledge about organizational and clinical activities from both inside and outside the organization
- Current and relevant data, such as the number of patients receiving diagnostic imaging examinations per month, the department repeat rate, and the number of practicing providers
- Availability of resources such as funds, staff time, and equipment

Measure. A **measure** is defined by TJC as a collection of valid and reliable data to demonstrate the effectiveness and efficiency of care and performance improvement. The first step in the measurement process is to identify and develop the measures or indicators, along with any thresholds. A quality improvement plan should include a description of the measurement process and methods, including data required and data availability, or the need for new data collection methods. These data can be collected by various means, including focus groups and quality improvement teams.

Assess. **Assessment** is defined by TJC as translating data collected during measurement into information that can be used to change processes and improve performance. This is the process of assigning meaning or determining the significance, implications, and conclusions of data that have been collected. This is used to improve activities, identify gaps, and plan for improvement. Based on the assessment of data, the next step can be determined, which may include (1) continue the process as is, with the same measures/indicators and data monitoring; (2) continue the process with modifications (implement additional interventions/strategies); (3) add new measures/indicators; or (4) stop monitoring. Proper assessment usually requires comparing data with a reference point or standard. This includes the following:

Internal:

- *Historical patterns of performance in the organization* (also called *baseline performance*). This is a comparison of current performance levels with those occurring previously, such as comparing current department repeat rates with those of the previous year. This should also include identification of best practices and problems (gaps) with prioritization of problems and actions to take.
- *Desired performance limits*. The patient population and referring providers expect a certain level of performance. This should be compared with the level achieved as indicated by the current data. The healthcare organization also may establish its own control limits, targets, and specifications that can be compared with the data obtained.

External:

- *Practice guidelines and parameters*. These procedures, developed by professional societies, expert panels, or in-house practitioners, represent a consensus of the best practices for a given diagnosis, treatment, or procedure. These are usually described in the form of a **critical path** that documents the basic treatment or action sequence in an effort to eliminate unnecessary variation. A critical path defines the optimal sequence and timing of intervention by healthcare practitioners for a particular diagnosis or process.

- *Performance measurement system*. A performance measurement system is an entity consisting of one or more automated databases that facilitates performance improvement in healthcare organizations through collection and dissemination of process or outcome measures of performance, or both. These systems allow an organization to compare its performance with that of other organizations using information such as patient outcomes, costs, lengths of stay for certain treatments, and mortality and morbidity rates. Examples are the TJC Indicator Measurement System and databases maintained by federal and state governments and third-party payers.
- *Benchmarking*. **Benchmarking** involves comparing one organization's performance standards with that of another; however, it focuses on the other organization's key processes that achieve performance rather than the numbers and statistical data obtained in an aggregate external reference database. Two main types of benchmarking exist: internal and external. Internal benchmarking compares performance with the best practices within one's own organization. External benchmarking compares an organization's performance with that of other organizations. External benchmarking can be further broken down into two types, competitive and world class. Competitive external benchmarking involves comparing an organization to competitors marketing the same product or service. The American College of Radiology publishes a National Radiology Data Registry that contains regional and national benchmarks for various diagnostic imaging modalities. This can be accessed online at http://nrdr.acr.org/. World-class external benchmarking involves benchmarking against organizations outside of one's specific industry. A good example might be comparing the billing and collection practices of a healthcare organization with those of a bank or department store. Another commonly used benchmarking site is available from the LeapFrog Group, which will allow you to compare your hospital to other hospitals in terms of assessing quality, resource use, and efficiency.

Improve. Once knowledge is gained through measurement and analysis, action can be taken to improve processes by refining or redesigning a process to improve its level of performance. This cycle of design, measure, assess, and improve should be continuously repeating in a CQI program (Fig. 2.15).

Other Quality Management/Quality Improvement Models

The following are some of the other specific quality management/quality improvement models that are currently in use:

- Evangelical Health Systems CQI Monitoring System
- Focus Analyze Develop Execute (FADE), created by Organizational Dynamics, a private consulting firm (Fig. 2.16)
- A five-stage plan developed by Joiner and Associates, a quality consulting group

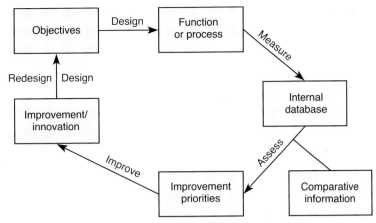

Fig. 2.15 Cycle for improving performance, showing the important steps, including inputs and outputs, of a systematic approach to improvement. (*From Joint Commission Resources:* Forms, charts, & other tools for performance improvement, *Oakbrook Terrace, IL, 1994, JCAHO. Reprinted with permission.*)

FADE

Phases of FADE problem solving

Focus–

Choose a problem and describe it

Analyze–

Learn about a problem by collecting and analyzing pertinent data

Develop–

Develop a solution and a plan

Execute–

Implement the plan, monitor the results, adjust as needed

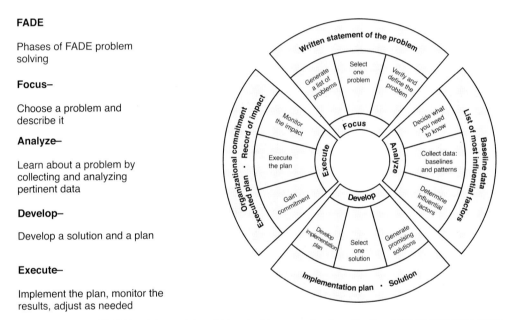

Fig. 2.16 Phases of FADE problem-solving. (*Printed with permission from* Quality action teams: team members workbook, *Organizational Dynamics, Inc., 1987,* www.odionline.com.)

The SWOT analysis, developed at Stanford Research Institute in California from 1960 to 1970, analyzes the internal and external environment of a healthcare organization. The environmental factors internal to the organization can be classified as strengths (**S**) or weaknesses (**W**), and those external to the organization can be classified as opportunities (**O**) or threats (**T**). The SWOT analysis provides information that can be helpful in matching a healthcare organization's resources and capabilities to the competitive environment in which it operates. The four components are placed into a matrix (see Fig. 2.17), and the factors are then placed into each category. The organization's strengths are its resources and capabilities, such as a good reputation among customers, expertise of providers and staff, or advanced equipment, that may not be available at competing imaging departments. Weaknesses are usually the absence of certain strengths such as a poor reputation among customers or lack of availability

of the latest equipment and procedures. The Strengths and Weaknesses boxes of the matrix contain attributes of the organization (internal in origin). Opportunities for growth might include obtaining the latest equipment or hiring providers with advanced skills. Threats to the healthcare organization may include competition from a nearby facility or new

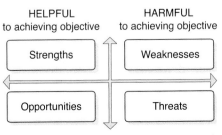

Fig. 2.17 SWOT analysis matrix.

regulations or reimbursement procedures. The Opportunities and Threats boxes contain attributes from the environment (external in origin).

The FOCUS-PDCA (Fig. 2.18) approach was developed by the Hospital Corporation of America in the 1980s, which adapted the "plan, do, check, and act" (PDCA) cycle used by Deming in Japanese industry. The PDCA cycle was initially developed by Walter A. Shewhart at Bell Laboratories in the 1930s, and may be referred to as either the Shewhart cycle, Deming cycle, or PDCA cycle. Shewhart originally used the term *PDSA* or *Plan, Do, Study, Act*. The Hospital Corporation of America included the preliminary steps of FOCUS. This model consists of the following tenets:

- **F** Find a process to improve or a problem to solve.
- **O** Organize a team that knows the process and work on improvement.
- **C** Clarify the problem and current knowledge of the process.
- **U** Understand the problem and the causes of process variation.
- **S** Select the method to improve the process.
- **P** Plan to implement a new method to improve the process.
- **D** Do the implementation and measure the change.
- **C** Check the results of the change.
- **A** Act to hold the improvements and continue further improvements.

The whole FOCUS-PDCA approach focuses on the answers to the following questions:
1. What are we trying to accomplish?
2. How will we know when this change is an improvement?
3. What changes can we predict will make an improvement?
4. How shall we pilot test the predicted improvement?
5. What do we expect to learn from the test run?
6. As the data come in, what have we learned?
7. If we get positive results, how do we hold on to the gains?
8. If we get negative results, what needs to be done next?
9. When we review the experience, what can we learn about doing a better job in the future?

- A failure mode and effects analysis (FMEA) is a procedure for analysis of potential failure within a system, classifying the severity or determining the failure's effect upon the system and helping determine remedial actions to overcome these failures. It was first used by the US armed forces in the late 1940s and expanded by the National Aeronautics and Space Administration in the 1960s to help put an astronaut on the moon. In the late 1970s, the Ford Motor Company implemented FMEA into the automotive industry. Before conducting FMEA, it is necessary to describe the process or system being evaluated. This is best done by using a flowchart (described in the next chapter). The analysis itself occurs in three steps:

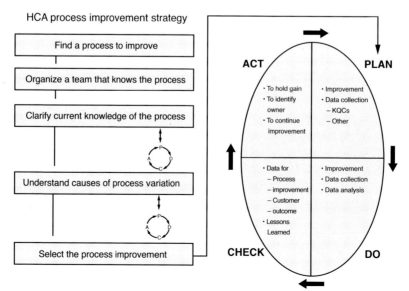

Fig. 2.18 The FOCUS-PDCA model. *HCA*, Hospital Corporation of America; *KQC*, Key Quality Characteristics. (*Reprinted with permission from Hospital Corporation of America, Nashville, TN, 1989.*)

Step 1: Severity. Determine all failure modes and their effects. Each effect is given a severity number (S) ranging from 1 (no danger) to 10 (important). If the severity of an effect has a number of 9 or 10, actions are considered to eliminate the failure mode (such as using only nonionic contrast media). A severity rating of 9 or 10 is usually reserved for effects that would cause injury or result in litigation.

Step 2: Occurrence. In this step, it is necessary to look at the cause of a failure and how often it occurs. All potential causes for failure should be identified and documented. A failure mode is given a probability number (O), which also ranges from 1 to 10. Actions need to be determined if an occurrence is high (meaning greater than 4 for nonsafety failure and greater than 1 when the severity number from step 1 is 9 or 10).

Step 3: Detection. Whenever actions are taken to minimize failure, it is important to see how efficiently failures can be detected in the system to prevent further failure. Each combination from the first two steps receives a detection number (D), which represents the ability of tests and inspections to detect failure modes. Once these three steps are completed, risk priority numbers (RPN) are calculated by multiplying the numbers from each step: RPN = S × O × D. This number is generally used as a threshold value in the evaluation of any action to reduce failure.

- Six Sigma is an approach to quality improvement that seeks to identify and remove the causes of errors in business processes. A key focus of Six Sigma is the use of statistical tools and analysis to identify and correct the root causes of variation. The focus is on using data, reducing variation, and eliminating defects or deviations in processes. It was originally developed by Motorola in 1986 and is now used in a variety of applications, including healthcare management.

The term is derived from statistics (discussed in the next chapter), where the word *Sigma* (the lowercase Greek letter σ) is used to represent the standard deviation (a measure of variation) of a statistical population. Six Sigma comes from the concept that if there are three standard deviations on either side of the mean of a process and the nearest limit (covering 99% of all variables), then there will be virtually no items that fail to meet the specifications. It allows you to measure how many errors you may have in a process so you can systematically figure out how to eliminate them. Six Sigma starts with process mapping to identify elements that are critical to quality and then focuses on changing these elements. This procedure was inspired by Deming's PDCA cycle and consists of the five steps of DMAIC:

Define process improvement goals and outcomes that are consistent with customer demands and the institution's strategy.

Measure key aspects of the current process and collect relevant data.

Analyze the data to verify cause-and-effect relationships. Determine what the relationships are, and attempt to ensure that all factors have been considered.

Improve or optimize the process based on data analysis by removing defects so that future performance is controlled.

Control the process to ensure that any deviations from the target are corrected before they result in errors or failure.

- Lean process improvement or lean methodology (which is sometimes referred to as the Toyota Production System) is defined as a systematic approach to identifying and eliminating waste, where waste is defined as any nonvalued tasks. The eight types of wastes most commonly found in healthcare organizations can be found in the following table:

Type of Waste	Description	Examples
1. Defects	Not meeting specified requirements or producing and correcting defects	Medication errors, wrong patient, wrong procedure, missing or incomplete information, misdirected results
2. Overproduction and production of unwanted products	Ties up more resources than necessary	Extra laboratory tests, computed tomography screening for coronary disease, magnetic resonance imaging for lower back pain, antibiotics for common cold
3. Waiting	Increases wait time, work in process, and delays response time to the customer	Waiting for test results, records, transport, examination room cleaning, patients, staff, or discharge
4. Not utilizing employees	Any ideas that are not considered and implemented	Patient experiences as seen through the caregiver
5. Transport (movement of materials or people)	The unnecessary movement of material, people, or a patient adding time and consuming space	Moving patients, transport between departments, medications, samples, or equipment
6. Inventory	Ties up capital and invites risk of obsolescence and damage	Drugs, supplies, equipment, specimens awaiting analysis
7. Motion (movement by workers)	Poor labor efficiency because of work layout or material not in easy reach	Searching for patients, medications, contrast media, charts, supplies, paperwork
8. Extra processing	Creates delays without adding any benefit and invites more defects in the process	Bed moves, retesting, repeat paperwork, repeat registration, readmit

There are five guiding principles of lean process improvement:

1. Value—specify value from the perspective of the customer
2. Value stream—characterize the value stream (set of activities) for each product/process while removing waste
3. Flow—progressive achievement of value-creating steps with minimal queues and no stoppages or backflows of product, information, or services
4. Pull—a system in which nothing is produced by a supplier until the customer signals a need
5. Perfection—always compete against perfection, not just your current competition

Lean process improvement is often used in conjunction with Six Sigma for analyzing, reducing, and eliminating waste in healthcare processes. One of the most common lean process improvement problem-solving, communication, and continuous improvement tools is known as A3. This gets its name from the fact that it originally utilized 11-inch × 17-inch legal paper (which is known as ISO Series A, size 3 paper and was the largest size that could be faxed at the time) to create a problem-solving template shown in Fig. 2.19. This form is based on the PDCA/PDSA model for continuous improvement, discussed earlier in this chapter.

Team Strategies and Tools to Enhance Performance and Patient Safety

One strategy that can support healthcare organizations in implementing a model of quality improvement is Team Strategies and Tools to Enhance Performance and Patient Safety (TeamSTEPPS). TeamSTEPPS is an evidence-based training program designed to improve quality and safety by enhancing communication and teamwork skills among healthcare professionals. The program was developed jointly by the Department of Defense and the AHRQ.

TeamSTEPPS teaches techniques to improve team structure, communication, leadership, understanding of what is happening ("situation monitoring"), and mutual support among team members. Together, these factors have a strong influence on quality improvement and quality of care. Organizations can also use TeamSTEPPS to "coach coaches" or "train the trainer."

Quality Improvement Coaches

A common challenge for department administrators or provider practices is not having the expertise, time, or capacity to focus on designing and implementing a quality improvement program. To help overcome that problem, organizations can seek help from quality improvement coaches, sometimes referred to as practice facilitators or practice enhancement assistants.

Quality improvement coaches are full- or part-time personnel hired or contracted to help medical practices evaluate and build organizational capacity for CQI. The functions of a quality improvement coach can include:

- Analyzing and evaluating performance, customer/patient feedback, or patient experience surveys
- Recommending changes and supporting internal teams with implementation
- Training clinicians and staff in quality improvement methods
- Team building
- Disseminating best practices and innovative ideas
- Providing specific materials and resources (flowcharts, computer training, etc.)
- Assisting with enhancing communication and technology, promoting adherence to best practices, and creating the capacity to participate in and benefit from research

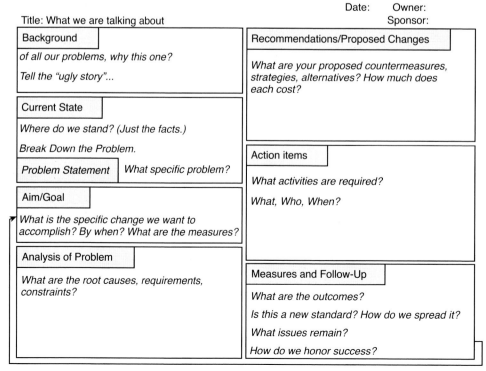

Fig. 2.19 Lean methodology A3 template.

SUMMARY

Quality management programs must incorporate quality improvement tools and procedures to be successful. This requires a basic knowledge of statistical concepts as well as knowing how to create a quality improvement plan. A key part of the quality improvement plan is to identify and analyze potential as well as actual problems so that effective solutions can be created and implemented. This includes being able to perform RCA studies as well as being able to utilize a process improvement model that effectively communicates these solutions to all involved parties.

REVIEW QUESTIONS

1. Which of the following terms best describes the entire set or group of items being measured?
   a. Population
   b. Sample
   c. Frequency
   d. Central tendency
2. Which of the following terms best describes the average set of observations?
   a. Mean
   b. Median
   c. Mode
   d. Variance
3. Which of the following terms best describes variables that have only two values or choices?
   a. Continuous variables
   b. Dichotomous variables
   c. Stochastic variables
   d. Statistical variables
4. A cause-and-effect diagram is also known as which of the following?
   a. Fishbone chart
   b. Pareto chart
   c. Trend chart
   d. Scatterplot
5. Which of the following terms best describes a chart that pictorially demonstrates whether key indicators are moving up or down over a given period of time?
   a. Histogram
   b. Pareto chart
   c. Trend chart
   d. Scatterplot
6. The distribution of continuous data can best be demonstrated by the use of which of the following?
   a. Histograms
   b. Control charts
   c. Scatterplot diagrams
   d. Pareto charts
7. Which of the following is not a tool for data presentation?
   a. Control charts
   b. Brainstorming
   c. Pareto charts
   d. Cause-and-effect diagrams
8. How many basic steps are involved in the creation of a TPM?
   a. 3
   b. 5
   c. 7
   d. 10
9. A procedure to identify potential failure within a system is
   a. SWOT
   b. FMEA
   c. Six Sigma
   d. FOCUS-PDCA
10. Which of the following groups is usually responsible for implementing the solutions that the focus groups have determined will improve a particular process?
    a. Quality circle
    b. Work team
    c. Quality improvement team
    d. Problem-solving team

3

Image Quality

OBJECTIVES

At the completion of this chapter, the reader should be able to do the following:

- Explain the factors affecting pixel brightness in digital imaging
- Describe the various units used to measure the brightness of light in photometry
- Describe the difference between illuminance and luminance
- Explain the factors affecting image contrast in digital imaging
- Describe the concept of contrast resolution

- Describe the various sources of noise in diagnostic imaging
- Distinguish between signal-to-noise ratio and contrast-to-noise ratio
- Explain the factors affecting spatial resolution in digital imaging
- Explain the various methods that can be used to evaluate spatial resolution in digital imaging
- Describe the concept of detective quantum efficiency
- Explain the difference between the concepts of accuracy, sensitivity, and specificity

KEY TERMS

Contrast resolution
Contrast-detail curve
Contrast-to-noise ratio
Detective quantum efficiency
Detector elements
Discrimination
Dynamic range
Edge spread function
Foot-candle
Full-width half maximum
Illuminance
Interpolation

Line spread function
Luminance
Lux
Modulation transfer function
Matrix size
Negative predictive value
Nit
Nyquist frequency
Photometry
Point spread function
Positive predictive value

Prevalence
Quantum mottle
Receiver operator characteristic curve
Sensitivity
Signal-to-noise ratio
Spatial resolution
Specificity
Steradian
Visibility of detail
Window level
Window width

The majority of diagnostic imaging in the 21st century is digital in nature. Regardless of the modality that is being utilized, there are certain common image quality characteristics that all of them have in common. The next several chapters of this text mentions many of these qualities and therefore requires the reader to have a basic understanding. These common image quality characteristics are discussed in this chapter. The first of these common characteristics is image or pixel brightness.

IMAGE OR PIXEL BRIGHTNESS

Since digital images are viewed on a display monitor, each pixel in the matrix will be assigned a brightness level (black, white, or gray shade) by the computer to demonstrate patient anatomy. This would be comparable to the optical density of film-based images. Pixel brightness is affected by:

1. Quantity and or quality of energy reaching the image receptor/detector. Depending on the modality, the amount and/or energy that reaches the image receptor/detector can determine the shade of each pixel that is displayed in the final image. In imaging systems that utilize X-rays (radiography, fluoroscopy, and computed tomography [CT]) systems), the amount and energy of the X-rays striking the detector array or imaging plate will help to determine the brightness of each pixel and therefore the overall brightness of the image displayed. In magnetic resonance imaging (MRI), the strength and frequency of the radio waves that return from the patient's body are interpreted by the computer and help determine pixel brightness. In ultrasound, the strength of the return echo received by the transducer elements determines the pixel brightness. In nuclear medicine scans, the amount of radiation emitted from a particular organ or tissue of the body helps to determine the brightness value of each pixel.

2. Software manipulation. The amount and energy of radiation exiting the patient during diagnostic imaging studies can create thousands of possible gray shades in the image, far more than the human eye can distinguish (generally 32–64). Because the range of stored shade values is so much wider than the visual range, any digital image is only a small part of the total data obtained by the computer. Each image is only a "window" on the total range of data. The range between the largest possible signal intensity, or frequency, divided by the smallest possible signal value that a system can process or display is called the *dynamic range* (similar to film latitude). The dynamic range of the digital signal carrying data to the computer will be far wider (digital radiography [DR] has a dynamic range of 10,000:1 compared with film, which has 40:1) than the range of grayscales in the image on the monitor (500:1). In simplistic terms, dynamic range is described as the number of gray shades that can be represented in an image. It can also be defined as the range of exposures over which a detector can acquire image data. The gray shades that make the image on the monitor are called the *window*. The computer can easily change the level and width of the display window by mathematical recalculations. The *window level* controls image brightness in digital modalities. The window level is the level within the signal that produces the center brightness level in the window (see Fig. 3.1). When the window level is increased, the image brightness will increase (direct relationship). Information outside of the chosen range will not appear in the image on the monitor. Since pixel brightness is determined by the amount of light emitted from a pixel location on a display monitor, a basic knowledge of photometry is required before we can go any further in our list of image quality characteristics. Photometry is the branch of science that deals with the measurement of the intensity of light.

PHOTOMETRY

The radiant energy that strikes or crosses a surface per unit of time or radiant energy emitted by a source per unit time is called *radiant flux* and is measured in watts (W). The watt is defined as the number of joules (J) of energy per second or 1 W = 1 J/s. Radiant flux, evaluated with respect to its capacity to evoke the sensation of brightness, is called *luminous flux*. The unit of luminous flux is the lumen and is affected by both the radiant flux (the amount of radiant energy per second) and the wavelength (color) of the light (yellow can appear brighter than purple or violet, even with the same number of light photons in the beam). One standard candle radiates about 12.5 lumens. The luminous intensity of a light source is the amount of luminous flux that is emitted per viewing area (such as a viewbox or digital display device), and is represented by the equation:

$$I = \frac{dF}{d\omega}$$

where I = luminous intensity, dF = luminous flux in lumens, and $d\omega$ = solid angle in steradians, and where ω is equal to the area on the surface of a sphere divided by the square of the

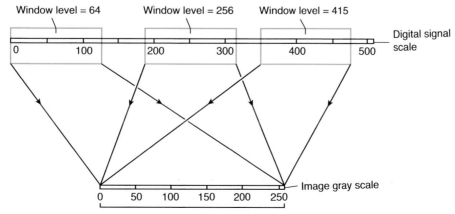

Fig. 3.1 Concept of window level. The same window width (128) has been used, but window levels of 64, 256, and 415 have been selected.

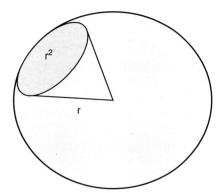

Fig. 3.2 A steradian is as area on the outside of a sphere equal to the square of the radius of the sphere.

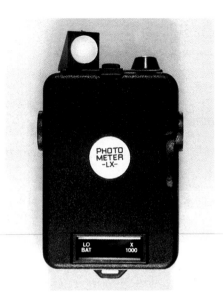

Fig. 3.3 Photographic light meter (photometer) for viewbox evaluation. (Courtesy Nuclear Associates, Carle Place, NY.)

radius of that sphere. A steradian is the area on the surface of a sphere that is equal to the square of the radius of that sphere see Fig. 3.2). There are 12.5 steradians in one sphere. This value of lumens per steradian is also called the *candle*, or *candela* (cd), and is the SI unit of luminous intensity. One candle or candela corresponds to 3.8×10^{15} photons per second being emitted from a light source through a cone like field of view.

The actual brightness of a particular area or source can be evaluated by one of two values, illuminance and luminance.

ILLUMINANCE

Illuminance is the amount of luminous flux incident per unit area, or the amount of light that is projected onto a given surface. It is not the amount of brightness of a light source, but rather the result of that light source in illuminating a particular area. For example, if we are reading a paper book or magazine, we are often more interested in the intensity of light falling on the page than we are in the brightness of a light source (which we would be if looking at a computer screen). The brightness of the page that you are reading is the illumination; the brightness of a particular light source is the luminance. The illumination that you obtain depends not only on how bright the source is (the luminance), but also on how far away it is (light intensity follows the inverse square law). Illuminance can be measured in units of lux (lumens per square meter) or foot-candles (ft-cd) (lumens per square foot). Conversion of foot-candles to lux can be accomplished by the following conversion values:

1 lux = 0.093 ft-cd or 1 ft-cd = 10.8 lux

The illuminance of the interior of a typical home, office building, or classroom from artificial light is approximately 1000 lux or 100 ft-cd. The light-localizing variable-aperture collimator must be able to illuminate a minimum of 15 ft-cd or 160 lux onto the X-ray table at a 100-cm source image distance (SID), according to Food and Drug Administration guidelines (discussed in Chapter 5). Viewbox brightness can be measured with illuminance (because the light bulb is illuminating the acrylic plastic [Plexiglas] front), but luminance is more accepted. If illuminance is used, standard viewboxes will have a value of about 5000 lux, 500 ft-cd, or 13 Exposure

Value (EV). A photodetector that is covered with both a photometric filter and a cosine diffuser is required for the measurement of illuminance (see Fig. 3.3). Table 3.1 shows various illuminance values.

LUMINANCE

Luminance is the luminous intensity per unit of projected area of source, or the amount of light that is emitted or scattered from a particular source. In other words, luminance measures the brightness or intensity from a particular light source. Luminance is the preferred method of measuring viewbox brightness in film/screen imaging as well as the brightness of digital display devices. Units that can measure luminance include candles or candela per square meter (also known as nit), candles per square centimeter, or candles per square foot. The range of human vision is from 6×10^{-6} nit to $10 \times 10 = 6$ nit. The optimum range is from about 1000–10,000 nit. The average viewbox for viewing film images has an average brightness level of 2000 nit, and a 36 W fluorescent tube has a brightness level of 8000 nit. Another set of units also can be used for measurement of luminance and is $1/\pi$ as great as

TABLE 3.1	Illuminance Values	
Setting	**Ft-cd**	**Lux**
Digital image reading room	1	10.8
Twilight	5	54
Corridor	20	216
Waiting room	30	324
Laboratory	100	1080
Tennis court	200	2160
Cloudy day	1000	10,800
Surgery	3000	32,400
Sunny day	10,000	108,000

Ft-cd, Foot-candles.

TABLE 3.2	Photometric Quantities and Units	
Quantity	**Unit**	**Abbreviation**
Luminous flux	Lumen	lm
Luminous intensity	Lumen/steradian or candela	cd
Illuminance	Lumen/ft² (foot-candle)	ft-cd or fc
	Lumen/m² (lux)	lx
Luminance	Candela/m² (nit)	nit

those mentioned earlier. These units are the lambert, foot-lambert (often used to measure television and computer monitor brightness), and meter-lambert.

$$1\ lambert = 1/\pi cd\ /cm^2$$
$$1\ foot\text{-}lambert = 1/\pi cd\ /ft^2$$
$$1\ meter\text{-}lambert = 1/\pi cd\ /m^2$$

For conversion of nit to foot-lamberts, the following equation can be used:

$$1\ cd/m^2(nit) = foot\text{-}lambert \times 3.43$$
$$(because\ 1\ foot\text{-}lambert = 3.43\ nit)$$

Primary display monitors should have a luminance greater than 170 nit (50 foot-lamberts) with 300 nit (90 foot-lamberts) preferred, and secondary display monitors should have a luminance greater than 100 nit (30 foot-lamberts).

For the luminance and illuminance units to be equated (because both can be used to measure display monitor brightness), 1 lux of illuminance may be thought of as the reflectance of a perfectly diffusing surface to 1 cd/m² (nit) of luminance (or 1 lux = 1 nit).

Table 3.2 summarizes the various photometric quantities and units.

IMAGE CONTRAST

Image contrast is defined as the difference in pixel brightness values between the various areas of the image. Images with a relatively small number of gray shades in addition to black and white shades are classified as having high contrast (because of the high or large difference between shade values) or short-scale contrast (because of the small range or scale of shade values). Images that have a relatively large number of gray shades in addition to black and white are classified as having low contrast (because there is a low or small difference between one shade value and the next) or long-scale contrast (because of the many gray values in addition to black and white). Image contrast is determined by a number of factors including:

1. Quantity and or quality of energy reaching the image receptor/detector. As with pixel brightness, imaging modalities may also use the amount and/or energy that reaches the image receptor to help determine the range of pixel brightness values (gray, black, or white shades) that are displayed in the image.
2. Subject contrast. This refers to the distribution of tissue densities and/or physiological changes that are present in the anatomical part undergoing the diagnostic study. Depending on the modality, subject contrast can be altered by utilizing a contrast agent, changing the pulse sequences used in MRI, or changing the angle of the ultrasound transducer during Doppler flow studies.
3. Computer software. Image contrast can be manipulated in digital imaging by using a factor called the *window width*. This is the range of shades or grayscale values displayed in the image on the monitor. A computer can expand or compress the range of signal values that can be used to produce the image window (see Fig. 3.4). When the window width is increased, image contrast will decrease (inverse relationship), showing more gray shades and vice versa. An extremely wide window can cause subtle changes to be missed, while an extremely narrow window width requires the computer to ignore a large amount of data outside of the chosen range. All pixels with values below the range register as black and all those above as white.
4. Computer hardware. Image contrast is also affected by the number of bits in the computer hardware that controls the numerical value that is stored at each pixel (each numerical value stored at a pixel location determines the black,

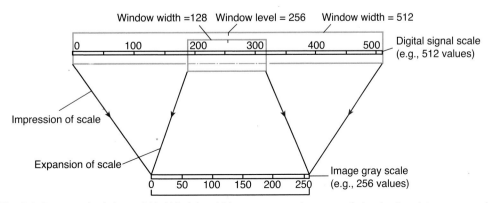

Fig. 3.4 Concept of window width. Window width compresses the range of signal values into a gray scale range that can be displayed on a monitor.

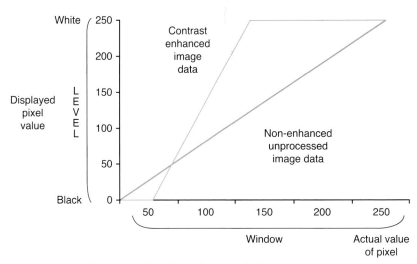

Fig. 3.5 Lookup table adjustment for image contrast.

white, or gray shade that is displayed at that pixel location on the display monitor). This number of bits is known as bit depth, grayscale bit depth, or the number of bits per pixel. A bit (contraction of binary digit) is the smallest unit of digital information that a computing device handles. It is also an electronic switch that can be on or off (1 or 0), and 8 bits = 1 byte. A byte is a grouping of 8 bits used to represent a character or numeric value. By stringing bits together, a pixel can produce various shades of gray. The number of gray shades a pixel can produce (dynamic range) can be calculated by 2^n (n = bit depth). For example, a 1-bit computer memory could only light up a pixel as either black or white. Digital projection radiographic systems have bit depths of at least 12, 14, or 16. 2^8 (1B) = 256 shades, 2^{10} = 1024 shades, 2^{12} = 4096 shades, 2^{14} = 16384, 2^{16} (2B) = 65,536 shades. Adding a bit doubles the number of gray shades, whereas removing a bit cuts the number in half. Increasing bit depth allows for more gray shades to be available in the image.

The downside of increasing the bit depth is that it adds to the file size of the digital image, which increases the storage requirement of the image in the picture archiving and communication systems. The dynamic range of a display monitor is much less than that of most computers used in image processing. Therefore a lookup table is utilized to transform the number of shades in the computer matrix to one that can be displayed on a monitor (Fig. 3.5).

CONTRAST RESOLUTION

Contrast resolution is the ability of an imaging system to distinguish structures with similar tissue density or thickness as separate entities and affects the visibility of detail in the image. The visibility of detail refers to how well structures appear in the image (i.e., is noise present, is the image too light or dark). This concept will be covered in more detail later in this chapter. In other words, separate shades of gray (contrast) should appear so that one structure stands out from the other. Digital radiographic systems (both computed radiography [CR] and

DR) have superior contrast resolution to film/screen radiographic systems (discussed in Chapter 8). MRI can demonstrate the best contrast resolution of all diagnostic imaging modalities. Contrast resolution is affected by the sensitivity of the image receptor (speed) and the amount of noise present. If the amount of noise is increased, the contrast resolution decreases. The amount of noise present is determined by the modality of image system used. There are several types of noise that can occur in imaging systems including:

- *Grain, random,* or *stochastic noise.* This is caused by the size of the silver grains that create the image in film-based imaging.
- *Anatomical noise.* This is caused by anatomy that is present in the image but is not of diagnostic interest and may interfere with the visualization of the anatomy of interest.
- *Structured* or *nonstochastic noise.* This is caused by the construction of the image receptor system, such as the array configuration in DR systems. This construction can cause a type of noise known as toiling, and discussed in greater detail in Chapter 8.
- *Quantum noise.* This is caused by quantum mottle, which is the statistical fluctuation in the number of photons per unit area that contribute to image formation. The quantum noise that is perceived in the image is normally stated as a percentage and determined by the following equation:

$$\text{Quantum noise} = \frac{100 \times \sigma}{N}$$

N is the mean number of photons per unit area, and σ is the standard deviation that measures the width of the distribution about that mean and is equal to the square root of *N*. For example, if a mean of 100 photons exposes an image receptor, the σ is 10 and the quantum noise is 10%. If a mean of 100,000 photons exposes an image receptor, the σ is 316, but the quantum noise is only 0.3%; therefore, as the total number of photons increases, the quantum noise perceived in the image decreases. The number of X-ray photons used to create a radiographic image is approximately $10^5/\text{mm}^2$ of image receptor. Care must be taken with very fast-speed image receptor systems because lower milliampere-seconds (mAs) values are required. This decrease in the number of photons increases the quantum noise, which manifests as a blotchy appearance to the image and decreased contrast resolution. Contrast resolution can be measured with a value known as the signal-to-noise ratio (SNR).

$$SNR = Signal/Noise$$

It is a mathematical way of understanding the difference between the stuff you want (patient anatomy) and the stuff you do not (noise). The signal value in diagnostic imaging is the contrast, or gray scale, of the image (image data). Because this value should be relatively large and the noise should be relatively small, a large SNR indicates high-contrast resolution. Increasing the SNR in radiographic imaging can be accomplished by increasing the milliampere-seconds (mAs) (which can increase patient exposure and heat created in the X-ray tube), increasing the kilovoltage peak (which can decrease radiographic contrast), increase scintillator phosphor layer thickness (which may degrade spatial resolution), or increase the X-ray attenuation capability of the phosphor material used in the scintillator. A high SNR indicates a low amount of noise in the image. The effect of noise is similar to film grain and base + fog in film images.

The higher the noise (lower SNR), the lower the image contrast (inverse relationship). The SNR value is more commonly used when television and digital images are described. An electronic signal that has a noise of 2 mV is 10% of a 20 mV signal, but only 0.01% when compared with a 20 V signal. For this reason, the concept of signal-to-noise ratio is used to describe the relationship between the signal amplitude and the size of the noise.

In radiography, both the signal and the noise must be measured in the same units, relative exposure for a film image, electric potential (volts) for an electronic image, or photon fluence (or exposure, etc.) for a radiographic signal. Once both are measured in the same units, they can be divided by one another to estimate the SNR. An SNR greater than 5 indicates that a lesion is almost certain to be detected.

The noisiest component of most digital systems is usually the display monitor (especially cathode ray tube (CRT) monitors). Commercial televisions often have an SNR of 200, with high-resolution monitors having a range of between 500 and 1000.

Most DR systems use a value known as detective quantum efficiency (DQE) to measure the lack of noise or cleanliness of the image. DQE refers to how well the imaging system converts SNR^2 incident on the detector into SNR^2 in the image. $DQE = SNR^2_{out}/SNR^2_{in}$. The SNR^2_{in} is the mean photon fluence (number of photons/unit area) incident upon the imaging system. The SNR^2_{out} is a function of how well an imaging system processes signal and noise in the image. DQE values range from 0 to 1, with 1 being the best. This value is best used in X-ray detection systems to indicate how efficient the system is in converting the amount of radiation received by the detector into a useful image, or in other words, it is a measure of X-ray absorption efficiency. Fig. 3.6 shows a graph of DQE as a function of X-ray energy for various image receptor capture elements. The DQE for DR systems should be at least 65% (0.65) at 0 line pairs per millimeter (lp/mm). The DQE is different from *quantum detection efficiency*, which measures how well a detector is able to absorb X-rays and create a signal.

Contrast resolution also can be described using a value known as contrast-to-noise ratio (CNR). As with the SNR, the CNR is defined as the contrast seen in the image, divided by the amount of noise existing in the image. The main difference between CNR and SNR is that the size and shape of the test object used to create the image is included in the SNR calculation, while CNR does not. CNR is most accurate when a homogenous test object is used. Increasing the contrast and reducing image noise will increase the CNR and therefore improve image quality and increase the ability to detect a lesion (especially in mammographic images). Contrast can be improved by reducing the amount of scattered radiation, reducing all causes of fogging, or using a contrast

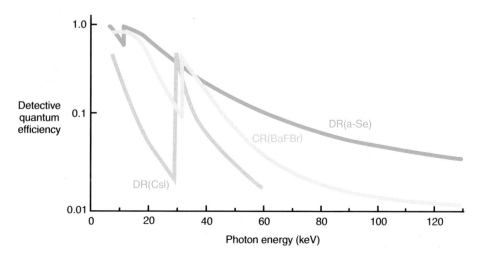

Fig. 3.6 Detective quantum efficiency as a function of X-ray energy for various image receptor capture elements. (*a-Se*), Amorphous selenium; (*BaFBr*), barium fluorobromide; *CR*, computed radiography; (*CsI*), cesium iodide; *DR*, digital radiography; *keV*, kiloelectron volt.

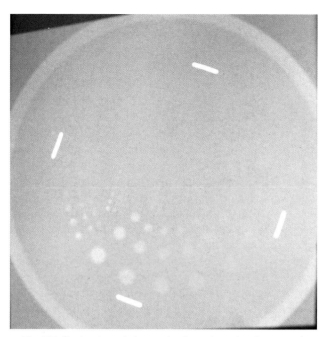

Fig. 3.7 Contrast resolution evaluation using a Leeds test tool.

TABLE 3.3 Matrix Size for Various Imaging Modalities

Imaging Modality	Matrix Size
Digital mammography	4096 × 6144
CR and DR	3520 × 4280
Digital fluoroscopy	1024 × 1024
Computed tomography	512 × 512
Multislice CT	512 × 512
Ultrasound	512 × 512
MRI	256 × 256
Nuclear medicine	128 × 128

CR, Computed radiography; *CT,* computed tomography; *DR,* digital radiography; *MRI,* magnetic resonance imaging.

agent. Reducing image noise can be obtained by reducing quantum mottle (accomplished by increasing the number of photons used to make the radiographic image) or by image postprocessing in digital imaging.

Digital imaging systems generally have superior contrast resolution to film/screen systems. MRI possesses the greatest contrast resolution capability of all current imaging modalities. An image of a contrast resolution test tool for radiographic systems is shown in Fig. 3.7.

SPATIAL RESOLUTION

Spatial resolution (also known as high-contrast resolution) is the ability of an imaging system to create separate images of closely spaced high-contrast (black-and-white) objects. It can also be thought of as how well the digital system can define an edge. In other words, do the two objects appear sharp and clear, or do they blur together? This is determined by a number of factors:

1. Matrix size of the computer. The matrix size of the computer refers to the total number of pixels that will be used to create the image. The larger the matrix size (number of pixels), the greater the spatial resolution (or sharper image). This is because the size of each pixel would also have to be smaller to fit into a matrix of the same dimensions. A smaller pixel size is comparable to having to use a smaller paintbrush to paint a scene containing fine detail, whereby a larger pixel size would be like trying to paint with a larger-size brush. The disadvantage to having more pixels in a matrix is that it will increase the storage requirement of the image data in the picture archiving and communication systems.

2. Matrix size of the image receptor/detector. Like computer matrix size, the number of pixels in the image receptor/detectors has the same effect on spatial resolution. More

detectors present in the image receptor/detector matrix means that spatial resolution would increase for a given image receptor size because each pixel would have to be smaller to fit more into the matrix. The number of pixels in an image matrix is determined by multiplying the number of horizontal pixels (M) × vertical pixels (N) in the image receptor/detector array. For example, if a CT image is created with 512 horizontal pixels and 512 vertical pixels, the total number of pixels in the image matrix would be 262,144. Pixel size can then be calculated when the number of pixels and the dimensions of the matrix (sometimes referred to as the field of view) is known.

Pixel size = dimension of matrix/# of pixels. For example, if the pixel size in millimeters of a 512 × 512 matrix is 200 mm (20 cm), the pixel size would be determined by:

200 mm/512 = 0.4 mm.
Therefore matrix size determines pixel size.

Table 3.3 shows the matrix size for various modalities. From the table, you can see that nuclear medicine images would display the least amount of spatial resolution, and digital mammography images would display the greatest spatial resolution.

3. Display monitor. Like computers and image receptors, digital display monitors have a built-in matrix made up of a specific number of pixels, and the more pixels in a specific matrix size, the smaller each pixel and the greater the spatial resolution in the displayed image. Display monitors are discussed in greater detail in Chapter 8, but monitors are usually sold with a specific number of pixels (expressed in megapixels), and the greater the number of megapixels, the greater the spatial resolution. Table 3.4 compares the number of pixels of various display monitors.

Standard computer monitors are used in *landscape* display modes, while those in CR and DR are used in *portrait* mode. Most monitors for digital radiographic and fluoroscopic systems have a matrix size of 2560 × 2048 (5 MP), while 2 MP are used for other modalities such as CT and MR. A 1 K × 1 K (1 MP) monitor would only have half the spatial resolution of a 1 K monitor. Since the matrix size of the computer and the matrix size of the monitor may differ, a process known as interpolation must be carried out.

TABLE 3.4 Pixels in Television and Computer Monitors

Format	4:3 Aspect Ratio	16:9 Aspect Ratio	Megapixels (MP)
Standard definition (SDTV)	640 × 480	720 × 480	0.3
High definition (HDTV1)	NA	1280 × 720	0.9
High definition (HDTV2)	NA	1920 × 1080	2.0
Ultra-high definition (UHD)	NA	2840 × 2160	4.0
Computed radiography and digital radiography monitor	NA	3520 × 4280	15.0
Digital mammography monitor	NA	4096 × 6144	25.0

N/A, Not applicable.

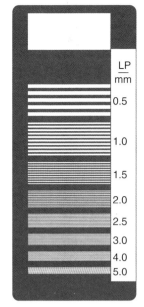

Fig. 3.8 Line pairs per millimeter resolution chart.

Interpolation is the mapping of an image of one matrix size to a display device of another size. For example, if a 2 K × 2 K image is displayed on a 1 K × 1 K monitor, interpolation requires that 4 pixels from the image matrix of the computer be mapped to each pixel of the matrix of the monitor. This can help to compensate for dead pixels in the original image. Monitors used by radiologists to view for diagnosis are called primary viewing monitors and those used by technologists are called secondary monitors.

4. Aperture size, detector size, or sampling frequency. The aperture size refers to the number of detectors per millimeter in the image receptor (i.e., number of detector elements in a DR active matrix array or number of detectors in the CT gantry). This can also be referred to as the sampling frequency. The smaller the detectors used, the more can be placed per millimeter in an array, which will yield a greater sampling frequency and therefore greater spatial resolution. In most cases, the number of detectors per millimeter will often match the number of pixels per millimeter in the image matrix of the computer.

The most common method of measuring spatial resolution in diagnostic imaging is to use a value known as *spatial frequency*. The unit of spatial frequency is the lp/mm and is obtained with a resolution chart (Fig. 3.8). A line pair includes an opaque line and a radiolucent space. In the resolution chart, 1 lp/mm would have a 0.5-mm lead bar separated by 0.5 mm of radiolucent material. Two lp/mm would have 0.25-mm lead bars separated by 0.25 mm of radiolucent material, and so on (see Table 3.5). The greater the lp/mm value, the smaller the object that can be imaged and the better the spatial resolution. The *limiting spatial resolution* (also known as the Nyquist frequency) is the maximum number

TABLE 3.5 Comparison of Spatial Resolution and Line Size

Spatial Resolution (lp/mm)	Line or Space Width (mm)
1	0.5
2	0.25
3	0.167
4	0.125
5	0.10
6	0.083
7	0.071
8	0.063
9	0.056
10	0.050

lp/mm, Line pairs per millimeter.

of lp/mm that can be recorded by the imaging system. This is determined by the following equation: Nyquist or maximum spatial frequency = one-half of the sampling frequency (number of pixels per millimeter). For example, a sampling frequency of 2 pixels per millimeter has a limiting resolution of 1 lp/mm (1 mm containing 2 pixels can display no better than only one black and one white pixel, or 1 lp/mm). If we want a spatial resolution of 5 lp/mm, we would need 10 samples (or pixels) per millimeter (i.e., 5 pairs of bright pixels next to 5 bands of dark pixels) (Fig. 3.9). With 10 pixels per millimeter, the spacing is then 0.1. If sampling occurs less than twice per cycle, information is lost and a fluctuating signal is produced (known as aliasing). A wraparound image that appears as two superimposed images that are slightly out of alignment results in a moiré effect (see Chapter 6).

The resolving power of the unaided human eye is approximately 30 lp/mm when inspecting an image up close, and at normal reading distance (about 25 cm), it is about 5 lp/mm.

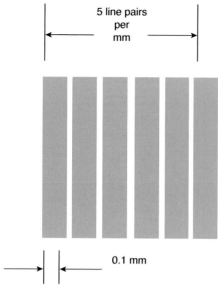

5 line pairs per mm

0.1 mm

Fig. 3.9 Line pairs in resolution chart.

Pixel Pitch (Sampling Pitch)

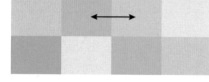

- The physical distance between adjacent DEL's or between data samples.
- Pixel pitch determines the maximum spatial resolution.
  - Nyquist's frequency.

Fig. 3.10 Concept of pixel pitch. *DEL,* Detector element.

Most radiographic systems cannot provide this level of spatial resolution. Nonscreen film holders that were once used in radiography could yield up to 100 lp/mm (but at a price of an extremely high radiation dose to the patient). Spatial resolution should be evaluated with a resolution chart or specialized phantom containing a resolution chart upon acceptance and then yearly.

Other methods of measuring spatial resolution include pixel pitch, point spread function (PSF), line spread function, and edge spread function.

Pixel Pitch

The pixel pitch is the physical distance between adjacent detector elements (Fig. 3.10). It can be determined by measuring the distance from the center of one pixel to the center of the next adjacent pixel. The smaller the pixel pitch, the better the spatial resolution. Typical DR systems should have a pixel pitch of between 100 and 150 μm.

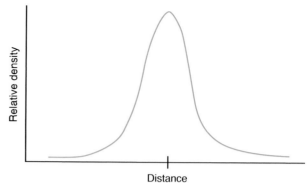

Fig. 3.11 Point spread function graph.

Optimum for DR systems is 3–5 lp/mm or 100–160 μm; 3 lp/mm = 160 μm pp and 5 lp/mm = 100 μm pp.

Point Spread Function

Point spread function is a graph that is obtained with a pinhole camera and a microdensitometer. The pinhole camera creates a black dot in the center of a film, and a microdensitometer is used to take readings of this point. These values are plotted on a graph versus the distance from the center of the point, as shown in Fig. 3.11. The narrower the peak on the graph, the better the spatial resolution and quality of the image. The width of the peak (in millimeters) of the PSF graph can be measured to yield a numerical value to indicate spatial resolution (the smaller the number, the better the spatial resolution and vice versa). The width is usually measured at half the maximum value and is termed full width–half maximum (FWHM). The limiting spatial resolution in lp/mm may be estimated by using the following equation:

$$1 / (2 \times FWHM)$$

For example, if the PSF has an FWHM value of 0.1 mm, the limiting resolution would be 1/(2 × 0.1 mm) or 5 lp/mm.

Line Spread Function

Line spread function is a graph that is more accurate and easier to obtain than the PSF graph. It requires an aperture with a slit that is 10 μm wide instead of the pinhole camera. Density readings of the centerline are taken and plotted (Fig. 3.12). FWHM values also can be obtained from this graph and interpreted much the same way as discussed with PSF.

Edge Spread Function

Edge spread function requires a sheet of lead to be placed on a cassette and exposed. Density readings are taken at the border between the black and white areas and plotted on a graph (Fig. 3.13).

The resolution test tool (see Fig. 3.8) can be imaged with an image receptor on acceptance and then yearly to evaluate any variation.

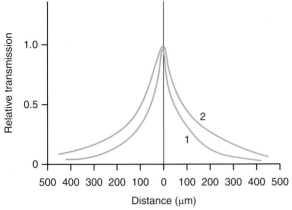

Fig. 3.12 Line spread function graph.

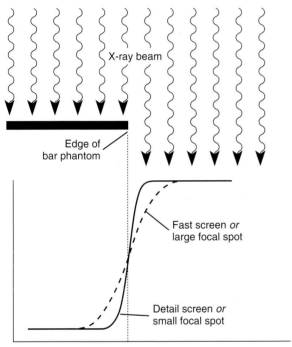

Fig. 3.13 Edge spread function graph.

Contrast-Detail Curve

A method for evaluating both contrast resolution and spatial resolution simultaneously is to construct what is known as a contrast-detail curve (Fig. 3.14). The curve plots the object contrast percentage on the y-axis and the just perceptible size that is visualized on the x-axis. A test tool made up of rows and columns of holes of various sizes and depths is required (Fig. 3.15). The curve shows that when the object contrast is high (i.e., large differences in size or thickness), small objects can be imaged. If object contrast is low (small differences in size or thickness), objects must be large to be visualized.

VISIBILITY OF DETAIL

As mentioned previously, the visibility of detail refers to how well the image can be seen or clarity of the image, and is affected by image brightness/darkness, contrast resolution, and DQE, which have been previously discussed. A common way to measure the visibility of detail is to measure the modulation transfer function (MTF).

Modulation Transfer Function

Modulation transfer function is a numeric value that is used to measure the visibility of detail and is obtained

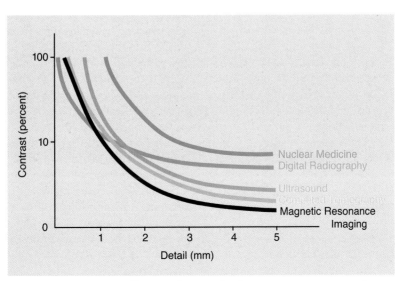

Fig. 3.14 Contrast-detail curve.

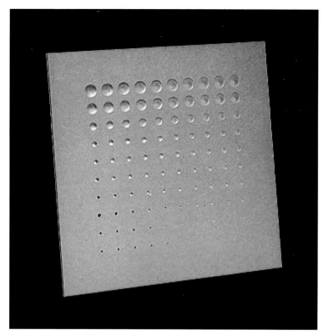

Fig. 3.15 Contrast-detail test tool.

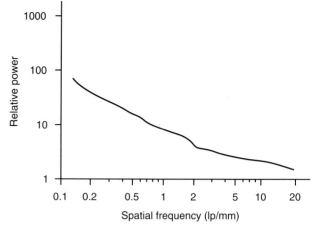

Fig. 3.16 Weiner spectrum indicating the modulation transfer function.

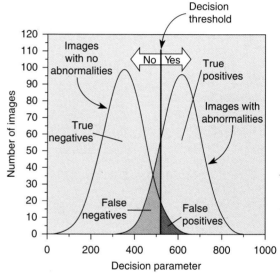

Fig. 3.17 Graph showing patients with disease versus healthy patients.

with a mathematic process known as *Fourier transformation*. Just as a mathematic number (slope) can be obtained from a linear graph, Fourier transformation can obtain a number from a curve. This number ranges from 0 to 1 (0%–100%), with 1 being the maximum spatial frequency. An easier way to think of MTF is demonstrated by the following equation:

$$MTF = \frac{\text{Information recorded in an image}}{\text{Information available in the part}}$$

If all of the patient information is recorded in the image, a value of 1 is obtained. For example, an MTF value of 0.5 indicates that 50% of the patient's anatomy is recorded. The total MTF of an imaging system is obtained by combining all of the component MTF values.

$$MTF_{total} = MTF_1 \times MTF_2 \times MTF_3, \text{ and so on}$$

For example, if a film can demonstrate 80% of the patient anatomy on an image (MTF = 0.8) and a screen can demonstrate 70% (MTF = 0.7), the total system MTF equals 0.8 × 0.7, or 0.56. A Weiner spectrum graph is sometimes used to demonstrate the relationship of MTF and spatial frequency (Fig. 3.16). DR systems should deliver an MTF of at least 30% (0.3) at 2 lp/mm and 60% (0.6) at 1 lp/mm.

The resolution test tool (see Fig. 3.8) can be imaged with an image receptor on acceptance and then yearly to evaluate any variation.

DIAGNOSTIC PERFORMANCE MEASUREMENT

The main outcome of a diagnostic imaging examination is an accurate diagnosis of a patient's condition so that proper treatment can be administered. This is affected by factors such as image quality (for which the technical staff is responsible) and the competency of the radiologist to interpret the image (determining whether the anatomy demonstrated in the image is healthy). In images of certain anatomic structures, the distribution of healthy patients follows a bell-shaped normal distribution. The distribution of patients with diseases also follows a normal distribution but with a different mean value (which can be larger or smaller depending on the patient population studied). Fig. 3.17 shows the distribution of these two groups. The two means are relatively far apart, so it should be easy to distinguish between the two.

The region where the two groups overlap indicates less of a distinction between them, and accurate diagnosis is more difficult. A diagnostic cutoff or threshold level is placed to distinguish a healthy diagnosis from a diagnosis of disease. Patients in whom disease has been diagnosed are considered positive. If a test result (such as a biopsy) reveals that the diagnosis is correct, a designation of *true positive* (TP) is given. Patients are designated as *false positive* (FP) if further

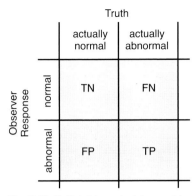

Fig. 3.18 Truth table or decision matrix.

study indicates that they do not have the disease despite the positive finding from the image. Healthy patients with no disease present are considered negative. If a diagnosis of negative is determined from an image and supported by followup studies, it is designated as *true negative* (TN). If a negative diagnosis is given to a patient who later is found to have the disease, then a designation of *false negative* (FN) is assigned. This information can be obtained from patient medical records and should be determined for high-risk studies such as angiographic procedures. A decision matrix or truth table can be used to demonstrate these values (Fig. 3.18). The FDA mandates that this information be derived for mammographic procedures. From this information, the values of accuracy, sensitivity, and specificity; prevalence; positive predictive value; and negative predictive value can be obtained.

Accuracy

Accuracy is the percentage or fraction of cases that are diagnosed correctly; it can be determined by the following equation:

$$\text{Accuracy} = \frac{(N_{TP} + N_{TN})}{N_{Total}} \times 100$$

N designates the number of cases. For example, if 210 mammograms are performed in 1 month, and the number of TNs is 167 and the number of TPs is 36, then the accuracy rate of the image diagnosis is 0.967, or 96.7%.

Sensitivity

Sensitivity also is referred to as the *TP fraction* and indicates the likelihood of obtaining a positive diagnosis in a patient with the disease (or the ability to detect disease). A sensitive test has a low FN rate. Sensitivity is determined by the following equation:

$$\text{Sensitivity} = \frac{N_{TP}}{(N_{TP} + N_{FN})}$$

If a department demonstrates 36 TPs and 3 FNs, then the sensitivity is 0.92, or 92%.

Specificity

Specificity is also known as the *TN fraction* and indicates the likelihood of a patient obtaining a negative diagnosis when no disease is present. A specific test has a low FP rate. Specificity is determined by the following equation:

$$\text{Sensitivity} = \frac{N_T}{(N_{TN} + N_{FP})}$$

A department receiving 167 TNs and 4 FPs has a specificity of 0.97, or 97%.

Positive Predictive Value

The positive predictive value is the probability of having the disease given a positive test and is determined by the following equation:

$$\frac{N_{TP}}{N_{TP} + N_{FP}}$$

A department having 36 TPs and 4 FPs will have a positive predictive value of 0.9, or 90%.

Negative Predictive Value

The negative predictive value is the probability of not having the disease given a negative test and is determined by the following equation:

$$\frac{N_{TN}}{(N_{TN} + N_{FN})}$$

A department having 167 TNs and 3 FNs will have a negative predictive value of 0.98, or 98%.

The ideal for all of the previous values is 100%. In general, the diagnostic performance will depend on the disease prevalence (also known in mammography as abnormal interpretation rate), which is determined by the following equation:

$$\frac{[N_{TP} + N_{FN}]}{[N_{TP} + N_{FP} + N_{TN} + N_{FN}]}$$

A diagnostic imaging department is responsible for establishing its own threshold of acceptability for each value, with both internal and external factors being considered (see Chapter 2). Departments that want to improve accuracy, sensitivity, and specificity can use special statistical phantoms for radiographic, mammographic, and fluoroscopic analysis (Fig. 3.19). These specialized phantoms allow for the position of the phantom components (e.g., test wires, simulated bone fragments, low-contrast objects) to be moved to different parts of the phantom each time it is used. This can eliminate the problem of "familiarity," whereby the observer is familiar with the phantom test pattern and begins to expect or predict that the objects are appearing at the appropriate location. By varying the location each time, the observer has to actually "see" the object at its location for the phantom testing to be valid. Many diagnostic imaging departments also use "double read" as a method to improve accuracy. With this method, two radiologists separately read the same case, and if their diagnoses differ from each other, they confer and decide conclusively. The previously given values can be used to create a receiver operator characteristic curve (ROC) that incorporates both the quality of the image created as well as the skill of the interpreting physician.

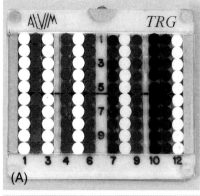

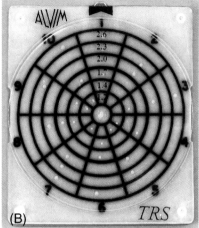

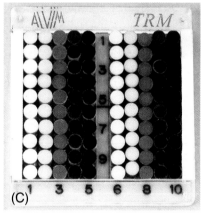

Fig. 3.19 Statistical phantoms for radiographic (A), mammographic (B), and fluoroscopic (C) images. (Courtesy Nuclear Associates, Carle Place, NY.)

Receiver Operator Characteristic Curve

A receiver operator characteristic curve, also known as a *relative operator characteristic curve*, is a plot of the TP probability or sensitivity versus the FP probability, which also can be described as (1-specificity) as the threshold criterion is relaxed (Fig. 3.20). It shows the tradeoff between

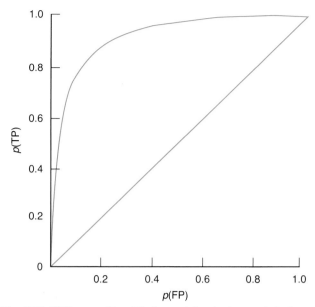

Fig. 3.20 ROC curve. The 45° diagonal line in the graph indicates pure guesswork by the observer. The curve on the left-hand side of the graph depicts an accurate imaging procedure. ROC, Receiver operator characteristic.

sensitivity and specificity (any increase in sensitivity will be accompanied by a decrease in specificity). Threshold criteria for accepting a positive diagnosis can range from strict to lax and represents different compromises between the need to increase sensitivity while minimizing the number of FPs. An ideal image would yield a TP probability of 1 (100%) and an FP probability of 0. Data points that would fall toward the upper left-hand corner of an ROC curve would indicate an accurate diagnosis. If data points fall on a line that is at a 45-degree angle within the graph, it would indicate random guessing by the observer. The area under the ROC curve is a measure of overall imaging performance and has a maximum value of 1 (100%). This area measures discrimination, that is, the ability of the test to correctly classify those with and without the disease. If random guessing occurs, the ROC curve is a straight line through the points (0,0) and (1,1). The area under the random guessing line (area under the ROC curve) is 0.5 (50%). As image quality and performance improve, the curve will move toward the upper left-hand corner, which increases the area under the curve to a maximum of 1.0 (100%). Radiologists or other readers of diagnostic images with low sensitivities as well as low FPs would be categorized as "underreaders" and image readers with very high sensitivities as well as correspondingly high FPs would be categorized as "overreaders." ROC evaluations of image readers can be used to establish the relative merits of a diagnostic imaging test.

SUMMARY

Implementing a quality management program requires more than just equipment monitoring and maintenance. The outcomes assessment of diagnostic images also must be performed to evaluate the success of the procedure. In this way, future problems may be avoided by analyzing current causes of repeat images and artifacts. Continuous improvement of image quality and customer satisfaction can occur when diagnostic image quality and diagnostic accuracy are monitored on a routine basis.

REVIEW QUESTIONS

1. Which of the following terms best describes the amount of light that is emitted from or scattered by a surface?
   a. Photometry
   b. Luminance
   c. Illuminance
   d. Optical density
2. Which of the following terms is the unit most commonly used to measure luminance?
   a. Lux
   b. Nit
   c. Foot-candle
   d. Lumen
3. Which of the following terms best describes the ability of an imaging system to create separate images of closely spaced high-contrast objects?
   a. Screen speed
   b. Spatial resolution
   c. Contrast resolution
   d. Quantum mottle
4. Which of the following terms also is referred to as the TP fraction?
   a. Accuracy
   b. Sensitivity
   c. Specificity
   d. None of the above
5. A DR flat panel detector element size will help to determine which of the following?
   a. Contrast resolution
   b. DQE
   c. Spatial resolution
   d. Dynamic range
6. If the bit depth of an MRI scanner is 12 bits, how many gray shades can be present in the image?
   a. 1024
   b. 2048
   c. 4096
   d. 8192
7. DQE is a measure of which of the following?
   a. Contrast resolution
   b. Image noise
   c. Spatial resolution
   d. X-ray absorption
8. The window width setting in a digital imaging system is used to manipulate which of the following values?
   a. Pixel brightness
   b. Spatial resolution
   c. Temporal resolution
   d. Image contrast
9. The type of contrast that is caused by variations in the tissue density within the anatomical part to be imaged defines which of the following?
   a. Image contrast
   b. Subject contrast
   c. Inherent contrast
   d. None of the above
10. Which modality generally displays the greatest spatial resolution?
    a. Nuclear medicine
    b. MRI
    c. DR radiographs
    d. Digital mammography

Film/Screen Image Receptor Systems

OBJECTIVES

At the completion of this chapter, the reader should be able to do the following:

- State the function and characteristics of a darkroom used for diagnostic imaging
- Explain the importance of proper safelight type and function
- Perform a safelight evaluation test
- Perform an evaluation of white light leakage and processing area condition
- Explain the conditions for proper film and chemical storage
- Discuss the importance of proper viewbox illuminator function on image quality
- Perform a viewbox quality control test

- Explain the evaluation process of image duplicators
- Explain the factors affecting screen speed
- Describe the importance of spectral matching of intensifying screens and film
- Describe the main differences between manual and automatic film processing
- List the main components of the developer and fixer solutions, and state the function of each component
- Explain the proper mixing procedure for developer and fixer concentrate solutions
- State the chemical safety procedures for the safe handling of processing chemicals as described by the Occupational Safety and Health Administration (OSHA)

- Describe the basic tests for determining the archival quality of processed images
- List the six main systems of automatic film processors and state the function of each system
- Describe the methods of installing film processors in a darkroom
- Understand the importance of a processor quality control program in diagnostic imaging
- List the main components of a processor quality control program in diagnostic imaging

- Describe the factors that affect chemical activity
- Indicate the proper processor cleaning procedures
- Describe the basic types of processor maintenance and appropriate maintenance procedures
- Perform sensitometric tests to monitor processor function and chemical activity performance
- Describe the importance of quality control in daylight systems

KEY TERMS

Agitation	Hyporetention	Relative speed
Archival quality	Illuminance	Safelight
Base + fog	Incident light	Screen speed
Bromide drag	Intensification factor	Sensitometer
Chemical activity	Latensification	Sensitometry
Contrast indicator	Latent image	Solarization
Darkroom	Locational effect	Spectral matching
Daylight systems	Luminance	Speed indicator
Densitometer	Luminescence	Static electricity
Developer	Manifest image	Synergism
Fixer	Nit	Temperature
Flood replenishment	Orthochromatic	Time-of-day variability
Flow meters	Oxidation/reduction reaction	Transmitted light
Fluorescence	Panchromatic	Ultraviolet
Foot-candle	Phosphorescence	Ventilation
Humidity	Photometry	Viewbox illuminator
Hydrometer	Psychrometer	Volume replenishment

Despite the digital revolution that has occurred in diagnostic imaging, many radiographic images may still be produced using film/screen image receptors. Since digital radiography systems have a high capital cost, film/screen radiography may still be in use (despite the fact that Medicare and Medicaid reimbursement is 20% less). Even with digital imaging, hard copy imaging may be desired, and this necessitates the use of silver-based film. Because all traditional film is light sensitive, it must be handled in a safe area where no light or ionizing radiation is present. Most diagnostic imaging departments use a darkroom area for this purpose, whereas other non-digital departments may use some form of a daylight system. Even departments with daylight systems usually have a traditional darkroom that can be used for duplicating existing radiographs or used as a backup in case of a malfunction in the daylight system.

DARKROOM FUNCTION

The function of a radiographic darkroom is to protect the film from white light and ionizing radiation during handling and processing. After a film has been exposed to light or ionizing radiation (such as in a cassette during a radiographic examination), it can be as much as two to eight times more sensitive to

subsequent exposure than an unexposed film (depending on the type of emulsion). This increase in sensitivity is formally known as latensification. As a result of this phenomenon, any accidental exposure from an unwanted source (such as a darkroom light leak) can destroy a diagnostic image. Film can also be affected by excess heat, humidity, static electricity, pressure, and chemical fumes. All of these variables must be carefully controlled to obtain a diagnostic quality image. If they are not controlled, the most common result is the presence of fog on the manifest image. Fog is defined as noninformational optical density that occurs because silver grains are formed and do not represent any of the anatomic structures within the patient.

DARKROOM ENVIRONMENT

A darkroom is considered a scientific laboratory by common practice standards and the Occupational Safety and Health Administration (OSHA), and should meet all of the requirements and possess all of the equipment of a laboratory. It also should be clean, well ventilated, well organized, and safe. Eating, drinking, and smoking must be prohibited in the darkroom because bits of food or ashes from cigarettes can get into image receptors as they are being loaded and unloaded. These can cause artifacts on the image that can mimic pathologic conditions (especially in mammography cassettes) or otherwise degrade the diagnostic quality of the image. These artifacts are discussed in detail in Chapter 6.

Darkroom Characteristics

Countertops or other work surfaces and rubber floor mats should be grounded to reduce the risk of static electricity. Static electricity creates sparks that emit white light (all colors of the visible spectrum). Because all imaging films are sensitive to some portion of the visible light spectrum, this light creates artifacts that appear on the processed image. The types of static artifacts are tree, crown, and smudge (see Chapter 6). In addition to the work surfaces being grounded, static can be minimized by the following:

1. Handle film properly. Proper film handling, placing a film into and out of a cassette or onto a film tray rather than sliding it, reduces the risk of static electricity because friction is a primary cause of static electricity.
2. Wear natural-fiber clothing (cotton) versus synthetic-fiber clothing (e.g., nylon, polyester).
3. Maintain a proper humidity range (30%–60% relative humidity). Moisture in the air absorbs the buildup of static charges. This is why static is less of a problem in the summer, when the relative humidity is greater. In some darkrooms, installation of a humidifier or ion generator may be necessary to maintain the recommended level of humidity. A psychrometer, which measures humidity, should be available or installed in the darkroom. A psychrometer is a type of hygrometer (a device that measures atmospheric humidity) for calculating relative humidity (Fig. 4.1). It

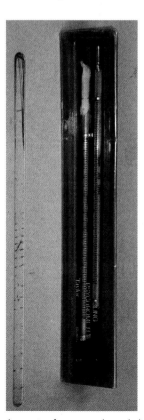

Fig. 4.1 Psychrometer for measuring relative humidity.

consists of a thermometer with wet and dry bulbs, the readings of which are compared, giving the rate of evaporation of water, from which the water vapor saturation of the atmosphere can be calculated. At low relative humidity, moisture evaporates from the wet bulb more rapidly, causing the wet bulb to have a lower reading than the dry bulb. The temperature difference between the two bulbs is used to calculate the relative humidity. Excessive humidity could cause the films to stick together, and the emulsion from the films could be removed when they are pulled apart. Excessive humidity also could cause a condensation problem, and the result could be artifacts (see Chapter 6).

4. Clean screens regularly with an antistatic nonabrasive cleaner. Appropriate screen cleaners are available from the manufacturer from whom the screen is purchased (it is important to match these products to the particular brand of screen). The proper procedure for cleaning intensifying screens is covered later in this chapter. This is especially critical with film/screen mammography cassettes because any dirt or debris in the cassette can leave artifacts that can mimic microcalcifications (an early sign of breast cancer).

The darkroom must be well ventilated to prevent buildup of heat and humidity, which degrade the film. Proper ventilation also removes excessive fumes from the processing solutions that may sensitize film emulsions. The presence of these fumes also can cause condensation of processing chemicals onto work surfaces in the darkroom (e.g., underneath cabinets or shelves). Over time, the residue created by this condensation may fall into open cassettes, causing artifacts to appear in the final images. Removing these fumes, along with periodically wiping these areas with a damp cloth, should minimize the occurrence of these artifacts. Temperature should be maintained in a range of 65–75°F (18–24°C). The fumes from the processing solutions are considered toxic, corrosive, and potentially carcinogenic by OSHA, the Environmental Protection Agency, and the Department of Transportation. OSHA maintains a listing of permissible exposure limits (PELs), which are the chemical levels to which employees can be exposed in the workplace without risk or harm. An environmental engineer can be consulted to monitor the level of a darkroom area. The following are PELs for some of the components found in processing solutions:

- Acetic acid: 25 mg/m³ (10 parts per million [ppm])
- Ammonium thiosulfate (as ammonia): 35 mg/m³ (50 ppm)
- Hydroquinone: 2 mg/m³ (0.44 ppm)
- Phenol: 19 mg/m³ (5 ppm)
- Sulfur dioxide: 13 mg/m³ (5 ppm)
- Glutaraldehyde: 0.7 mg/m³ (0.2 ppm)
- Silver: 0.01 mg/m³

The values just listed were established in 1968, and discussion to revise these figures is taking place. In recent years, many technologists and darkroom technicians have complained of hypersensitivity to darkroom chemicals, a condition sometimes called *darkroom disease,* which manifests in a variety of symptoms ranging from hives to severe fatigue and impairment of the immune system. The Society of Toxicology and the American Society of Radiologic Technologists are currently collecting data on this phenomenon. Proper ventilation in a darkroom should keep the levels of chemical vapors well below PELs and should include a source of fresh air, slight positive air pressure (so that chemical fumes are not sucked out of the processor), and ventilation to the outside atmosphere. *This should yield about 8–10 room changes of air per hour.* A ventilator duct should be placed near the floor, in either the lower portion of the entrance door or the wall.

Many darkrooms have interior walls that are mistakenly painted black, and these walls can make the room too dark. Instead, darkroom walls should be painted in pastels and light colors to increase the reflectance of the light emitted from the safelight. Enamels or epoxy paints are best because they are easy to clean and more durable. However, a matte finish must be used because a high-gloss finish could reflect and amplify light leaks. Should any darkroom wall lie adjacent to a radiation area (e.g., radiographic room, nuclear medicine area), proper lead shielding that is appropriate to the type and energy of radiation used must be present in the walls to protect darkroom personnel and prevent fogging of the film.

The processing of most diagnostic images requires a large quantity of clean water. Today, in most automatic film processors, only cold water is used because the processors have built-in heating systems to regulate solution temperatures. Adequate drainage must be in place to remove the dirty water and used chemicals after processing is completed. *Adequate drainage* is generally defined as the capacity to handle 2.5 times the maximum outflow of the processor when all drains are open. For most automatic film processors, this is about 10 gallons per minute (38 L/min). A floor drain is generally desired for maximum efficiency, with a 3-inch-diameter cast iron or plastic (polyvinylchloride) pipe. Local building codes should be referenced before choosing polyvinylchloride pipe because some municipalities have restrictions on its use. Copper or brass pipes and fittings should be avoided because of the corrosive effect of the processing chemicals. These drains should be dedicated only to film processors and should not share a common line with sinks and toilets to reduce the chance of blockage. They also must be cleaned on a regular basis with a commercial drain cleaner because buildup forms over time. This is especially important when metallic replacement silver recovery units are used. Flooring around the drain must be easy to clean and moisture resistant and of a light color to allow identification of objects that may have been dropped in the dark.

Darkrooms should have adequate storage space for film and chemicals. Film must be stored in an upright position (with no heavy objects or other boxes of film stacked on top) to avoid pressure marks. Open boxes of film should be kept in a metal film bin (usually mounted under the work counter) to minimize the chance of being exposed to white light (Fig. 4.2). Passboxes, also known as *film transfer systems,* also should be present to prohibit white light from entering. These are special boxes whereby one side has a door inside of the darkroom and the other side of the passbox has another door on the outside. If one of the doors is open, the other cannot be opened. This allows a person on the outside to place a cassette

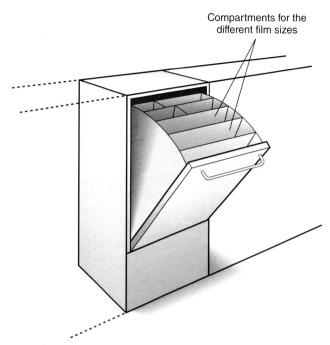

Compartments for the different film sizes

Fig. 4.2 Standard darkroom film bin.

in the box and close the door, and then the person inside of the darkroom can open the door without allowing light into the darkroom. The darkroom door should be double interlocked or revolving, or a lightproof maze can be installed if floor space permits.

Darkroom Lighting

A darkroom should have two types of lighting, overhead lights and safelights.

Overhead Lighting

Overhead lighting is the standard white light that normally illuminates the interior rooms of hospitals and clinics. This standard lighting is necessary for cleaning, maintenance, and possible emergencies (e.g., darkroom personnel becoming ill). Proper overhead lighting normally requires a standard fluorescent fixture (two to four 48-inch fluorescent tubes) per 8 ft^2 (0.74 m^2) of floor space. The overhead light should be interlocked with the film bin(s) so that if a bin is open, the light cannot be energized. If this is not practical, a cover should be placed over the switch to prevent accidental activation. Film bin alerts also are available (at a minimal cost) that sound a continuous alarm while the film bin is open to prevent accidental exposure to white light.

Safelight

A safelight is a light source that emits wavelengths to which particular types of film are not sensitive. Ordinary room light (known as white light) is really a mixture of all of the colors in the visible light spectrum mixed together, as shown in Fig. 4.3. Each individual color is determined by the wavelength of the light photon, which is measured in units called angstroms (Å). One angstrom is equal to 10^{-10} m of 10^{-8} cm. Wavelengths range from about 4000 Å for violet light to 8000 Å for red

Red	Orange	Yellow	Green	Blue	Indigo	Violet

Fig. 4.3 Visible light spectrum.

light. In comparison, the wavelengths of diagnostic radiographs generally range from only 0.1 to about 0.5 Å.

Even the best safelight emits some white light (only lasers emit a pure light of one specific wavelength), and so it is important not to leave film in safelight indefinitely. Also, remember the concept of latensification, whereby a film that has been previously exposed is more sensitive than film that has not been exposed. A typical radiographic film (exposed) should be able to remain in safelight for at least 40 seconds without becoming fogged. Mounting safelights at least 3–4 feet from feed trays or loading counters also helps minimize safelight fog.

The type of film to be processed in the darkroom determines the type of safelight to be used.

Blue-violet-sensitive film. Blue-violet-sensitive film is a common type of film used in screen cassettes, and, as its name implies, is primarily sensitive to the colors blue, indigo, and violet. An amber-colored safelight (a mixture of red, orange, and some yellow) is normally used, with two options available. For the average-sized darkroom, a fixture type of safelight containing either a 7.5-watt (W) or 15-W light bulb is sufficient (Fig. 4.4). A 7.5-W bulb is recommended for single-emulsion film. The light bulb is covered by a colored piece of plastic or glass called a *filter.* The most common types of filters for blue-violet-sensitive film are the Kodak Wratten 6B or the Kodak Mor-Lite (which is slightly brighter). Both of these filters emit an amber-colored or brownish-colored light. The other option, called a *sodium vapor lamp* (Fig. 4.5), is used in a large darkroom or when bright safelight conditions are desired. This works on the same principle as mercury streetlights; however, sodium yields a bright amber color when energized, instead of the bright white color of the mercury lamps. These lights are large and expensive and require a long warmup time to reach maximum brightness. They must be mounted on the darkroom ceiling (at least 6 feet above counters and film bins) because of their brightness level and to provide indirect lighting. Shutter or door openings on top are adjusted with a pull chain to regulate the level of brightness.

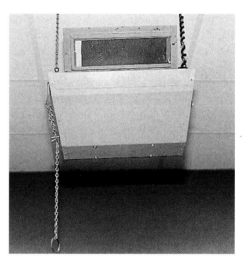

Fig. 4.5 Sodium vapor lamp darkroom safelight.

Orthochromatic film. Orthochromatic film is mainly sensitive to the green portion of the visible spectrum, in addition to the blue-violet portion. A red or magenta dye is added to the film emulsion to increase the absorption of green light by the silver halide crystals. Amber is a mixture of red, orange, and yellow, and the safelights discussed previously are not compatible with this type of film because orange and yellow are too close to green in the spectrum. It is therefore necessary to use a safelight with the same fixture and light bulb combination mentioned previously, but to use a safelight filter that emits light that is pure red. The most common of this type is the Kodak GBX Series of all-purpose filters (GBX stands for green/blue/X-ray). In addition, all Kodak duplicating film requires a GBX-2 filter. An older type of safelight filter that is still acceptable for orthochromatic film is the Kodak 2 filter, which is dark red. Another option is an LED safelight, which uses a light-emitting diode that consumes low power and can last up to 15 years. These safelights are perfectly compatible for use with blue-violet-sensitive film but are not as bright as safelights with amber filters. Facilities should avoid the use of red-colored light bulbs such as those found in Christmas decorations. Although considerably less expensive than actual safelight fixtures, they can emit too much white light, resulting in safelight fog.

New modality film. New modality film is designed to obtain images from either a cathode-ray tube (multiformat camera) or a laser camera (often used in computed tomography, sonography, nuclear medicine, magnetic resonance imaging, and older digital radiographic systems [hence the name]). The light source for many of these devices usually emits light that is red or amber colored, and so the film emulsion is designed accordingly (it is also sensitive to infrared). A fixture and light bulb combination safelight with a dark green filter (Kodak Number 7) can be used with these emulsions.

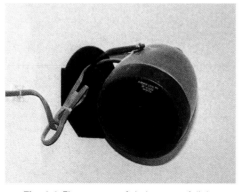

Fig. 4.4 Fixture type of darkroom safelight.

This filter is dark and some time is necessary for the eyes of technologists or darkroom personnel to adapt. Some types of new modality film are panchromatic (sensitive to all colors of the visible spectrum) and therefore cannot be exposed to any safelight. It is best to consult the literature accompanying the box of film or the manufacturer's technical representative before dark green safelight is used. The dry laser printer has virtually replaced the need for this type of film.

Other film types. Most other types of film (e.g., duplicating, subtraction, spot, industrial) can be processed in darkrooms with the safelights just discussed. It is best to consult the film manufacturer to determine the correct type of safelight for these films. Cine film that has been used in cardiac catheterization studies is black-and-white motion picture film (panchromatic) and cannot be exposed to safelights. It normally requires its own dedicated processor (see Chapter 9).

Dry laser printer film. Film used in dry laser printers (discussed in Chapter 8) may need to be handled in darkroom conditions, depending on whether or not it has a special dye added to the top-coating layer. If present, this dye will block ordinary room light from exposing the emulsion (the laser from the printer can still penetrate the dye), and so the film can be loaded into the printer in ordinary room light. Film that does not have this coating will have to be loaded under darkroom conditions.

Light and Leakage Testing

Safelight Testing

Safelights may become unsafe over time as a result of cracks or pinholes in the filter (resulting from expansion and contraction with heat), the wrong wattage of the bulb being installed, or the doors on a sodium vapor lamp being open too far. Therefore a safelight test should be performed at least semiannually or more frequently if problems are discovered. Testing also should be performed when the safelight bulb or filter is changed. Safelights that are turned on for 24 hours a day, 7 days a week, should have their filters changed annually. If safelights are turned on an average of 12 hours a day, 7 days a week, the filter should be changed every 2 years. Testing requires a sensitized film (preexposed) because this makes it more sensitive to safelight fog.

Safelight testing (Fig. 4.6) can be accomplished by either of the procedures discussed in the following boxes.

PROCEDURE: SAFELIGHT TESTING

This procedure is performed with a penetrometer (step wedge) on dual-emulsion films only.

1. Use a tape measure to verify the proper distance from the safelight to the work counters or feed trays. Also check the wattage of light bulbs and inspect the filter for cracks or pinholes. Ensure that the filter type matches the film type.
2. Load an 8 inch × 10 inch (20 cm × 25 cm) cassette with film from a fresh box of film. If more than one type of film is used by the facility, a separate test should be performed for each type of film.
3. Take the loaded cassette to a radiographic room and center the cassette on a radiographic table at a source-to-image distance (SID) of 40 inches (100 cm). Place a penetrometer (step wedge) in the center of the cassette, aligning the long dimension of the wedge with the long axis of the cassette. Collimate the light field to the edges of the step wedge.
4. Expose the cassette at approximately 70 kilovolts (peak) (kVp) and 5 milliamperes-second (mAs). Ideally, the image of the step wedge on the film should have an optical density of approximately 1 when measured with a densitometer. The kilovolt (peak) and milliampere-second can be adjusted depending on the speed of the image receptors that are used.
5. Bring the cassette back into the darkroom, lay the exposed film on the counter, and cover one-half of the film with an opaque material such as cardboard. Be sure to bisect the latent image of the penetrometer into right and left halves and not top and bottom.
6. Expose the film to normal safelight conditions for 2 min, and then process the film.
7. Place the film on a viewbox illuminator and observe whether there is a defined line or break between the halves (see Fig. 4.6). If there is no defined line between the halves, then there is no safelight fog because the human eye can observe differences of as little as 0.01 optical density units. If a discernible line is present, use a densitometer to measure the optical density on each side of the line. The difference between the two sides is a measure of darkroom fog. Because the difference in optical density measurements varies for each step, the step with the maximum density difference must be found. Record the density difference value and the step on which it was measured. This same step should be used for all future safelight tests. The maximum density difference (or darkroom fog level) should be less than 0.05 optical density units. Levels in excess of this value indicate serious safelight fog, which can reduce the image contrast of any films that are exposed to these conditions. If the fog levels are greater than 0.05, readjusting the position of the safelight, replacing the safelight filter, checking to see that the proper wattage bulb has been installed into the safelight, or closing the shutters on a sodium vapor lamp can usually correct the situation.

PROCEDURE: SAFELIGHT TESTING

This procedure is performed with a sensitometer and is acceptable for both single-emulsion (which is usually slower speed) and dual-emulsion film if one does not want to use the previous procedure.

1. In the darkroom (in complete darkness with the safelights turned off), remove a sheet of film from a fresh box of film.
2. Expose this sheet of film with a sensitometer and place it on the counter in the darkroom. Place an opaque card over one-half of the exposed wedge pattern on the film, just as in the first procedure.
3. Expose the film to normal safelight conditions for 2 min, and then process the film.

Continued

PROCEDURE: SAFELIGHT TESTING—cont'd

4. Use a densitometer to determine the step that will have an optical density closest to 1.4 optical density units (using the side that was covered with the opaque card).
5. Determine the maximum density difference (the difference in optical density between the covered side and the uncovered side) for this step and record for future use. For dual-emulsion films, the maximum density difference should not exceed 0.05 optical density units (as in the first procedure). For single-emulsion films, the maximum density difference between the halves cannot exceed 0.02 optical density units. Because single-emulsion film generally has a lower inherent contrast, it is vitally important to keep any additional fogging (which reduces contrast even further) to a minimum.

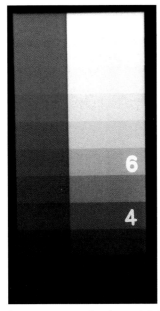

Fig. 4.6 Image of penetrometer showing safelight fog. (Courtesy Nuclear Associates, Carle Place, New York.)

Leakage Testing and Processing Area Condition

While safelights are tested, a check for light leaks, other extraneous light sources (e.g., indicator lights on processors, duplicators, luminous dials on a clock), and processing area conditions usually also can be performed.

PROCEDURE: DARKROOM LEAK TESTING

1. Turn on all white lights in the area surrounding the darkroom. Enter the darkroom and shut off all safelights and overhead lights.
2. After eyes adapt to the dark (about 5 min), check for white light leaks, especially near the processor, darkroom doors, water pipes, ventilation ducts, and suspended ceiling tiles. Light leaks can cause artifacts and reduce image contrast.
3. Turn on the overhead lighting and inspect the countertops and processor feed tray for foreign objects, dampness, cleanliness, and sharp edges. These conditions can cause artifacts if not corrected.
4. Locate the reserve fixer and developer tanks. Check to ensure that they are properly ventilated and that the temperature of the area is within accepted limits. Excessive temperature can cause a deterioration of the processing solutions.
5. Locate the film storage area and verify that the boxes of film are being stored vertically and under the proper temperature conditions. Also check the age of the film and the visibility of the expiration date. The oldest boxes of film should be positioned so that they will be used first. Artifacts can result if these conditions are not within proper parameters.
6. Correct any problems or deficiencies.

Film and Chemical Storage

Film should be stored at a temperature range between 55 and 75°F (14–24°C), whether in the darkroom (only open boxes of film, kept in the film bin), storage closet, or warehouse. Excessive heat can cause age fog, and too low of a temperature can lead to moisture condensation on the film, resulting in artifacts. Humidity also must be controlled (30%–60% relative humidity), especially with film in which the moisture-proof inner seal has been opened. As previously mentioned, static artifacts can appear if the air is too dry. Premature aging of the film, condensation, and films sticking together could be a problem in high humidity conditions. Film can be stored in a refrigerator or freezer to prolong the shelf life, provided that the inner seal is unopened. If kept in a freezer at 0°F or below, the deterioration or aging process stops and the expiration date can be extended for any time that the film was in the freezer. After removal, a 24-hour warmup period is required before the inner seal can be opened and the film used. This is to prevent condensation and the associated artifacts from appearing on the film.

Chemicals should be stored in a well-ventilated area with a temperature range between 40 and 85°F (5–30°C). The temperature should not exceed 70°F (21°C) for a prolonged period. The area should be darkened or have minimal lighting because the developer solution can degrade if exposed to bright light. It is best not to store film and chemicals near each other because film chemistry contains quantities of potassium, a percentage of which is in the form of potassium-40, which is a naturally occurring radioactive isotope that can fog film over time. Most film manufacturers recommend that background radiation not exceed 7 microroentgens (μR)/h. Levels near large quantities of processing chemicals can reach 12 μR/h. Most manufacturers of film and processing chemicals give a 12-month expiration date on the basis of an ambient temperature of 68°F (20°C).

VIEWBOX QUALITY CONTROL

Viewbox Illuminators

Most diagnostic images are transparencies and therefore require an illuminator to view the final image. Proper functioning of the viewbox illuminator is essential in maintaining image quality because it has a direct effect on the contrast. Over time, heat from the fluorescent bulb inside can discolor the plastic front of the viewbox. Dirt and dust can form on both the inside and outside of the plastic viewing surface, as well as the outside surface of the fluorescent bulb. This can reduce light output by as much as 10% per year, and the image contrast is decreased. For this reason, the bulbs should be changed every 2 years (especially viewboxes used in mammography), even though the typical fluorescent bulb has a rated life of 7500–9000 hours. With multiple viewboxes, replace all lamps at the same time with bulbs of the same manufacturer, production lot, and color temperature to maintain consistency. All viewboxes should be cleaned weekly with an antistatic, nonabrasive cleaner, and the intensity of all viewboxes within the department should be checked for consistency. A viewbox quality control test should be performed on acceptance and then at least once a year (weekly for those used in mammography).

Viewbox Quality Control Test

The viewbox quality control test requires a screwdriver and either a photographic light meter or a 35-mm camera with a built-in light meter (Fig. 4.7).

IMAGE DUPLICATING UNITS

Film duplicating units, or copiers, are standard pieces of equipment in diagnostic imaging darkrooms (Fig. 4.8). Because legal considerations make hospitals reluctant to release original images, copies are made so that patients can

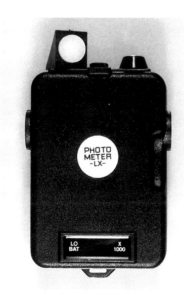

Fig. 4.7 Photographic light meter (photometer) for viewbox evaluation. (Courtesy Nuclear Associates, Carle Place, New York.)

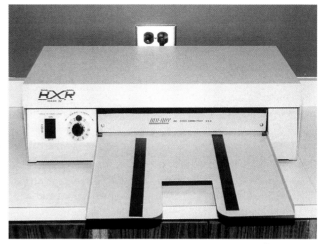

Fig. 4.8 Duplicating unit for copying diagnostic images.

consult with specialty providers without having to repeat the examinations. Most units emit ultraviolet (UV) light using special black light bulbs. UV light is more penetrating than visible light; thus it can penetrate the darker areas of a processed image, and so the image can be duplicated. The copy film is single-emulsion film sensitive to UV light, and so a standard safelight can be used. The emulsion side of the film should be placed against the original image during the duplication process. The emulsion of duplicating film is more unstable than conventional film because of latensification. This is because it has been preexposed by the manufacturer to the point of solarization, or image reversal. For this reason, large quantities should not be stockpiled.

FILM/SCREEN IMAGE RECEPTORS

Most of the images recorded during conventional analog radiography are obtained with film/screen combination image receptors. Thomas Edison developed intensifying screens in 1896, and Michael Pupin first used a film/screen combination in radiography later that same year. The X-rays exiting the patient energize the phosphor crystals, and the result is the emission of light called luminescence. Luminescence can occur by one of two different processes, fluorescence or phosphorescence.

1. **Fluorescence** is the light of certain crystals emitted within 10^{-8} s after the crystals are exposed to radiation. This means that light is emitted promptly. This is the type of luminescence that is desired for use in intensifying screens.
2. **Phosphorescence** is the light of certain crystals emitted sometime after 10^{-8} s after the crystals' exposure to radiation, resulting in a delayed emission of light. This delayed emission of light is often called *afterglow* or *lag*. This is not desired for use in intensifying screens because the delayed emission of light fogs the film in the cassette before the radiographer can get it to the processor or daylight system. This type of luminescence is desired for the output phosphor of fluoroscopic image intensifiers and cathode-ray tube displays such as television and computer monitor screens.

PROCEDURE: VIEWBOX TESTING

1. Inspect the acrylic plastic (Plexiglas) front of the viewbox for discoloration, dust, and other artifacts. Clean or replace the acrylic plastic if necessary.

2. Unplug the viewbox and remove the acrylic plastic front with the screwdriver. Inspect the fluorescent light bulb for proper wattage, cleanliness, and discoloration; clean or replace if necessary. When finished, replace the acrylic plastic front and screws.

3. Determine the brightness level. This procedure requires a basic understanding of the concepts of **photometry**, which is the study and measurement of light. To measure the brightness level of viewbox illuminators, use a photographic light meter (photometer) (see Fig. 4.7), which ideally can measure both **luminance** and illuminance. The American College of Radiology recommends measuring the luminance in **nit**. The aperture of the photometer should be 9 inches away from the viewbox front when brightness is measured. This can vary slightly, depending on the manufacturer of the photometer (follow the manufacturer's instructions for your particular model). Make the first reading in the center viewbox. Conventional viewbox luminance should be at least 1500 nit, with 1700 nit being standard. Viewboxes used for viewing mammograms should have a luminance of about 3500 nit. If illuminance is used to measure brightness, the minimum illuminance should be 5000 lux or 500 **foot-candles** (ft-cd). The greater the brightness level of the viewbox, the greater the contrast observed in the viewed diagnostic image.

4. Determine viewbox uniformity. Once it has been determined that the viewbox has sufficient luminance (brightness level), then the uniformity of the brightness for each viewbox panel, each bank of viewboxes, and all viewbox banks within the entire radiology department must be determined. For an individual viewbox or a single-viewing panel (usually 14 inches × 17 inches) within a bank, mentally divide the viewing panel into quadrants. Hold the photometer 9 inches away (or per manufacturer's instructions) from the center of each quadrant and record the luminance. Compare this value with the center reading obtained in step 3. These readings should not deviate by more than ±10% of each other. To determine the uniformity of a single bank of viewboxes, hold a photometer 9 inches away from the center of each individual viewbox within the bank, record the readings, and compare with each other. These readings should not vary by more than ±15% of each other. The uniformity of each bank of viewboxes found in the entire radiology department also should be determined. This can be accomplished by taking the average of the center readings from each bank of viewboxes in the radiology department and comparing them with each other. These values should be within ±20% of each other. If a photometer is unavailable, a photographic light meter or a 35-mm camera with a built-in light meter can be substituted (this cannot be accepted during Mammography Quality Standards Act inspections). A photometer can measure only illumination and not luminance. If the camera uses an exposure value (EV) scale to measure light intensity, set the film speed indicator to ASA 100. Place the camera lens in contact with the center of the viewbox front, look into the viewfinder, and record the reading. Repeat this procedure for each quadrant to verify viewbox uniformity. An EV of 13 indicates 500 ft-cd of illumination (the minimum acceptable value for a standard viewbox). An EV of 14 indicates twice as much light (or 1000 ft-cd), and an EV of 12 is one-half as much (250 ft-cd). If the light intensity is doubled, the maximum optical density that can be viewed is also doubled. For example, if 500 ft-cd can illuminate a maximum optical density of 2.5 on the image, then 1000 ft-cd can illuminate a maximum optical density of 2.8. Some cameras have a light meter that does not use an EV scale but instead, indicates the shutter speed to use when taking the photograph and looking into the viewfinder. In this case, set the film speed indicator to ASA 64 and the shutter to f8. The denominator of the shutter speed indicated is the light intensity in foot-candles. For example, if the indicated shutter speed is 1/400 s, the light intensity is 400 ft-cd.

5. Measure the color temperature. The quality or spectrum of light that is emitted from a light source can be defined by its color temperature. This is the temperature at which a black body radiator emits light of a comparable color. A surface that absorbs all of the radiant energy that is incident on it would appear black and is called a *black body*. The color temperature is measured in kelvin (K) and measured with a color temperature meter (available from scientific supply companies). Standard viewboxes should have color temperatures ranging from 5400–10,000 K. Most viewbox manufacturers prefer a rating of 6250 K.

6. Measure the ambient light conditions. The ambient light is the light level of the viewing room and the radiologist's viewing area separate from the viewbox. This light must be less than that of the viewbox or a decrease in contrast level is observed in the image. To survey this level, turn the illuminators off and place the meter or camera 1 foot away from the viewbox to record the reading. The maximum ambient room light should be 30 ft-cd (320 lux) or 8 EV. For mammographic viewing areas, the maximum ambient light should be 4.5 ft-cd (50 lux) or less (equivalent to a moonlit night). Ambient light can vary considerably in various areas of a hospital. Operating rooms typically have a range of 300–400 lux, emergency department rooms about 150–300 lux, and staff offices about 50–180 lux.

Most units have an exposure level switch to regulate the quality of the copy image. Film duplicators should faithfully copy optical densities of up to 2.5 from the original image. To verify this, make a copy of a sensitometer film, use a densitometer to measure each step, and compare with the original image. They should be the same or within an optical density of 0.02 and should be evaluated on a weekly basis. To check the contact between the copy film and the original during duplication, use a radiograph of a wire mesh screen (used to evaluate film/screen contact) and make a copy. The copy should demonstrate the same sharpness level of the mesh pattern throughout the image. This should be performed monthly.

Images obtained with a multiformat camera or a laser camera can be particularly difficult to duplicate because of its single emulsion. An image from a Society of Motion Picture and Television Engineers test pattern or AAPM TG 18-QC test pattern (see Chapter 8) should be produced from the camera and then duplicated with the copier. Optical density readings from the same areas of the copy and the original should be taken with a densitometer and compared. Again, they should be the same or within a value of 0.02.

The fluorescent light from the crystals in the intensifying screen is used to expose the film (rather than for X-ray interaction) and creates 95%–98% of the optical density. This results in lower patient exposure (compared with a nonscreen exposure) because only a relatively small number of X-rays are necessary for the screens to emit a relatively large quantity of light. Proper application of intensifying screens is necessary to create adequate images. Because considerable variation can occur with the use of screens, proper quality control protocols should be in place. Several intensifying screen variables are discussed.

Intensifying Screen Speed

Intensifying screen speed refers to the amount of light emitted by the screen for a given amount of X-ray exposure. A screen that is designated as fast creates an increased amount of light compared with a screen designated as slow when both are exposed to identical kVp and mAs factors. Screen speed can be measured by intensification factor, relative name, or speed value.

Intensification Factor

The exposure required to create a certain optical density without a screen (direct exposure) is divided by the exposure required with a screen to create the same optical density, which determines the intensification factor.

$$\text{Intensifaction factor} = \frac{\text{Exposure without screens}}{\text{Exposure with screens}}$$

For example, if 100 mAs create an optical density of 1.0 on a direct exposure film and 5 mAs create the same optical density value with a film/screen combination, then that screen has an intensification factor of 20. The larger this value, the faster the speed of the screen.

Relative Speed Value

Relative speed is the most common method of designating screen speed and is used for all screens with rare earth phosphors. A mathematic number that is a multiple of 100 is used, with a larger number designating a faster speed. When one speed is changed to another, a change in mAs is required to maintain optical density. This can be calculated with the following equation:

$$\text{New mAs} = \frac{\text{old mAs} \times \text{old relative speed value}}{\text{New relative speed value}}$$

For example, if 10 mAs were used with a 100-speed screen, then 5 mAs would be used with a 200-speed screen.

Name of Screen

Older, non–rare earth screens use specific names such as *fast* or *slow* to designate screen speed. A listing of these older names, along with their relative speed values, is presented in Table 4.1.

TABLE 4.1 Older Names for Screen Speed

Name of Screen	Relative Speed Value
Ultrahigh or hi-plus	300
High or fast	200
Medium, par, or standard	100
Detail, slow, or high resolution	50
Ultradetail	25

Factors Affecting Screen Speed

Type of phosphor material. Many different phosphor materials have been used in screens since 1896. They are generally divided into two categories, rare earth and non–rare earth phosphors. The non–rare earth phosphors are the original type of screen material and emit light in the blue-violet portion of the color spectrum. Examples include calcium tungstate, barium strontium sulfite, and barium fluorochloride. The rare earth phosphors were developed in the early 1970s and are currently the most common type of intensifying screen material. The name *rare earth* is used because these materials have atomic numbers ranging from 57 through 71 and are known as the *lanthanide,* or *rare earth,* series from the periodic table of elements. These materials possess a greater detective quantum efficiency (the ability to interact with X-rays) and a greater conversion efficiency (the ability of screens to convert X-ray energy into light energy). The older calcium tungstate screens have a conversion efficiency of 4%–5%, whereas the newer rare earth screens have values ranging from 15% to 25%. Thus the rare earth phosphors are faster than the non–rare earth phosphors. Table 4.2 presents the more common rare earth phosphors and the color of light emitted.

The rare earth phosphors are mixed with materials called *activators* (the elements terbium, niobium, or thulium) that help determine the intensity and color of the emitted light.

Thickness of phosphor layer. A thicker layer of phosphor material causes the screen to emit more light because the extra material can absorb more X-rays. This decreases the resolution of the resulting image because of increased light diffraction or diffusion (Fig. 4.9). Rare earth screens generally demonstrate better resolution than non–rare earth screens because they have greater conversion efficiencies and therefore do not have to be placed in as thick a layer. The average range of phosphor thickness is from 150 to 300 µm.

TABLE 4.2 Emission Color of Common Rare Earth Phosphors

Name of Screen	Relative Speed Value
Gadolinium oxysulfide	Green
Lanthanum oxysulfide	Green
Yttrium oxysulfide	Blue-green
Yttrium tantalate	Blue-green
Lanthanum oxybromide	Blue
Lutetium tantalate	Blue

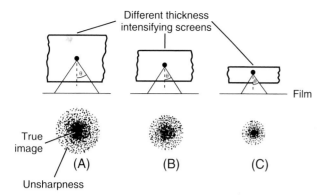

Fig. 4.9 Effect of screen active layer on light diffusion and image sharpness.

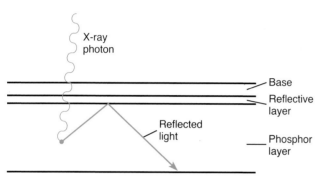

Fig. 4.10 Reflected light within phosphor layer.

TABLE 4.3 K-Shell Binding Energies for Some Phosphor Materials

Element	Atomic Number	K-Shell Binding Energy (keV)
Yttrium	39	17.5
Barium	56	37.4
Lanthanum	57	38.9
Gadolinium	64	50.2
Tungsten	74	69.5

keV, Kiloelectron volts.

Kilovolt (peak) selection. The phosphor material in a screen must interact with the X-ray photon for luminescence to occur. The greatest absorption of X-rays occurs when the X-ray photon energy and the binding energy of the K-shell electron are almost the same. This is called the *K-edge effect.* Because the kVp setting on the control panel regulates the X-ray photon energy and the phosphor material used controls the K-shell binding energy, care must be taken to match the kVp used in technique selection. For example, a dedicated mammography cassette usually has a lower K-edge value (15–20 kiloelectron volts [keV]) because lower kVp techniques are used. If one of these cassettes is used at 100 kVp instead, it functions much more slowly than if used at its proper kVp. Table 4.3 indicates the K-shell binding energies for different phosphor materials.

Quality Control Testing of Screen Speed

Quality control testing of screen speed should occur on acceptance and then yearly. First, one should evaluate whether similar cassettes marked with the same relative speed are the same using the following procedure.

Size of phosphor crystals. Using larger phosphor crystals increases the speed of the screen by allowing more absorption of incident X-rays but decreases image resolution because of increased light diffusion. Crystals that are needle-shaped help minimize this effect.

Reflective layer. When X-rays interact with the phosphor material of a screen, light is emitted isotopically (in all directions). Because the film is only on one side of the screen, light traveling away from the film is normally lost to the imaging process. Faster speed screens add a layer of titanium dioxide to reflect light back toward the film. This increases the speed but decreases the resolution because of the angle of the reflected light.

Light-absorbing dyes. Slower speed screens have light-absorbing dyes added to the phosphor layer to control reflected light (Fig. 4.10). This dye decreases speed but increases image resolution.

Ambient temperature. When the ambient temperature of an intensifying screen increases significantly above room temperature (above 85°F [30°C]), the screen may function slower than usual. The higher temperature gives the phosphor crystal more kinetic energy. This additional energy does not cause more light to be emitted but rather, increases the energy (and therefore the color) of the light emitted. Because the film may not be sensitive to this new color, the resulting radiograph appears underexposed.

PROCEDURE: SPEED UNIFORMITY

1. Make an exposure of a step wedge or homogenous phantom onto an image receptor so that the center of the image has an optical density of about 1.5.
2. Expose each image receptor to the same technical factors.
3. Process each radiograph and take optical density readings of the same center area in each. If the image receptors are all the same relative speed, the optical density readings should not vary by more than a value of ±0.05.

Cassettes also should be evaluated to ensure that the screen speed is uniform throughout the entire surface. Intensifying screens should be uniform in speed throughout the entire surface of the screen itself. In other words, the speed in the center should be the same as the speed at the outer edges or anywhere else on the screen. During manufacturing processes, inconsistencies may occur in which the phosphor layer is applied more thickly at one portion of the screen than at another. In addition, during screen cleaning, excessive rubbing may remove more of the phosphor layer at one point than at another. Therefore a test of screen uniformity should be performed on acceptance and then yearly.

1. Make an exposure of a homogenous phantom onto an image receptor that yields an optical density of approximately 1.5.
2. Process the radiograph and take optical density readings in the center and in each of the four quadrants of the image. These values should not vary by an optical density value of more than ±0.05. Any film/screen image receptors that exceed this limit should be removed from service.

Spectral Matching

Previously in this chapter, it is mentioned that various films are sensitive to specific colors of light and therefore require special-colored safelights to illuminate the darkroom. Because intensifying screen phosphors emit blue, blue-green, or green light, the film used inside the cassette should be sensitive to the corresponding color. This is known as spectral matching. Any blue-violet-emitting screen phosphor should be used with monochromatic blue-violet film, and green-emitting phosphors must be used with orthochromatic film. The non–rare earth screen phosphors tend to emit a broadband of light (Fig. 4.11), whereas rare earth phosphors emit specific colors of light, also known as *line emission* (Fig. 4.12).

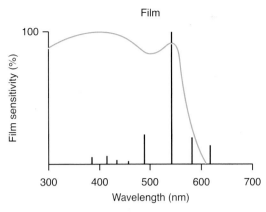

Fig. 4.12 Line spectrum from rare earth screen phosphor.

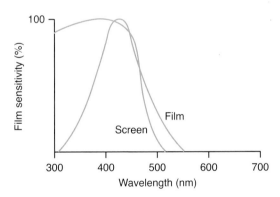

Fig. 4.11 Broadband spectrum from non–rare earth phosphor.

Film/Screen Contact

A close contact between the screen and film must be maintained to guarantee image sharpness. If poor contact exists, localized blurring of the radiographic image will occur (Fig. 4.18). Therefore cassettes should be tested regularly for poor film/screen contact using the wire mesh test. When placed on top of a cassette and exposed, the wire mesh pattern will be created on the resulting film. Areas of localized blurring will indicate bad contact (Fig. 4.13).

- Expose the wire mesh test tool that is placed on the cassette front, using exposure factors of 50 kVp and 5 mAs tabletop.
- Process the film and evaluate the resulting image. Areas of poor contact appear as localized blurring (see Fig. 4.14). Bent or warped cassettes, warped screens, and foreign objects inside the cassette are the most common causes of poor film/screen contact.

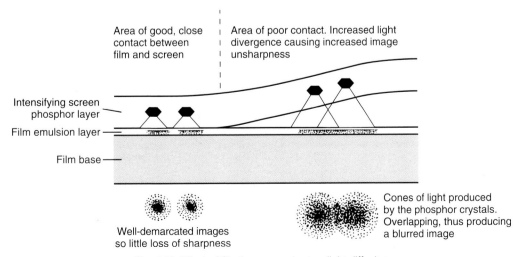

Fig. 4.13 Effect of film/screen contact on light diffusion.

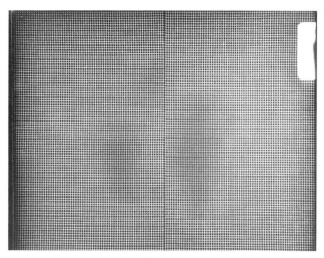

Fig. 4.14 Wire mesh image.

Screen Condition

Cassettes containing intensifying screens must function as designed to create optimum radiographic images. Errors to avoid include improper film position within the cassette, poor film/screen contact, and uneven closure of the cassette. Intensifying screens also must be free of dirt, stains, and defects to properly image anatomic structures. A regular schedule (at least every 6 months) of screen cleaning with an antistatic solution should be standard department policy because artifacts can mimic certain pathologic conditions. The end of the day is usually the best time to clean cassettes because of decreased demand for their use. A UV lamp can be used in the darkroom to examine the surface condition of the screens (Fig. 4.15). Be sure to remove the film from the cassette before turning on the UV lamp. The following is an accepted procedure for cleaning intensifying screens.

After a film has been exposed to radiation, the image it contains is still invisible to the human eye and is called a **latent image**. For the film to be converted to a visible image, or **manifest image**, the silver contained in the film must be changed from an ionized state (Ag^+) to a neutral, or reduced, state (Ag^0), in which the silver turns black. This conversion requires the film to be processed by various solutions that change the latent image to a visible one, and also preserves the image for permanent storage.

Automatic Film Processing

Automatic processing requires an electromechanical device called an *automatic film processor*. This processor transports the film from one solution to the next without any manual labor except for placing the film into the device. Automatic processing shortens the overall processing time, increases

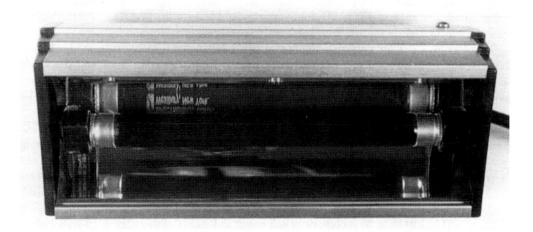

Fig. 4.15 Ultraviolet lamp for inspecting intensifying screens. (Courtesy Nuclear Associates, Carle Place, New York.)

the number of films that can be processed during a given period, and ensures less variability of overall film quality than manually processed films because processing time, solution temperature, and chemical replenishment are controlled automatically. The disadvantages of automatic processing include greater capital and maintenance costs, increased chemical fog resulting from greater processing temperatures, and transport problems that can damage or destroy images during processing. In a diagnostic imaging department that has not converted to digital imaging, the advantages of automatic processing versus manual processing far outweigh the disadvantages, and automatic film processing is virtually exclusive.

PROCESSING CHEMICALS

Developer

As mentioned previously, the developer is the most important processing solution; it converts the latent image to a manifest image. This process is accomplished by the developer solution, which carries out an oxidation/reduction reaction, or *redox*. When a chemical is oxidized (broken down), it releases electrons. These electrons are then available to convert another compound into a more simplified, or reduced, state (hence the term *oxidation/reduction reaction*). During film processing, the developer solution ingredients are oxidized and the silver halide crystals are reduced to black metallic silver. This chemical reaction can be summarized by the following equations that occur at different times during oxidation reduction.

The first occurs during exposure to radiation:

$$Ag^{++Br^{-}+radiation} \rightarrow Ag^{o} + Br^{-+Ag}$$

(five atoms, latent image)

The second occurs during immersion in developer:

$Ag^{++Developer} + Ag^{o}$ (five atoms, latent image) $\rightarrow$
Ag^{o} (10^{8} atoms, visible image) + oxidized developer

Developer Components

Developer is composed of developing or reducing agents, preservatives, accelerators or activators, restrainers, regulators, antifoggants or starters, hardeners, solvents, and sequestering agents. All these components act on the film.

Developing or Reducing Agents

Developing or reducing agents carry out the oxidation/reduction reaction that converts the latent image to a manifest image. Two different reducing agents are used in standard developer solutions: phenidone and hydroquinone.

Phenidone. Phenidone (elon or metol in manual developing) is fast acting and produces image optical densities of as much as 1.2. It is responsible for the minimum diameter

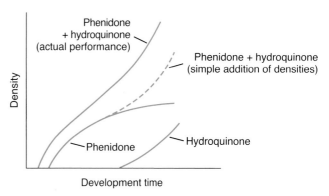

Fig. 4.16 Graph demonstrating the superadditivity effect of phenidone and hydroquinone.

(D_{min}) and speed indicators used during sensitometric testing (described later in this chapter).

Hydroquinone. Because hydroquinone acts more slowly than phenidone, the development process is completed and so image optical densities greater than 1.2 are visualized. Hydroquinone is responsible for the maximum diameter (D_{max}) and for contrast indicators used in sensitometric testing. These indicators are the first variables to show an indication of developer failure because hydroquinone is the processing chemical most sensitive to changes in temperature, concentration, pH, and exposure to light and heavy metals. Hydroquinone levels should be maintained in the range 20–25 g/L.

The overall optical density is created by the synergistic action of the two reducing agents. *Synergism* means that the action of the two agents working together is greater than the sum of each agent working independently. Synergism is also known as *superadditivity* (Fig. 4.16).

Preservative. The preservative, or antioxidant, protects the hydroquinone from both aerial oxidation (chemical reaction with air) and internal oxidation (chemical reaction with other developer ingredients). If the hydroquinone is oxidized, there is a decrease in the D_{max} and contrast indicators during a sensitometric test, along with a loss of the shoulder on the H and D curve. Oxidized developer causes the developer solution to turn from a clear brown liquid to one that is dark and muddy. If strongly oxidized, the solution also has the odor of ammonia because this is a byproduct of the oxidation chemical reaction. Most developer replenishment tanks have a floating lid inside the tank in addition to the main lid on the outside to minimize contact with the outside air. The chemicals sodium sulfite, potassium sulfite, and cycon can be used as developer solution preservatives.

Accelerator, activator, or buffering agent. The accelerator, activator, or buffering agent has two functions: to soften and swell the emulsion so that reducing agents can work on all the emulsion, and to provide an alkaline medium for the reducing agents. The developing agents must exist in an alkaline medium to have the free electrons available to reduce the silver to Ag^{o}.

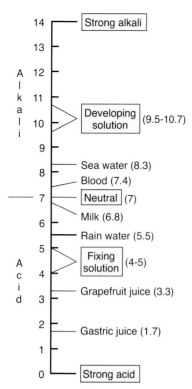

Fig. 4.17 Potential hydrogen (pH) scale.

An indicator known as *potential hydrogen,* or *pH,* is used to measure the alkalinity of a solution, and it refers to the exponential (p) value of hydrogen ions (H⁺) available for a reaction. Those chemicals with high hydrogen potential (H⁺) are called *acids;* those with a high alkaline or hydroxide potential (OH⁻)—and therefore a low hydrogen potential—are called *bases.* The pH scale ranges from 0–7 (acids) and from 7–14 (bases) (Fig. 4.17). This scale is based on the concentration of positively charged hydrogen ions (H⁺), measured in moles per liter. For example, a pH of 4 means that a particular solution contains one-ten-thousandth (10^{-4}) of a mole of hydrogen ions per liter. For this value to be converted to pH, the negative exponent (−4) is changed to a positive number (4). A solution with an H⁺ concentration of one-ten-millionth (10^{-7}) moles per liter has a pH of 7, and so on. Because the pH scale is logarithmic in nature, a change of one whole number on the pH scale can represent a 10-fold change from the previous concentration. A pH of 1 denotes 10 times more H⁺ ions than a pH of 2, a pH of 3 has 10 times fewer H⁺ ions than a pH of 2, and so on. Pure water is neutral and has a pH of 7. Fixer is an acidic solution; therefore care must be taken not to add it to developer solutions because only 0.1% contamination deteriorates the developer activity enough to compromise image quality. Chemicals that can be used as accelerators include sodium carbonate, sodium hydroxide, potassium carbonate, and potassium hydroxide.

Restrainer, regulator, antifoggant, or starter. The restrainer (regulator, antifoggant, or starter) holds back, or restrains, the action of the developing agents, and so they reduce only the silver halide crystals exposed to radiation. The chemical used in most brands of developer is potassium

bromide in the form of K⁺ Br⁻, which is similar chemically to Ag⁺ Br⁻. If the reducing agents become too active, they attack the potassium bromide instead of the silver halide. Potassium iodide can also be used as the restrainer. Overdiluting or underreplenishing can reduce the levels of restrainer and increase the speed indicator during a sensitometric test.

Hardener. When a film enters the warm developer solution, the gelatin emulsion begins to soften and swell, which causes the film to stick to the rollers of an automatic film processor. Therefore developer manufacturers add a weak hardener (a stronger one is present in fixer solutions) to control emulsion swelling and stickiness. If the amount of hardener is depleted because of underreplenishment, wet films, transport problems, and films that have not been cleared of undeveloped silver halide may result. The chemical agent used as a hardener is glutaraldehyde.

Solvent. The previously mentioned ingredients are mixed with a solvent to form developer solution. The most common and readily available solvent is water. The water should be drinkable and have the following characteristics: filtration to particles less than 40 μm, dissolved solids less than 250 ppm, a pH of 6.5–8.5, a hardness of 40–150 ppm, heavy metals less than 0.1 ppm, chloride less than 25 ppm, and sulfate less than 200 ppm.

Sequestering agent. Much of the developer used in hospital darkrooms is shipped in concentrated form and then mixed with tap water at the clinical site. Because impurities (e.g., calcium ions, metals such as iron and copper) can be found in tap water, many manufacturers add a sequestering agent called *ethylenediamine tetraacetic acid* (*EDTA*) or *edetate* to prevent impurities from interfering with the developer chemicals. EDTA is an oily substance that causes calcium and other mineral contaminants to stick together and dissipate to the bottom of processing tanks. EDTA also helps form stable chemical complexes with metallic ions.

Developer Activity

How well a developer functions is called *developer activity,* and it is governed by the following five factors: solution temperature, immersion time, solution concentration, type of chemicals used, and solution pH.

Solution temperature. The greater the solution temperature (Fig. 4.18), the more active the developing agents become, especially hydroquinone. A warmer solution temperature will increase the optical density of the resulting image and vice versa. If the temperature decreases to less than 60°F (15.5°C), the hydroquinone stops working, which causes the resulting images to decrease in optical density and contrast. At temperatures greater than 75°F (24°C), the developing agents become increasingly active, which increases the optical density of subsequent images. The optimum temperature range for developer solution is 68–72°F (20–22.2°C). However, automatic processing solutions may range from 85–105°F (29.4–40.5°C) to process images more rapidly.

Immersion time. The greater the length of time in the solution, or immersion time (Fig. 4.19), the greater the optical densities recorded on the processed image and vice versa.

85 °F　　　　　　　　90 °F

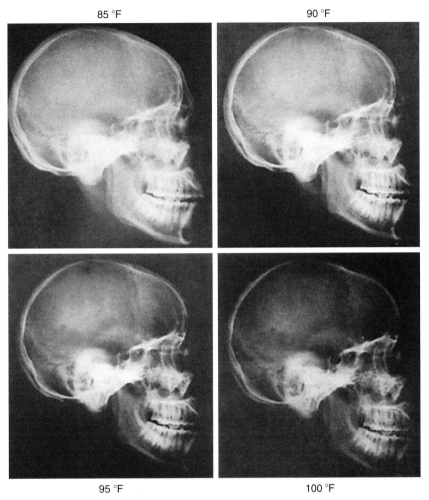

95 °F　　　　　　　　100 °F

Fig. 4.18 Radiographs showing the effect of solution temperature on optical density and contrast.

The reason for this is that the developing agents are in contact with the silver ions for a longer period and can reduce more silver ions to metallic silver.

Solution concentration. Solution concentration refers to the percentage of water versus other chemicals in the solution and is measured by specific gravity (the density of a liquid compared with water). An instrument called a *hydrometer* measures specific gravity, which ranges from 1.07 to 1.10 in typical developer solutions. The specific gravity should not vary by 14 ± 0.004 from the manufacturer's specifications.

Type of chemicals used. Developer solutions that contain elon or metol behave differently from those that contain phenidone. The DuPont Cronex HSD system uses an acid developer solution to process the film, and therefore it behaves quite differently from conventional developer solutions.

Solution pH. The developer solution should maintain a pH between 10 and 11.5 and should not vary by more than ±0.1 from the manufacturer's specifications. Excessive pH increases the optical density of a processed image or causes increased oxidation, whereas a pH value that is too low decreases the optical density of any resulting image.

Over time, the developer becomes exhausted and requires replenishment. Reasons for this replenishment include the following:

- Significant quantities of developer are consumed during the development process.
- The liberation of bromide and hydrogen bromide acid into the developer during development can lower the pH and cause a decrease in activity. These bromide levels should be maintained in the range 4–8 g/L to maintain proper pH.
- Aerial and internal oxidation begins as soon as the solution is mixed and developing agents are consumed.
- A certain volume of developer solution is removed by the film's emulsion each time a film is fed into the processor. The squeegee action of the crossover rack helps minimize this effect.

Developer Mixing Procedure

Developer solution is usually available in two forms: as a premix or as a concentrate.

Premix or ready-mix. As the name implies, a premix or ready-mix solution has all the ingredients combined with the solvent so that no mixing is required at the clinical site. The solutions are usually delivered in 5-gallon or 10-gallon

2 min   68 °F   4 min

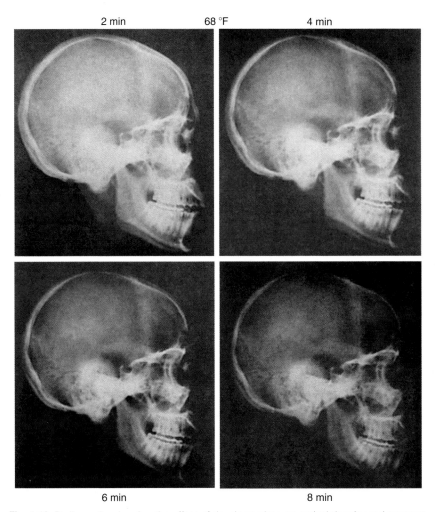

6 min   8 min

Fig. 4.19 Radiographs showing the effect of developer time on optical density and contrast.

containers and are poured directly into the replenishment tanks. The disadvantages of this method include a relatively short shelf life (from 2 weeks to 3 months) and greater cost (about 40% more than the concentrate). Therefore large quantities should not be stockpiled, and frequent deliveries must be made.

Concentrate. The main ingredients of the solution may also be shipped to the clinical site in a concentrated form and are mixed with water at the clinical site. This form is less convenient, but the cost is reduced significantly. The concentrate kit usually comes in three parts. Part 1 contains the hydroquinone, preservative, and accelerator, and has a pH between 11 and 12. Part 2 contains the phenidone and restrainer and has a pH of 3. Part 3 contains the hardener and has a pH of 3.

When solution from the concentrate is mixed, the proper amount of water should be present in the tank, and then each solution is added in the proper order. Large quantities of chemicals should be mixed electrically with a commercially available system. These systems use a propeller type of variable-speed mixer. The speed must be regulated because excessive speed introduces unwanted air into the chemicals, which can oxidize the developer. These systems are not practical for facilities that use only a small volume of developer each week.

Fresh chemistry should last 2 weeks and then be discarded. Concentrate lasts 1 year when stored at room temperature and away from direct sunlight. Excessive agitation (shaking of the bottles) during mixture and storage should be avoided because this may cause a decomposition of the chemicals, resulting in reduced activity of the solution.

Fixer

Fixer solutions remove all the unexposed and undeveloped silver halide crystals from the film. As soon as this happens, the film is said to be cleared. They are also responsible for halting the development process and hardening the emulsion for permanent storage.

Fixer Ingredients

Fixers are composed of the following six components: fixing agent, preservative, hardener or tanning agent, acidifier, sequestering agent, and solvent.

Fixing agent, clearing agent, or hypo. The fixing agent (clearing agent or hypo) removes the unexposed and undeveloped silver halide crystals from the film. The chemical ammonium thiosulfate is used in most modern fixing solutions (sodium thiosulfate has been used in manual solutions).

Hypo is a common name for thiosulfate compounds. It picks up unexposed silver atoms from the silver halide crystal to form ammonium thio-silver-sulfate. The fixing process is summarized by the following equation:

$$2AgX + Na_2S_2O_3 \rightarrow Ag_2S_2O_3 + 2NaX$$

where X designates the halide used in the film emulsion (either bromide or iodide).

The action of this agent is controlled by dilution, replenishment, and the use of a recirculating electrolytic silver recovery unit.

The effectiveness of the fixing agent is evaluated by a clearing time test.

PROCEDURE: CLEARING TIME TEST

1. Take a strip of undeveloped green film and dip it into the fixer solution. Use a stopwatch to measure the clearing time.
2. Film should clear in 10 seconds at room temperature and in less than 7 seconds at 90°F (32°C). If it does not, the fixing agents are not working properly and the problem may be the result of improper mixing (usually too much water), a pH that is too high, or expired solution. To correct this problem, dispose of the fixer, clean out the replenishment tank, and refill it with fresh solution. It is recommended that the clearing time test be performed again on the new solution to be sure that it is functioning according to accepted levels.

Preservative. The chemical sodium sulfite dissolves the silver out of the ammonium thio-silver-sulfate, and it is returned or recycled back to ammonium thiosulfate. In this way, sulfite is available to clear more of the undeveloped silver from the film. It can be depleted by excess developer carryin, underreplenishment, and the use of recirculating electrolytic silver recovery units, which deplete sodium sulfite. The concentration of this chemical should be maintained in a range 15–50 g/L.

Hardener or tanning agent. For the film to be stored permanently, the emulsion must be hardened to keep the image from fading or being scratched during handling. This process is called *tanning.* Potassium alum, chrome alum, and aluminum chloride are the more common chemicals used as fixer hardeners. When these materials combine with the gelatin proteins to form complex molecules, hardened emulsion results. These agents also help reduce water absorption during washing, and drying time is reduced.

Acidifier, activator, or buffer. The acidifier, activator, or buffer has two functions: neutralizing any developer remaining in the emulsion and providing an acid medium for the fixing agent. Just as the developing agents need an alkaline medium in which to function, the fixing agent can dissolve undeveloped silver only in an acidic solution. The acid allows the fixing agent to diffuse into the emulsion, which allows the necessary contact with the undeveloped silver ions to be made. Fixer pH should be maintained at a level between 4 and 4.5 and should not vary more than ±0.1 from the

manufacturer's specifications. Chemicals that help maintain pH are commonly known as *buffers.* Both acetic acid and sulfuric acid can be used as the acidifier.

Sequestering agent. Sequestering agents help prevent the development of aluminum hydroxide, which forms as the developer solution is carried into the fixer. Because aluminum hydroxide is an alkaline compound, its formation results in an increase in fixer pH. Carboxylic acids, boric acids, or borate salts may be used as sequestering agents in fixer solutions.

Solvent. Water is used as the solvent in which to suspend the other chemicals. The same standards listed for the developer solvent—water—also apply to the fixer. The concentration of fixer is measured by specific gravity and may range from 1.077–1.11. The specific gravity should not vary by more than ±0.004 from the manufacturer's specifications.

Fixer Mixing Procedure

The fixer solution may be purchased in either ready-mixed or concentrated form. The ready-mix may cost as much as 20% more but has the same convenience as ready-mixed developer. The concentrate must be mixed with water and usually comes in two parts. Part 1 contains the ammonium thiosulfate, preservative, and acidifier; part 2 contains the hardener in a strong acidic solution.

As with developer, one starts with water in the tank and mixes large quantities with a commercial mixing unit. It is recommended that the fixer be mixed before the developer because inadvertent splashing of fixer could contaminate the developer.

Washing

Washing is important for the archival quality of the film because it removes the fixer from the film emulsion before drying. If hyporetention is allowed to take place, the reaction of the thiosulfate with the silver in the emulsion produces Ag_2S, or silver sulfide, which can stain the image from pale yellow to dark brown. By law, films must be archived 5 years; groups such as the military require an archival time of 40 years after death, separation, or retirement. Commercial test kits are available to measure the amount of hyporetention (Fig. 4.20). One type of test kit involves the use of a specialized test strip that is placed in contact with a processed film after a drop of solution is applied to its surface, and the test strip changes color. An accompanying color guide then allows the matching of the color on the strip to the appropriate value on the guide, which then indicates the amount of hyporetention.

Another type of hyporetention test kit involves placing a drop of hypo test solution on a film and then judging the color of the resulting stain. The hypo test solution is a mixture of silver nitrate, acetic acid, and water, and it must remain in a dark container because it is light sensitive. When a drop of this solution is applied to a processed film, it causes a chemical reaction with any fixer that still remains. The result is a brown stain. The more fixer that remains on the film, the darker this stain becomes. A test strip containing different colored stains is supplied with the solution test kit and is then

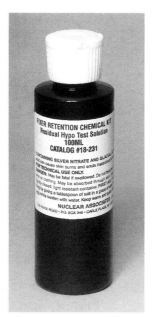

Fig. 4.20 Hyporetention kit for evaluating residual fixer in processed films. (Courtesy Nuclear Associates, Carle Place, New York.)

used to indicate the exact level of hyporetention. The solution is applied to a processed film in the darkroom and is allowed to stand for 2 min. After 2 min, the excess solution is blotted (not wiped) and the film is taken to the lightroom area for comparison with the test strip. The American National Standards Institute (ANSI) suggests the amount of hyporetention not exceed 2 $\mu g/cm^2$ for radiographic film images and 5 $\mu g/cm^2$ for mammographic film images. These ANSI tests should be performed at least semiannually (every 6 months) for radiographic images (preferably every 3 months) and must be performed quarterly (every 3 months) for mammographic images. If the level of hyporetention exceeds these values, determine whether the wash tank has the correct amount of water present (there should be a level mark on the side of the tank). If the amount of water is sufficient, then check the water flow rate to ensure that it is set to the processor manufacturer's standard.

The water used in washing should have the following characteristics: hardness of 40–150 ppm, pH of 6.5–8.5, dissolved solids less than 250 ppm, and a specific gravity of 1. Washing time should be at least 50%–100% of the developer time, and the temperature should be about 5°F (3°C) less than the developer temperature to help trigger the heater thermostat in the automatic processor. The water flow rate should be at a rate of 1–3 gal/min for removal of hyporetention, proper agitation, and prevention of algae and bioslime. If this is a problem, a few milliliters of laundry bleach (5% sodium hypochlorite) may be added to the wash tank at shutdown.

Chemical Safety

Because OSHA considers the darkroom a scientific laboratory, it has several safety requirements in place, including the implementation of hazard communication standards (HCS) and the use of personal protective equipment (PPE).

1. HCS (also known as right to know or RTK standards) were established by OSHA to ensure that both employers and employees have knowledge of all workplace chemical hazards, in addition to the appropriate protection procedures from these hazards. These standards were updated in 2012 and are now called HazCom 2012. In 2012, OSHA began aligning the HCS with the Globally Harmonized System of Classification and Labeling of Chemicals (GHS). The updated HCS enables companies and organizations to streamline their safety data sheets (SDS) and labels to comply with one system, the GHS. As of June 1, 2016, all companies must comply with the GHS. One important tool to help diagnostic imaging departments comply with these standards is the Safety Data Sheet (SDS) (formerly known as material safety data sheets or MSDS), which should be available for viewing by employees for all chemical compounds (i.e., processing solutions) used by employees (Fig. 4.21). These forms must be kept on file for each hazardous chemical compound and must be readily accessible to all employees. They also must contain the following items:
    1. Identification
    2. Hazard(s) identification
    3. Composition/information on ingredients
    4. First-aid measures
    5. Firefighting measures
    6. Accidental release measures
    7. Handling and storage
    8. Exposure controls/personal protection
    9. Physical and chemical properties
    10. Stability and reactivity
    11. Toxicologic information
    12. Ecological information
    13. Disposal considerations
    14. Transport information
    15. Regulatory information
    16. Other information (such as the date of preparation or last revision)

Sections 12–15 are needed to align with international requirements of the GHS system but fall outside the jurisdiction of OSHA in the United States.

Each SDS uses a rating scale to indicate the hazard level of various chemicals. A level 1 rating indicates a slight hazard, level 2 is a moderate hazard, level 3 is a serious hazard, and level 4 is a severe hazard. The SDS also must indicate the category of the hazard. OSHA categorizes hazardous chemicals as being either a physical hazard or a health hazard.

Chemicals that are a physical hazard are based on the physical or chemical properties of the product—such as flammability, reactivity, or corrosivity to metals. Examples include compressed gases (such as oxygen), oxidizers (such as chlorine bleach), combustible liquids (such as gasoline or kerosene), and flammable materials (such as cleaning solvents). The complete list of physical hazards is as follows:

Flammable gases
Flammable aerosols
Oxidizing gases
Gases under pressure

IDENTITY *(As Used on Label and List)*	Note: Blank spaces are not permitted. If any item is not applicable, or no information is available, the space must be marked to indicate that.

Section I

Manufacturer's Name	Emergency Telephone Number
Address *(Number, Street, City, State, and ZIP Code)*	Telephone Number for Information
	Date Prepared
	Signature of Preparer *(optional)*

Section II - Hazardous Ingredients/Identity Information

Hazardous Components (Specific Chemical Identity; Common Name(s))	OSHA PEL	ACGIH TLV	Other Limits Recommended	% *(optional)*

Section III - Physical/Chemical Characteristics

Boiling Point		Specific Gravity (H_2O = 1)	
Vapor Pressure (mm Hg)		Melting Point	
Vapor Density (AIR = 1)		Evaporation Rate (Butyl Acetate = 1)	
Solubility in Water			
Appearance and Odor			

Fig. 4.21 Material safety data sheet components. *OSHA*, Occupational Safety and Health Administration; *ACGIH TLV*, American Conference of Governmental Industrial Hygienists threshold limit values; *PEL*, permissible exposure limits; *LEL*, lower exposure limit; *UEL*, upper exposure limit; *NTP*, nucleoside triphosphates; *IARC*, International Agency for Research on Cancer.

Continued

Flammable liquids
Flammable solids
Self-reactive substances and mixtures
Pyrophoric liquids
Pyrophoric solids

Self-heating substances and mixtures
Substances and mixtures that, in contact with water, emit flammable gases
Oxidizing liquids
Oxidizing solids

Section IV - Fire and Explosion Hazard Data

Flash Point (Method Used)	Flammable Limits	LEL	UEL
Extinguishing Media			
Special Fire Fighting Procedures			
Unusual Fire and Explosion Hazards			

(Reproduce locally)   OSHA 174, Sept. 1985

Section V - Reactivity Data

Stability	Unstable		Conditions to Avoid
	Stable		
Incompatibility (Materials to Avoid)			
Hazardous Decomposition or Byproducts			
Hazardous Polymerization	May Occur		Conditions to Avoid
	Will Not Occur		

Section VI - Health Hazard Data

Route(s) of Entry:	Inhalation?	Skin?	Ingestion?
Health Hazards (Acute and Chronic)			
Carcinogenicity:	NTP?	IARC Monographs?	OSHA Regulated?
Signs and Symptoms of Exposure			
Medical Conditions Generally Aggravated by Exposure			
Emergency and First Aid Procedures			

Fig. 4.21, cont'd.

Section VII - Precautions for Safe Handling and Use

Steps to Be Taken in Case Material is Released or Spilled
Waste Disposal Method
Precautions to Be taken in Handling and Storing
Other Precautions

Section VIII - Control Measures

Respiratory Proctection *(Specify Type)*		
Ventilation	Local Exhaust	Special
	Mechanical *(General)*	Other
Protective Gloves		Eye Protection
Other Protective Clothing or Equipment		
Work/Hygienic Practices		

* U.S.G.P.O.: 1986 - 491 - 529/45775

Fig. 4.21, cont'd.

Organic peroxides
Corrosive to metals
Combustible dusts
Simple asphyxiants
Pyrophoric gases
Physical hazards not otherwise classified

Health hazards are based on the ability of the product to cause a health effect—such as eye irritation, respiratory sensitization (may cause allergy or asthma symptoms or breathing difficulties if inhaled), or carcinogenicity (may cause cancer). The complete list of health hazards is as follows:

Acute toxicity
Skin corrosion/irritation
Serious eye damage/eye irritation
Respiratory or skin sensitization
Germ cell mutagenicity
Carcinogenicity
Reproductive toxicity
Specific target organ toxicity—single exposure
Specific target organ toxicity—repeated exposure
Aspiration hazard

Biohazardous infectious materials
Health hazards not otherwise classified

An SDS should be included with each shipment of processing solution. If not, one can be obtained by contacting the manufacturer. OSHA's HCS also include information on hazard evaluation, the proper labeling of containers, the maintaining of lists of chemicals used by the facility, and employee training, which were discussed in Chapter 1. The complete OSHA SDS standards can be found in 29 CFR 1910.1200(g).

2. OSHA developed PPE standards to ensure that employees have proper protection from workplace hazards. These standards include selecting the appropriate PPE, training employees in the proper use of the PPE, maintaining the PPE in a safe and sanitary condition, and replacing the PPE when it becomes damaged or defective. Safety equipment such as eye protection (preferably full-face or nonvented goggles) must be available to personnel who handle, mix, transport, or use processing chemicals. The equipment must meet or exceed the requirements of ANSI Standard Z87.1-1989, "American National Standard Practice for Occupational and Educational Eye and Face Protection." In case of

failure or nonuse of the PPE, an eyewash station should be located prominently in the area where chemicals are in use. Should any amount of processing solution come in contact with the eye, the employee should wash the eye copiously and contact a provider immediately. For protection of the rest of the body, chemically resistant aprons composed of neoprene (chemically resistant) or similar material should be provided. In addition, shower facilities should be available to remove any chemical that has come in contact with the skin. For hand protection, gloves made of neoprene or a similar material should be available for employees who handle processing solutions. OSHA's PPE standards require gloves whenever employees' hands are exposed to potential absorption of harmful substances (such as processing solutions). Training programs for personnel also must be established, and attendance of participants documented. Only trained personnel should perform mixing, cleaning, or maintenance work. The complete OSHA PPE standards are available in 29 CFR 1910.

The Environmental Protection Agency (EPA) also has regulations concerning the use and disposal of processing chemicals. The EPA-SARA Title III (Superfund Amendments and Reauthorization Act of 1986) requires all users of developer solution to report the quantity used. The Resource Conservation and Recovery Act of 1987 governs waste management practices and limits liquid waste containing silver to a level of no more than 5 mg/L, or 5 ppm, which limits the amount of used processing chemicals and wash tank water that can be placed in public sewers and private septic systems before a special permit is required. Waste management may also come under the jurisdiction of the Clean Water Act of 1977, which is a 1977 amendment to the federal Water Pollution Control Act of 1972, which set the basic structure for regulating discharge of pollutants to water in the United States. The act prohibits the discharge of pollutants into any surface water unless strict standards are in place and a special National Pollution Discharge Elimination System (NPDES) permit has been filed with the EPA. Any medical facility that discharges directly to any surface water must have an NPDES permit. The EPA describes a local wastewater treatment facility as a publicly owned treatment works (POTW), which must also have an NPDES permit. If the wastewater from the diagnostic imaging department is discharged to the local POTW and has a silver concentration of 5 ppm or more, and more than 15 kg/month is being discharged, the facility must submit a one-time written notification to the local POTW, the EPA, and the state hazardous waste authority. Material with a pH between 5.5 and 10 can be disposed of safely down the drain; all three parts of the concentrated developer and both parts of concentrated fixer are disqualified. A shipment of scrap film, a silver-laden fixer, and silver recovery cartridges from the clinical site to a refiner or treatment plant also require a special permit from the EPA or the Department of Transportation or both.

The developer solution is considered the most dangerous processing chemical because of its high alkalinity, which makes it especially dangerous to the eyes (hence OSHA's requirement for eye protection) and skin. A main component of film emulsion is gelatin (a form of collagen), which is an organic form of protein that is broken down by chemicals with a high pH. Because human soft tissue contains collagen, the skin and eyes are at risk if contact is made with developer. Hydroquinone can be absorbed through the skin and is corrosive to the eyes and nasal membranes. Glutaraldehyde is a tanning agent (made to harden collagen-based material) and therefore is a skin irritant. Wearing eye protection, rubber gloves, and an apron should always be standard operating procedure when pouring or mixing developer. Fixer is a strong acid that can burn the eyes and irritate the skin. As with developer, proper safety apparel should be worn when pouring and mixing fixer. Wash immediately any skin that has been in contact with processing solutions.

AUTOMATIC PROCESSOR MAIN SYSTEMS

All automatic film processors have six main systems: transport, temperature control, circulation, replenishment, drying, and electrical.

Transport System

The transport system is responsible for transporting the film through the various steps in processing and for controlling development and total processing times. This system also plays a minor role in solution agitation and concentration. It is the largest and most complex system in an automatic processor. Because it has many moving parts, it is also the system most likely to break down. The transport system is made up of three smaller subsystems: the roller subsystem, the transport rack subsystem, and the drive subsystem.

Roller Subsystem

The rollers are responsible for "grabbing" the film and transporting it through the various stages of processing. They also provide a squeegee action that helps prevent too much solution carryover. There are three main types of rollers:

1. *Entrance rollers* are primarily serrated rollers made of rubberized plastic, which enables these rollers to grip the film better as it enters the processor (Fig. 4.22).
2. *Transport, or planetary, rollers* are responsible for the transportation of film and often have a diameter of 1 inch. They usually are mounted in pairs, either staggered or directly opposite to each other (Fig. 4.23).
3. *Master, or solar, rollers* are larger rollers, with a 3-inch diameter. These rollers are found at the bottom of each solution tank, where the film must bend and turn back upward.
4. Rollers can be made of acrylic plastic (Plexiglas), stainless steel, polyester plastic, rubberized plastic, and phenolic resin.

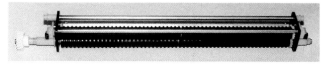

Fig. 4.22 Entrance rollers for automatic film processor.

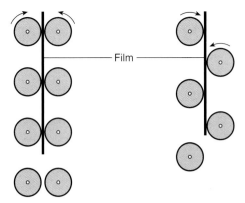

Fig. 4.23 Transport rollers for automatic film processor.

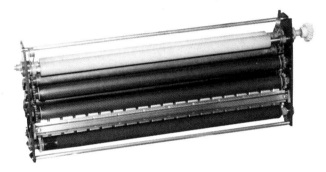

Fig. 4.24 Vertical rack assembly.

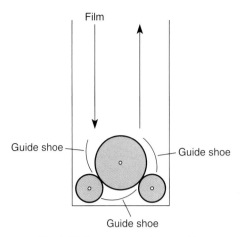

Fig. 4.25 Turnaround rack assembly.

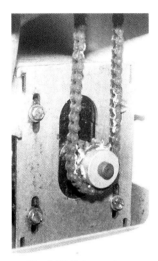

Fig. 4.26 Drive system.

The phenolic rollers are orange-brown and wooden. Care must be taken when cleaning phenolic rollers (no abrasive pads). Because these rollers are made of relatively soft material that can be scratched, liquid can be absorbed into the roller and warping can occur. For these reasons, rollers made of phenolic resin are usually found in the dryer section.

Transport Rack Subsystem

The transport rack subsystem is the rack or frame that contains the rollers, guide shoes, and associated hardware. There are four types of transport racks:

1. *Entrance rack.* The entrance rack contains the entrance rollers, guide shoes, and a microswitch to activate the replenishment system (in volume replenishment systems) (see Fig. 4.22).
2. *Vertical or deep racks.* Vertical or deep racks contain the transport rollers that transport the film into or up out of the tank (Fig. 4.24). Side plates and tie bars hold the rollers in place. The side plates and tie bars can expand and contract over time and may cause misalignment.
3. *Turnaround rack.* The turnaround rack is found at the bottom of the tank and contains a master roller, transport rollers, and two to three guide shoes (Fig. 4.25).
4. *Crossover rack.* Crossover racks move from developer to fixer, from fixer to wash tank, and from wash tank to dryer. The crossover rack for the wash tank to dryer transition is often called a *squeegee rack* because it helps remove water from the film, and faster drying occurs. Usually, these racks contain a master roller, transport rollers, and two guide shoes, but they can vary from

manufacturer to manufacturer. These racks are not in solution and therefore must be cleaned before use because chemical residue can crystallize on the rollers during downtime. If the processor is on standby for longer than 2 hours, then the crossover racks should be cleaned before use.

Drive Subsystem

The drive subsystem is the portion of the transport system that supplies the mechanical energy to move the film (Fig. 4.26). This subsystem includes the following:

1. *Drive motor.* The drive motor is a 1/20-hp to 1/8-hp electric motor that runs at 1725–1750 rpm.
2. *Main drive chain.* The main drive chain is a No. 25 chain that attaches the drive motor to the gear system (similar to a bicycle chain). It is located on the side of the deep racks.
3. *Gear reduction mechanism.* The gear reduction mechanism is a series of gears of different sizes that reduce the speed to between 10 and 20 rpm.
4. *Gears.* Gears transfer the mechanical energy from the motor to the rollers. The two types of gears are "drive" gears, which normally are attached to the ends of the rollers, and "worm" gears, which are located on the main drive

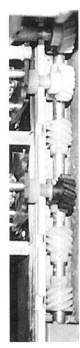

Fig. 4.27 Worm and drive gears.

shaft and are used to power the drive gears (Fig. 4.27). The gears can be made of plastic or metal.

5. *Main drive shaft.* The main drive shaft connects the gear reduction mechanism to the drive gears with a system of worm gears.

Gears out of solution may be coated lightly with grease. Sprockets and chains out of solution require a light coating of oil, but care must be taken to avoid getting petroleum-based products in chemical solutions or on rollers. In the dryer section, lubricants must be avoided; therefore the gears must be kept clean to minimize friction.

The average transport system speed for a 90-second processor is about 60 inches of film per minute.

Temperature Control System

The temperature control system is also called the *tempering system* and regulates the temperature of each solution. The two basic types of this system currently in use are water-controlled systems and thermostatically controlled systems.

Water-Controlled System

The water-controlled system is often called a *warm-water processor.* It uses the wash water temperature to regulate the solution temperature by circulating the water around the outside of the stainless-steel processing tanks. This method requires a large supply of hot water and a mixing valve to regulate water temperature (Fig. 4.28).

Thermostatically Controlled System

Processors with a thermostatically controlled system are often called *cold-water processors* because they require only cold wash water to enter the unit. These systems use either an electronic heater for each tank or a heat exchanger, with a thermostat to

regulate the system. The heat exchanger is a thin walled stainless steel tube located at the bottom of each tank (Fig. 4.29). When a heat exchanger is used, the dryer air is used to heat the solutions in each tank. Because the dryer air temperature can exceed 120°F (49°C), the cooler wash water is pumped through the heat exchanger tube to keep the solution temperature in the proper range (typically 85–95°F or 29–35°C). This system is much more practical than the others because it does not require the large hot-water heater and associated utility costs to maintain the supply necessary for the water-controlled system. For this reason, most of the newer processors are of this type. Regardless of the type of temperature control system used, the system must maintain the developer temperature to within ±0.5°F (0.3°C) of the manufacturer's specifications.

Circulation System

The circulation system is also referred to as the *recirculation and filtration system.* It uses a series of pumps to circulate the solution continuously in each tank and serves the following functions:

1. *Ensures complete chemistry mixing.* During processor downtime, chemicals inside the tanks may begin to separate, with the water rising to the top and the chemicals dissipating to the bottom (a condition known as *stratification*). Swirling of the solutions by the circulation system ensures uniform concentration.
2. *Provides uniform temperature.* Because the heating or heat-exchanging elements are typically on the bottom of the tank, uneven regions of temperature can develop unless the solutions are being circulated continuously.
3. Provides the equivalent of agitation performed in manual processing.

During manual film processing, the halide ions that have been separated from the silver leave the emulsion in the form of bromine gas, which can cause a layer of bubbles to form on the outside surface of the film. This layer may block developing agents from reaching the inner portion of the emulsion, and areas of uneven development called *streaking* occur. Agitation in manual processing involves "jiggling" the film every 30 seconds to shake this layer of bubbles on the film. With the developer swirling over the surface of the film in an automatic processor, the layer of bubbles is removed in much the same way as agitation in manual processing.

A 25-μm filter is often located in the developer loop of this system to remove gelatin and other impurities that become dissolved in the developer during processing (Fig. 4.30). This filter must be replaced periodically as part of processor maintenance. Most manufacturers recommend replacement of this filter on a monthly basis or after the processing of 5000 films. A filter is not required for the fixer portion of this system. The circulation rate of this system is roughly 3–5 gal/min for the developer tank and 1–3 gal/min for the fixer. Failure of this system usually results in uneven development of the resulting image.

Replenishment System

The replenishment system is also called the *regeneration system* and it is responsible for replenishing processor solutions. It

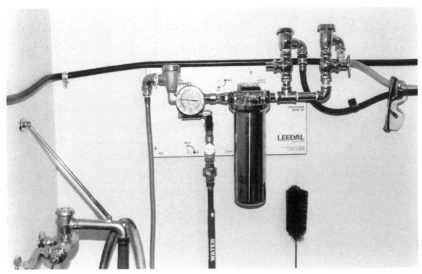

Fig. 4.28 Mixing valve for warm-water automatic processors.

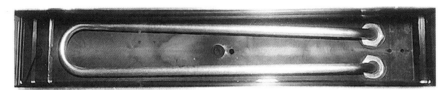

Fig. 4.29 Heat exchanger located at the bottom of the water tank in a thermostatically controlled temperature system.

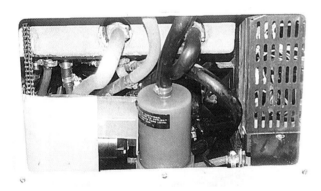

Fig. 4.30 Developer circulation system filter.

consists of a series of pumps, plastic tubing, and plastic storage tanks. The plastic tubing linking the replenishment solution storage tanks to the processor should be inspected periodically because it may become pinched or twisted, which blocks the flow of fresh solution (resulting in underreplenishment). The two different types of replenishment systems available in film processors are volume replenishment and flood replenishment.

Volume Replenishment

With the volume replenishment system, the most common type of replenishment system, a volume of chemicals is replaced for each film that is fed into the processor. A micro-switch is placed usually at either end of the entrance rack that senses the film and then activates the system, and so the size of the film controls the amount of replenishment that takes place.

The average replenishment rates for this system are as follows:
1. *Developer:* 4–5 mL/in of film, or roughly 60–70 mL/sheet of 14-inch × 17-inch film (35 cm × 43 cm)
2. *Fixer:* 6–8 mL/in, or roughly 100–110 mL/sheet of 14-inch × 17-inch film

The volume replenishment system is used for relatively busy processors that process at least 25–50 sheets of 14-inch × 17-inch film or the equivalent per 8-hour workday.

Flood Replenishment

Flood replenishment is also called *timed replenishment* or *standby replenishment* and is used for processors that are not in constant use or that process less than 25–50 sheets of 14-inch × 17-inch film or equivalent per day. With the low volume of patient films processed per day, there may be a considerable gap in time between films entering the processor, which allows the developer solution inside the automatic processor to become oxidized, and subsequent films are under-developed. This situation prompts the radiographer either to increase technical factors (the result is a greater patient dose) or to increase the replenishment rate of a volume replenishment system (the results are greater department costs). With a flood replenishment system, the replenishment is controlled by a timer, which replenishes the solutions periodically, regardless of the number of films processed. This system was developed by Donald E. Titus of the Eastman Kodak Company. The replenishment pump should operate for approximately 20 seconds every 5 minutes and deliver about 65 mL of each solution. These variables maintain a total replenishment rate of 780 mL/h. All developer in the processing tank should be replaced every 16 working hours.

Most processors include a replenishment rate indicator, and so monitoring is easy. In the case of other types of processors, special test paper is available for testing certain concentrations in the developer and fixer.

For developer, the special test paper estimates the levels of bromide ions dissolved in the solution. Stable developer should have a bromide level of about 6 g/L. Levels greater than 8 g/L indicate underreplenishment, which can cause underdevelopment and lead to a lack of optical density and contrast of the resulting image. Underreplenishment is caused most often by a pinched or blocked replenishment line, pump failure, microswitch failure, or failure of the timer circuit during flood replenishment. Levels less than 4 g/L indicate overreplenishment, which can result in overdevelopment that causes increased optical density and fogging. Overreplenishment is caused most often by either a microswitch or a pump that does not shut off.

Fixer replenishment can be estimated with silver estimating paper, which estimates the dissolved silver content in the solution. Normal fixer contains about 4–6 g/L (0.4–0.6 troy oz/gal). Levels greater than 8 g/L indicate underreplenishment (which causes a lack of clearing and a possible lack of hardening in the resulting film), whereas levels less than 4 g/L indicate overreplenishment, which does not affect film quality adversely but does waste fixer (and therefore money).

Drying System

The dryer system consists of two or three heating units between 1500 and 2500 W that are used to dry the film. The system draws at least 10 A of electric current, which means that the system consumes 60%–80% of the electrical power going into the processor. A hot-air blower moves the air at a rate between 100 and 300 ft³/min over the film. A series of air fins and air tubes are used to direct the air onto the film (Fig. 4.31). These fins and tubes must be kept clean for maximum efficiency. Most automatic processors also require

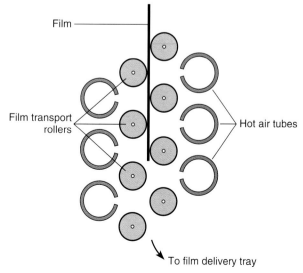

Fig. 4.31 Dryer air tubes.

an exhaust tube (which is similar to one found on a clothes dryer) to empty the hot air out of the processing area. This air can have a temperature exceeding 100°F (37.8°C) and relative humidity values between 25% and 100%, which are not conducive to proper film storage.

Electrical System

The electrical system consists of a solid-state circuit board or microprocessor that distributes electrical power to the other systems. In some newer processors, the microprocessor can be accessed to disclose quality control information such as solution temperature and replenishment rate. It usually handles 4–5 kW/h and between 15 and 25 A of current. This system requires periodic replacement because of the heat, humidity, and corrosive environment inside of the processor.

TYPES OF AUTOMATIC PROCESSORS

Automatic processors are of several types and they usually are named according to the time it takes to process the film completely, often called the *dry-to-drop time.*

1. *Seven minutes:* The original Kodak automatic processor from the 1950s; processes about 100 films/h.
2. *Three minutes:* Also called a *double-capacity processor* because it processes 200 films/h.
3. *Ninety seconds:* Also called a *fast-access processor* because the film is available in 90 seconds and the processor has a capacity of 300 films/h; developed by Kodak in the mid-1960s and still the most commonly used film processor.
4. *Sixty seconds:* A newer type of processor that can process up to 350 films/h.
5. *Forty-five seconds:* The newest type of processor; requires special film and chemistry to function properly.
6. *Variable speed:* Processing time can be varied according to the type of film used. In other words, the radiographer may select a 90-second processing time, a 180-second processing time, and so on. An example of this is the "extended processing" used in mammography, which increases normal processing time to increase the film contrast. This is covered more completely in Chapter 9. Some processors also have a standby option that is useful for low-volume facilities. The drive system and dryer blower are shut off and the water flow rate is reduced, but the chemical and the dryer temperatures are maintained. This activity occurs when 2 min pass without a film entering the unit.

Processor Size

Automatic film processors come in three basic sizes according to the number of films processed during a given period: the floor-size processor, the intermediate-size processor, and the tabletop-size processor.

Floor-Size Processor

The floor-size processor is the largest processor and, as its name implies, it sits on the floor of the darkroom or lightroom. It has heavy-duty rollers, gears, and a drive motor, and so it can handle a high volume of operation. This size processor is found primarily in the main radiology department of hospitals.

Intermediate-Size Processor

The intermediate-size processor is a smaller version of the floor-size processor and usually sits on four support legs. It is about the size of a single laundry sink. This processor costs less than the floor-size model and is often found in providers' offices and clinics, and in specialized areas of hospitals, such as surgery.

Tabletop-Size Processor

The tabletop-size processor is the smallest and least expensive processor. It is designed for low-volume operation, such as in a mobile facility, and is small enough to fit on the countertop of a darkroom.

Processor Location

A processor can be installed in the darkroom in one of four methods: totally inside, bulk inside, bulk outside, or totally outside.

Totally Inside

With totally inside installation, the processor is completely inside the darkroom, and noise, heat, and humidity are generated. Therefore this is the least desirable method of installation. An advantage of this method, however, is easy retrieval of film that has jammed in the processor because it can be removed in safe lighting.

Bulk Inside

With bulk inside installation, most of the processor is inside the darkroom and only the drop tray is on the outside. This method minimizes the heat and noise in the darkroom but still allows easy retrieval of jammed film.

Bulk Outside

Bulk outside installation places the feed tray inside the darkroom but all other components outside. This method eliminates the heat, noise, and humidity inside the darkroom but makes retrieval of films more difficult because they must be removed in white light.

The minimum space on all sides of the processor must be 24 inches, to allow for servicing.

Totally Outside

Daylight processing systems and processors are designed to eliminate the need for a darkroom, and so they are located totally outside any darkroom area.

PROCESSOR QUALITY CONTROL

The most important part of a quality management program in departments using film/screen image receptors is the quality control of the film processor, resulting primarily from the large degree of variability that can occur with processing systems. Daily monitoring of processor operation and function is required to keep these variables from degrading the image

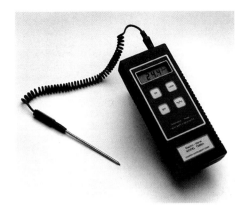

Fig. 4.32 Digital thermometer for monitoring solution temperatures. (Courtesy Gammex/RMI, Middleton, Wisconsin.)

quality. There are four components to a processor quality control program: chemical activity, cleaning procedures, maintenance, and monitoring.

CHEMICAL ACTIVITY

As mentioned earlier in this chapter, chemical activity refers to how well the processing chemicals are functioning. Many variables affect chemical activity, including the solution temperature, processing time, replenishment rate, solution pH, and specific gravity and proper mixing.

Solution Temperature

Variations in developer temperature can affect image contrast, optical density, and the visibility of recorded details significantly. Therefore developer temperature should not vary by more than ±0.5°F (0.3°C) from the manufacturer's recommendations. It should be monitored at the beginning of the workday and then periodically throughout the day. Many film processors have either an analog thermometer or a light-emitting diode indicator of solution temperature built into the front panel. If this is unavailable, a digital thermometer with a remote probe (Fig. 4.32) is the best instrument to monitor solution temperature because it is the most accurate and works quickly. A glass alcohol-filled thermometer is an adequate alternative. A mercury thermometer should never be used because mercury is a toxic substance, and it poses a difficult and potentially hazardous cleanup problem in the event of breakage. Mercury can also sensitize film, even in small quantities. The accuracy of any built-in thermometer should be checked monthly with a digital thermometer and should be within ±0.5°F (0.3°C).

Fixer activity is not as temperature sensitive as developer activity, but the temperature should be maintained within ±5°F (3°C) of the developer temperature to avoid reticulation marks (discussed in Chapter 6) and to clear the film properly. Wash water temperature should be the same as that of the fixer to complete washing.

To check the solution temperatures, place the probe in each tank, starting with the developer. Be sure that the probe is clean to avoid contamination. Next, check the wash water

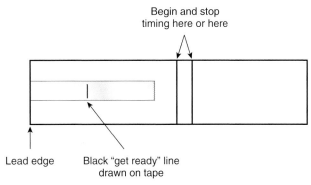

Fig. 4.33 Time-in-solution test tool.

temperature and then the fixer temperature. Afterward, rinse the probe with water so that it is ready for the next inspection.

Processing Time

Variations in developer time can have the same effect on image quality as solution temperature. Therefore developer time should be maintained to within ±2%–3% of the manufacturer's specifications. As mentioned earlier in this chapter, the transport system is responsible for maintaining processing time. Most of this system is made up of moving parts (and experiences the most wear and tear of any system), and so it is subject to the most variability and breakdown. Processing time should be checked daily at the beginning of each workday (or more often if a malfunction is suspected) and can be determined with a stopwatch or digital timer. To establish developer time, feed the film into the processor with the top open. When the leading edge of the film enters the solution, start the timer; when the leading edge first emerges from the solution, stop the timer. For a 90-second processor, the time should be between 18 and 22 seconds, with a margin of error of roughly 0.5 seconds. Total processing time is evaluated using a stopwatch to measure the time when the leading edge of the film enters the processor to when it begins to appear in the drop section; then, compare that time with the manufacturer's specification. For help with this procedure, a time-in-solution test tool is available (Fig. 4.33). The tool consists of a strip of clear film base with two white tape strips that form the letter *T*. A black line is drawn about halfway on the first strip as a "get ready" line to alert the person performing the test to prepare to start the stopwatch. Timing begins when the cross of the *T* enters the solution.

Replenishment Rate

As film is processed during the course of the workday, the processing solutions are being depleted. If they are not replenished adequately, a decrease in image contrast and optical density occurs. Excessive replenishment has the opposite effect. Most film processors have replenishment rate flow meters that indicate the replenishment rate for each solution. The values indicated should be within ±5% of the manufacturer's specification for the type of replenishment system in use (volume replenishment vs. flood replenishment). These values for most processors are described earlier in this chapter. The amount of replenishment also should be within 5%

of these values. A stopwatch and a graduated cylinder can be used to verify replenishment rate and flow meter accuracy. With the top of the processor open, an 8-inch × 10-inch (20-cm × 25-cm) film should be fed into the processor lengthwise. The graduated cylinder should be placed under the opening of the replenish line so that the fresh solution pumps directly into the cylinder. When the film passes through the entrance rack, the replenishing pump shuts off, stopping the flow of solution. When this happens, the volume of solution in millimeters should be divided by 10 to get the milliliter-per-inch value (or divided by 25 to obtain milliliters per centimeters) and then compared with the manufacturer's values.

Solution pH

Most developer solutions must function in a pH range between 10 and 11.5 to convert the latent image to a visible image. A developer pH that is too low (caused by underreplenishment or contamination) decreases image contrast and optical density, whereas excessive pH has the opposite effect. Fixer solutions should maintain a pH between 4 and 4.5 for proper clearing. Although not as critical as the other factors affecting chemical activity, pH should be checked daily to avoid potential problems. A digital pH meter is recommended for evaluating pH because of its accuracy. If one is not available, litmus paper or similar commercially available test strips are an inexpensive alternative. The strips are dipped into the solution, and they change color to indicate the pH value. Care should be taken (by wearing rubber gloves) not to get processing chemicals on one's skin when using this method.

Specific Gravity and Proper Mixing

Processing chemicals must be mixed to the manufacturer's concentration specifications to function within operating parameters. The easiest method to evaluate solution concentration is to measure the specific gravity.

$$\text{Specific gravity} = \frac{\text{Density of X liqiud}}{\text{Density of water in equal amount}}$$

A **hydrometer** is the instrument used to measure specific gravity. It resembles a large glass thermometer (Fig. 4.34). When placed in a liquid, the hydrometer sinks to a certain depth in the solution, and the level of the liquid indicates the specific gravity on the stem of the hydrometer. Measure the developer first, and then rinse the hydrometer with water and measure the fixer. Developer specific gravity should be in the range 1.07–1.1 and should not vary by more than ±0.004 from the manufacturer's specifications. Fixer solutions should be in the range 1.077–1.11 and should not vary by more than ±0.004 from the manufacturer's specifications.

PROCESSOR CLEANING PROCEDURES

Processors that are dirty—the most common cause of processor breakdown—cannot function according to established parameters. Therefore proper cleaning procedures should be performed daily, monthly, quarterly, and yearly.

PROCEDURE: DAILY PROCEDURE

1. Open the top of the processor to determine whether the crossover racks were removed the previous night (which should be the case, as shown later in this section). Use of the processor may have been necessary during the night on an emergency basis. If the racks are present, remove the splash guards and crossover racks and rinse them with water. Be sure that the rollers and guide shoes are free of dirt, debris, gelatin, or crystallized processing chemicals. Use a soft sponge or plastic cleaning pad for cleaning; avoid using steel wool pads or other metallic scrubbers. Turn the rollers by hand so that all surfaces can be reached.
2. Remove the deep transport racks from each solution and rinse with water. Take care not to drip one solution into another—especially the fixer into the developer—when lifting the racks out of the solution tanks. Remove stubborn dirt or residue with a soft sponge or plastic scrubber. Inspect the rollers and gears for any obvious defects. Replace the racks back into the solutions carefully while avoiding contamination.
3. Activate the transport system and observe the rollers and gears for asymmetry, rotation, and hesitation during operation. Replace the crossover racks and again observe the rollers and gears during operation. Replace any defective parts (especially gears and roller tension springs) and be sure that all mounting screws are tightened.
4. Observe the level of processing solutions to be sure that they are within 1 mm of specified levels. Activate the replenisher pump or add fresh solution from the storage tank if the level is low.
5. After shutdown, remove the crossover racks and store them adjacent to the processor (if practical) to minimize the formation of chemical residue. Raise the top of the processor so that a 2-inch to 4-inch gap exists to allow chemical fumes to escape and to avoid condensation of chemicals onto the various processor components.

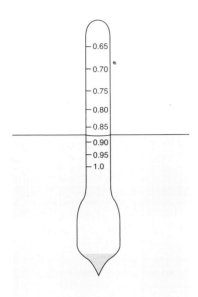

Fig. 4.34 A floating hydrometer is used to measure specific gravity. In this particular instance, the specific gravity indicated by the hydrometer is 0.87 g/cm³.

Daily

These procedures should be performed daily at startup.

The procedure just mentioned normally requires 15–20 min daily to complete and can add several years to the life expectancy of the processor in addition to eliminating most processor artifacts.

Monthly

PROCEDURE: MONTHLY PROCEDURE

1. Drain all processing tanks and wash the inside with water. Use a soft sponge or plastic scrubber to remove stubborn dirt or residue.

2. Rinse all tanks with water and refill them with the proper amount of chemical solution. The developer solution must be "seasoned" before any films can be processed because typical replenisher solution is too concentrated. Seasoning involves adding starter solution, which is stabilized potassium bromide. This addition raises the bromide level to between 4 and 8 g/L, which is the normal level for developer solution while processing films. Fresh developer replenisher used to refill the tank has levels far less than this, which can increase the fog level of the film. The amount of starter solution required is about 100 mL/gal solution.

Quarterly

PROCEDURE: QUARTERLY PROCEDURE

1. Drain, wash, and rinse all replenishment tanks with water. Be especially careful to remove the oxidized developer from the sides of the developer replenisher tank.
2. Refill tanks with fresh solution and check the specific gravity with a hydrometer.

Yearly

Replenisher and circulation system pumps and tubing can experience a buildup of dirt and chemical residue that can reduce the efficiency of these systems and therefore some manufacturers suggest the use of a system cleaner to reduce these deposits. The developer system cleaner has an acidic pH level to counteract the alkaline developer, whereas the fixer system cleaner has an alkaline pH to counteract the acidic fixer. Remove the transport racks before a system cleaner is used because phenolic and soft rubber rollers can absorb the cleaner and contaminate future processing solutions slowly. Most system cleaners are either chlorine based (which can break down hydroquinone) or sulfamic based (which also breaks down hydroquinone and dissolves metallic silver). Take great care to flush systems with water to remove residual cleaner. Some manufacturers do not recommend the use of a system cleaner in their processors because of the risk of contamination, and so it is best to check with a technical representative.

PROCESSOR MAINTENANCE

Poorly maintained processors (in addition to dirty ones) cannot function according to established parameters and can degrade image quality. They also can lead to premature replacement of the processor, which is a large capital expense ($5000 to $50,000). A film processor should last for at least 10,000 hours of operation or a minimum of 5 years. Therefore a proper maintenance schedule must be maintained by the diagnostic imaging department to ensure continued satisfactory operation of the film processor. Keep a log of any maintenance procedures to document care. There are three types of processor maintenance: scheduled, preventive, and nonscheduled.

Scheduled Maintenance

Scheduled maintenance includes procedures that are performed daily, weekly, and monthly. For automatic film processors, scheduled maintenance includes proper lubrication of moving parts; observation of all moving parts; replacement of filters in the water and developer circulation system; adjustment or replacement of tension springs, pulleys, and gears; and correction of any mechanical problems.

Preventive Maintenance

Preventive maintenance is a planned program that details specific parts of the processor to be replaced regularly. Items such as gears and rollers should be replaced after a certain number of hours of operation.

Nonscheduled Maintenance

Nonscheduled maintenance is required when a system failure occurs. The need for this type of maintenance can be minimized by proper cleaning of the processor, along with performing scheduled and preventive maintenance procedures.

Suggested Scheduled Maintenance Procedures

A processor maintenance schedule should include maintenance procedures daily at startup; daily during operation; daily at shutdown; and weekly, monthly, quarterly, and yearly.

Daily at Startup

PROCEDURE: DAILY STARTUP MAINTENANCE

1. Follow the daily cleaning procedures listed earlier in this chapter.
2. Ensure that the processor feed tray and darkroom countertops are clean.
3. Feed four 14-inch × 17-inch (35-cm × 43-cm) green unprocessed films into the processor to clean the rollers of any

residual matter and to assess transport system operation. Do not use preprocessed radiographs because they may contain residual fixer and have a hardened emulsion, which causes extra stress on the transport system. Any residual fixer also may contaminate the developer solution.

Daily During Operation

PROCEDURE: DAILY MAINTENANCE DURING OPERATION

1. Assess any changes in the normal operation of the processor, including noise level, vibration, odors, indicator buzzer, and film-feeding characteristics.
2. Shut down the unit after 2 hours if no films have been processed (unless the system is equipped with a standby option). If the unit has been shut down for 30 min or longer, run another 14-inch × 17-inch piece of green film through the system to clean the rollers.

Daily at Shutdown

PROCEDURE: DAILY MAINTENANCE AT SHUTDOWN

1. Follow the cleaning procedures for shutdown listed previously (item 5 in the section on daily processor cleaning procedures).
2. Note any obvious problems or changes in the unit such as abnormal odors or residues.

Weekly

PROCEDURE: WEEKLY MAINTENANCE

1. Use a thermometer to evaluate the solution temperature and dryer thermostats for accuracy. Compare the value on the thermostat with the value indicated on the thermometer. Solution temperatures must be maintained at previously mentioned parameters. The dryer thermostat should be accurate to within ±5°F (3°C).
2. Evaluate replenishment rates for accuracy using the previously mentioned procedure.
3. Lubricate the main driveshaft bearings, motor, and drive chain with motor oil.
4. Inspect replenishment system microswitches on the entrance rack for proper operation on units equipped with volume replenishment.
5. For units equipped with flood replenishment, drain the developer tank, rinse it with water, and fill it with fresh solution.
6. Inspect and service the silver reclamation unit.

Monthly

PROCEDURE: MONTHLY MAINTENANCE

1. Follow the monthly cleaning procedures listed earlier in this chapter.
2. Use a large bottlebrush to remove and clean all dryer air tubes.

PROCEDURE: MONTHLY MAINTENANCE—cont'd

3. Replace the filter in the developer circulation. This filter removes dissolved gelatin and other impurities larger than 75 μm from the developer. Before installing the filter, soak it in fresh developer solution to remove any air from the system.
4. Replace the water filters if the flow rate decreases by more than 10% of the accepted amount.
5. Flush the floor drain with a commercial drain cleaner.
6. Perform a safelight test.

Quarterly

PROCEDURE: QUARTERLY MAINTENANCE

1. Follow the quarterly cleaning procedure listed earlier.
2. Inspect all transport racks, rollers, gears, and guide shoes for wear or malfunction.
3. Check the integrity of all electrical connections and remove any dirt or corrosion.
4. Perform a hyporetention test on processed films using an American National Standards Institute test kit to evaluate the archival quality of images.

Yearly

PROCEDURE: YEARLY MAINTENANCE

1. Disassemble each transport rack and replace worn rollers, gears, or mounting springs.
2. Disassemble the drive motor and gearbox, lubricate the internal components, and replace worn parts.
3. Disassemble all replenishment and circulation system pump heads and replace worn parts, including rubber diaphragms and seals.
4. Replace the tubing in the circulation and replenishment system with one-eighth-inch clear polyvinyl chloride tubing. Install new clamps to mitigate the corrosive environment in the processor.

PROCESSOR MONITORING

Processor monitoring is accomplished with the performance of daily sensitometric tests that evaluate the performance of both the processor systems and processing chemicals. **Sensitometry** measures the relationship between the intensity of radiation absorbed by the film and the optical density produced. Two British amateur photographers, F. Hurter and U. Driffield, developed the current system of comparing these quantities (hence the Hurter and Driffield curve, which demonstrates film contrast). The following equipment is required to perform sensitometric tests: a sensitometer, a **densitometer**, either a control chart or graph paper, and quality control film.

Sensitometer

The **sensitometer** is an instrument designed to expose a reproducible, uniform, optical step-wedge pattern onto a film

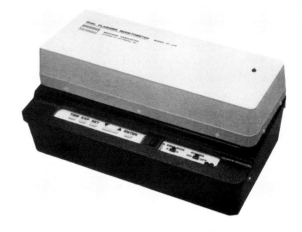

Fig. 4.35 Sensitometer. (Courtesy Gammex/RMI, Middleton, Wisconsin.)

(Fig. 4.35). It contains a controlled-intensity light source with a standardized optical step-wedge image (also called a *step tablet*). These patterns are available in 11-step and 21-step versions (Fig. 4.36). The 11-step pattern increases the optical density by a factor of 2 (100%) between each step. The 21-step pattern increases optical density by a factor of 1.41 (41%) between each step and is more useful in sensitometric tests. A radiograph taken with an aluminum step wedge or penetrometer should not be used in processor sensitometric tests because X-ray generators are subject to too much variation from day to day, and the origin of any differences in radiographic images cannot be determined (i.e., the problem could be with the processor or with the X-ray generator). The controlled light source of the sensitometer eliminates these variations.

X-Rite®
1
2
3
4
5
6
7
8
9
10
11
12
13
14
15
16
17
18
19
20
21
TIME: DATE: ID NO

Fig. 4.36 Twenty-one-step sensitometry film image. (Courtesy Nuclear Associates, Carle Place, New York.)

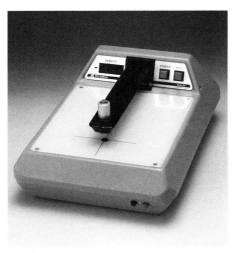

Fig. 4.37 Densitometer, which is used to measure optical density. (Courtesy Gammex/RMI, Middleton, Wisconsin.)

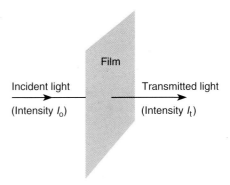

Fig. 4.38 Diagram of incident and transmitted light. *Io*, Original intensity; *It*, transmitted intensity.

Most sensitometers have settings that allow the selection of blue-violet light emission or green light emission to match the spectral response of the film being tested. They also should have an option for exposing single-emulsion film or double-emulsion (duplitized) film. These settings must be selected properly to match the type of film to be used. Sensitometers remain fairly consistent in their operation until the light bulb burns out. The main concern for quality control technologists is to ensure that the exposure window of the sensitometer (where the light exposes the film) is kept clean—free of dirt and dust. Do not touch these windows or wipe them with any type of cloth or gauze pad because they are fragile. Instead, purchase a can of compressed air (which is free of moisture and therefore prevents condensation) from an office supply store and use it to remove any dirt or debris.

Densitometer

The densitometer, also known as *a transmission densitometer,* measures the optical density of a portion of an image using a zero-point to 4-point scale (Fig. 4.37). It is a photographic light meter that measures the amount of light transmitted (transmitted light) through a portion of film and compares it with the original amount of light incident on the film (Fig. 4.38). A value of 0–4 points is then calculated with the following equation:

$$\text{Optical density} = \log_{10} \frac{\text{Incident light}}{\text{Transmitted light}} \text{ or } \log_{10} \frac{I_i}{I_t}$$

If the transmitted light were 10% of the incident light, the optical density would be 1 because the equation would be the following:

$$\text{Optical density} = \log_{10} \frac{100}{10}$$

Because the incident light is the full amount of light striking the film, it has a relative value of 100%. The $\log_{10}$ symbol (meaning log to the base 10) in the equation asks the question: Ten to what power equals the number in the equation? Because 100 divided by 10 equals 10, the $\log_{10}$ of the number 10 is 1 ($10^1 = 10$); therefore if only 1% of the incident light is transmitted through the film, that portion of the image has an optical density of 2 because $100/1 = 100$ and $10^2 = 100$. A difference in the optical density scale of 0.3 is equivalent to a difference of two times in the amount of light transmission through the film because $10^{0.3} = 2$. This means that an optical density of 1.3 is twice as dark as an optical density of 1, and so on. The anatomic structures displayed on a diagnostic image usually have optical density values ranging from approximately 0.25 to 2.5 when measured with a densitometer; this is known as the *diagnostic range*. Optical densities outside this range do not contain diagnostic information when viewed on a standard viewbox illuminator.

Control Chart

A control chart is a graph that has predetermined upper and lower thresholds indicated (see Chapter 2) and is used to plot the data obtained during the sensitometric test (Fig. 4.39). Most control charts are designed to have these data recorded each day for an entire month.

Before sensitometric tests are performed, ensure that the processor is clean and functioning properly; that fresh, properly mixed chemicals are available; and that a safelight test has been performed with satisfactory results. The processor also should be in operation for at least 20 min so that the temperatures are at optimal levels.

After all the previously mentioned values are determined, they should be plotted on a control chart (see Fig. 4.39). This chart helps monitor chemical activity and processor performance, and documents the quality control activities for accreditation or government agencies. Because control charts have data plotted for an entire month, any trends in processor performance may appear and need to be addressed. The minimum number of data points in one direction that constitutes a trend that should be investigated is five for general radiography and three for mammographic processors. A processor quality control documentation form and daily sensitometric test form are included on the accompanying Evolve website. If a processor quality control program has not been implemented previously, the accepted operating level or base control number for each indicator has to be established. This established operating

PROCEDURE: SENSITOMETRIC TESTING

1. Place an 8-inch × 10-inch (20-cm × 25-cm) sheet of unexposed film in the sensitometer and expose it according to the manufacturer's instructions.
2. Feed the exposed film into the processor as soon as possible. Avoid variability by keeping the time between the exposure of the sensitometer film and the processing consistent. Be sure to feed the film into the processor correctly (see "Locational effect" discussed in the following list). This helps avoid the following variables:
   - **Bromide drag**, also called *bromide flow* or *directional effect,* is caused by the release of halide ions by the emulsion during development and their subsequent coating of the trailing areas of the film, which decreases the optical density of these areas. To minimize this effect, feed the least dense end of the sensitometric strip first, with the long axis of the wedge pattern parallel to the entrance rollers. The steplike image created by the sensitometer is usually created at the edge of one side of the film, along the 10-inch (25-cm) dimension, as shown in Fig. 4.36. The opposite side of the film is unexposed and should be fed into the processor first to reduce the number of halide ions that are "dragged" over the remainder of the film.
   - **Locational effect** results from a difference in the location of the test film insertion into the processor. To minimize this effect, always try to insert the film on the same side of the feed tray each time a sensitometric test is performed.
   - **Time-of-day variability** is important because chemical activity and processing system parameters can vary considerably throughout the course of the workday. Therefore sensitometric test films should always be processed at the same time each day, preferably early in the morning, after the processor has reached optimum operating levels.
3. After the film is processed, optical density readings of each of the 21 steps and the clear portion of the image should be measured with a densitometer and recorded. After the first day, when the operating parameters of the processor are established, it is not necessary to measure all 21 steps for succeeding days' test films.
4. From these optical density readings, the following indicators of processor performance are established:
   - *Base + fog.* Often abbreviated B + F, **base + fog** is the optical density of the clear portion of the image and is the result of the blue tint added to the base of the film and any black metallic silver grains that were created by aging of the film or background radiation exposure. The B + F value for most film ranges from 0.1 to 0.2 and should never exceed 0.25. When the accepted operating level is established, it should never vary by more than an optical density value of ±0.05 for dual-emulsion films and 0.03 for single-emulsion films during subsequent days' sensitometric test films. An above-normal developer temperature, an above-normal developing time, overreplenishment, contaminated solution, improper film or solution storage conditions, improper safelights, an incorrect starter solution in the developer, and fogged film can increase the B + F value above accepted limits.

   - *Speed indicator* or *middensity point* (MD). MD is a measure of the amount of exposure energy necessary to produce an optical density of one greater than the B + F. After the B + F is determined, find the step with an optical density closest to one greater than this value. The value of this step is always measured and recorded as the speed indicator, regardless of the value obtained. For example, if the B + F is 0.2 on the first day, and step 8 of the sensitometry image yields an optical density of 1.2 on the same day, then the optical density of step 8 is always used to determine the speed indicator for all future days' tests. This value should not vary by an optical density of ±0.15 from the accepted operating level. Increased developer temperature, increased developer time, overreplenishment, excessive concentration of developer or replenisher (usually resulting from developer mixed incorrectly; not enough water is added to the concentrate), no starter solution in fresh developer, or a contaminated solution can increase this value above established limits. A reversal decreases the speed indicator below accepted limits.
   - *Minimum density* (D_{min}) or *low density* (LD). D_{min}, or LD, is the optical density of the step closest to 0.25 greater than the B + F, which approximates the low end of the diagnostic range of optical densities. Again, after this indicator is established, the same step is used in future days' testing, regardless of the optical density reading. The optical density of this step should not vary by more than ±0.05 for dual-emulsion films and 0.03 for single-emulsion films from the accepted operating level during any future test. The optical density value of this indicator is created primarily by the action of phenidone, which is less sensitive to variability than hydroquinone. Essentially, the same factors affecting the B + F indicator also affect D_{min}.
   - *Maximum density* (D_{max}) or *high density* (HD). D_{max}, or HD, is the optical density of the step closest to two greater than the B + F, which is close to the upper value of the diagnostic density range. This value should stay within ±0.15 from the accepted operating level. This optical density value is created primarily by hydroquinone, which is more sensitive to variability than phenidone. An increase in developer time, temperature, or pH; overreplenishment; or overconcentration of developer solution can increase this value above the upper limit and vice versa.
   - *Contrast indicator or relative density difference* (DD). Because *contrast* is defined as the difference among optical densities on the processed image, a **contrast indicator** can be obtained by calculating the difference between the D_{max} and D_{min} values during each day's sensitometry test. When the accepted operating level is determined initially, it should not vary by more than ±0.15 during any subsequent tests. Increased developer temperature or developer time, overreplenishment, or overconcentration of developer solution can increase the contrast indicator above the upper limit. A decrease below the lower limit occurs if the given factors are decreased.

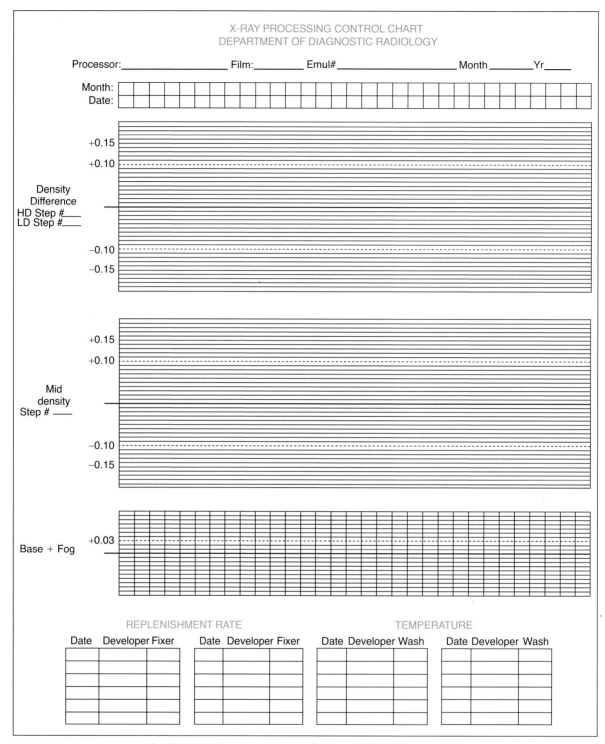

Fig. 4.39 Processor control chart. *HD,* High density; *LD,* low density.

level is the value plotted at the center line of the control chart for each indicator. To establish the accepted operating level for each indicator, establish the control box of film (see the later discussion on quality control film) and expose a sheet of film with a sensitometer for 5 consecutive days. Determine the B + F, MD, and DD for each day. At the end of the fifth day, average the B + F, MD, and DD values for all 5 days. These averages are the accepted operating levels or base control numbers used on the control chart.

Quality Control Film

When a processor quality control program is implemented, a fresh box of film should be selected and dedicated to sensitometric testing only. This box of film is known as the *control box* and should be labeled clearly and stored under ideal conditions (e.g., no light, ionizing radiation, or chemical fumes). When all but a few sheets of film in the control box have been used, a crossover procedure to a new box of control

CROSSOVER WORKSHEET

Site		Date	
Film type		Technologist	

New Emulsion # | | | | | **Old Emulsion #** | | | |

Film #	Low Density (LD) Step #____	Mid Density (MD) Step #____	High Density (HD) Step #____	B+F	Film #	Low Density (LD) Step #____	Mid Density (MD) Step #____	High Density (HD) Step #____	B+F
1					1				
2					2				
3					3				
4					4				
5					5				
Average					Average				
Average Density Difference: DD = HD − LD =					Average Density Difference: DD = HD − LD =				

MD difference between new and old film (New MD − Old MD)	
DD difference between new and old film (New DD − Old DD)	
B+F difference between new and old film (New − Old)	

	MD	DD	B+F
Old operating levels			
Difference between new and old film			
New operating levels			

CROSSOVER WORKSHEET
EXAMPLE

New Emulsion # 24578 | | | | **Old Emulsion #** 23456 | | | |

Film #	Low Density (LD) Step #10	Mid Density (MD) Step #11	High Density (HD) Step #13	B+F	Film #	Low Density (LD) Step #10	Mid Density (MD) Step #11	High Density (HD) Step #13	B+F
1	0.49	1.25	2.39	0.18	1	0.46	1.27	2.33	0.17
2	0.50	1.23	2.43	0.18	2	0.48	1.30	2.30	0.17
3	0.49	1.26	2.40	0.17	3	0.46	1.27	2.28	0.18
4	0.53	1.28	2.41	0.18	4	0.48	1.28	2.32	0.17
5	0.49	1.28	2.43	0.18	5	0.47	1.31	2.35	0.18
Average	0.50	1.26	2.41	0.18	Average	0.47	1.29	2.31	0.17
Average Density Difference: DD = HD − LD = 1.91					Average Density Difference: DD = HD − LD = 1.84				

MD difference between new and old film (New MD − Old MD)	−0.03
DD difference between new and old film (New DD − Old DD)	+0.07
B+F difference between new and old film (New − Old)	+0.01

	MD	DD	B+F
Old operating levels	1.34	1.90	0.17
Difference between new and old film	−0.03	+0.07	+0.01
New operating levels	1.31	1.97	0.18

Fig. 4.40 Crossover worksheet for determining new operating levels. *B + F*, Base + fog.

film should be performed to minimize any variation that may occur from one batch of film to another (Fig. 4.40).

CHARACTERISTIC CURVE

In addition to the control chart, many diagnostic imaging departments may also benefit from the daily creation of a characteristic curve (also known as the *sensitometric curve, Hurter & Driffield curve, H & D curve,* or *D log E curve*) to monitor processor performance. Because the characteristic curve demonstrates film contrast, changes in the curve from day to day can indicate problems in the processing solutions or

PROCEDURE: CONSTRUCTING A CHARACTERISTIC CURVE

1. Remove a sheet of 8-inch × 10-inch (20-cm × 25-cm) film from the film bin and expose it with a sensitometer. Process the film.
2. Using a densitometer, take optical density readings of each step of the 11-step or 21-step pattern.
3. On a sheet of graph paper, plot the optical density of each step on the y-axis and the step number (beginning with the least dense step) on the x-axis. Connect the points on the graph. The resulting curve should have the characteristic *S* or sigmoidal shape (see Fig. 4.41).

Continued

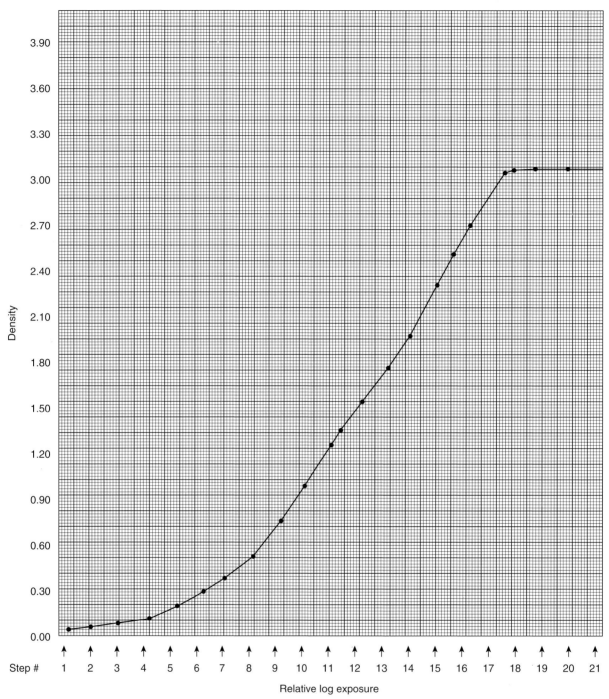

Fig. 4.41 Sample plotting of a characteristic curve.

PROCEDURE: CONSTRUCTING A CHARACTERISTIC CURVE—cont'd

4. Calculate the average gradient (slope) of the straight-line portion of the curve using the optical density points of 0.25 and two greater than the B + F. This yields the contrast indicator of DD. The speed indicator or MD step also should be plotted as the step closest to one more than the B + F. These values should not vary by more than ±0.15 from the established value.

processor system performance. The characteristic curve also demonstrates B + F and film speed or sensitivity (Fig. 4.41).

PROCESSOR TROUBLESHOOTING

As mentioned earlier in this chapter, an automatic film processor is subject to considerable variability during the course of operation, resulting in visible changes in image quality. The troubleshooting guide in Table 4.4 identifies specific processor problems, conditions, or both, and details the necessary corrective action.

TABLE 4.4   Processor Control Chart Troubleshooting Guide

Processor Problem	Trend in Graph	Image Appearance	Corrective Action
Unsafe darkroom	Sharp increase in B + F with a sudden decrease in the contrast indicator but no change in developer temperature	Increased fog level	Check safelight filter, check for light leaks, check film type and safelight type, check film storage conditions
Developer temperature too high	Sharp increase in speed and contrast indicators, with a smaller increase in B + F	Excessive optical density	Check incoming water temperature or developer thermostat setting
Developer temperature too low	Slight decrease in B + F, with sharp drops in speed and contrast indicators	Optical density too low	Check incoming water temperature or developer thermostat setting
Developer concentration or pH too high	Sharp increase in speed and contrast indicators, with a smaller increase in B + F	Excessive optical density	Check replenishment rates, mix fresh solutions, or both
Developer concentration or pH too low	Sharp increase in speed and contrast indicators, with a smaller increase in B + F	Optical density too low	Check replenishment rates, mix fresh solutions, or both
Underreplenishment	Gradual decline in contrast and speed indicators, with normal values for B + F and developer temperature	Decreased fog level and overall decrease in optical density	Check replenishment rates
Overreplenishment	Increase in B + F level and speed indicator, with a decrease in contrast indicator	Increased fog level and decrease in image contrast	Check replenishment rates
Oxidized developer	Slight increase in B + F, with a decrease in speed and contrast indicators	Loss of image contrast	Drain developer tank and mix fresh solution; add correct amount of starter solution

B + F, Base + fog.

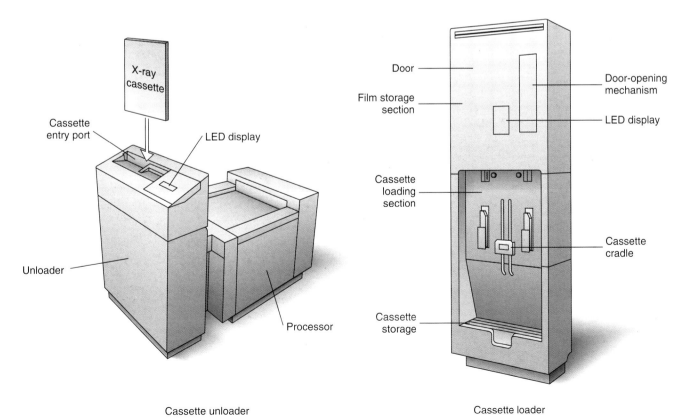

Cassette unloader   Cassette loader

Fig. 4.42 Daylight systems. *LED*, Light-emitting diode.

1. Expose and process five films from the old and new boxes of film with a sensitometer. Do this at the same time, processing the films one after the other. Be sure to identify which five films are from the old box and which five are from the new box.
2. From each film, determine the B + F, MD value, and DD indicators as described previously. Determine an average of these values for the old box of film and the new box of film (see Fig. 4.40).
3. Determine the difference between the boxes of film by subtracting the average of the old box of film from the average of the new box of film.
4. Determine the new operating level for each indicator (B + F, MD, or DD) to be used as the accepted value by taking the original operating level (the accepted value of each indicator used for the original box of film) and adding to it the difference between the boxes determined in step 3. In other words, the new indicator operating level equals the original operating level plus the difference.

DAYLIGHT SYSTEMS

Many diagnostic imaging departments have eliminated traditional darkrooms in favor of daylight systems, which load cassettes automatically with fresh sheets of film and unload exposed cassettes directly into a processor (Fig. 4.42). Because the film is loaded and unloaded from the cassette mechanically, a regular maintenance program is essential for continued proper operation. This program includes cleaning and lubrication of moving parts and replacement of parts as needed. Excessive dirt or dust in the loading section of these systems may enter the cassettes, causing artifacts to appear on subsequent images. It also may result in excessive friction between the sheets of film and the inside of the cassette. Improper loading may occur, and films may become stuck inside the system. Keep the cassette-unloading section of these systems clean and free of dirt so that films unload properly and do not become stuck in the unit (white light exposure may ruin any image present). Create separate areas for loaded and unloaded cassettes and label them clearly. Clean, maintain, and monitor the processing section the same way as conventional film processors. When performing sensitometric tests, create a sensitometry image in a darkroom area as discussed previously. Then, place the film manually into a cassette (obviously, in the darkroom) and unload it into the system so that it can be processed by the daylight system's automatic film processor. At this point, the indicators of processor performance (e.g., B + F or D_{min}) are determined. Maintain temperature and humidity in the area where the daylight system is in use according to the manufacturer's specifications because high humidity results in films sticking together and jamming inside the unit. Humidity that is too low could result in static artifacts on the resulting images.

SUMMARY

Maintaining proper darkroom conditions and procedures is essential to achieving the desired film-based radiographic image. These images also must be displayed with the use of proper viewing conditions for optimum diagnostic capability. Quality control procedures must also be performed for film/screen image receptors and film-based image duplicator units. All radiographers also should have knowledge of image receptor factors such as spatial resolution, contrast resolution, and signal-to-noise ratio, as these factors are also important in discussing image quality with digital image receptors. An established processor quality control program should reduce image variability to a minimum, which should also reduce the number of repeat images required and maintain the acceptable level of image quality established by the facility.

Refer to the Evolve website at https://evolve.elsevier.com for Student Experiments 4.1: Darkroom Fog Check and Viewbox Illuminations; 4.2: Measurement of Spatial Frequency; 4.3: Hyporetention Test; 4.4: Automatic Processor Inspection; 4.5: Quality Control of Mechanized Processors; and 4.6: Daily Processor Quality Control.

REVIEW QUESTIONS

1. Which of the following is the main reason to prohibit food and drink in a film darkroom?
   a. Avoid contamination of processor solutions
   b. Prevent artifacts
   c. Prevent pressure marks on the film
   d. Prevent static artifacts
2. Which of the following terms best describes the amount of light that is emitted from or scattered by a surface?
   a. Photometry
   b. Luminance
   c. Illuminance
   d. Optical density
3. Which of the following names a device that can be used to measure darkroom humidity levels?
   a. Sensitometer
   b. Densitometer
   c. Hydrometer
   d. Psychrometer
4. Proper darkroom ventilation should include how many room changes of air per hour?
   a. 3–5
   b. 6–8
   c. 8–10
   d. 10–12

5. What is the margin of error for the specific gravity of processing solutions?
   a. 0.002
   b. 0.004
   c. 0.006
   d. 0.1
6. When is the best time to process sensitometric films?
   a. Morning, after the processor is warmed up
   b. Late morning or midday, after the peak-demand period
   c. Late afternoon, during the low-demand period
   d. Evening, during the lowest-demand period
7. Which of the following values is the maximum variation allowed for the contrast indicator in daily sensitometric films?
   a. ±0.01
   b. ±0.05
   c. ±0.15
   d. ±0.2

8. Which of the following is located at the bottom of each processing tank?
   a. Entrance rack
   b. Vertical rack
   c. Turnaround rack
   d. Crossover rack
9. Which of the following materials are used in the construction of an entrance roller?
   a. Acrylic plastic (Plexiglas)
   b. Stainless steel
   c. Polyester
   d. Rubberized plastic
10. Hydrogen ions (H^+) that constitute one-ten-thousandth of a molar of a liquid would have which of the following pH values?
   a. 2
   b. 4
   c. 6
   d. 8

Quality Control of X-ray Generators and Ancillary Radiographic Equipment

OBJECTIVES

At the completion of this chapter, the reader should be able to do the following:

- Explain the difference between single-phase, three-phase, and high-frequency X-ray generators
- Recognize the voltage waveform characteristics of the three types of X-ray generators
- List the voltage ripple values for the three types of X-ray generators
- Calculate the power output rating for the three types of X-ray generators
- List the three main parts of a quality control program for radiographic equipment
- List and describe the performance tests for radiographic equipment
- List the main components of an automatic exposure control system
- Perform quality control testing of various automatic exposure control parameters
- Describe the quality control parameters for conventional and digital radiographic tomographic systems
- Discuss the importance of grid uniformity and alignment on image quality
- Explain the quality control tests performed on mobile equipment

KEY TERMS

Actual focal spot
Air kerma
Automatic exposure control
Comparator
Coulomb per kilogram
Detector
Effective focal spot
Focal spot blooming

Gray
Grid latitude
Grid uniformity
Half-value layer
High-frequency
Homogenous phantom
Ion chamber
Kilowatt rating

Law of Reciprocity
Linear tomography
Line focus principle
Linearity
Mobile X-ray generator
Objective plane
Photodetector
Pluridirectional tomography

Portable X-ray generator
Reciprocity
Rectification
Reproducibility

Roentgen
Sensor
Single-phase
Solid-state detector

Three-phase
Voltage ripple

Several of the previous chapters have addressed film/screen image receptors (digital image receptors are discussed in a later chapter) and the importance of quality control testing to avoid poor-quality images. However, many other components of diagnostic imaging departments are subject to variability and must have separate quality control protocols established to ensure safe operation and function. One such component is the equipment used to convert electrical energy into electromagnetic energy (X-rays), commonly called the X-ray unit or X-ray machine. Components of the X-ray machine include the X-ray generator, the control or operating console, a high-voltage generator, and the X-ray tube, tube accessories, and patient support assembly.

X-RAY GENERATOR

The X-ray generator is the largest component of the radiographic unit. It contains the high-voltage transformers, rectifiers, timing circuitry, and milliampere-second (mAs) and kilovolt (peak) (kVp) selectors. Single-phase, three-phase, and high-frequency X-ray generators are available.

Single-Phase Generator

A single source of alternating current is used to power the generator in a single-phase (1Φ) (Greek letter phi) generator. A representation of single-phase alternating current is shown in Fig. 5.1.

The graph in Fig. 5.1 plots the voltage on the y-axis versus time on the x-axis. The peaks in the graph represent the flow of electricity changing direction throughout the circuit. Voltage values range from 0 V to a peak value (hence the term *kilovolts* [*peak*]) and back to 0 V. The two types of single-phase generators used in diagnostic radiography are half-wave rectified and full-wave rectified.

Half-Wave Rectified

Before going any further, we must first define the term *rectification* as it is used in describing different types of X-ray generators. Rectification is the process of changing alternating

current into a pulsating direct current. All types of X-ray machines must carry out rectification because the transformers require alternating current to properly function and X-ray tubes will only function properly with direct current.

In a half-wave rectified generator (sometimes known as a one-pulse, or self-rectified X-ray generator), one-half the normal alternating current wave is used to power the X-ray tube and the other half is shut off by the addition of one or two rectifiers. This design causes the normal single-phase alternating current waveform graph to appear as shown in Fig. 5.2.

Because the standard frequency of alternating current in the United States is 60 Hz, or 60 cycles per second (a cycle represents the current flowing in each direction one time), only 60 pulses of electricity per second (or one pulse per cycle) can be used to create X-rays. This means the X-rays are emitted in pulses, or spurts, and therefore a longer amount of time is required to obtain a specific quantity of X-rays. For this reason, half-wave rectified units are generally used in dental X-ray units and some small portable X-ray units.

Full-Wave Rectified

Full-wave rectified or two-pulse generators use a combination of four rectifiers to channel all the pulses through the X-ray tube during X-ray production. The resultant waveform through the X-ray tube contains two pulses per cycle or 120 pulses per second. The resulting waveform graph for this type of unit appears in Fig. 5.3.

Because 120 pulses of electricity per second can be used to create X-rays, twice as many X-rays can be created per mAs as compared with the half-wave unit. This fact allows full-wave rectified units to be used for many conventional radiographic procedures. However, the X-rays are still emitted in pulses (as demonstrated by the number of times the pulses reach 0 V on the waveform graph) and therefore still require some time to achieve a specific quantity of X-rays. The shortest exposure time available for single-phase X-ray generators is 1/120 second. For this reason, full-wave rectified units are seldom

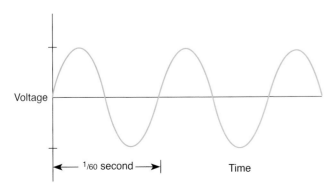

Fig. 5.1 Voltage waveform graph of a single-phase alternating current.

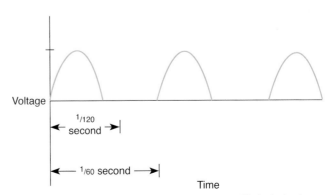

Fig. 5.2 Voltage waveform graph of a half-wave rectified, single-phase current.

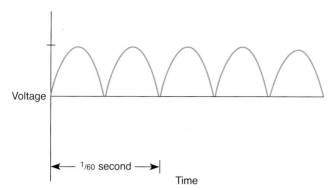

Fig. 5.3 Voltage waveform graph of a full-wave rectified single-phase current.

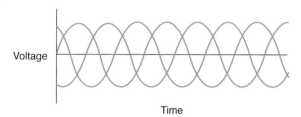

Fig. 5.4 Voltage waveform graph of a three-phase alternating current.

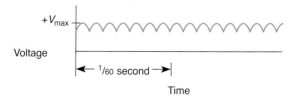

Fig. 5.5 Voltage waveform graph of a three-phase, six-pulse current. V_{max}, Peak voltage across the X-ray tube during X-ray production.

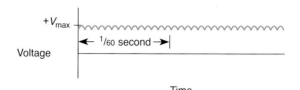

Fig. 5.6 Voltage waveform graph of a three-phase, 12-pulse current. V_{max}, Peak voltage across the X-ray tube during X-ray production.

found in larger hospitals but may be found in doctors' offices and small clinics.

Three-Phase Generator

Three-phase (3Φ) X-ray generators are powered by three separate sources of alternating current that are staggered so they are "out of phase" with one another by 120 degrees, or one-third of a cycle. The voltage waveform graph for three-phase alternating current appears in Fig. 5.4.

By the time one pulse of current begins to drop toward 0 V, another pulse is heading back up to the maximum value, so the voltage never reaches 0 V and X-rays are produced constantly (eliminating the pulsed effect of single-phase units), which allows exposure time values as low as 1/1000 second (1 ms). The X-rays created with three-phase units also have a greater average energy than those of single-phase units because the voltage is near the peak value for a greater percentage of the time during X-ray production (which can lower patient dose compared with single-phase units). The main disadvantages of three-phase equipment are greater capital cost (at least twice as expensive as a single-phase unit) and the size of the unit (because of the additional electronic components required). In general, the advantages outweigh the disadvantages, and the three-phase X-ray generator has been the most common type of unit in major hospitals and medical centers up until the year 2000. The two types of three-phase generators are six-pulse and 12-pulse generators.

Three-Phase, Six-Pulse Generators

The six-pulse type of three-phase unit uses six rectifiers and one-half the three-phase alternating current pulses. The resulting voltage waveform appears in Fig. 5.5.

As mentioned previously, one cycle of single-phase alternating current refers to one pulse of electricity traveling each direction one time so that two pulses comprise one cycle. Because 60 cycles occur each second, one cycle requires a time of 1/60 second. In a three-phase, six-pulse X-ray generator, six pulses of electricity exist during the same cycle or 1/60-second time interval (instead of two pulses per 1/60 second in single phase), hence the name *three-phase, six-pulse*. This means that 360 voltage pulses are now available per second.

Three-Phase, 12-Pulse Generators

The three-phase, 12-pulse type of X-ray generator uses 12 rectifiers (four rectifiers per phase) that direct all the three-phase alternating current pulses through the X-ray tube during X-ray production. This action yields 12 pulses of electricity per one-cycle (1/60-second) time interval, for a total of 720 voltage pulses available per second. This unit is more efficient than the three-phase, six-pulse unit but is more expensive in capital cost. The voltage waveform for a three-phase, 12-pulse X-ray generator appears in Fig. 5.6.

High-Frequency Generator

Developed during the late 1970s, high-frequency X-ray generators were the newest generators available. They are sometimes referred to as *medium-frequency generators*, depending on the design and manufacturer. These units can be supplied with either a single-phase or three-phase source of alternating current that is first fed into a microprocessor circuit before entering the high-voltage section. This microprocessor changes the frequency of the alternating current from the standard 60 Hz to as much as 100,000 Hz in some of the more recent models. It is then rectified and smoothed with capacitors before application across the X-ray tube, which causes the pulses to merge together and results in a voltage waveform such as the one that appears in Fig. 5.7.

High-frequency generators and three-phase generators produce similar voltage waveforms. However, the capital cost and power requirements for high-frequency units are far less than those for three-phase units. The transformers in

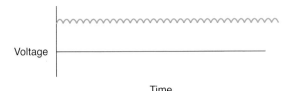

Fig. 5.7 Voltage waveform graph showing the resulting current through the X-ray tube in a high-frequency X-ray generator.

high-frequency units can be smaller because they are much more efficient at higher frequencies (according to Faraday's Law of Electromagnetism), which accounts for the lower capital cost. The transformers also reduce the space requirement for installation. Because these units yield most of the advantages of a three-phase unit but at a fraction of the cost, they have become the most commonly utilized X-ray systems in hospitals, medical centers, clinics, and doctors' offices.

Voltage Ripple

Voltage ripple is a term used often to distinguish the voltage waveforms of each type of X-ray generator. A voltage ripple is the amount of variation from the peak voltage that occurs during X-ray production. The voltage ripple value is determined by the following equation:

$$\% \text{voltage ripple} = \left(V_{max} - V_{min}\right) / V_{max} \times 100$$

V_{max} is the peak voltage across the X-ray tube during X-ray production, while V_{min} is the lowest voltage across the tube during X-ray production. For single-phase units, the voltage ripple is considered to be 100% because the voltage drops from its peak all the way to 0 V before increasing again, so 100% of all possible voltages are obtained. For three-phase equipment, the voltage does not decrease all the way to 0 V. One pulse increases as soon as the previous one falls, which yields a voltage ripple of 13% for a three-phase, six-pulse generator and a ripple of 3.5% for a three-phase, 12-pulse unit. High-frequency generators can create voltage ripple values between 1% and 15%, which are comparable with those of three-phase units.

Power Ratings

The power output of an X-ray generator is used to measure the capacity of X-ray production from the individual unit. This value is measured in kilowatts (kW) and is called the **kilowatt rating**. It is usually calculated by determining the maximum combinations of kVp and milliamperes (mA) that can be achieved by a particular generator at an exposure time of 100 ms. These two values are then placed into the following equations:

$$\text{Three-phase and high-frequency kW} = \frac{kVp \times mA}{1000}$$

$$\text{Single-phase kW} = \frac{kVp \times mA \times 0.707}{1000}$$

The rippling effect of the single-phase alternating current requires that the 0.707 multiplier be added to the equation.

The greater the power rating of the X-ray generator, the higher the purchase price of the system.

CONTROL OR OPERATING CONSOLE

The control or operating console contains all the various controls to operate the X-ray machine (e.g., kVp selector, mAs selector) and various meters to monitor the production of X-rays. Guidelines by the US Food and Drug Administration mandate that diagnostic X-ray machine operating consoles must indicate the conditions of exposure (kVp, mAs) and when the X-ray tube is energized. The conditions of exposure usually are indicated by the mAs and kVp selection mechanism (i.e., the mAs or kVp buttons or computer touch pad keys that are pushed). There is also either an analog or a digital milliamp-second meter to indicate the quantity of X-rays produced by the X-ray unit. These meters also are used to indicate energized X-ray tubes and to detect lights or audible signals. Characteristics for the control booth area, which houses the operating console of a radiographic X-ray unit, include the following:

1. The floor of the control booth must be 7.5 ft² or larger.
2. The exposure switch should be fixed within the booth at a position at least 30 inches from any open edge of the booth wall and should be closest to the examining table.
3. X-ray photons must scatter at least twice before they can enter any opening in the control booth. Each time an X-ray photon scatters, its intensity from the scattering object is 1/1000 of the original intensity at a distance of 1 m.
4. The control booth window must have the same shielding requirements as the walls (usually a 1.5-mm lead equivalent), be at least 1 ft² in size, and be mounted at least 5 feet above the floor. There should be no obstructions blocking the view of the patient table.
5. The wall of the control booth, facing the radiographic examination table, must be at least 7 feet high and fixed to the floor.
6. Any door on the control booth that is an entrance to the examination room should be interlocked with the control panel so that an exposure cannot be made unless the door is closed.

HIGH-VOLTAGE GENERATOR

The high-voltage generator of the radiographic unit is responsible for converting the relatively low-voltage values supplied by the power companies (usually 220–440 V) to the kilovolt levels necessary for the production of diagnostic radiographs. Included in this generator is a high-tension transformer, which is a shell-type step-up transformer that increases the voltage level selected using an autotransformer to the kilovolts selected on the control console. Also included in the high-voltage generator is a filament (step-down) transformer that feeds a stepped-down voltage level to the filament of the X-ray tube. This area also may contain rectifiers that convert the alternating current of the incoming power supply to a pulsating direct current that is fed to the X-ray tube for X-ray production. The number of rectifiers ranges from 4 to 12 depending on the type of X-ray generator and are usually solid state in nature. The high-voltage generator is normally housed in a metal box that may be found in the X-ray room or in a nearby area, such as the control booth. High-voltage cables (one going to the cathode of the X-ray tube and another to the anode) connect the high-voltage generator to the X-ray tube.

X-RAY TUBE, TUBE ACCESSORIES, AND PATIENT SUPPORT ASSEMBLY

The third main part of any radiographic X-ray unit is a combination of the X-ray tube, X-ray tube support mechanism, patient support assembly (i.e., X-ray examination table), and X-ray tube accessories such as the collimator and added filtration. Most radiographic X-ray tubes are rotating anode X-ray tubes that can withstand greater kVp and mAs combinations than the stationary anode X-ray tubes used in dental offices and in small portable X-ray machines. The X-ray tube must be equipped with a metal housing to prevent leakage of radiation. This housing must confine the leakage amount to less than 100 mR per hour (1 mGy per hour air kerma) when measured at a distance of 1 m away from the housing. The X-ray tube must also be equipped with a variable-aperture collimator to control the size of the X-ray field (discussed in detail later in this chapter). The X-ray tube support mechanism that holds the X-ray tube in position over the bucky device must have the following characteristics (the bucky device contains the image receptor and is taught to X-ray students on the first day of the program):

1. The support mechanism must be strong because the X-ray tube, insulating coil, collimator, and metal housing are heavy.
2. The support mechanism should be counterbalanced to help offset the weight of the X-ray tube and accessory devices. This design makes the assembly more stable and allows it to be moved more easily during patient positioning.
3. Immobilization locks must be incorporated into the support mechanism to hold the X-ray tube in position.
4. In relation to the image receptor, the X-ray tube position must be indicated clearly (source-to-image distance [SID] indicator) and must be accurate to within 2% of the SID.

In addition, if a radiographic examination table is present (as opposed to an upright bucky or chest unit), the maximum tabletop thickness over the bucky assembly is 1 mm of aluminum equivalent to prevent the tabletop material from absorbing excessive amounts of radiation before reaching the image receptor (which would, therefore increase the patient dose).

QUALITY CONTROL PROGRAM FOR RADIOGRAPHIC UNITS

When the X-ray equipment has been installed successfully and has passed all acceptance tests, it needs to be monitored periodically to ensure it continues to perform according to the manufacturer's specifications. This periodic testing is the quality control testing of the equipment. The main goal of this quality control program is to ensure consistent, high-quality diagnostic images, minimize radiation exposure to both

patient and department staff, and help in cost effectiveness by reducing downtime and waste. The three parts of a quality control program for radiographic equipment are visual inspection, environmental inspection, and performance testing. These tests should be performed upon acceptance of new equipment (or after a major repair of existing equipment) and then at least annually. Any items that are found to not meet manufacturer's specifications will need to be corrected or repaired. Most states and accrediting agencies require that all records of corrections or repairs be maintained for inspection. In addition, records of quality control testing should also be maintained in either written form or in a computerized database.

Visual Inspection

Visual inspection includes checking the main components of the equipment to ensure that there are no hazardous, inoperative, out-of-alignment, or improperly operating items in the system. This inspection should be performed at least annually (monthly for American College of Radiology accreditation), with a checklist for documentation. An example of this checklist is provided on the Evolve website. The inspection should include the control console, overhead tube crane, radiographic table, protective lead apparel, and miscellaneous equipment.

Control Console

The control console contains all the selectors for controlling X-ray production (mAs, kVp, and the various meters that monitor the operation of the generator). Control console inspection includes verifying the proper function of X-ray tube heat sensors and the overload protection indicator (discussed later in this chapter). The proper functioning of all panel lights, meters, and switches must be verified as well. The exposure switch must be at least 30 inches from any opening and fixed to the control console. The inspection should ensure a proper view of the exposure room through the window (an unobstructed view of the examination table) and the presence of an up-to-date technique chart that is displayed near the control panel. A technique chart provides technical factors, anatomical examination, patient thickness for examination being performed, proper exposure indicator ranges for the digital imaging system in use, and SID needed to make clinical radiographs when the radiographic system is in manual mode. Most states as well as accrediting agencies require that a technique chart relevant to the particular X-ray machine shall be provided or electronically displayed in the vicinity of the control panel and used by all operators.

Overhead Tube Crane

The overhead tube crane is the mounting bracket that holds the X-ray tube over the X-ray table. Items to evaluate in this section include the condition of the high-voltage cables and other wires (are they discolored or frayed?); the condition of the cable brackets, clamps, or tie-downs (are they intact and functioning normally?); the stability of the system; proper movement; SID and angulation indicator function (discussed later in this chapter); detent operation; lock function;

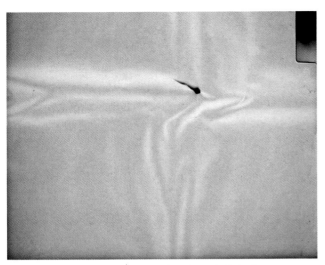

Fig. 5.8 Image of lead apron with a large hole in the center.

the bucky center light; collimator light brightness (discussed later in this chapter); and interlock function. Also, ensure that there are no oil leaks around the X-ray tube and generator, and that these are free from dust.

Radiographic Table

A patient is usually in contact with the X-ray table throughout the diagnostic procedure, so it must be kept clean and safe. Items to inspect include surface condition and cleanliness of the tabletop, power top and angulation switches, bucky tray and cassette locks, stability, table angulation indicator (use a protractor to verify the indicator is accurate to within ±2 degrees), and the condition of any footboard or shoulder braces. The tabletop material over the bucky area should not absorb more than 1.0 mm of aluminum equivalent.

Protective Lead Apparel

Lead aprons and gloves should be present in the radiographic room and should have a minimum 0.25 mm of lead-equivalent thickness. Standards set forth by accrediting agencies dictate that healthcare organizations must perform routine inspections on protective lead apparel for defects such as holes, cracks, and tears on an annual basis. These checks may be performed by visual or tactile means or X-ray imaging. If X-ray imaging is utilized, they can be radiographed or viewed fluoroscopically (with remote fluoroscopy if possible) on acceptance and then every 6 months thereafter to determine whether any cracks or holes are present (Fig. 5.8). If a defect is found, protective devices shall be replaced or removed from service until repaired. Keep a record of when these inspections are performed, as well as the results and any corrective action as documentation for accrediting agencies. Software programs are available for maintaining these inspection reports. When not in use, protective lead apparel should be properly hung on clothing hangers to prevent cracks. Lead vinyl sheets and gonadal shields also should be evaluated in the same manner. If a piece of lead protective apparel is no longer usable, it must be disposed of in an appropriate manner. According to the Health Physics Society, lead and other heavy metals meet the criteria for hazardous materials under the Resource Conservation and Recovery Act. The best option for disposal is to recycle the protective apparel so the lead can be reused.

Miscellaneous Equipment

A measuring caliper should be present in radiographic rooms in which the manual technique is used along with a technique chart to establish the correct exposure factors. Ensure that positioning sponges and other patient position aids are clean and free of contrast media. Check the manual integrity of any stepstools or intravenous fluid stands as well.

Environmental Inspection

Environmental inspection should be performed at least annually (it may need to be performed more frequently with older equipment), and it involves general observation of mechanical and electrical integrity and stability. Often, it can be performed along with the visual inspection.

- Mechanical Integrity—Key items to look for are the presence of loose or absent screws, bolts, or other structural elements that may have been improperly installed or have worked loose due to use. The functioning of meters, dials, and other indicators should be checked.
- Mechanical Stability—Of key importance from the equipment side are the stability and stiffness of the X-ray tube support and image receptor (i.e., table bucky or wall-mounted cassette holder). The mechanical condition of the X-ray tube counterweights and tracks (especially in overhead tube stands) must also be included in the environmental inspection. Lubricate the moving parts. The availability and adequacy of patient support devices such as the table or immobilizing devices should also be checked. In addition, it is important to check the reproducibility of positioning of the source and image receptor that may be indicated or controlled by physical marks or detents. A check of the accuracy of angulation scale should be made. As part of the check of structural stability, an inspection of the electrical and/or mechanical locks on the machine should be carried out.
- Electrical Integrity—One item included in this portion of the environmental inspection is evaluation of the condition of the X-ray tube high-tension cables, which is accomplished by checking the covering on the outside of the cables (or any other wires that are visible on the outside of the unit). Any discoloration of the outside insulation, especially where the wire or cable bends, could be an indicator of internal heat and a potential short circuit. Check to make sure that the retaining rings at the termination points are tight and that there are no breaks in the insulation. It is important to observe the "lay" of the cables. If they do not hang properly, they can interfere with the positioning of the tube and may fail prematurely. Consult a biomedical engineer, medical physicist, or vendor service technician if discoloration is present.
- Electrical Safety—Electrical safety is critical for both the patient and the equipment operator. The system should be checked by a safety engineer. This involves a physical

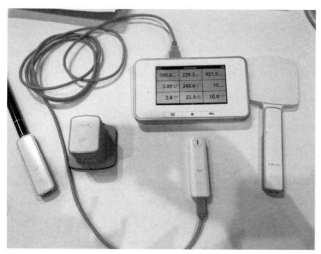

Fig. 5.9 The noninvasive evaluation of radiation output system is a microprocessor that can be programmed to acquire and analyze exposure data, providing quality control test results for numerous parameters.

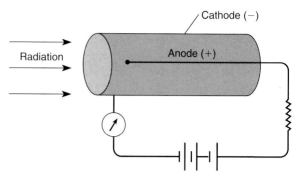

Fig. 5.10 Schematic diagram of an ion chamber.

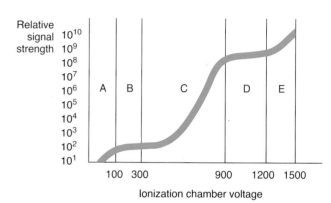

Fig. 5.11 Graph showing how the intensity of the signal from a gas-filled detector increases as the voltage across the chamber increases. (A) Region of recombination; (B) ionization region; (C) proportional region; (D) Geiger–Müller region; (E) region of continuous discharge.

inspection of the electrical wiring. Key areas where problems often occur include the power cord to light indicators in the beam limitation system, the wires to the exposure hand switch, and other similar power hookups. Verify that all elements are well grounded (to each other and to the ground). All radiographic equipment should be electrically grounded, and all obvious electrical connections should be intact.

Should the possibility of a short circuit exist, never touch an electrical device with one hand while the other hand is touching any type of conductor; doing so directs the flow of electricity through the heart. If someone is experiencing an electric shock, do not grasp the person directly. Instead, either open the main switch (turn off the power) or use some type of insulator (dry wooden board) to separate the person from the source of the electricity. A good rule of thumb to remember when dealing with electric current is that the combination of high voltage and low amperage tends to throw a person, whereas a combination of low voltage and high amperage tends to hold a person and is potentially more dangerous. For older equipment or equipment that has a history of problems with electrical safety, a biomedical engineer, medical physicist, or vendor service technician should be consulted for environmental inspections (you may also wish to have them accompany you during these inspections). Many states require that an electrical inspection record be posted on the equipment.

Performance Testing

Performance testing evaluates the performance of the X-ray generator and X-ray tube with specialized test instrumentation, which can range from simple phantoms and test tools to sophisticated computerized systems such as the RaySafe X2 X-ray Measurement System (Fig. 5.9) or similar devices available from various manufacturers. These computerized systems make the data gathering for performance evaluations quick and easy, but they can cost thousands of dollars. It is more common for facilities to use several smaller devices to gather the necessary data. The results of these tests must be documented for both governmental and accreditation agencies. Most states and accreditation agencies require these performance tests be performed by a medical physicist. However, radiographers should know how the tests are performed and how to interpret the results. Sample forms for many of these tests are provided on the accompanying Evolve website.

Radiation Measurement

Much of the data obtained during performance testing include radiation measurement; therefore some type of radiation detector is a standard piece of equipment for many of these tests. The more common type of detector used in performance testing is the gas-filled chamber. As radiation enters this chamber, it ionizes the gas along its path (Fig. 5.10), which produces a trail of ions that allows the flow of current through the chamber for a split second. This current is converted to a voltage pulse that is amplified and counted. The size of the voltage pulse is proportional to the energy expended in the chamber by the incident radiation. A quenching material may be added to the chamber to speed the return of ions to a stable state. There are three types of gas-filled chamber detectors, which vary according to the chamber voltage (Fig. 5.11): the ion chamber, the proportional counter, and the Geiger–Müller counter.

Ion chamber. With 100–300 V placed on it, the ion chamber is the least sensitive of the three chambers. The ion chamber is useful for measuring X-rays because a high sensitivity is not required for their detection; ion chambers are often used

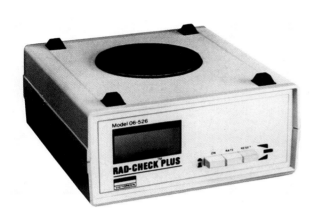

Fig. 5.12 Digital dosimeter. (Courtesy Gammex/RMI, Middleton, Wisconsin.)

in performance testing. They usually are available as pocket ionization chambers (also called *pocket dosimeters*) and analog or digital dosimeters (Fig. 5.12). They also can be used as the sensor in automatic exposure control (AEC) systems and as the detectors in computed tomographic scanners.

Proportional counter. A voltage of 300–900 V placed on the chamber increases the sensitivity. Proportional counters are often used in stationary laboratory counters to measure small quantities of radioactive material.

Geiger–Müller counter. A voltage of 900–1200 V placed on the chamber yields the greatest sensitivity. Geiger–Müller counters often are used for contamination control in nuclear medicine departments.

Some newer types of radiation-monitoring devices use a solid-state or semiconducting detector instead of an ionization chamber. These models incorporate a crystal of either silicon or germanium with selected impurities (such as lithium) added to detect the incident radiation. When the crystal is attached to an electric current, little or no current can flow through the crystal because no free electrons are available.

If the crystal is exposed to radiation, electrons are dislodged within its matrix and electric current can flow through it. The increase in current is proportional to the amount of radiation incident on the crystal and is registered with an analog or digital meter. This type of detector is relatively small and accurate but usually costs more than ionization chambers. It is also more sensitive than a gas-filled chamber. In most gases, an average energy of 30–40 electron volts (eV) is expended per ion pair produced. In a silicon semiconductor, an ion pair is produced for each 3.5 eV deposited by the incident radiation. For germanium detectors, only 2.9 eV are required to produce an ion pair, which means many more ion pairs are produced in semiconductor detectors (compared with ion chambers) for a given amount of energy absorbed.

The value obtained from the radiation detector is most often the radiation intensity, which can be measured in a special unit called the Roentgen (R), in an International System of units called coulomb per kilogram (C/kg), or in air kerma,

which uses an International System or units called the Gray (Gy). KERMA is an acronym for **k**inetic **e**nergy **r**eleased in **ma**tter and measures the amount of kinetic energy transferred into charged particles (such as electrons) by X-rays or gamma rays. It is expressed in units of joules per kilogram or gray. Air kerma is often used instead of the traditional SI unit of C/kg to express radiation intensity. 1 R = 8.76 mGy of air kerma.

K_{air} (Gy) = 0.00876 (Gy/R) × (R), so 1 Gy is approximately equal to 100 Roentgen.

$$1\,mR = 0.01\,mGy$$
$$1\,R = 2.58 \times 10^{14}\,C/kg$$
$$1\,C/kg = 3.88 \times 10^{3}\,R$$

Because both units measure a relatively large amount of radiation, smaller increments of milliroentgens (mR) or microcoulombs per kilogram (μC/kg) are most often obtained during performance testing. Some detectors are designed so that the exposure rate (intensity of radiation per unit of time) can be displayed in addition to the radiation intensity, and they are known as *rate meters*. Detectors also can be calibrated to measure absorbed dosage in rads or grays. One rad is equivalent to 0.01 Gy or 1 cGy.

Reproducibility of Exposure

An X-ray generator should always produce the same intensity of radiation each time the same set of technical factors is used to make an exposure. For example, if 80 kVp, 500 mA, and 0.02 second yields 100 units of radiation when measured with a dosimeter, then at any future time when the same technical factors are entered into the same X-ray generator, the yield, when tested, should also be 100 units. This concept is known as reproducibility. *The maximum variability allowed in reproducibility is ±5% according to (1020.31(b)), 21 Code of Federal Regulations Subchapter J.* Evaluation of reproducibility variance requires a dosimeter, unless a computerized noninvasive system is used. Reproducibility testing should be performed after equipment installation, after a major system repair, and then annually.

PROCEDURE: REPRODUCIBILITY OF EXPOSURE

1. Place a lead apron on top of a radiographic tabletop with the center of the lead apron in the approximate center of the tabletop. Place a dosimeter on top of the lead apron. The lead apron absorbs backscatter from the tabletop material, which reduces the accuracy of any readings obtained. If a lead apron is unavailable, substitute a sheet of lead vinyl. Center the central ray of the X-ray beam on the dosimeter using a SID of 40 inches. Collimate the beam so that the X-ray field is just slightly larger than the dosimeter or remote probe.

2. Make a series of three to five separate exposures of the dosimeter at 80 kVp and 10 mAs. Clear the dosimeter (reset to zero) after each exposure. Record each reading on some type of documentation form, such as the Radiographic Survey Form found on the Evolve website.

Continued

3. With the readings obtained, use the following equation to determine reproducibility variance:

$$\text{Reproducibility variance} = \frac{(\text{Exposure or air kerma}_{max} - \text{exposure or air kerma}_{min})}{(\text{Exposure or air kerma}_{max} + \text{exposure or air kerma}_{min})}$$

where exposure or air kerma$_{max}$ is the maximum amount of milliroentgens or µC/kg air exposure or mGy of air kerma, and exposure$_{min}$ is the minimum amount of milliroentgens or µC/kg air exposure or mGy of air kerma.

The calculated variance should be less than 0.05 (5%) for a properly functioning X-ray generator. This test should be performed after installation of new equipment and then annually or when service is performed on the X-ray generator or X-ray tube. Variations in X-ray generator performance (e.g., kVp selector, milliamp (mA) selector, rectifier failure) or X-ray tube operation (e.g., filament evaporation, arcing) can cause the reproducibility variance to exceed accepted limits, which produces radiographs of inconsistent quality and necessitates repeat patient exposure to radiation.

X-ray Beam Quantity

X-ray generators should emit a specific amount of radiation (measured in milliroentgens or milligray air kerma) per unit of X-ray tube current and time (mAs). In addition, similar types of X-ray generators and tubes in a department should emit the same values of milliroentgens per mAs, microcoulombs per kilogram per mAs, or milligray per mAs of air kerma, so that technique charts can be valid in all rooms and the number of repeat examinations can be reduced. The original value of milliroentgens per mAs, microcoulombs per kilogram per mAs, or milligray per mAs is determined after installation of the unit or at the start of the quality control program. This original value is usually obtained at 80 kVp, 100-cm SID, and 2.5-mm aluminum total filtration. The beam quantity (also known as radiation output) is then measured annually and compared with this original value. The original installation value and future values should be within ±10% of each other in a properly functioning X-ray generator. In addition, values obtained in different radiographic rooms with similar X-ray generators and tubes also should be compared and should fall within ±10% of each other to establish room-to-room consistency. If these rooms exceed the 10% variation limit, they should have separate technique charts provided for each room. The beam quantity for single-phase generators should be approximately 4.0 ± 0.8 mR/mAs (1.0 ± 0.2 µC/kg/mAs) (0.04 ± 0.08 mGy/mAs air kerma) at 80 kVp, 100-cm SID, and 2.5-mm aluminum total filtration, whereas three-phase and high-frequency units should be approximately 2.5 mm 6.0 ± 1 mR/mAs (1.5 ± 0.25 µC/kg/mAs) (0.06 ± 0.01 mGy/mAs air kerma) at 80 kVp, 100-cm SID, and 2.5-mm aluminum filtration.

Many states and The Joint Commission require the posting of this value to guarantee the X-ray generator does not emit excessive amounts of radiation exposure for a given combination of kVp per mAs. These values are also important to

help achieve diagnostic reference levels and achievable doses discussed in Chapter 1.

X-ray Beam Quality

X-ray beam quality refers to the energy or penetrating power of the X-ray beam. When discussing beam quality, there are two types that are important. The maximum beam quality refers to the highest energy X-rays within the beam and is determined by the kVp. This is why kVp accuracy is a performance test and is discussed later in this chapter. The other type of beam quality is the average beam quality, which refers to the average of all the different X-ray energies in a beam. It is affected by the type of X-ray generator and the amount of filtration in the beam. Since filtration significantly effects average beam quality, it can be used as a measurement of radiation quality at a specific kVp and X-ray generator type.

Proper filtration is necessary to remove low-energy photons from the X-ray beam (1020.30(m), 21 CFR Subchapter J). A patient's skin dose can increase by as much as 90% if the photons are not removed. This test should be performed after installation and then annually or whenever service is performed on the X-ray tube or collimator. The best method to determine whether adequate filtration exists is to measure the half-value layer (HVL), which is the amount of filtration that reduces the exposure rate to one-half its initial value, because it is not usually possible to measure inherent filtration. The reason the measurement is not easily acquired is a result of filament evaporation that takes place continually, which adds a layer of tungsten to the inside of the X-ray tube window. By measuring the HVL (which measures beam quality) instead of the total amount of filtration, it does not matter how much material is in the path of the beam as long as sufficient beam quality is measured and obtained. Using HVL for determining sufficient filtration is also relatively easy and is noninvasive. The HVL should not vary from its original value (which is established after installation) or its value at the beginning of the quality control program. It is dependent on the kVp used, the total beam filtration, and the type of X-ray generator (Fig. 5.13, Table 5.1).

1. Place a dosimeter on the radiographic tabletop on top of a lead apron or sheet of lead vinyl, with an SID of 40 inches or 100 cm (just as in step 1 of the procedure to determine reproducibility).
2. Make an exposure at 80 kVp, 100 mA (large focal spot), and 100 ms (10 mAs). Some physicists recommend that the dosimeter be placed under a homogenous phantom of aluminum or acrylic plates or in the bucky for this measurement; any of these is satisfactory, but the test must always be performed the same way so the values can be compared for variation.
3. Divide the radiation measurement recorded from the dosimeter by 10 mAs to obtain the value of milliroentgens per mAs, microcoulombs per kilogram, or milligray of air kerma per mAs. Record this value and repeat the test at least annually (with the same procedure and exposure factors).

PROCEDURE: X-RAY BEAM QUANTITY—cont'd

Compare the current and previous readings, then determine the percent variation with the following equation:

$$\text{Percent variation} = \frac{(\text{Exposure or air kerma}_{max} - \text{Exposure or air kerma}_{min}) \times 100}{\text{Exposure or air kerma}_{max}}$$

The original installation value and future values should be within ±10% of each other in a properly functioning X-ray generator. In addition, values obtained in different radiographic rooms with similar X-ray generators and tubes also should be compared and should fall within ±10% of one another to establish room-to-room consistency. If these rooms exceed the 10% variation limit, they should have separate technique charts provided for each room. Variation in milliroentgens per mAs (microcoulombs per kilogram per mAs or milligray per mAs of air kerma) for a single room can occur over time as a result of problems in X-ray generator calibration, timer circuit inaccuracy, and filament evaporation from the cathode of the X-ray tube (some of the tungsten from the filament is deposited on the inside of the window of the X-ray tube, which causes additional filtration of the beam).

A quick test to determine whether adequate filtration is present can be performed in cases in which HVL measurements cannot be made. However, this quick test indicates the presence of adequate filtration only and not the actual amount of filtration; therefore it should not take the place of HVL measurements during formal quality control testing. Using this method, a dosimeter and a 2.3-mm-thick aluminum plate are used.

TABLE 5.1 Minimum HVL for Diagnostic X-ray Units

X-RAY TUBE VOLTAGE (KILOVOLT [PEAK])		MINIMUM HVL (mm ALUMINUM)	
Designed Operation Range	Measured Operating Potential	Specified Dental Systems	Other X-ray Systems
<50	30	1.5	0.3
	40	1.5	0.4
	49	1.5	0.5
50–70	50	1.5	1.2
	60	1.5	1.3
	70	1.5	1.5
>70	71	2.1	2.1
	80	2.3	2.3
	90	2.5	2.3
	100	2.7	2.7
	110	3.0	3.0
	120	3.2	3.2
	130	3.5	3.5
	140	3.8	3.8
	150	4.1	4.1

HVL, Half-value layer.

Kilovolt (Peak) Accuracy

The X-ray tube voltage (measured in kVp) has a significant effect on image contrast, optical density, and patient dose. Therefore the kVp stated on the control panel should produce an X-ray beam with a comparable and consistent amount of energy. ***Variations between the stated kVp and the X-ray beam quality must be within ±5%.*** For example, if 80 kVp is selected on the control panel, the maximum X-ray beam energy should fall within ±4 kVp of this value. The kVp accuracy can be determined using a specialized test cassette (film/screen departments only), such as the Wisconsin Test Cassette (Fig. 5.14), Ardan and Crook's cassette, or a digital kVp meter (Fig. 5.15), according to the respective manufacturers' instructions. The digital meters are usually more accurate and easier to use (because when they are exposed, the measured kVp appears automatically with a light-emitting diode [LED] readout) but are more expensive than the test cassettes. The test cassettes require that a film be placed inside and exposed to a specific set of technical factors. The resulting image is then analyzed visually or with a densitometer to obtain the measured kVp. Whichever device is used for this test, it should estimate the peak voltage at various kVp stations available for the particular X-ray generator being evaluated. This process should be done in 10- to 20-kVp increments, usually beginning with 50 kVp. This test should be performed after installation and then annually or when service is performed on the X-ray generator or tube. Variations in kVp output may be caused by variations in the line voltage supplying the X-ray generator, by faulty high-voltage cables, or by problems with the autotransformer/kVp selection circuitry.

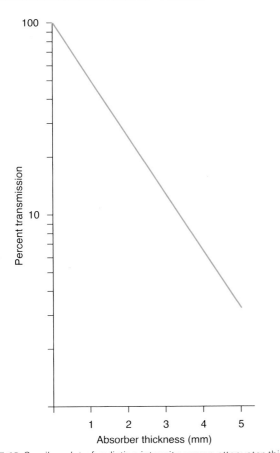

Fig. 5.13 Semilog plot of radiation intensity versus attenuator thickness for determination of the half-value layer.

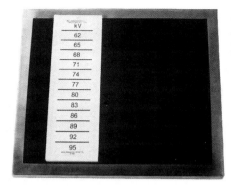

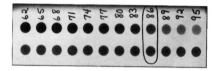

Fig. 5.14 Wisconsin Test Cassette. (Courtesy Gammex/RMI, Middleton, Wisconsin.)

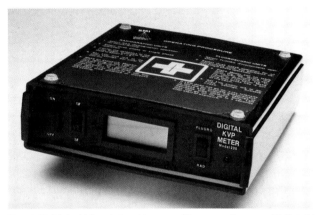

Fig. 5.15 Digital kilovolt (peak) meter. (Courtesy Gammex/RMI, Middleton, Wisconsin.)

PROCEDURE: HALF-VALUE LAYER

1. Place a dosimeter on the radiographic tabletop on top of a lead apron or lead vinyl (to prevent backscatter).
2. Adjust the tube-to-dosimeter distance to between 60 and 80 cm and collimate the X-ray beam to an area slightly larger than the dosimeter.
3. Make an exposure at 80 kVp and 50 mAs and record the amount of radiation from the dosimeter on a documentation form such as the HVL Evaluation Form found on the Evolve website.
4. Clear the dosimeter and add a 1-mm-thick aluminum plate between the bottom of the collimator and the dosimeter and expose it. Record the reading and clear the dosimeter. Repeat this procedure, adding aluminum plates in 1-mm increments until a total of 6–8 mm are in place.
5. Use semilog graph paper and plot a graph of X-ray intensity (dosimeter readings) on the y-axis versus absorber thickness on the x-axis (see Fig. 5.13). Draw in a curve by connecting the dots in the graph. The HVL is determined by taking one-half the maximum dosimeter reading and then

drawing a line from this point on the y-axis to the curve, then drawing another line from this point on the curve down to the x-axis. This value on the x-axis represents the HVL, and it should be greater than 2.3 mm or more because this is the minimum HVL at 80 kVp, according to the Food and Drug Administration. HVL amounts at various kVp values are given in Table 5.1.

PROCEDURE: FILTRATION QUICK TEST

1. Place the dosimeter on the radiographic table on top of a lead apron.
2. Make an exposure at an SID of 40 inches at 80 kVp and 50 mAs, and record the reading.
3. Clear the dosimeter and make a second exposure using the same technical factors but with the aluminum plate between the detector and the X-ray source.
4. Place the readings obtained into the following equation:

$$\frac{\text{Exposure with aluminum plate}}{\text{Exposure without aluminum plate}}$$

If adequate filtration is present, the number obtained from the equation should range from 0.5 to 0.75. If the number is less than 0.5, beam filtration is inadequate. If the number is greater than 0.75, excessive filtration exists, which is legally acceptable but can be an indicator of pending X-ray tube failure because of excessive tungsten deposits on the X-ray tube window resulting from filament evaporation.

Voltage Waveform

As discussed previously, each type of X-ray generator creates a distinctive voltage waveform. If the waveform could be displayed on an oscilloscope screen during X-ray production, considerable information could be obtained concerning kVp accuracy, timer accuracy, rectifier malfunctions, loading characteristics, contact or switching problems, and high-voltage cable or connector arcing (Fig. 5.16) because these variables affect the size or shape of the waveform. An oscilloscope is hooked up electronically (only by personnel with an extensive electronics background such as physicists, biomedical engineers, or service engineers) to specific areas of the X-ray generator, or it can be attached to a commercially available X-ray output detector (Fig. 5.17). This detector is placed in the X-ray beam, and the output cable is connected to the oscilloscope input. Newer versions of the output detector can be attached to a laptop computer, iPad, or similar device to view the output waveform. The display is then analyzed for potential problems and is documented for future reference. These waveforms should appear to be stable to within ±5% from initiation to at least 100 ms and should show no spikes or dropouts during any exposure. The rise time (when voltage increases from 0 V to the peak voltage) should represent less than 1% of the total exposure time, whereas the fall time (when the voltage decreases from the peak back to 0 V at the end of the exposure) should represent less than 10% of the total exposure time. This test should be performed on installation and then annually or

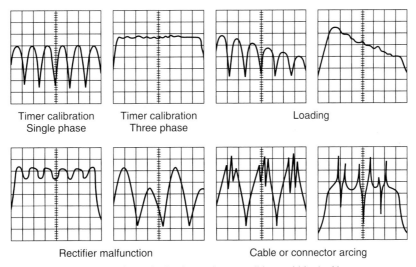

Timer calibration
Single phase

Timer calibration
Three phase

Loading

Rectifier malfunction

Cable or connector arcing

Fig. 5.16 Voltage waveforms indicating various conditions within the X-ray generator.

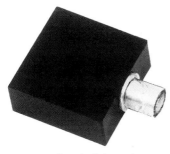

Fig. 5.17 Output detector for obtaining voltage waveforms. (Courtesy Nuclear Associates, Inc., Carle Place, New York.)

Timer Accuracy

On systems with separate mA and time selection, exposure time directly affects the total quantity of radiation emitted from an X-ray tube; therefore an accurate exposure timer is critical for acquiring properly exposed image receptors and reasonable patient radiation exposure. ***The variability allowed for timer accuracy is ±5% for exposure times longer than 10 ms and ±20% for exposure times less than 10 ms.*** Timer accuracy should be determined on installation and then annually, or when service is performed on the X-ray generator or if technique problems arise suddenly. The easiest method to validate timer accuracy is the use of a digital X-ray timer available from various manufacturers (Fig. 5.18). These timers usually incorporate a solid-state detector that measures the total time of X-ray production and then displays the time by means of a digital LED readout. These devices cost several hundred dollars, so other lower-cost methods can be used. One of the oldest methods is the spinning top test, which includes a spinning top consisting of a metal disk with a hole or slit cut into the outside edge. If a single-phase X-ray unit is being evaluated, a

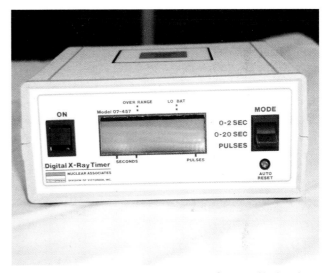

Fig. 5.18 Digital timer for radiographic units. (Courtesy Nuclear Associates, Inc., Carle Place, New York.)

manual spinning top can be used (Fig. 5.19). Single-phase generators emit X-rays in pulses, and therefore each pulse creates a dot on the radiograph made of the spinning top (Fig. 5.20). The number of dots appearing on this radiograph is then compared with the number that should, theoretically, appear at the particular time station selected on the control panel for each exposure. The shortest exposure time available on most single-phase X-ray units is 1/120 second (8.3 ms). The number of dots that should, theoretically, appear is determined by the following equations:

Half-wave rectified:

$$\text{Correct number of dots} = \text{Exposure time (second)} \times 60$$

Full-wave rectified:

$$\text{Correct number of dots} = \text{Exposure time (second)} \times 120$$

Exposures should be made at 1/10, 1/20, 1/30, and 1/40 of a second for single-phase equipment.

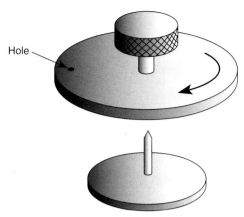

Hole

Fig. 5.19 Manual spinning top.

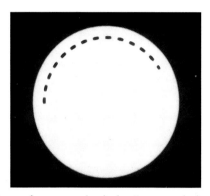

Fig. 5.20 Image from manual spinning top on a single-phase X-ray generator.

For three-phase and high-frequency generators, X-ray production is constant, so a solid line or arc appears instead of a series of dots. For this reason, a manual spinning top cannot be used; a synchronous or motor-driven spinning top is used instead (Fig. 5.21). The synchronous spinning top is also used to evaluate single-phase equipment. The electric motor in the synchronous spinning top rotates at a constant speed of 1 revolution per second so that at the end of 1 second, a 360-degree circle is made. When placed on an image receptor and exposed with a three-phase or high-frequency X-ray generator, this device creates an arc on the processed image that is some fraction of 360 degrees at exposure times less than 1 second. These X-ray units are capable of creating exposure times as short as 1/1000 second (1 ms). The arc size on the image is measured with a protractor (Fig. 5.22) and then inserted into the following equation to determine the actual exposure time (as a fraction) that occurred:

$$\text{Actual exposure time} = \frac{\text{Arc size}}{360}$$

For example, if the image yields an arc size of 72 degrees, 72/360 equals a 1/5-second exposure time (0.2 seconds or 200 ms). At least four different time stations should be tested for three-phase equipment.

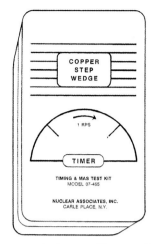

Fig. 5.21 Synchronous spinning top. (Courtesy Nuclear Associates, Inc., Carle Place, New York.)

Many of the newer high-frequency units come equipped with mAs timers instead of separate milliampere and time stations. Because the exposure time is regulated by the internal microprocessor circuitry, the actual time is unknown to the radiographer. A digital mAs meter must be used instead of the digital timer or spinning top test. These devices have electrical probes that must be attached to the circuitry of the unit to obtain a reading. Only a person with adequate training on the use of these devices should attempt to access the circuitry.

Another option to determine timer accuracy is to use an oscilloscope to display the voltage waveform, which was discussed in the previous section.

Milliampere, Exposure Time, and Milliampere-Second Linearity and Reciprocity

The milliampere selector in an X-ray generator is used to regulate the X-ray tube filament temperature which, along with the exposure time, ultimately determines the quantity of X-rays in the X-ray beam. Therefore the accuracy of the milliampere selected is equally important to the accuracy of the exposure timer. One method of testing milliampere accuracy is to make a 1-second exposure while watching the mAs meter on the control panel. A better method is to determine the milliampere **reciprocity** and linearity. Reciprocity refers to the same mAs being selected but with different combinations of milliamperes and exposure times. This parameter is only applicable to those X-ray units that have separate mA and time selection on the control console.

The radiation output should be the same as long as the kVp is kept constant. For example, an exposure of 70 kVp, 50 mA at 1 second should produce the same amount of radiation as an exposure of 70 kVp, 100 mA at 1/2 second because both yield 50 mAs. ***Any variation in reciprocity must be ±10%.***

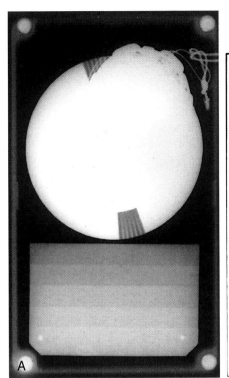

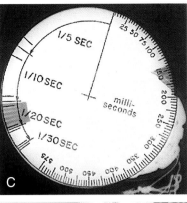

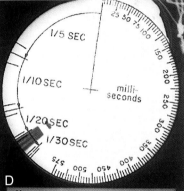

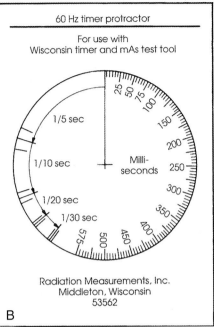

Fig. 5.22 (A) Radiograph produced at 200 mA and a 1/20-second exposure. (B) RMI protractor template. (C) Radiograph A with template showing acceptable results for a 1/20-second exposure. (D) Radiograph produced at 200 mA and 1/30 of a second showing unacceptable results. *mAs*, Milliampere-second. (From Ballinger PW: *Merrill's Atlas of Radiographic Positions and Radiologic Procedures*, 9th ed. Mosby; 1999.)

PROCEDURE: RECIPROCITY

1. Place a dosimeter 40 inches from the focal spot on the radiographic tabletop on top of a lead apron or lead vinyl.
2. Make three to five exposures at 80 kVp and 20 mAs. Each exposure should be at a different milliamperes and time combinations. Be sure to reset the dosimeter after each exposure.
3. Record the dosimeter readings from each exposure and then divide each by 20 mAs to yield the milliroentgens per mAs, microcoulombs per kilogram per mAs, or milligray per mAs air kerma value.
4. The minimum, maximum, and average of three to five of these values are then used to determine the reciprocity variance with the following equation:

Reciprocity variance =
$$\frac{(\text{Exposure or air kerma}_{max} - \text{exposure or air kerma}_{min}) \div 2}{\text{Exposure or air kerma}_{average}}$$

Adequate reciprocity exists when the variance is less than 0.1 (10%).

If a dosimeter is unavailable, images of an aluminum step wedge or homogenous phantom made of aluminum or acrylic can be created with the use of a similar procedure to the one described earlier. Using a 10-inch × 12-inch image receptor, make three to five exposures at 80 kVp and 5 mAs (be sure to use lead vinyl strips so you can fit all three to five images on a single image receptor). If a film/screen image receptor is used, take optical density readings of the same area from each of the three to five images with a densitometer and then compare them. The readings should be within an optical density value of ±0.1. If a computed radiology (CR) or digital radiography (DR) image receptor is used, measure the pixel brightness value of the same area. The values should be within 20% of each other.

Linearity means that sequential increases in mAs should produce the same sequential increase in the exposure measured. In other words, if factors of 70 kVp and 10 mAs produced 50 units of exposure on a dosimeter, then 70 kVp and 20 mAs on the same X-ray generator should produce an exposure of 100 units if the X-ray generator is calibrated correctly. ***Any variation must be within ±10% according to (1020.31(c)), 21 CFR Subchapter J*** and can be evaluated in a manner similar to reciprocity.

PROCEDURE: LINEARITY

1. Place the dosimeter on the radiographic table on a lead apron or strip of lead vinyl, just like in the reciprocity procedure.
2. For mA or mAs linearity, make four exposures using 70 kVp, 0.1 seconds (100 ms), at milliampere stations of 50, 100, 200, and 400. These yield mAs values of 5, 10, 20, and 40 (each exposure twice the previous one). These factors can be modified if the X-ray generator does not have these milliampere stations. If only mAs selection is available on the control console, you can make the four exposures at 5, 10, 20, and 40 mAs.
3. To determine timer linearity (for units with separate mA and exposure time selection only), repeat step 2 using the same mA and exposure times that are double the previous exposure.
4. Record each reading and determine the exposure or air kerma/mAs value for each exposure, along with the maximum, minimum, and average exposure or air kerma/mAs values, then determine mA and timer linearity (on units that have separate mA and time stations) or mAs linearity (for units with only mAs selection available) using the following equation:

Linearity variance =

$$\frac{(\text{Exposure or air kerma}_{max} - \text{exposure or air kerma}_{min}) \div 2}{\text{Exposure or air kerma}_{average}}$$

Adequate linearity exists when the variance is less than 0.1 (10%). This variance also can be determined without a dosimeter, with a step wedge or homogenous phantom and image receptor. Make an exposure of the phantom or step wedge onto an image receptor using the previously mentioned technical factors. If a film/screen image receptor is used, compare the optical density readings of the same area to determine whether they are within ±0.1 of each other. If CR or DR is used, measure the pixel value of each area. These values should not vary by more than 20%. Problems with the X-ray generator, such as the milliampere selector, timer circuitry, transformers or rectifier failure, can cause the linearity variance to exceed accepted limits.

Focal Spot Size

The area of the anode bombarded by projectile electrons is called the *focal spot*. Because these projectile electrons lose their kinetic energy at this point, this spot is also the source of X-ray photons in the X-ray tube. This area can be viewed from two perspectives: the actual rectangular surface on the target where electrons strike, called the actual focal spot, and the actual focal spot viewed from the perspective of the image receptor, called the effective (apparent or projected) focal spot. The effective focal spot always appears smaller than the actual focal spot because of the angle of the line focus principle (Fig. 5.23). This effect is the result of the angle of the anode surface (the smaller the anode angle, the smaller the effective focal spot size). The effective focal spot size has a significant impact on the amount of recorded detail and spatial resolution in a radiographic image because an increase in the effective focal spot size decreases the amount of recorded detail and spatial

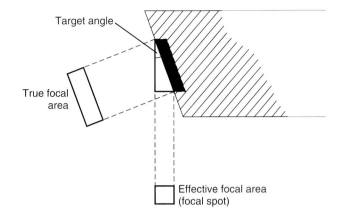

Relationship between true and effective focal areas

$$\text{Sine of target angle} = \frac{\text{Opposite}}{\text{Hypotenuse}}$$

Fig. 5.23 Line focus principle.

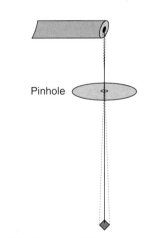

Fig. 5.24 Concept of the pinhole camera.

resolution. Therefore focal spot size should remain relatively constant throughout the life of the X-ray tube. However, focal spot size can increase with age and use and with increases in the milliampere station selected. This phenomenon is known as focal spot blooming. Several performance tests are used to evaluate the degree of focal spot blooming.

Pinhole Camera

As shown in Fig. 5.24, a pinhole camera is made up of a plate of gold platinum alloy with a tiny hole of a specified shape and size cut into its center. A 0.03-mm hole is used for measuring focal spots smaller than 1 mm. A 0.075-mm hole is used for measuring focal spot sizes from 1 to 2.5 mm, and a 0.1-mm hole is used for measuring focal spot sizes greater than 2.5 mm. When placed on a stand over an image receptor (preferably a fine-grain film placed in a nonscreen holder or an extremity cassette) and then exposed, an image of the focal spot is projected on the film and can be measured with a ruler or micrometer after processing. The image is then compared with the stated, or nominal, focal spot size supplied by the X-ray tube manufacturer.

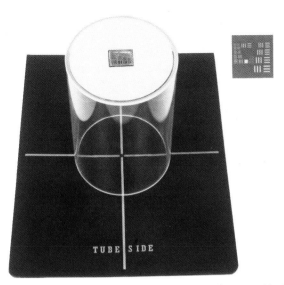

Fig. 5.25 Image from the focal spot test tool. (Courtesy Nuclear Associates, Inc., Carle Place, New York.)

Focal Spot Test Tool

As shown in Fig. 5.25, an image of this test tool is obtained, and the resulting image is compared with a chart supplied by the manufacturer (Table 5.2).

Resolution Chart

Resolution charts are tools that project a chart pattern of various shapes or lines onto a film when radiographed. These charts can be used to estimate focal spot size. The two basic types are star charts (Fig. 5.26) and slit charts. Slit charts usually yield the amount of spatial resolution in line pairs per millimeter, which then correspond to a certain focal spot size used to create the image (discussed in detail in Chapter 3 because this also determines the spatial resolution of imaging systems). When a star pattern resolution chart is used, the

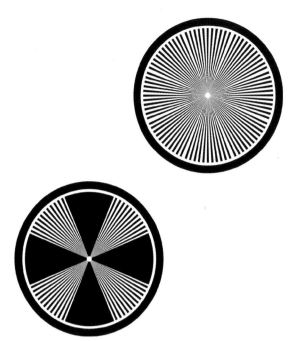

Fig. 5.26 Star resolution patterns.

pattern is imaged on a fine-grain film (preferably in a non-screen holder) and the image diameter (D_i) is measured from the resulting film. When this is compared with the actual diameter of the star pattern (D_o), the magnification factor (M) can be calculated with the following equation:

$$M = \frac{D_i}{D_o}$$

TABLE 5.2 Guide to Accompany Focal Spot Test Tool

Smallest Group Resolved	Group (lp/mm)	Dimension of Effective Focal Spot (mm)
1	0.84	4.3
2	1	3.7
3	1.19	3.1
4	1.41	2.6
5	1.68	2.2
6	2	1.8
7	2.38	1.5
8	2.83	1.3
9	3.36	1.1
10	4	0.9
11	4.76	0.8
12	5.66	0.7

lp/mm, Line pairs per millimeter.
*The accuracy of this test is limited to 16% because the group sizes change by steps of 16%.

PROCEDURE: FOCAL SPOT EVALUATION WITH PINHOLE CAMERA

1. Place the pinhole camera stand on the radiographic tabletop and align it with the central ray and image receptor. If CR is used, set preprocessing image data recognition to fixed mode (the CR image receptor will act like a film/screen cassette).
2. Adjust the pinhole-to-image receptor distance and SID to obtain the proper enlargement factor. For focal spots less than 2.5 mm, an enlargement factor of two should be selected. This means the pinhole-to-image receptor distance should be 60 cm and the X-ray source-to-pinhole distance should be 30 cm. For focal spots larger than 2.5 mm, the enlargement factor should be one, which is obtained with a source-to-pinhole distance of 40 cm and a pinhole-to-image receptor distance of 40 cm.
3. Expose the image receptor to 75 kVp and 50 mAs (100 mAs if a nonscreen image receptor is used). These factors should yield an optical density between 0.8 and 1.2 on the resulting image.
4. Measure the pinhole area on the processed image with a ruler or calipers along both the x-axis and the y-axis (with the long axis of the X-ray table and transverse to the long axis of the X-ray table). If CR or DR is used, use the measuring software or print a hard copy of the image using a dry laser printer.
5. Divide the measurements by the enlargement factor obtained in step 2 to obtain the dimensions of the focal spot.

TABLE 5.3   National Electronics Manufacturers Association Values for Nominal Focal Spot Size Variation

Stated Focal Spot Size (mm)	Focal Spot Blooming Variation Allowed (%)
≤0.8	50
0.8–1.5	40
≥1.6	30

The diameter of the blur zone, or zero contrast band, in millimeters is measured from the image with a ruler (the diameter measured in both the x and y dimensions can be used to obtain the exact dimensions of the focal spot). This is the diameter of the center of the pattern where the lines appear blurred. A smaller focal spot size should be able to image lines that are closer together (such as in the center of the star pattern) so that the blur zone is smaller in diameter. After the diameter of the blur zone is obtained, the following equation can be used to calculate the focal size:

$$\text{Focal spot size (in mm)} = \frac{\theta D}{M - 1}$$

where θ is the spoke angle of the star pattern in radians (radians equals degrees multiplied by π, then divided by 180) obtained from the star pattern. D is the diameter of the blur zone measured in millimeters, and M is the magnification factor. Both the x and y dimensions of the focal spot size should be calculated.

The focal spot size should be determined on installation, and then evaluated annually. The maximum degree of focal spot blooming that is allowable is determined by the National Electronics Manufacturers Association. The values for nominal focal spot size variation are listed in Table 5.3.

For example, if a focal spot size is stated to be 0.5 mm by the manufacturer but measures 0.75 mm during an evaluation test, is it within the National Electronics Manufacturers Association

guidelines? The answer is yes. Because its stated size is 0.5 mm, it is allowed as much as 50% variation, and 50% of 0.5 mm is 0.25 mm. Therefore the maximum focal spot size is 0.75 mm, which is just within the variation allowed.

Beam Restriction System

The beam restriction system is responsible for regulating the size of the X-ray field area. It therefore plays a significant role in patient dosing (because it controls the amount of patient anatomy exposed to radiation) and image contrast (because an increase in the area of the field increases the production of scattered radiation). Performance of the beam restriction system should be evaluated on installation and then at least annually or whenever work is performed on the system. Older systems may require more frequent evaluation. The factors to evaluate in the beam restriction system include light field–radiation field alignment (congruence), positive beam limitation systems, accuracy of the x–y scales, and illuminator bulb brightness, and are covered in (1020.31(e), (f), (g), 1020.32(b)), 21 CFR Subchapter J.

Light Field–Radiation Field Alignment (Congruence)

The light field–radiation field congruence value measures how well the collimator regulates the field size and whether the area illuminated by the positioning light and the area exposed by X-rays are the same. The collimator is made up of two sets of lead shutters that can be opened and closed, along with a small light bulb mounted on the outer edge and a mirror mounted in the center to reflect the light from the bulb through the shutter opening (Fig. 5.27). Over time, this mirror may shift or the mechanism that moves the shutters can malfunction, causing improper performance, which leads to greater patient dosing and repeat images. *The edges of the light field and the radiation field must be congruent to within ±2% of the SID. Evaluation can be performed by using either a collimator test tool with the manufacturer's instructions or the eight-penny (or nine-penny) test* (Figs. 5.28 and 5.29).

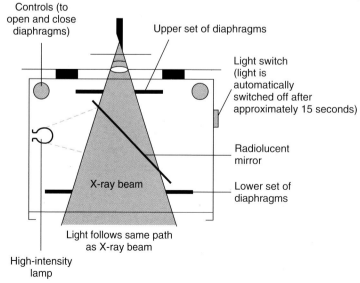

Fig. 5.27 Schematic of variable-aperture collimator.

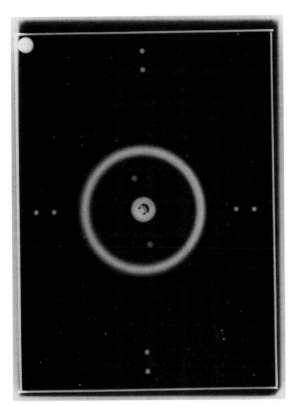

Fig. 5.28 Image obtained with a collimator test tool showing that the collimator is within accepted limits.

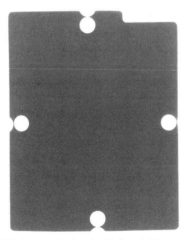

Fig. 5.29 Image obtained with the eight-penny test.

Positive Beam Limitation Systems

The image receptor–radiation field alignment value must be determined for X-ray units equipped with positive beam limitation or automatic collimation. These systems have sensors in the bucky tray that detect the size of the image receptor and then adjust the collimator shutters automatically to match. Malfunctions in this system can occur with age and use, and can be evaluated with a collimator test tool placed on top of the tabletop, with an image receptor in the bucky. An image is created with the previously described procedure for the collimator test tool, light field–radiation field congruence. Testing should be done in both the vertical and horizontal positions if

the X-ray tube is used in both positions. ***Variation between the X-ray field and either the length or width of the image receptor must not differ by more than 3% of the SID.*** An override switch should be in place to disconnect the positive beam limitation in case of malfunction. ***The sum of the length and width differences should be no more than ±4% of the SID used in taking the measurement.*** For example, you could be off by a maximum of 3 cm (3% of the 100-cm SID) in either the 24-cm or 30-cm dimension of the image receptor and still be in compliance. However, you could not be off by 3 cm in both directions at the same time, as this would exceed the 4% limit.

PROCEDURE: LIGHT FIELD/X-RAY FIELD CONGRUENCE

Collimator Test Tool

The collimator test tool requires an image to be created with the use of an image receptor.

1. Place an image receptor on top of a radiographic table with the X-ray beam centered to the center of the image receptor. Next, place the test tool on top of the image receptor according to the manufacturer's instructions. If CR is used, set preprocessing image data recognition to fixed mode (the CR image receptor acts like a film/screen cassette).
2. Adjust the collimators to the area outlined on the test tool. Make an exposure using the technical factors supplied by the test tool manufacturer.
3. Process the image and determine visually whether the X-ray field and radiation field are congruent (see Fig. 5.28).

PROCEDURE: LIGHT FIELD–X-RAY FIELD CONGRUENCE

Eight-Penny (Nine-Penny) Test

1. The eight- or nine-penny test involves laying eight pennies on a 10-inch × 12-inch (25-cm × 35-cm) cassette placed on a tabletop but collimated to an 8-inch × 10-inch field size at a 40-inch SID.
2. Four of the pennies are placed on the inside edge of the light field at the center of each dimension, and the other four are placed on the outside edge, in contact with the inner pennies, meeting at the edge of the light field. A ninth penny may be included (hence the alternate name, *nine-penny test*), and may be placed in the light field toward the cathode end of the X-ray field to demonstrate on the resulting image the direction of any error in X-ray field–radiation field congruence (see Fig. 5.29). If CR is used, set preprocessing image data recognition to fixed mode (the CR image receptor acts like a film/screen cassette).
3. When a radiograph is made and the image is processed, the collimation line of the X-ray field also should fall between the pairs of pennies or at least within the shadow of the pennies, because the diameter of a penny is 0.8 inches (which is exactly 2% of 40 inches).

Accuracy of the X–Y Scales

Modern collimators have two knobs, or dials, on the front that allow radiographers to control the X-ray field size during manual collimation. These knobs also have some type of indicator that shows the size of the x and y dimensions of the X-ray field. ***The indicated size on the collimator of the x and y dimensions and the actual field size measured on the film must correspond to within ±2% of the SID.*** The accuracy of the collimator x–y indicators permits proper sizing of the X-ray field when the collimator light is nonfunctional or poorly visualized due to patient positioning or anatomy. This accuracy can be tested with a collimator test tool or a 14-inch × 17-inch (36-cm × 45-cm) cassette placed on a 40-inch SID tabletop.

PROCEDURE: ACCURACY OF COLLIMATOR X-Y SCALE ADJUSTMENT

1. Set the x–y control knobs on the collimator to a 10-inch × 12-inch field size (25 × 33 cm) and expose a 14-inch × 17-inch image receptor. If CR is used, set preprocessing image data recognition to fixed mode (the CR image receptor acts like a film/screen cassette).
2. Process the image and use a ruler to measure the black rectangle in the center of the image. The dimensions should be within 0.8 inches of 10 inches × 12 inches.

Illuminator Bulb Brightness

The beam restriction system must be equipped with a positioning light and mirror, according to the Center for Devices and Radiological Health (1020.31(d)(2)(ii)) 21 CFR Subchapter J. The distance from the light bulb to the center of the mirror should equal the distance from the X-ray tube focal spot to the center of the mirror. ***The illumination of the light source must be at least 15 foot-candles or 160 lux when measured at a 100-cm (40-inch) distance.*** A photometer such as the one described in Chapter 3 for evaluation of image display monitor brightness or a photographic light meter should be used.

PROCEDURE: ILLUMINATOR BULB BRIGHTNESS

1. Bring a photometer or photographic light meter into the radiographic room. Set the meter to record luminance in lux or foot-candles. Adjust the ambient light to the level used routinely in the room during diagnostic procedures.
2. Set the X-ray tube-to-tabletop distance at 40 inches (100 cm) and turn on the illuminator light. Collimate to a 10-inch × 12-inch field size.
3. The crosshairs should appear in the light field. Divide the light field into four equal quadrants. Place the photometer or light meter in the exact center of each quadrant of the light field and record the brightness (be sure to avoid dark bands such as those from the crosshair images). The reading should be at least 15 foot-candles or 160 lux.

An illuminator bulb with an inadequate level of brightness may lead to positioning errors and subsequent repeat images. This problem is usually corrected by replacing the light bulb or cleaning the mirror inside the collimator.

X-ray Beam Alignment

The X-ray tube must be mounted properly in its metal housing so that the central ray of the X-ray beam is aligned to the center of the image receptor in the bucky tray. If there is misalignment, image cutoff occurs. Beam alignment should be evaluated on installation and then annually with a beam alignment test tool (Fig. 5.30). Items to evaluate in this category include perpendicularity and X-ray beam–bucky tray alignment.

Perpendicularity

The X-ray tube must be mounted in its housing so that the central ray of the X-ray beam is within 1 degree of perpendicular. If not, the image demonstrates shape distortion. With age and use, the X-ray tube can shift in its housing, causing a lack of perpendicularity (mainly from the heat inside the housing causing a breakdown of the rubber O-rings that support the X-ray tube on either side). Rough handling of the housing during X-ray examinations can also cause the X-ray tube to shift slightly within its housing.

PROCEDURE: PERPENDICULARITY

Beam Alignment Tool
1. Place an image receptor on the radiographic tabletop and center the X-ray beam, using a 40-inch SID.
2. Place the beam alignment tool on top of the image receptor and collimate to the area on the template.
3. Make an exposure using 60 kVp and mAs appropriate to the speed of the image receptor being used. If CR is used, set preprocessing image data recognition to fixed mode (the CR image receptor acts like a film/screen cassette).
4. Process the image. Within the test tool, a steel ball is mounted in the center of a disk at each end of the 15-cm-tall plastic container. When the balls are positioned over one another and at a right angle to the image receptor, their images appear as one if the central ray is perpendicular to the image receptor. If the image of the upper steel ball (which is magnified because it is farther away from the image receptor) intersects the image of the first disk (appears as a ring), the central ray is approximately 1.5 degrees away from perpendicular.

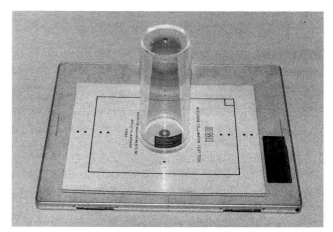

Fig. 5.30 Beam alignment tool.

X-ray Beam–Bucky Tray Alignment or Central Ray Congruency

The center of the bucky tray and the center of the X-ray beam must be aligned to avoid clipping important anatomy and to avoid grid cutoff. *X-ray beam–bucky tray alignment must be within 1% of the SID.* The same beam alignment tool used to determine perpendicularity also can be used to evaluate this alignment (Fig. 5.31).

Source-to-Image Distance and Tube Angulation Indicators

All medical X-ray units must be equipped with SID and tube angulation indicators, according to the Center for Devices and Radiological Health, because they influence patient dose, optical density, recorded detail, size distortion, and shape distortion. *The SID indicator must be installed so it is accurate to within ±2% of the SID. The tube angulation indicator must be accurate to within ±5 degrees.* The accuracy of the tube angulation indicator can be checked with a protractor. SID indicator accuracy is determined with a simple tape measure or the triangular method and should be checked on installation and then annually or when service is performed

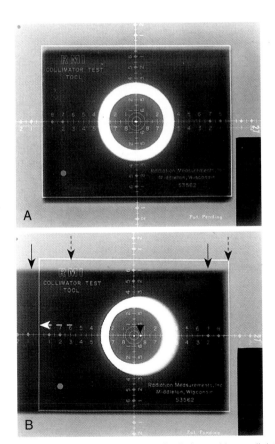

Fig. 5.31 (A) Acceptable beam perpendicularity and beam–light field alignment. (B) Unacceptable beam perpendicularity and beam–light field alignment. Radiation beam (*arrows*) does not agree with collimator light field (*broken arrows*). Perpendicularity is out of alignment. Note the top head is shifted to the right (*arrowhead*). (From Ballinger PW: *Merrill's Atlas of Radiographic Positions and Radiologic Procedures,* 9th ed. Mosby; 1999.)

on the X-ray tube. When evaluating with the triangulation method, use the following procedure.

Overload Protection

Most X-ray generators are equipped with an overload protection mechanism to prevent excessive temperatures inside the X-ray tube during a single exposure. *The overload protection mechanism should not permit an exposure that exceeds 80% of the tube capacity for a single exposure.* This exposure level can be determined by selecting a kVp and milliampere combination that exceeds this 80% limit and then engaging the rotor button, which should cause a tube overload indicator light to appear on the control panel; some systems do not allow the rotor to engage in this situation. Should either of these fail to occur, the user should call a service technician to repair the system. No one should engage the expose button because serious X-ray tube damage can result if the overload protection system is malfunctioning. The overload protection mechanism should be evaluated at installation and then annually or when service is performed on the X-ray generator.

PROCEDURE: X-RAY BEAM/BUCKY TRAY (IMAGE RECEPTOR) ALIGNMENT

Beam Alignment Test Tool

1. With the X-ray tube centered by means of the centering detent lock, place an image receptor in the bucky tray and slide it into its proper place. If CR is used, set preprocessing image data recognition to fixed mode (the CR image receptor acts like a film/screen cassette).
2. Position the test tool so the metal washer is in the exact center of the X-ray field using the crosshairs from the positioning light, then expose the image receptor.
3. Process and then analyze the resulting image visually. The image of the washer should be in the center of the film or within 0.4 inches (or ≈1 cm) of the center (see Fig. 5.31). A service engineer should be called if the alignment is off by more than this amount.

PROCEDURE: X-RAY BEAM/BUCKY TRAY (IMAGE RECEPTOR) ALIGNMENT

Washer or Coin Method

If a beam alignment tool is unavailable, the following procedure also can be used to determine X-ray beam–bucky tray alignment.

1. Bring a metal coin, a steel washer, or a lead number zero, along with an 8-inch × 10-inch image receptor, into a radiographic room. If CR is used, set preprocessing image data recognition to fixed mode (the CR image receptor acts like a film/screen cassette).
2. Place the image receptor in the bucky tray (with the long axis of the image receptor in the same direction as the long axis of the radiographic table) and center the X-ray field to the image receptor. Set the SID for 40 inches (100 cm).
3. Turn on the positioning light and place the coin, lead zero, or steel washer in the center of the crosshairs. Place another coin or some other lead number in the light field, near the edge closest to where you are standing. This allows you

Continued

PROCEDURE: X-RAY BEAM/BUCKY TRAY (IMAGE RECEPTOR) ALIGNMENT—cont'd

to determine in which direction the alignment may be off when analyzing the resulting image.

4. Make an exposure using 50 kVp and 1 mAs (you may have to increase this amount, depending on the image receptor speed). Process the image.

5. Using a ruler, measure the distance from the middle of the outside of the long axis of the image to the washer, coin, or lead zero (with CR or DR systems, use the electronic measuring software). If proper beam alignment exists, the distances are exactly the same. If they are not the same, the image of the washer, coin, or lead zero should be within 0.4 inches of the center of the image, or a service technician should be notified to repair the system.

X-ray Tube Heat Sensors

As just mentioned, most X-ray generators are equipped with overload protection circuits to prevent excessive tube heat in a single exposure. In general, they do not protect against cumulative heat buildup that can occur when several exposures are made within a relatively short period. To guard against this accumulated heat, radiographers can rely on anode cooling charts or housing cooling charts supplied by the tube manufacturer. Use of these charts is especially critical during fluoroscopy and angiography, during which considerable heat can be produced quickly. Many newer units are equipped with X-ray tube heat sensors that provide an LED readout of the percentage of heat capacity remaining inside the X-ray tube housing. ***Heat sensors should provide a warning when anode heat reaches 75% of the maximum***. These devices should be checked at installation and then every 6 months. Checking involves taking several exposures at a known heat unit value and then comparing the total with the known maximum heat capacity of the X-ray tube provided by the manufacturer.

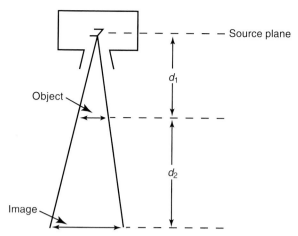

Fig. 5.32 Similar triangle configuration for determination of source-to-image distance. d_1 is the distance from the focal spot to the object; d_2 is the distance from the object to the image receptor.

ANCILLARY EQUIPMENT

The creation of diagnostic radiographs in a modern radiology department requires more than just an X-ray generator, X-ray tube, and X-ray table. Several types of ancillary equipment are also involved in the imaging chain to help create or enhance the radiographic image, regulate X-ray production, and protect the patient and radiographer, including AEC systems, conventional tomographic systems, grids, and portable and mobile X-ray generators. Because variation in this equipment can occur during use, quality control protocols must be in place to minimize repeat examinations.

Automatic Exposure Control Systems

The AEC system has been used in radiography since the 1960s. It functions as a regulator for the exposure time and provides constant exposure to the image receptor, regardless of the kVp or mAs selected or thickness of the part being imaged. This type of system involves some type of radiation detection device that measures the quantity of X-rays received by the patient or image receptor. When this exposure reaches a level corresponding to a predetermined value, the system causes the X-ray generator to terminate the exposure. This value is set by a service engineer on the basis of the image receptor system used in the department. A postreading mAs indicator should be present on the control console and should display accurately the total mAs delivered during the exposure. An AEC system has two main parts, the detector and the comparator.

Detectors

The **detector**, also known as the **sensor**, is a radiation detector that monitors the radiation exposure at or near the patient and produces a corresponding electric current proportional to the quantity of X-rays detected. Detectors are sometimes referred to as *cells* or *chambers*. Normally, three detectors are available for use by the radiographer, one in the midline and one on either side of the midline (Fig. 5.33). Units also are available with one or as many as five detectors. The X-ray machine control console should have indicators present that

PROCEDURE: SOURCE-TO-IMAGE DISTANCE INDICATOR ACCURACY

1. Place a radiopaque object (e.g., a metal plate about 2 inches long) at a distance from the focal spot mark on the X-ray tube housing. Measure and record the exact distance from the focal spot to the object. This value is known as d_1 (Fig. 5.32). Also measure and record the exact size of the object.

2. Using a 40-inch SID, make an image of the object using an image receptor. If CR is used, set preprocessing image data recognition to fixed mode (the CR image receptor acts like a film/screen cassette). Make sure the object is positioned in the beam so that it is covered completely by the beam and the image receptor is large enough to contain the image produced.

3. Process the image and measure the size of the radiopaque object recorded in the image. The SID ($d_1 + d_2$) can then be calculated using the similar triangles equation and inserting the measured values of d_1, object size, and image size:

$$\frac{d_1}{\text{Object dimension}} = \frac{d_1 + d_2 \,(\text{SID})}{\text{Image dimension}}$$

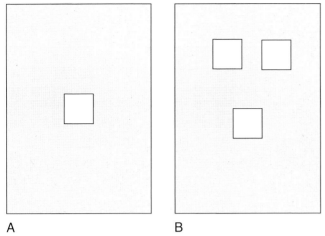

A   B

Fig. 5.33 Sensor cell location for automatic exposure control systems. (A) Single-cell option. (B) Three-sensor option.

reflect which detectors are active. Three different types of radiation detectors have been used in AEC systems: photodetectors, ion chambers, and solid-state detectors.

Photodetectors

The photodetector, or photocell, uses a scintillation crystal (usually sodium iodide) coupled with a photomultiplier tube (Fig. 5.34). When radiation interacts with the crystal, light is created and enters the photomultiplier tube. This light then releases electrons through the process of photoemission. The electrons multiply in number and form an electric current proportional to the original amount of radiation that struck the photocell. The photodetector was the original detector used as a sensor and was marketed under the name *phototimer*. This name is still used commonly to describe AEC systems, although the photodetector is seldom used in modern systems. These sensors are placed behind the image receptor to measure the exposure because they are not radiolucent. Care must be taken with these systems so that the lead in the back of the cassettes (normally present to control backscatter) is not excessive.

Ion Chambers

The ion chamber (discussed earlier in this chapter) consists of a gas-filled chamber. It is smaller than a photocell and can

be made of a radiolucent material, which allows it to be placed between the grid and the front of the image receptor so that any type of cassette design can be used. An ion chamber is the most common type of sensor found in current AEC systems and is often marketed under the name *ionomat*.

Solid-State Detectors

The solid-state detector uses a small silicon or germanium crystal, which is more sensitive but also more expensive than photocells or ion chambers. The crystals are radiolucent and can be placed between the grid and image receptor. The solid-state detector is often marketed under the name *autotimer*.

Comparator

The comparator is an electronic circuit that receives the current signal sent by the sensor. An internal capacitor stores a voltage as long as this current is flowing. When the voltage in the capacitor becomes the same as a preset reference voltage, a switch is opened that terminates the exposure. Changing the density selector switch changes this reference voltage and, therefore the quantity of radiographs produced by the generator. Each step on the density selector should change the radiation exposure by 25%–30%. Typical selector settings are shown in Fig. 5.35. The radiographer also must select the proper chamber and kVp, verify the properly positioned patient and X-ray tube, and verify backup time/mAs in case of system failure.

Quality Control for Automatic Exposure Control

It is very common for radiographic examinations to be performed with AEC systems. It is estimated that more than 60% of all hospital radiology departments have radiographic equipment that uses an AEC system or anatomically programmed units (which contain a microprocessor circuit with preprogrammed technical factors). The advantage of AEC is that it delivers consistent image receptor exposure over a wide range of patient thickness and kVp settings. Proper system performance should therefore be monitored through quality control procedures at installation and then semiannually or whenever work is performed on the system. Items that should be monitored include backup time/mAs, or maximum exposure time

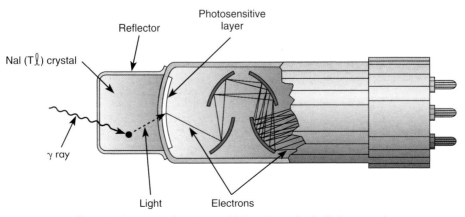

Fig. 5.34 Schematic for photomultiplier tube and scintillation crystal.

Density setting

Weak, very young Very old, debilitated	−2
Thin Easy to penetrate	−1
Average Normal build	0/Neutral
Muscular	+1/+2

Fig. 5.35 Automatic exposure control density selector settings.

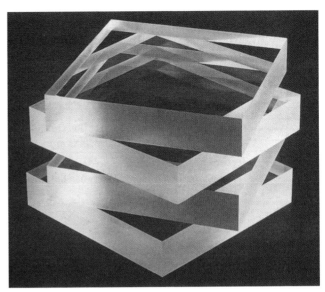

Fig. 5.36 Automatic exposure control test tool consisting of acrylic sheets of varying thickness. (Courtesy Nuclear Associates, Inc., Carle Place, New York.)

and minimum exposure time. Results should be recorded as pass or fail on a documentation form. A sample form for AEC system evaluation is available on the Evolve website.

Backup, or Maximum Exposure, Time/Milliampere-Seconds

Because the exposure is controlled by the sensor and comparator combination instead of a conventional timer, care must be taken to avoid excessive patient exposure and heat in the X-ray tube in the case of system failure or during the examination of an extremely large patient. This is accomplished by setting a backup time (or backup mAs on systems with only mAs selection) on the control console. *The backup system should terminate the exposure within 6 seconds or 600 mAs, whichever comes first,* and can be checked with the following procedure.

PROCEDURE: BACKUP TIME OR MILLIAMPERE-SECONDS

1. Place a lead apron over the AEC detector cells and make an exposure at 70 kVp and 100 mA.
2. Watch the mAs meter on the control panel in addition to using a stopwatch to determine whether the backup system terminates the exposure within the 6-second or 600-mAs limit. If not, release the expose button so the X-ray tube is not damaged.

Minimum Exposure Time/Milliampere-Seconds

The detector and comparator combination requires a certain period to detect the radiation, compare it with the preset value, and then terminate the exposure (usually around 10 ms). If a particular X-ray examination requires an exposure less than this amount, the AEC system cannot respond in time and the resulting image is overexposed. For this reason, distal extremity radiographs are, in general, not performed with AEC. Certain lung diseases such as emphysema can also require less than the minimum exposure time, so it is important to lower the milliamperes before making the exposure. The manufacturer's literature should be checked regarding the minimum exposure time available, and then the technologist should be instructed regarding which radiographic examinations and kVp and milliampere combinations can and cannot be used with AEC.

Consistency of exposure with varying milliamperes or milliampere-seconds. The AEC system should be able to adjust the exposure time and maintain image receptor exposure with any changes in milliamperes (or mAs on systems with only mAs selection available) on the control panel. *Any variation cannot exceed ±10%.* To evaluate this parameter, use the following procedure (Fig. 5.36).

PROCEDURE: CONSISTENCY WITH VARYING MILLIAMPERES OR MILLIAMPERE-SECONDS

1. Obtain a homogenous phantom, which is uniform in thickness, made of acrylic plastic (Plexiglas or Lucite) that is at least 10 cm in thickness (see Fig. 5.36).
2. Make a series of four radiographs of the phantom on a 10-inch × 12-inch (25-cm × 30-cm) image receptor using 70 kVp, a 40-inch SID bucky, and a normal density setting, with at least four different milliampere stations (or 4 mAs stations on systems with only mAs selection available on the control console). If CR is used, set preprocessing image data recognition to fixed mode (the CR image receptor acts like a film/screen cassette).
3. Process each radiograph. If a film/screen image receptor is utilized, use a densitometer to measure the optical density of the center of each image. For CR or DR images, print a hard copy of the image using a dry laser printer, or measure the pixel brightness at the center of the image. *The optical density values should measure the same or be within an optical density of ±0.2, or no more than a 30% difference in pixel brightness*. If not, inconsistent image receptor exposure in the resulting radiographs can occur, leading to repeat exposures. This is usually the result of a malfunctioning comparator.

Consistency of exposure with varying kilovolts (peak). The AEC system should be able to adjust the exposure time and maintain image receptor exposure with any changes in kVp on the control panel. Consistency can be evaluated with the same homogenous phantom mentioned previously.

Consistency of exposure with varying part thickness. The AEC system should be able to adjust the exposure time and maintain the same image receptor exposure with any changes in part thickness. System evaluation again uses a homogenous phantom.

PROCEDURE: CONSISTENCY OF EXPOSURE WITH VARYING KILOVOLTS (PEAK)

1. Make four exposures of the phantom on a 10-inch × 12-inch image receptor using 100 mA, a normal density setting, a 40-inch SID bucky, and values of 60, 70, 80, and 90 kVp. If CR is used, set preprocessing image data recognition to fixed mode (the CR image receptor acts like a film/screen cassette).
2. Process the four radiographs and take optical density readings of the center of each image using a densitometer. For CR or DR images, print a hard copy of the image using a dry laser printer, or measure the pixel brightness at the center of the image. ***The optical density values should measure the same or be within an optical density of ±0.3, or no more than a 50% difference in pixel values with digital systems.***

PROCEDURE: CONSISTENCY OF EXPOSURE WITH VARYING PART THICKNESS

1. Make three exposures on separate 10-inch × 12-inch image receptors at 70 kVp, 100 mA, a normal density setting, and a 40-inch SID bucky. Make each exposure with a phantom thickness of 10, 20, and 30 cm. If CR is used, set preprocessing image data recognition to fixed mode (the CR image receptor acts like a film/screen cassette).
2. Process each image and take density readings of the center. For CR or DR images, print a hard copy of the image using a dry laser printer, or measure the pixel brightness at the center of the image. ***The optical density values should measure the same or be within an optical density of ±0.2, or no more than a 30% difference in pixel values.***

Consistency of exposure with varying field sizes. The AEC system should be able to compensate for changes in the area of field provided the detector remains in the field. Radiographs of the homogenous phantom can also be used to evaluate this parameter.

Consistency of automatic exposure control detectors. Most AEC systems use a configuration of three detectors. Each detector should provide the same exposure or exposure time as the other two. For evaluation, use the following procedure.

PROCEDURE: CONSISTENCY OF EXPOSURE WITH VARYING FIELD SIZES

1. Make a series of three exposures of the phantom using 70 kVp, 100 mA, a normal density setting, and 40-inch SID. If CR is used, set preprocessing image data recognition to fixed mode (the CR image receptor acts like a film/screen cassette).
2. Make each exposure with a different field size of 6-inch × 6-inch, 10-inch × 10-inch, and 14-inch × 14-inch, with an appropriate image receptor size. Be sure the X-ray beam is centered on the detector chamber.
3. Process the images and record the optical density from the center of each. For CR or DR images, print a hard copy of the image using a dry laser printer, or measure the pixel brightness value at the center of the image. ***The optical density values should measure the same or be within an optical density of ±0.1, or no more than a 20% difference in pixel values.***

PROCEDURE: CONSISTENCY OF AEC DETECTORS/CELLS

1. Make a series of three radiographs of the homogenous phantom using a different detector selection for each. Be sure the phantom is placed over the appropriate detector. Use exposure factors of 70 kVp, 100 mA, a normal density setting, and a 40-inch SID bucky. If CR is used, set preprocessing image data recognition to fixed mode (the CR image receptor acts like a film/screen cassette).
2. Process the radiographs. For film/screen image receptors, compare the optical density readings from the center of each image. For CR or DR images, print a hard copy of the image using a dry laser printer, or measure the pixel brightness at the center of the image. ***The optical density values should measure the same or be within an optical density of ±0.2, or no more than a 30% difference in pixel values.***

Reproducibility

Exposures made at the same kVp and mAs settings of the same phantom thickness should produce the same image receptor exposure each time. This is referred to as reproducibility.

PROCEDURE: AUTOMATIC EXPOSURE CONTROL REPRODUCIBILITY

1. Make three exposures of the homogenous phantom using 80 kVp, 200 mA, a normal density setting, a 10-inch × 12-inch image receptor size, and a 40-inch SID bucky. If CR is used, set preprocessing image data recognition to fixed mode (the CR image receptor acts like a film/screen cassette).
2. Process each radiograph. For film/screen image receptors, compare the optical density readings taken from the center of each image. For CR or DR images, print a hard copy of the image using a dry laser printer, or measure the pixel brightness at the center of the image. ***The readings should be within an optical density of ±0.10 of each other, or no more than a 20% difference in pixel values.***

An alternative method of evaluating reproducibility is to make the same three exposures but not to use an image receptor to record an image. Instead, place a radiation detector and homogenous phantom over the appropriate sensor chamber and record the readings obtained in each exposure. For valid results, the radiation detector should be radiolucent. The reproducibility variance can then be calculated with the equation used earlier in this chapter. *The reproducibility variance must be within 0.05 (5%).*

Density or Signal-to-Noise Ratio Control Function

The density (for film/screen image receptors or signal-to-noise ratio [SNR] (for digital image receptors) selection should allow for changes in radiation exposure allowed to the image receptor of 25%–30% for each increment. Depending on the manufacturer of the systems, the density/SNR selector can range as follows:

| −2 | −1 | 0 or N | +1 | +2 |
| −1/2 | −1/4 | 0 or N | +1/4 | +1/2 |

The 0 or N selection is most often used for normal-sized patients. Choosing a negative value reduces the exposure to the image receptor, while positive values increase the exposure allowed to the image receptor. Accuracy can be evaluated by the following procedure.

PROCEDURE: DENSITY/SIGNAL-TO-NOISE RATIO EXPOSURE FUNCTION

1. Make a series of five radiographs of the homogenous phantom using 70 kVp, 100 mA, and a 40-inch SID bucky, and using the density/SNR selector settings of normal (0/ neutral), +1, +2, −1, and −2 (these settings vary according to manufacturer). Be sure to mark each image with a lead number or some other identifier. If CR is used, set preprocessing image data recognition to fixed mode (the CR image receptor acts like a film/screen cassette).
2. Take optical density readings from the center of each of the processed images and compare. For CR images, print a hard copy of the image using a dry laser printer, or measure the pixel brightness at the center of the image. **Each should increase in optical density by a value of 0.2–0.25 (30% difference in pixel values), from the lowest to the highest density/SNR setting (−2 to +2)**.

Reciprocity Law Failure

The Law of Reciprocity states that the same amount of radiation should be created at any mAs value regardless of the milliampere/time combination used; therefore, the image receptor exposure should also be the same. Film/screen image receptor systems can experience reciprocity failure at very short exposure time values (<10 ms) and very long exposure time values (>1 second). This phenomenon does not occur in digital systems.

- Phantom images of either a homogenous phantom or an anthropomorphic (lifelike) phantom should be made at 70 kVp, a normal density setting, a 40-inch SID bucky, and the lowest milliampere station possible on the control panel (so that a long exposure time is used).
- Another image should be made with the highest milliampere station available (to yield a short exposure time).
- Optical density readings should be obtained from the center of each image and compared. If reciprocity failure exists, the optical density of the images varies by more than a value of ±0.2.

Conventional Tomographic Systems

Many radiographic units are equipped with a conventional tomographic system that is used to image certain "slices" of the body, whereas all other slices are blurred. This system helps remove superimposition and improves radiographic contrast in the area of interest. There are two basic types of conventional tomography: linear tomography and pluridirectional tomography.

In linear (sometimes called *rectilinear*) tomography, the X-ray tube and image receptor move longitudinally in opposite directions during the exposure (Fig. 5.37). The plane through the fulcrum or pivot point remains in focus, whereas structures that are above and below this plane are blurred by the motion of the tube and film. This plane is called the objective plane or tomographic section. The fulcrum level determines the level of the objective plane and is measured from the radiographic tabletop upward. For example, a 5-cm tomographic section means the objective plane is 5 cm above the tabletop. The thickness of the tomographic section is determined by the tomographic angle, which is the angle between the central ray at the beginning of the exposure and at the end of the exposure. The greater the tomographic angle, the thinner the tomographic section because of the greater motion of the tube and film (Fig. 5.38).

In pluridirectional tomography, the X-ray tube and film move in a variety of patterns such as circular, elliptical,

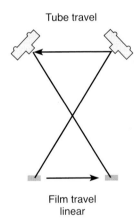

Fig. 5.37 Principle of linear tomography.

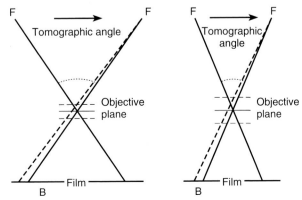

Fig. 5.38 Effect of tomographic angle on section thickness. *F*, Focal spot; *B*, bucky.

hypocycloidal, and trispiral (Fig. 5.39). These units produce sharper images than rectilinear units because of the increased motion of the tube and film. Because of this complexity of motion, pluridirectional units are dedicated usually only to tomographic imaging, which has limited their use on a wide-spread basis because most radiology departments cannot afford to have a room dedicated solely to this type of unit with a relatively small number of patients who might benefit.

Quality Control of Tomographic Systems

Because tomography involves motion of the X-ray tube and image receptor, considerable variation can occur in the performance of these systems with age and use. In addition, most X-ray generators for tomographic systems may not be calibrated for the extremely low milliampere/long exposure time combinations used during these procedures. Mechanical instabilities can manifest in the tube system as a result of the large mass of the X-ray tube and housing. This manifestation can cause inconsistencies in the exposure and asymmetry in tube motion and can lead to poor image quality; therefore, specific quality control tests should be performed at installation and then annually. Specialized test tools and phantoms should be used for these evaluations (Fig. 5.40). Factors to

evaluate include visual observation of tube/bucky assembly motion, section level, section thickness, level incrementation, exposure angle, spatial resolution, section uniformity and beam path, and patient exposure.

Observation of tube/Bucky assembly motion. The motion of the X-ray tube–Bucky assembly should be evaluated for correctness of motion and stability during movement. In particular, the movement of the Bucky assembly should be smooth relative to the motion of the X-ray tube. As the system ages, it may become necessary to evaluate the motion stability more frequently to maintain acceptable performance.

Section level. The level of the tomographic section (fulcrum level) indicated on the equipment and the actual level of the tomographic section imaged above the tabletop should be the same or within ±5 mm (some manufacturers suggest ±1 mm for pluridirectional units). Evaluation is made with a test tool that has a series of lead numbers at various depths that are imaged on the image receptor (Fig. 5.41). A tomographic exposure is made of the test tools at various fulcrum levels. The resulting image is then analyzed for the number that appears the sharpest. For example, if the fulcrum for the exposure is set for 5 cm, the number 5 should be the sharpest number visible.

Section thickness. The thickness of the tomographic section depends on the tomographic angle. Table 5.4 lists the

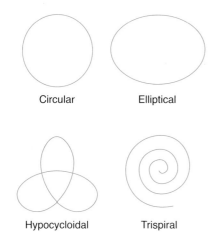

Circular   Elliptical

Hypocycloidal   Trispiral

Fig. 5.39 Pluridirectional tomographic patterns.

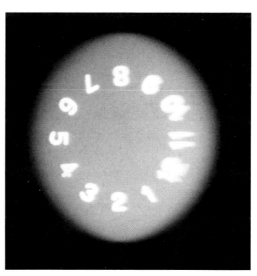

Fig. 5.41 Image from a tomographic test tool indicating the level of tomographic section.

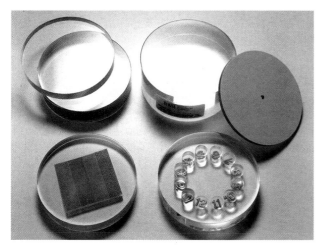

Fig. 5.40 Tomographic test tool. (Courtesy Gammex/RMI, Middleton, Wisconsin.)

TABLE 5.4 **Section Thickness at Various Tomographic Angles**	
Tomographic Angle (degrees)	**Section Thickness (mm)**
50	1.1
40	1.4
30	2
10	6
5	11
0	—

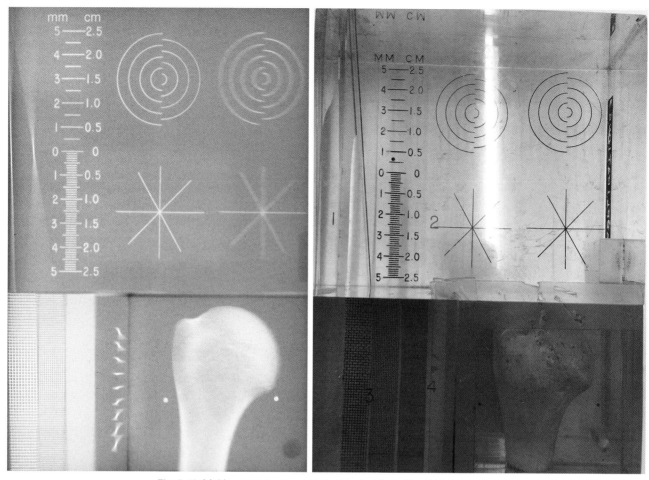

Fig. 5.42 Multipurpose tomographic test tool with section thickness ruler.

section thickness at various tomographic angles. Evaluation is made with a special multifunction test tool according to the manufacturer's instructions (Fig. 5.42).

Exposure angle. The exposure angle determines the thickness of the tomographic section so it can be used as an alternative to measuring section thickness. ***It is important that the value indicated on the equipment and the actual angle be the same or within ±5 degrees for units operating at angles greater than 30 degrees. For exposure angles less than 30 degrees, the maximum variation allowed is ±2 degrees.*** Accurate measurement of this variable is difficult and is best accomplished by evaluating the section thickness with the appropriate phantom. Variations in section thickness are usually the result of improper exposure angles.

Level incrementation. All tomographic units have some type of ruler or other device to indicate the level of the tomographic section. ***A ruler should be constructed so that changing from one tomographic section to the next is accurate to within ±2 mm.*** Evaluation can be accomplished with the same test phantom and procedure used in section-level determination.

Spatial resolution. Spatial resolution in tomographic imaging is the ability of the tomographic system to resolve objects within the tomographic section. The structures within the tomographic section must be demonstrated with sufficient spatial resolution to make an accurate diagnosis

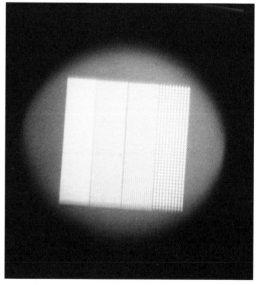

Fig. 5.43 Image from a tomographic test tool indicating the resolution pattern.

possible. Fig. 5.43 shows an image of a tomographic resolution test tool with brass or copper wire mesh patterns of 20 holes per inch (0.8 holes/mm), 30 holes per inch (1.2 holes/mm), 40 holes per inch (1.6 holes/mm), and

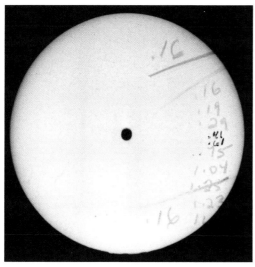

Fig. 5.44 Lead aperture of a tomographic test tool.

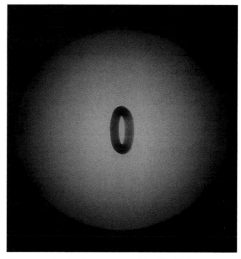

Fig. 5.46 Image of a lead aperture with elliptical motion. (Courtesy Central DuPage Hospital, Winfield, Illinois.)

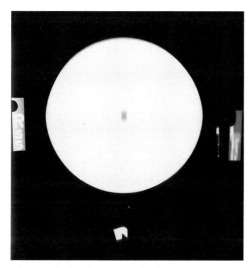

Fig. 5.45 Image of a lead aperture with linear tomography.

50 holes per inch (2 holes/mm). Most tomographic units should be able to resolve a mesh screen pattern of at least 40 holes per inch. Variations in resolution are usually the result of asymmetry in tube motion.

Section Uniformity and Beam Path

The amount of radiation emitted should be consistent throughout the tomographic exposure so the optical density of the image is uniform. Consistency can be evaluated with a test tool consisting of a lead aperture (Fig. 5.44). When an exposure is made on a linear tomographic unit, a thin line should appear on the resulting image (Fig. 5.45). Optical density readings should be taken throughout the line and compared. *Any variation should be within an optical density value of ±0.3.* This same device can also be used for evaluation of beam path. Any asymmetry in motion or inconsistencies in the exposure alters the normal shape of the beam path. Linear units should demonstrate a straight line, as shown in Fig. 5.45. Pluridirectional units should create images that are appropriate to the pattern selected. Fig. 5.46 shows an image

created with an elliptical pattern. *Path closure in pluridirectional units should be within ±10% of the path length.*

Patient Exposure

As the X-ray tube and film move in opposite directions during tomography, different patient thicknesses exist at various points within the exposure; therefore the number of mAs is greater during conventional tomography than with conventional radiography of the same view. The tomographic exposure should not exceed two times the nontomographic exposure for the same part. For example, if 50 mAs is required for an anteroposterior projection of the kidneys, an anteroposterior tomographic cut of the same kidneys should be obtained at 100 mAs or less. For departments equipped with more than one tomographic unit, patient exposure should not vary by more than 20% if the units have comparable X-ray tubes and generators. Evaluation can be made by exposing an abdomen or skull phantom to create both tomographic and nontomographic images.

PROCEDURE: TOMOGRAPHIC MILLIAMPERES-SECOND

1. Using either an abdomen or skull phantom, make a nontomographic exposure with an appropriate-size image receptor and the kVp and mAs specified for your particular unit. If CR is used, set preprocessing image data recognition to fixed mode (the CR image receptor acts like a film/screen cassette).
2. Using the same phantom, make a tomographic image at the same kVp and appropriate mAs specified for your particular unit.
3. Process the images and use a densitometer to obtain density readings of the same anatomic structure from each image (e.g., middle of the L4 vertebra and middle of the sella turcica). For CR or DR images, print a hard copy of the image using a dry laser printer, or measure the pixel brightness at the center of each image. **The readings should be**

Continued

PROCEDURE: TOMOGRAPHIC MILLIAMPERES-SECOND—cont'd

the same or within an optical density value of ±0.1, or no more than a 20% difference in pixel values.

4. If the optical density readings are similar, compare the mAs values used for each exposure. The tomographic exposure should not be more than double the mAs required for the nontomographic exposure.

Digital Radiographic Tomosynthesis

Conventional tomographic systems are being replaced by digital radiographic tomosynthesis (DRT). This technology combines digital image capture and processing with simple tube/detector motion as used in conventional radiographic tomography. This process is commonplace in mammographic exams but is being used to replace conventional tomography for other parts of the body. DR image receptors are required for DRT systems because they provide rapid readout. This requires about 10 static exposures at slightly different central ray angles through the region of interest. Depending on the system, either a continuous sweep or stop-and-shoot motion of the tube can be utilized. Each examination requires a specific sweep angle that can range from 100 to 50 degrees. Larger sweep angles provide better separation of structures and resolution but suffer more elongation. Postacquisition image processing permits reconstruction of any desired plane through the exposed area. Postacquisition software can also modify blur, image brightness, contrast, and resolution. The primary advantage over conventional tomography is that the resulting images can be manipulated as well as re-created in various planes without reexposing the patient.

Quality control testing for these systems is currently determined by the equipment manufacturers and test phantoms are available.

Grids

The grid is the most common device for controlling scattered radiation (assuming collimation to the appropriate field size has been performed). Improper use of a grid can cause grid cutoff (resulting in an underexposed radiograph) or grid artifacts (e.g., grid lines and moiré patterns). These artifacts are discussed in detail in Chapter 6. Grid artifacts also occur because of imperfections during the manufacturing process or mishandling during clinical use (dropping the grid). Barium or other contrast media also create artifacts and must be removed. The grid variables to be evaluated are grid uniformity and grid alignment, which should occur at installation and then annually.

Grid Uniformity

All the lead strips in the grid must be spaced uniformly or a mottling effect may appear in the image, which can mimic a pathologic condition. Nonuniformity occurs from manufacturing defects or by dropping a grid on its edges. For evaluation of **grid uniformity**, the following procedure may be used.

PROCEDURE: GRID UNIFORMITY

1. Place an image receptor under a grid and make an image of a homogenous phantom (made of either aluminum Lucite or a pan of water), using a kVp comparable for use with the grid ratio and enough mAs to create an optical density of 1.5.
2. After processing, take optical density readings of the center and the four quadrants (and any suspicious areas) of the image and compare. **All density readings should be within an optical density value of ±0.10 for proper uniformity**. For CR or DR systems, measure pixel brightness in each of the previously mentioned areas. There should not be more than a 20% difference in pixel brightness. Stationary grids on grid cassettes may require more frequent evaluation.

Grid Alignment

Grids that are misaligned attenuate more of the primary X-ray beam, and this attenuation results in a loss of image quality and greater patient dosing. Proper alignment refers to centering the X-ray field with the focused grid and maintaining the proper grid focusing distance. Grid focusing distance is the proper distance from the X-ray source that a focused grid can be used because the angle of the lead strips in the grid and the angle of divergence of the X-ray photons being emitted match at a specific range of distance values only. Alignment is more critical with greater grid ratios such as 10:1, 12:1, and 16:1 because grid latitude is less. **Grid latitude** is the margin of error in centering the X-ray beam on the center of the grid before significant grid cutoff appears in the resulting image. The alignment must be within the grid latitude specified by the manufacturer (usually within 1 inch). The grid latitude value is found either on the grid front or in the literature supplied by the manufacturer. A commercial grid alignment tool is available (Fig. 5.47) and should be used according to the manufacturer's specifications.

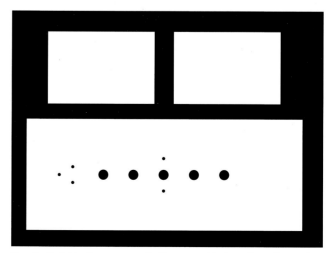

Fig. 5.47 Grid alignment tool. (Courtesy Nuclear Associates, Inc., Carle Place, New York.)

TABLE 5.5	Comparison of Mobile Radiographic Units		
Direct Power	**Capacitor/Discharge**	**Battery Powered**	**High Frequency**
Single-phase output	Constant potential (X-ray production constant)	Constant potential (X-ray production constant)	Constant potential (X-ray production constant)
Limit of 15 mA	Limited to short exposure time	Unit is relatively large and heavy	Unit is small and lightweight
Subject to power fluctuations	No power fluctuation	No power fluctuation while battery is being charged	High kilovolts (peak) and milli-ampere-seconds available
Requires standard outlet in immediate area of operation	Requires standard outlet in immediate area of operation	No need for outlet in immediate area of operation	Requires standard outlet in immediate area of operation

mA, Milliampere.

Portable and Mobile X-ray Generators

Many radiographic examinations must be performed with mobile X-ray generators in hospitals and medical centers because patients' conditions may prevent them from being transported to the main X-ray department. Most of the variables mentioned earlier in this chapter, such as reproducibility, linearity, and focal spot size, can be tested with the same test tools and procedures used for standard radiographic equipment. Testing should occur upon acceptance and then annually (some states require semiannual inspection) or when service is performed Additional tests need to be performed annually on all systems, including testing of brakes, visual inspections of protective bumpers, drive speed control, and correct functionality of the forward/reverse switch. Electrical safety and grounding are critical for the safe operation of mobile equipment. A policy also must be in place regarding the storage of the keys that are required to operate this equipment. Federal and state regulations prohibit leaving keys in mobile equipment when this equipment is not in use and stored in a public area. This is a safety indicator of The Joint Commission. Some type of lockbox with a combination lock, a key storage area within the radiology department, and a key allotment policy for radiographers are just some of the possible ways to address this concern. A distinction should be made between portable and mobile X-ray generators.

Portable X-ray Generator

A portable X-ray generator is small enough to be carried from place to place by one person. It consists of an oil-filled metal tank or casing that contains a stationary anode X-ray tube and transformers. A smaller control unit, containing the exposure switch and timer circuitry, attaches to the casing by means of a 6-ft (1.8-m) cord. A metal stand or tripod holds the casing in place. The maximum output for portable units is 75 kVp and 15 mA, so use is confined generally to chest and extremity examinations in nursing homes, to battlefield use by the military, and to field veterinary use.

Mobile X-ray Generator

A mobile X-ray generator is a smaller version of a radiographic unit that is mounted on wheels and pushed from one location to the next. Mobile units are most often found in hospitals for the examination of patients who are too ill or injured to be taken to the main radiology department. Often, mobile units are mistakenly called "portables." There are several types of mobile X-ray generators (Table 5.5).

Direct-power units. Direct-power units are usually equipped with stationary anode X-ray tubes and have a plug that is placed into a standard 110/120-V outlet. The maximum output for most of these units is 100 kVp and 15 mA. These units are subject to power fluctuations in line voltage.

Capacitor discharge units. Capacitor discharge units are equipped with a high-tension capacitor that must be precharged before each exposure. For the unit to operate properly, it must be plugged in to the main power supply, and the appropriate kVp and mAs are selected. A charge button is then activated on the control panel that allows the capacitor to charge up to the selected value, which usually takes about 10 seconds. A green light indicates a full charge. The X-ray exposure should be made immediately after the indicator light appears because the charge on the capacitor begins to leak. If the kVp drops below 2 kVp of the selected value, the green light deactivates and no exposure can be made until the unit is recharged. Because the voltage drops during the exposure (at about 1 kV/mAs), the exposure time should be kept short to keep the kVp at the desired level. This effect also makes testing for kVp variation difficult for these units; therefore an average kVp/mAs value should be established on installation and then maintained throughout the life of the unit. *Any variation of the kVp/mAs value must be within ±5%. X-ray output is constant, much like that of a three-phase or high-frequency X-ray generator.* These units should also be checked for radiation that may be emitted from capacitor energy storage equipment in standby status. Radiation emitted from the X-ray tube when the exposure switch or timer is not activated shall not exceed a rate of 2 mR per hour or 0.02 mGy per hour at 5 cm from any accessible surface of the diagnostic source assembly with the beam-limiting device fully open.

Cordless, or Battery-Powered, Mobile Units

Cordless, or battery-powered, mobile units use a series of lead or nickel-cadmium wet-cell batteries (usually three) that must be kept charged when the unit is not in use (with a built-in charger that is plugged into the main power supply). The batteries are used to power a drive motor that propels the unit and a polyphase electric generator that produces the electric current that energizes the X-ray tube. These units can usually attain a maximum output of 100 kVp and 25 mA, with a constant X-ray output. The batteries should be removed from the unit, cleaned, discharged completely, and then recharged every 6 months to maintain a continued optimum charge. The X-ray output (in milliroentgens or milligrays of air kerma) per mAs should be determined when the unit is fully charged and again after it has been driven for a distance comparable to what would be expected in clinical use. Radiation output should decrease by no more than 20% under these conditions.

High-Frequency Mobile Units

Like their larger counterparts, high-frequency mobile units are equipped with a microprocessor circuit that increases the frequency of the alternating current to create a nearly constant potential. Some systems are plugged into a standard outlet, whereas others have batteries that must be kept charged. These systems usually achieve as much as 133 kVp and 200 mAs, with a minimum exposure time of 3 ms. For battery-powered systems, the milliroentgen/mAs output should be determined when the unit is fully charged and again after it has been used for a length of time comparable with what occurs during clinical use. Radiation output should decrease by no more than 20% between the two values.

SUMMARY

Through visual inspections, environmental inspections, and performance testing, variation in the functioning of radiographic equipment can be kept to a minimum, which should increase department efficiency, lower the repeat rate, and reduce the number of unnecessary exposures. In addition, ancillary equipment used in conjunction with radiographic units must function within specific parameters to obtain consistent and acceptable quality images. Therefore quality control testing is also required to monitor this level of performance.

Refer to the Evolve website at https://evolve.elsevier.com for Student Experiments 5.1: Radiographic Unit Visual Check; 5.2: Half-Value Layer Measurement and Filtration; 5.3: Milliampere and Exposure Time Linearity; 5.4: Reproducibility, Milliampere-Second Reciprocity, and Milliroentgen per Milliampere-Second; 5.5: Collimation, Beam Alignment, and Perpendicularity; 5.6: Automatic Exposure Control Reproducibility; 5.7: Automatic Exposure Control and Patient Positioning; and 5.8: Grid Alignment.

REVIEW QUESTIONS

1. The indicated level of the tomographic section and the actual level of the section must correspond to within _____mm.
   a. 2
   b. 5
   c. 10
   d. 15

2. A three-phase X-ray generator can operate at a maximum of 100 kVp and 500 mA at 100 ms. What is the kilowatt rating of this generator?
   a. 5
   b. 35
   c. 50
   d. 500

3. The backup system for an automatic exposure control should terminate the exposure at _____ second(s) or _____ mAs, whichever comes first.
   a. 1; 100
   b. 3; 300
   c. 6; 600
   d. 9; 900

4. How large of an arc appears during a spinning top test of a three-phase X-ray generator at 50 ms?
   a. 18 degrees
   b. 20 degrees
   c. 36 degrees
   d. 90 degrees

5. Which of the following should a quality control program for radiographic equipment include: (1) visual inspection, (2) environmental inspection, or (3) performance testing?
   a. 1 and 2 only
   b. 2 and 3 only
   c. 1 and 3 only
   d. 1, 2, and 3

6. The minimum HVL for X-ray units operating at 80 kVp is _____ mm of aluminum.
   a. 1.3
   b. 1.5
   c. 2.3
   d. 2.5

7. The maximum variability allowed for the reproducibility of exposure is ±_____%.
   a. 2
   b. 5
   c. 10
   d. 20

8. Any variations between the stated kVp on the control panel and the measured kVp must be ±_____%.
   a. 2
   b. 5
   c. 10
   d. 20

9. The variability allowed for timer accuracy in exposures less than 10 ms is ± _____%.
   a. 2
   b. 5
   c. 10
   d. 20

10. The variability allowed for mAs linearity is ± _____%.
    a. 2%
    b. 5%
    c. 10%
    d. 20%

6

Radiographic Image Artifacts

OBJECTIVES

At the completion of this chapter, the reader should be able to do the following:
- Explain the importance of repeat analysis studies in quality management
- Determine the causal repeat rate of a diagnostic imaging department
- Determine the total repeat rate of a diagnostic imaging department
- Identify artifacts that may appear in radiographic images
- Explain the corrective action required for elimination of the appearance of image artifacts

KEY TERMS

Artifacts
Chatter
Dropped pixels
Histogram error
Reject or repeat analysis program (RAP)
Repeat analysis
Reticulation marks

The desired outcome of a diagnostic imaging study is the creation of a high-quality diagnostic image, a correct diagnosis by the interpreting physician, and the satisfaction of all internal and external customers (e.g., the patient, referring provider, third-party payer). Most of the material in the previous chapters has involved a discussion of quality management processes and quality control testing to ensure that the equipment delivers optimal image quality. However, quality control testing can minimize only the risk of obtaining subquality images but cannot prevent them entirely; therefore a quality management program also must include looking at the final outcome of a diagnostic X-ray procedure (e.g., image quality, correct diagnostic) and determining the quality of the outcome to see whether further improvement can be achieved. Steps involved in this outcome assessment include a repeat analysis of images (to avoid future repeats) and an artifact analysis of images (to identify the cause and prevent future occurrence).

REPEAT ANALYSIS

An important aspect of a quality management program for diagnostic imaging departments is the performance of a reject, retake, or repeat analysis procedure. The difference between reject and repeat images is as follows:

Rejects: All rejected images, including repeats (retakes)

Repeats: Patient images repeated, resulting in additional patient exposure

A reject or repeat analysis program (RAP) is a systematic process of cataloging rejected images and determining the nature of the repeat so that repeat images can be minimized or eliminated in the future. Repeat analysis provides important data about equipment and accessory performance, departmental procedures, and the skill level of the technical staff. With this knowledge, solutions can be found to minimize repeats and also document the effectiveness (or lack thereof) of quality control and quality management protocols. Table 6.1 lists the information required for an effective RAP according to the American Association of Physicists in Medicine, Task Group 151.

ADVANTAGES

The main advantages of lower department repeat rates are improved department efficiency, lower department costs, and lower patient doses for modalities that utilize ionizing radiation.

Improved Department Efficiency

With the number of repeated images kept low, the amount of time that patients must spend undergoing diagnostic procedures decreases. This increases patient (customer) satisfaction and allows the department to service more patients in the same period.

Lower Department Costs

Whereas the cost of film and processing is no longer relevant in a fully digital environment with soft-copy reading, other concerns remain. Having a technologist tying up a procedure room to repeat an image lowers department efficiency and increases the cost of labor. Repeat images also cause depreciation of equipment (such as shortening tube life in radiography and computed tomography), which can add significant costs to diagnostic imaging departments through repair and/or replacement.

Lower Patient Doses

A diagnostic image that is unacceptable results in the repeat of that particular view or procedure, which means that the patient must be reexposed to ionizing radiation (except for sonography and magnetic resonance imaging studies). As an example, a lumbar spine series performed on a 200-speed imaging system yields an entrance skin exposure of approximately 600 mrad (6 mGy). A repeat of this study would obviously double this amount of radiation.

CAUSAL REPEAT RATE

An important piece of data to obtain from a repeat analysis is the causal repeat rate, which is the percentage of repeats that occur from a specific cause. In repeat analysis studies performed in departments that use film/screen radiography and do not have quality control procedures for the darkroom, processor, and equipment, 45% of all repeats were caused by exposure errors. With quality control protocols in place, studies have demonstrated that most repeats are caused by positioning errors. Digital departments with quality control procedures also show positioning errors as the number one cause of repeat exposures.

For a causal repeat rate to be determined, a worksheet such as the one included in Fig. 6.1 for digital radiography departments should be used so that the proper statistical information is obtained and recorded. The American College of Radiology

TABLE 6.1	Information Required for an Effective Repeat Analysis Program (AAPM TG 151)	
Field	**Function**	**Required/Optional**
Acquisition station/digitizer	Identify specific stations with problems	Required
Accession number	Links study through RIS	Required
Examination date and time	Temporal sorting of data	Required
Body part/view	Sorting	Required
Exposure indicators	Exposure analysis/troubleshooting	Required
Reject category	Allows reject analysis	Required
Technologist ID	Linking technologist and study	Required
Reject comments	Further clarifies reason for rejection-free field	Optional
Technique factors	Troubleshooting	Optional
Thumbnail image	QC of reason for rejection	Optional

AAPM, American Association of Physicists in Medicine; *QC*, quality control; *RIS*, radiology information system.

CR/DR Repeat Analysis Form

Room # _____   Date: _____   Technologist: _____

Patient ID	Exam	positioning	overexpose	underexpose	motion	wrong exam code	collimation	artifact	No exposure	Double expose	No marker	Marker over part	Wrong exam code	other

Fig. 6.1 Repeat analysis worksheet (CR/DR). *CR*, Computed radiography; *DR*, digital radiography.

is a good source for worksheets for other modalities. In radiography departments that are still film/screen, reject film images are saved for silver reclamation purposes, so sorting them daily and recording the data on the worksheet can be done on a regular basis. In digital departments, the database of most computed radiography (CR) and digital radiography (DR) systems can be accessed to yield repeat analysis data. Most departments tabulate the data monthly to obtain a large enough statistical sample (at least 250 patients) for reliability. It is recommended that the same individual be responsible for performing the analysis because image viewer differences can affect the outcome of the repeat analysis study. The worksheet should include the radiographic procedures performed in the department, along with the possible causes of rejection such as positioning, overexposure, underexposure, motion, artifacts, and miscellaneous causes. Once the data have been recorded for the specified period, the causal repeat rate and the total department rate should be determined. The causal repeat rate is the percentage of repeats from a specific cause such as positioning error or technique error and is calculated with the following equation:

$$\text{Causal repeat rate} = \frac{\text{Number of repeats for a specific cause}}{\text{Total number of repeats}} \times 100$$

For example, if a radiography department has a total of 185 repeat images during a 1-month period and 67 of the 185 are the result of positioning errors, then the percent of repeats caused by positioning error is 36%. Many radiology information systems can calculate the causal repeat rate when department staff enter the number and cause of repeat images into the system.

TOTAL REPEAT RATE

Once the causal repeat rate worksheet is completed, the next important piece of data in a repeat analysis study is to obtain the total repeat rate for the entire department. The total department repeat rate is determined with the following equation:

$$\text{Total repeat rate} = \frac{\text{Number of repeat images}}{\text{Total number of views taken}} \times 100$$

For example, if a department performs a total of 1160 views during a 1-month period and 132 are rejected and must be repeated, then the total department repeat rate is 11.4%. Some automatic film processors have a counting device that records the total number of images processed that can be used as the "total number of views taken" in the equation (most CR and DR systems have software that can access the total number of images processed during a given period to obtain the same information). Many factors influence this rate, such as the quality of the equipment, the competence of the technical staff, the patient population, data collection method, shift (weekend, evening, or day shift), and the number of images accepted by radiologists to diagnose.

- Data from the repeat analysis are used to identify which of these factors is a major contributor to the overall repeat rate. If a particular piece of equipment is often identified as being at fault for repeat images, data from the repeat analysis can be used to justify repair or replacement costs. If certain employees demonstrate an abnormally high number of repeats, additional in-service education or other corrective action can be used to help alleviate the problem. Ideally, total repeat rates in radiography departments should be between 1% and 3% for digital departments. The average in the United States is approximately 10% in film/screen departments and 4%–8% in digital departments.

Repeat rates for radiographic procedures should not exceed 8% for general radiography and 5% for pediatric radiography, according to the American Association of Physicists in Medicine, Task Group 151. Both the American Association of Physicists in Medicine and the American College of Radiology suggest a repeat rate in excess of 10% for general radiography and 7% for pediatric radiography as thresholds for investigation and corrective action. The total repeat rate for mammography should be 2% or less, but a rate of 5% is probably adequate if the radiologist and medical physicist agree that this is a reasonable level. In addition, mammographic repeat rates cannot change by more than ±2% each quarter. If greater than this amount occurs, the change should be investigated and corrective action taken if necessary. However, this may not be practical in all departments when the amount of variation that may be present in imaging equipment, technologist experience level, institutional image quality acceptance standards, and patient population is considered. Generally, department repeat rates that are too high should be investigated and corrective action taken. A department repeat rate that is too low may signal problems with compliance or acceptance of poor-quality images.

ARTIFACT ANALYSIS

One cause of rejected images listed in the repeat analysis worksheet is the presence of image artifacts. An artifact is anything on a finished radiograph that is not part of the patient's anatomy. Artifacts can contribute significantly to the total repeat rate. Therefore a thorough knowledge of artifacts and their possible causes is necessary so that corrective action can be taken. The remainder of this chapter will focus on artifacts found in radiography.

Analog (Film/Screen) Radiography

Image artifacts found in film/screen radiography can be placed into one of three categories: processing artifacts, exposure artifacts, and handling and storage artifacts.

Processing Artifacts

Processing artifacts are caused by or occur during the processing of diagnostic images.

Emulsion Pickoff

In emulsion pickoff, the emulsion is removed from or "picked off" of the film base. This occurs when two images are stuck

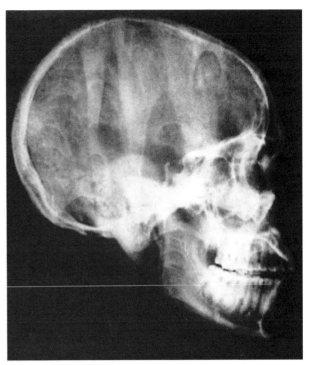

Fig. 6.2 Curtain effect.

together before or during processing and then pulled apart afterward. It also occurs with single sheets of film that are processed in underreplenished developer, which results in glutaraldehyde failure. Because glutaraldehyde is the weak hardener added to the developer solution that keeps the film from sticking to the rollers, failure of this ingredient will cause the emulsion to be removed from the film and deposited on the rollers.

Gelatin Buildup

Emulsion that has been removed from earlier images and either stuck on processor rollers or dissolved in the developer solution can be deposited on subsequent images. The primary cause is underreplenished developer solution or failure of the developer circulation system filter.

Curtain Effect

Solution dripping on, or "running down," a film can form patterns on the film that resemble a lace curtain (Fig. 6.2). This is more common in manually processed images but can occur in automatically processed images if the wash water is dirty or if a film has jammed and must be removed from the processor before passing through the dryer section.

Chemical Fog

Chemical fog is an overdevelopment of the film that results in excessive base + fog and minimum diameter (D_{min}) values with sensitometry images and excessive optical density with radiographic images (Fig. 6.3). The main cause is developer temperature, time, pH, or concentration above the manufacturer's specifications. It

Normal fog

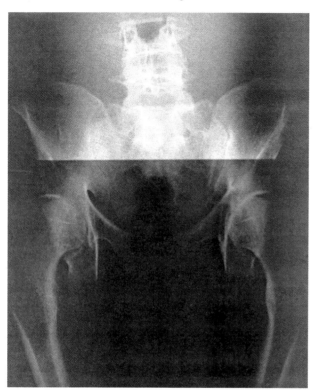

Severe fog

Fig. 6.3 Chemical fog.

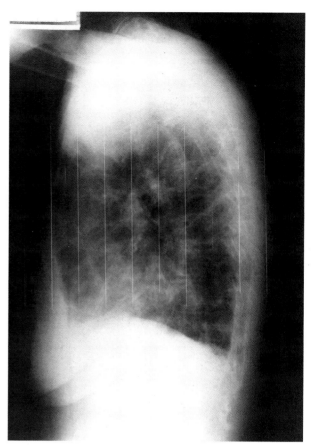

Fig. 6.4 Guide shoe marks.

also may occur with overreplenishment of the developer solution.

Guide Shoe Marks

Guide shoe marks are scratches on images made by the jagged edges of the guide shoes because they may be bent, worn, damaged, incorrectly installed, or incorrectly adjusted. They also may occur with improperly seated transport racks or rollers (Fig. 6.4). Guide shoe marks caused by crossover assemblies usually occur at the top surface of the film. Guide shoe marks from turnaround assemblies tend to occur at the bottom surface of the film. These scratches run parallel to (in the same direction as) the direction of film travel.

Pi Lines

Pi lines are artifacts that occur relative to the circumference of a roller and therefore occur at regular intervals (Fig. 6.5). These marks run perpendicular to the direction of film travel and are usually caused by dirt or debris on the rollers.

Chatter

Chattering artifacts appear as bands of increased optical density that occur perpendicular to film direction. Chatter is caused by inconsistent motion of the transport system, usually because the drive gears or drive chain slips. Chemical buildup on gears or gears not seated properly can cause chatter marks that are approximately ⅛-inch apart. A rusty

or loose drive chain can cause chatter marks that are about ⅜-inch apart.

Dichroic Stain

The term *dichroic* refers to "two colors," brown and greenish yellow. The presence of brown stains on a radiograph could indicate a film processed in oxidized developer or hyporetention that has been present during several years of storage. The greenish yellow type of stain indicates the presence of unexposed and undeveloped silver halide crystals remaining on the film after processing and is caused by incomplete fixation.

Reticulation Marks

When uneven solution temperatures cause excessive expansion and contraction of the film emulsion during processing, the result is a network of fine grooves in the film surface (**reticulation marks**).

Streaking

Streaking is uneven development of the image that can be caused by the failure of agitation in manual processing or the failure of the circulation system in automatic processing (Fig. 6.6).

Hesitation Marks

Hesitation marks (also known as *stub lines*) are stripes of decreased optical density where transport rollers are left in contact with the film and further development is prevented

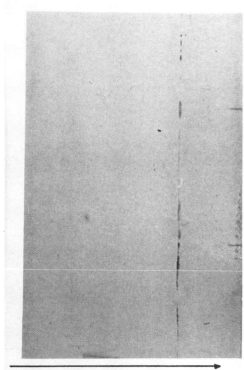

Direction of film transport

Fig. 6.5 Pi lines.

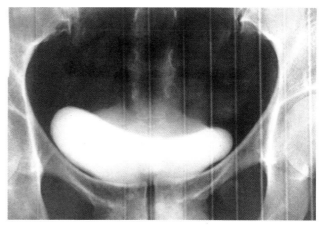

Fig. 6.7 Hesitation marks.

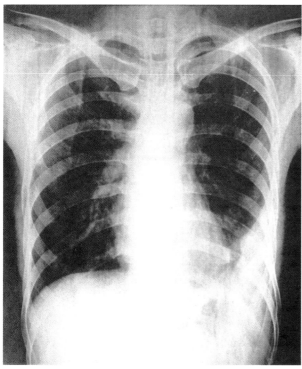

Fig. 6.6 Streaking.

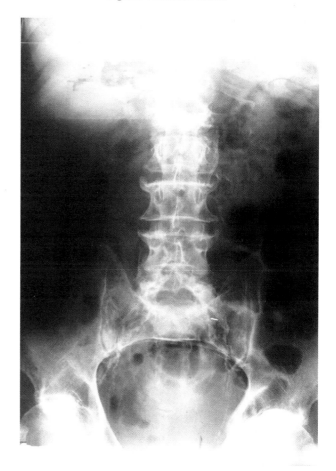

Fig. 6.8 Water spots.

Water Spots

Should water or other liquid come in contact with an unprocessed image, a pattern of increased optical density appears after processing (Fig. 6.8).

Wet-Pressure Sensitization

The entrance rollers on most processors are made of soft rubber with grooves on the surface to grab the film from the feed tray. Should these rollers or the film become wet before the film is introduced, the combination of the pressure and the water marks forms a series of dark stripes that match the

(Fig. 6.7). These artifacts occur when the processor is turned off or loses power while the film is in the developer section or if the film becomes jammed while in the developer section. They also can occur if the transport system speed decreases significantly.

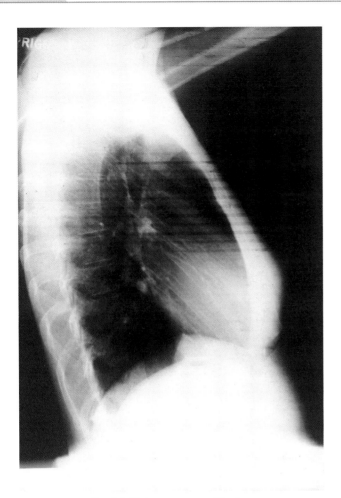

Fig. 6.9 Wet-pressure sensitization.

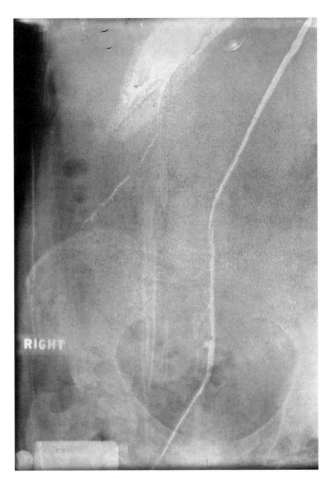

Fig. 6.10 Hyporetention.

grooves on the rollers (Fig. 6.9). The marks also may occur if the tension on the entrance rollers is too great. These marks run in the same direction as film travel. These artifacts also are known as *entrance roller marks.*

Hyporetention

Hyporetention is a white, powdery residue that remains on the film surface because of incomplete washing (Fig. 6.10). This residue forms when the fixer chemicals crystallize as the film dries. A lesser degree of hyporetention can result in brown dichroic stains, which were discussed previously.

Insufficient Optical Density

Images that lack sufficient optical density as a result of processing problems can occur because of the following conditions: developer temperature that is below accepted limits, insufficient developer time, underreplenished developer solution, a developer that is contaminated by the fixer, developer pH that is too low, or insufficient developer concentration.

Excessive Optical Density

Images with excessive optical density as a result of processing problems can occur because of the following conditions: the extension of the developer temperature's accepted limits, excessive developer time, overreplenishment, higher accepted limits of the developer pH, or excessive developer concentration.

Exposure Artifacts

Exposure artifacts are caused by the patient, the technologist, or the equipment during a diagnostic procedure.

Motion

A motion artifact is a blurring of the image caused by the motion of the patient, X-ray source, or image receptor. This results in a significant loss of recorded detail. Patient motion can be reduced with short exposure time, immobilization, and proper instructions to the patient.

Patient Artifacts

Patient artifacts are caused by items that can be either on or within the patient when a diagnostic procedure is performed. Examples of patient artifacts include buttons, snaps, necklaces, earrings, hairpins, wet hair, and body piercing jewelry.

Improper Optical Density

Improper selection of technical factors by the technologist or improper cell selection with automatic exposure control results in improper optical density.

Improper Patient Position or Missing Anatomy of Interest

Improper patient position or missing anatomy of interest is the result of improper patient, X-ray, or image receptor position by the technologist, or improper collimation, which can clip the anatomy of interest.

Quantum Mottle

Quantum mottle is a grainy appearance in a radiograph that is caused by statistical variations in the number of X-ray photons covering a specific area. This is usually present when there is an insufficient amount of radiation reaching the image receptor or detection device. This can occur with film/screen radiography, CR, DR, fluoroscopy, computed tomography, and nuclear medicine imaging. This is discussed later in this chapter under both Computed Radiography Artifacts and Digital Radiography Artifacts.

Poor Film-to-Screen Contact

Poor film-to-screen contact results in localized blurring of the radiographic image, which also may demonstrate slightly increased optical density in these regions.

Double Exposure

Double exposure occurs when an image receptor is exposed more than once before the image is processed.

Grid Artifacts

Improper use of a grid causes grid artifacts, which include grid lines, grid cutoff, and moiré effect.

Grid Lines

Grid lines are shadows of the lead strips that appear on the resulting image and are caused by failure of the grid to move during the exposure, improper grid-focusing distance, improper angulation of the central ray with respect to the grid lines, or improper centering (Fig. 6.11).

Grid Cutoff

Grid cutoff is a decrease in optical density caused by primary radiation being absorbed by (or cut off by) the grid (Fig. 6.12). Any improper use of a grid can cause grid cutoff.

Moiré Effect

Moiré effect, or zebra pattern artifact in film/screen radiography, is a double set of grid lines caused by the placement of a grid cassette in a bucky whereby two grids are above the image receptor (Fig. 6.13). This artifact also can occur in CR systems when a stationary grid having a grid frequency in the range of 85–100 lines per inch is used, and the grid lines are parallel to the CR reader scan lines. This is because of the scan frequency of the laser in the image reader device closely matching the grid frequency. To eliminate this particular cause of moiré effect, the following steps can be taken:

1. Ensure grids are moving during the exposure.
2. Use a grid with a higher grid frequency.
3. Use a crosshatch grid or a multihole grid.
4. Change the orientation of the grid so that the grid lines are perpendicular to the CR reader scan lines.

Handling and Storage Artifacts

Handling and storage artifacts occur during darkroom handling or during storage before use.

Fig. 6.11 Grid lines.

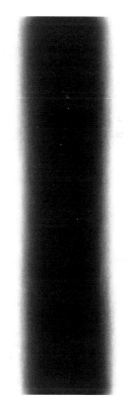

Fig. 6.12 Grid cutoff.

Light Fog

The light of any improper color that strikes the film before development fogs the film and therefore lowers the image contrast. Fog is any noninformational optical density present in a film image.

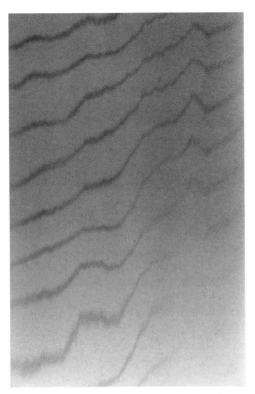

Fig. 6.13 Moiré effect, or zebra pattern, artifact.

Age Fog

Age fog may occur in film that has been processed beyond the expiration date or has been stored in a warm, humid environment. It results in a lower image contrast.

Safelight Fog

Safelight fog is caused by an improper safelight filter, cracks or pinholes in the safelight filter, incorrect wattage of the safelight bulb, incorrect distance between the safelight and work surfaces, or widely open sodium vapor lamp shutters.

Radiation Fog

Radiation fog appears in film that has been exposed to ionizing radiation before development.

Pressure Marks

Excessive pressure, such as a heavy object placed on the film before development, causes pressure marks, which are areas of increased optical density. Pressure marks occur because the pressure splitting the bond between the silver and the halide ion in the film emulsion results in the presence of black metallic silver after processing. Film should be stored vertically to minimize the risk of pressure artifacts.

Static

The sparks from static electricity expose film and produce three types of static artifacts: tree static, crown static, and smudge static (Fig. 6.14).

Tree Static

Tree static resembles trees or bushes without leaves and is usually caused by low-humidity conditions in the film processing area.

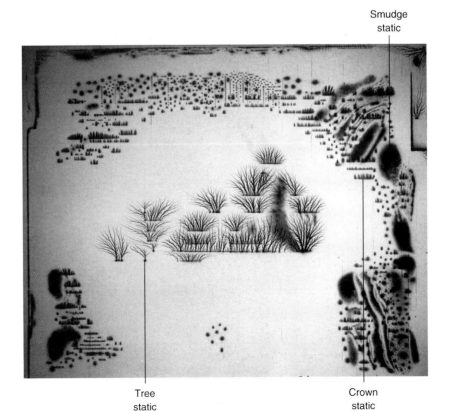

Fig. 6.14 Image demonstrating static artifacts.

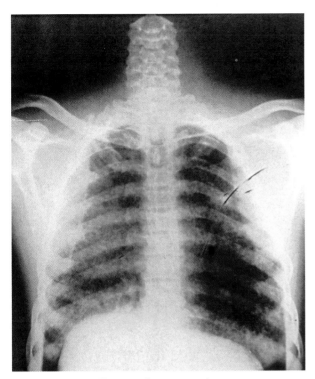

Fig. 6.15 Crescent marks.

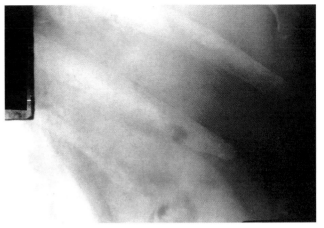

Fig. 6.16 Cassette marks.

Crown Static

Crown static marks radiate in one direction and resemble a crown. Excessive friction from the pulling of the film (such as in a daylight system, in which the film is "squeezed" too tightly between the intensifying screens) can produce these marks.

Smudge Static

Smudge static consists of dark areas where excessive amounts of light have exposed the film and is usually caused by rough handling in the film processing area.

Crescent or Crinkle Marks

Crescent or crinkle marks are half-moon-shaped marks of increased optical density caused by bending of the film before processing (Fig. 6.15). The bending of a processed film image can result in crescent marks that are of decreased optical density because some of the silver can be moved from the area where the bending has occurred.

Scratches

Scratches are areas where the emulsion has been removed by sharp objects such as fingernails or sharp points on surfaces.

Cassette Marks

Cassette marks are white specks on the image caused by dirt or debris inside the cassette. This foreign matter blocks the light from the screen from reaching the film. Regular cleaning of the screens with an antistatic cleaner can minimize these artifacts (Fig. 6.16).

Computed Radiography (CR) Artifacts

Even though liquid processing and film/screen image receptors are not used with digital radiographic systems, artifacts can still occur and therefore must have their sources recognized by radiographers to minimize their occurrence. This is in addition to the exposure artifacts listed earlier in the section on film/screen artifacts—these also will occur with CR and DR systems (except for poor film/screen contact). Artifacts occurring during preprocessing functions often cannot be corrected, whereas those occurring during postprocessing tend to be recoverable. CR system artifacts can be broken down into three main categories: image plate artifacts, plate reader and processing artifacts, and operator error.

IMAGE PLATE ARTIFACTS

Defects in the Imaging Plate

Scratches, scuff marks, or cracks in a CR image plate can mimic fractures and signs of pneumothorax (Fig. 6.17). Therefore image plates must be inspected periodically, and damaged plates must be removed from service.

Phantom Image Artifact

CR image plates must be properly erased before use, or data from previous images will interfere with current image data (Fig. 6.18). In DR imaging, this artifact is known as electronic memory artifact or "ghosting" and can be caused by exposures that are taken in too rapid a sequence, resulting in not enough time for each previous exposure to transfer the entire signal (e.g., the image receptor is not completely read out).

Foreign Objects

Dirt and debris can find their way to CR image plates and DR flat panels, causing light-colored specks similar to those that occur with dirty intensifying screens in film/screen radiography (Fig. 6.19).

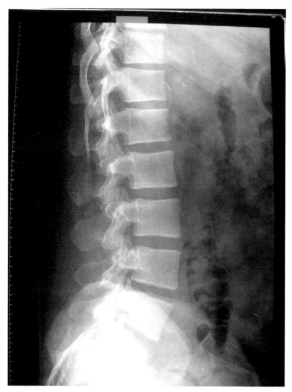

Fig. 6.17 Artifact caused by scratches on a computed radiography plate. (Courtesy Janet Petersen, Elmhurst Memorial Hospital, Elmhurst, Illinois.)

Background Radiation

The CR image plate can respond to an exposure as low as 10 µR (0.1 mGy air kerma). Background radiation can vary between 40 and 80 µR/day (0.4–0.8 mGy air kerma/day). It is recommended that CR plates be erased daily if not used to eliminate unwanted noise (Fig. 6.20).

Backscatter Lines

The dark line is caused by backscatter transmitted through the back of the cassette. The line corresponds to the cassette hinge where the lead coating was weakened or cracked. To reduce backscatter, the radiographer should collimate when possible.

Phosphor Wear

CR image plates are inserted into and out of the reader unit each time the plate is processed. Eventually, friction can start to remove the photostimulable phosphor crystal from the plate, which can impair image quality. The plate must be replaced if this begins to occur (Fig. 6.21).

PLATE READER AND PROCESSING ARTIFACTS

Electronic Noise

Noise created by the internal electronics of the CR reader system can occur in CR images. Noise suppression filters can usually eliminate this problem.

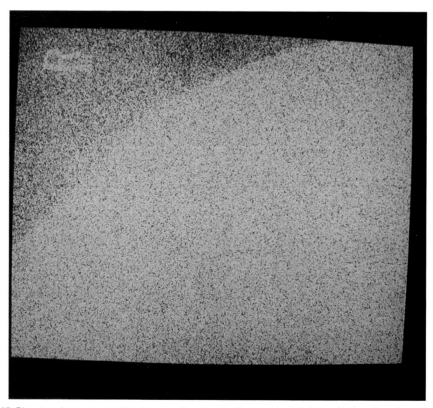

Fig. 6.18 Phantom image caused by incomplete erasure of computed radiography imaging plate. (Courtesy Janet Petersen, Elmhurst Memorial Hospital, Elmhurst, Illinois.)

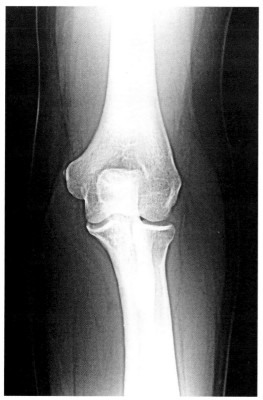

Fig. 6.19 Artifact caused by dirt on computed radiography imaging plate.

Fig. 6.21 Phosphor wear on computed radiography imaging plate.

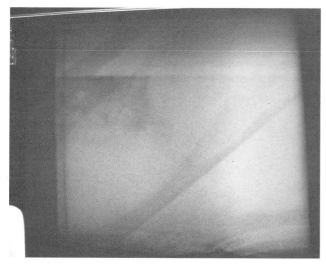

Fig. 6.20 This image was produced by background radiation on a computed radiography plate that had not been used for days. (Courtesy Barbara Smith Pruner, Portland Community College, Portland, Oregon.)

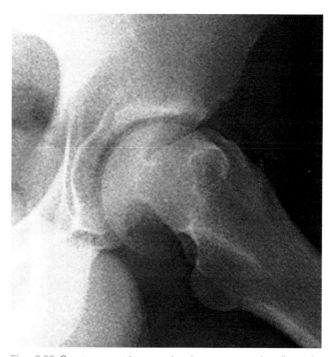

Fig. 6.22 Quantum mottle occurring in a computed radiography image.

Quantum Mottle

Just as with film/screen systems (or any imaging system that relies on photons to cover an area of interest), quantum mottle can occur with digital imaging systems and create the same "grainy" appearance. Often, it is even more common in digital systems, as radiographers may use lower milliampere-second values to decrease patient dose and then use computer software to correct image brightness (Fig. 6.22).

Increased Sensitivity to Scatter

Both CR and DR systems have image receptors that are much more sensitive to scattered radiation as a result of lower K-edge values. This means that the effects of scatter (and background radiation) can cause a decrease in image contrast that postprocessing software may not be able to correct.

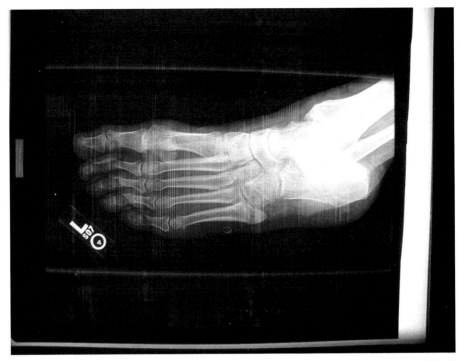

Fig. 6.23 Scan lines appearing on digital image. (Courtesy Janet Petersen, Elmhurst Memorial Hospital, Elmhurst, Illinois.)

Reader Malfunction

CR scanner malfunction can cause skipped scan lines, missing pixels, and distorted images (Fig. 6.23). These also can be caused by memory problems, digitization problems, or communication errors. Dust and debris also can collect on the rotating polygonal mirror or light collection optics in the image reader device. Lasers also have a limited life and must be replaced periodically.

Excessive Equalization

Normally, the exposure index ("S" value, exposure index (EI), log of median exposure (LgM), etc.) will indicate if the receptor exposure level was appropriate. However, the exposure index may not be correctly calculated if a histogram analysis problem has occurred. Equalization processing can make light areas darker and darker areas lighter.

Aliasing

Aliasing can occur if not enough samples are taken (fewer than twice per cycle), and the representation of the original signal will not be accurate after computer processing. This sampling error is referred to as aliasing and causes moiré pattern artifacts in the image (Fig. 6.24). A moiré or zebra pattern artifact can also occur if the grid frequency and scan frequency of the CR reader unit are similar and oriented in the same direction.

OPERATOR ERROR ARTIFACTS

Heat Blur

This is a blurring of the image that can occur when a CR system imaging plate is exposed to intense heat before being processed within the CR reader system.

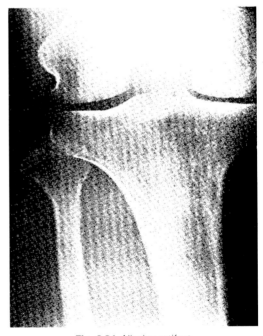

Fig. 6.24 Aliasing artifact.

Improper Image Brightness

When CR systems are used, improper image brightness (optical density when placed onto a hard-copy image) can occur when an incorrect preprocessing histogram is selected (e.g., an adult histogram for the radiography of a pediatric chest). This is known as **histogram error**. Improper image brightness with CR systems also can occur because of nonparallel collimation. For the histograms used by CR systems to

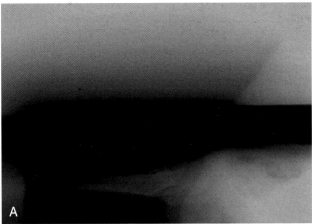

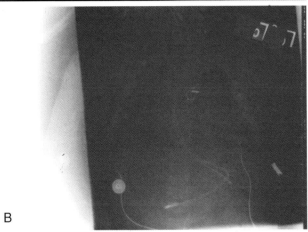

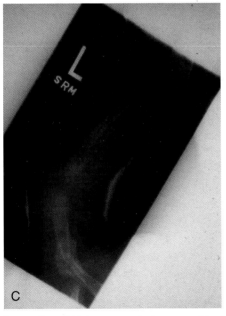

Fig. 6.25 A sampling of histogram analysis errors. (Courtesy Barry Burns, University of North Carolina, Chapel Hill, North Carolina.)

process the final image, the collimation edges of the radiation field should be parallel to the sides of the imaging plate (Fig. 6.25). This way, the preprogrammed histogram in the CR system, the histogram created by the imaging plate match, and the computer can assign the correct optical density values to the appropriate region of the image. When collimation is not parallel, the histograms do not match correctly and the system then may be unable to determine the appropriate image brightness value.

Double Exposure

As with film/screen image receptors, CR imaging plates can be double exposed, leading to both images being lost because data are entered during preprocessing functions (Fig. 6.26).

Improper Use of a CR Cassette

CR cassettes have both a front and a back and are not interchangeable. Fig. 6.27 shows an image taken with the CR cassette upside down.

Digital Radiography Artifacts

DR systems can experience artifacts that are very similar to some CR artifacts. The most common DR artifacts are as follows.

Dropped Pixels

Sometimes detector elements in an active-matrix array can stop functioning, which means that no data from that area are included in the final image (Fig. 6.28). Because each pixel is relatively small (40–100 μm) and there are five or more megapixels in the image, this usually will not be visible. If several detector elements in a specific area all stop at once, white specks can appear in the image that can mimic certain pathologies. Equalization (also known as flat-fielding) software can often correct for dropped pixels, but care should be taken with DR active-matrix arrays (especially cassette-based systems), because rough handling can damage them, causing dropped pixels.

Quantum Mottle

Just as with CR systems, quantum mottle can occur with DR systems and create the same "grainy" appearance. Often, it is even more common in DR systems, as they require lower milliampere-second values because of their higher detective quantum efficiency (see Fig. 6.22).

Increased Sensitivity to Scatter

Both CR and DR systems have image receptors that are much more sensitive to scattered radiation because of lower K-edge values. This means that the effects of scatter (and background radiation) can cause a decrease in image contrast that postprocessing software may not be able to correct.

Electronic Interference

Wireless DR image receptors can suffer from electronic interference from devices that draw large amount of electronic power or from cell phones, laptops, and the like. Care must be taken to avoid these sources of interference (Fig. 6.29).

Tiling Artifact

As mentioned in Chapter 8, DR system active-matrix arrays are constructed using a series of smaller thin film transistor

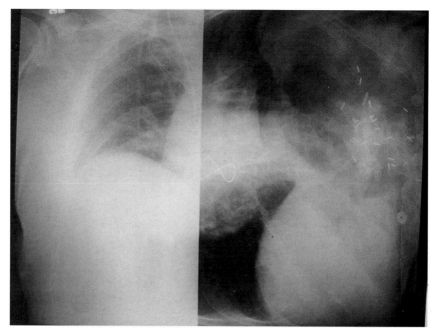

Fig. 6.26 Double exposure. (Courtesy Pamela Verkuilen, AMITA Saint Alexius Medical Center, Hoffman Estates, Illinois.)

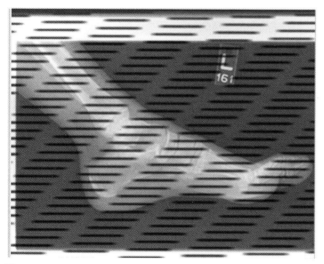

Fig. 6.27 Image taken with computed radiography cassette upside down.

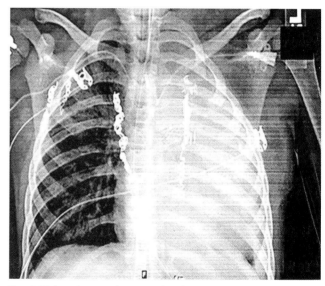

Fig. 6.29 Interference from nearby electrical equipment with wireless digital radiography cassette.

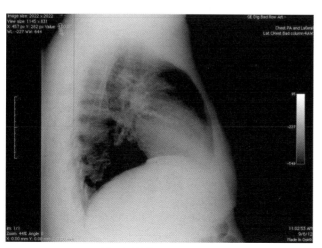

Fig. 6.28 Dropped pixels.

chips that are laid out in rows and columns (much like tiles on a wall or floor). Because each chip may have slightly different electronic connections, the current values from each of these chips may have slightly different electronic values that are fed back to the computer for processing. This can lead to slightly different brightness values that can be seen in the final image (Fig. 6.30). Equalization or flat-fielding software can usually eliminate this artifact.

Dirt or Foreign Matter

As with film/screen and CR image receptors, dirt or other foreign matter (such as contrast media) can cause white specks in the processed image (Fig. 6.31).

Fig. 6.30 Tiling artifact with digital radiography active matrix array.

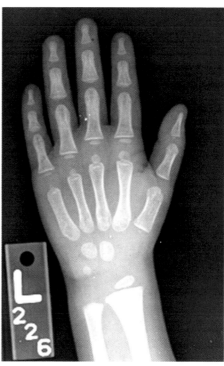

Fig. 6.31 Artifact caused by dirt on front of digital radiography image receptor.

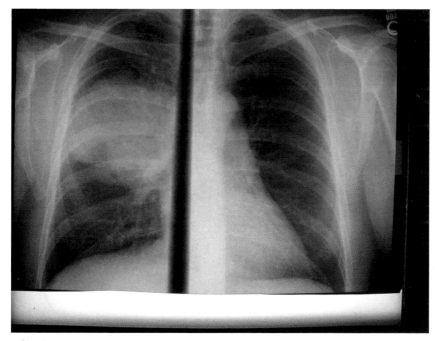

Fig. 6.32 Shading occurring during hard-copy printing. (Courtesy Pamela Verkuilen, AMITA Saint Alexius Medical Center, Hoffman Estates, Illinois.)

Printer Errors

Both CR and DR systems rely on dry laser printers to produce hard copies of images. Even though these devices are generally more reliable than wet film processors, they are still subject to problems, including incorrect density calibration, light leaks, transport problems, and laser misalignment. These can lead to artifacts such as shading, which results in dark areas in the image (Fig. 6.32), and the "corduroy effect" (Fig. 6.33), where scan lines caused by transport problems appear in the image. The corduroy artifact can also appear in DR images, where they are caused by a combination of uniformly spaced components within the detector and the sampling rate of the signal. Usually, a software update can change the sampling rate and eliminate the artifact.

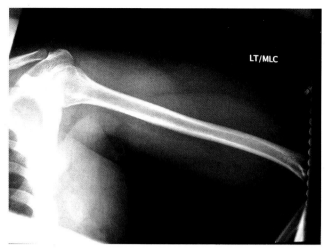

Fig. 6.33 Corduroy effect. (Courtesy Pamela Verkuilen, AMITASaint Alexius Medical Center, Hoffman Estates, Illinois.)

SUMMARY

Implementing a quality management program requires more than just equipment monitoring and maintenance. The outcomes assessment of diagnostic images also must be performed to evaluate the success of the procedure. In this way, future problems may be avoided by analyzing current causes of repeat images and artifacts. Continuous improvement of image quality and customer satisfaction can occur when diagnostic image quality and diagnostic accuracy are monitored on a routine basis.

Refer to the Evolve website at https://evolve.elsevier.com for Student Experiment 6.1: Reject-Repeat Analysis.

REVIEW QUESTIONS

1. In departments with a quality management program in place, the greatest number of repeat images is caused by which of the following?
   a. Equipment problems
   b. Image fog
   c. Patient motion
   d. Positioning error

2. If a department performs 1160 views during a 1-month period and 132 are repeated, the department repeat rate is which of the following?
   a. 9.5%
   b. 10.7%
   c. 11.4%
   d. 14.8%

3. Any repeat rate exceeding _____ should be seriously examined.
   a. 2%–4%
   b. 4%–6%
   c. 6%–8%
   d. 10%–12%

4. Which of the following processing artifacts run in the same direction as film travel?
   a. Pi lines
   b. Guide shoe marks
   c. Hesitation marks
   d. Chemical fog

5. Which of the following artifacts can occur in both CR and film/screen radiography?
   a. Static electricity
   b. Wet-pressure sensitization
   c. Moiré pattern
   d. Water spots

6. The types of static artifacts include (1, tree; 2, crown; 3, smudge):
   a. 1 and 2
   b. 2 and 3
   c. 1 and 3
   d. 1, 2, and 3

7. Which of the following is not a digital imaging artifact?
   a. Tiling
   b. Hyporetention
   c. Dropped pixels
   d. Electronic noise

8. Data for determining repeat rates should include at least _____ patients to obtain a statistical sample large enough for valid results.
   a. 100
   b. 150
   c. 250
   d. 500

9. Ghost images can appear when:
   a. Radiation fatigue is present.
   b. Dirt or foreign matter is on the front of the image receptor.
   c. Too low of a milliampere-second value is used.
   d. A DR image receptor is not completely read out.

10. Which of the following artifacts occurs as a result of patient motion during exposure?
    a. A processing artifact
    b. An exposure artifact
    c. A handling artifact
    d. No artifact

Quality Control of Fluoroscopic Equipment

OBJECTIVES

At the completion of this chapter, the reader should be able to do the following:

- List the main components of a modern fluoroscopic system
- Discuss how the brightness of fluoroscopic images is maintained

- Describe the various methods of monitoring fluoroscopic images
- Perform visual and environmental inspections of a fluoroscopic system
- List and describe the performance tests for fluoroscopic equipment

KEY TERMS

Air kerma
Air kerma rate (AKR)
Automatic brightness control
Automatic brightness stabilization
Automatic exposure rate control (AERC)
Automatic gain control
Brightness gain
Charge-coupled device (CCD)
Cinefluorography

Complementary metallic oxide semiconductor (CMOS)
Flat-panel sensor (detector)
Flux gain
High-contrast resolution
Image intensifiers
Image lag
Image-orthicon
Low-contrast resolution
Minification gain
Multifield image intensifier

Orthicon
Photoemission
Photofluorospot
Pincushion distortion
Plumbicon
Relative conversion factor
S distortion
Veiling glare
Vidicon
Vignetting

Fluoroscopic imaging is used widely in radiology to visualize the dynamics of internal structures and fluids. The image produced is a dynamic, or real-time, image compared with conventional radiography, which creates a static image. Because of the real-time image created, fluoroscopy is used widely for gastrointestinal (GI) studies, vascular and cardiac studies, and interventional procedures. Many of these studies and procedures involve a considerable length of X-ray exposure time for the patient. For this reason, fluoroscopy is considered one of the principal sources of medical radiation to the population of the United States. In particular, upper GI tract fluoroscopy is the most commonly conducted fluoroscopic procedure in the United States and contributes the greatest effective radiation dose to the US population.

Strict quality control guidelines and protocols should be in place to minimize variation in equipment performance so patient dose is as low as possible. Federal guidelines for fluoroscopic equipment are found in Title 21 of the Code of Federal Regulations Part 1020 (21 CFR 1020) Subchapter J, which uses input from the American College of Radiology, the American Association of Physicists in Medicine (AAPM), and various other groups. Many states have or will be adopting fluoroscopic protocols developed by the Nationwide Evaluation of X-ray Trends committee of the Conference of Radiation Control Program Directors. This chapter contains many of the mentioned guidelines and protocols, but regulations in the state of practice also must be checked.

INTRODUCTION TO FLUOROSCOPIC EQUIPMENT

The three main parts of a typical fluoroscopic unit are the X-ray tube and generator, the image intensifier, and the

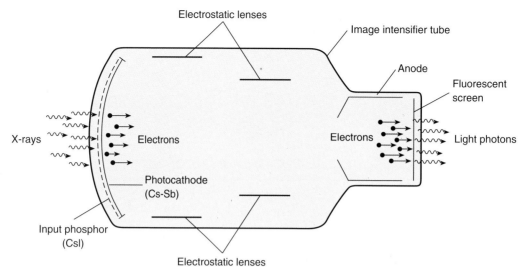

Fig. 7.1 Schematic of an image intensifier tube. *CsI,* Cesium iodide; *Cs-Sb,* cesium antimony.

video monitoring system. The X-ray generators in modern fluoroscopic units are most often high-frequency units for maximum efficiency. Fluoroscopic units equipped with cine mode require fast exposure times, on the order of 5–6 ms for a framing rate of 48 frames/s; therefore the X-ray generators must offer a high output—that is, a 130- to 200-kW power rating. The X-ray tubes are usually higher-capacity tubes (at least 500,000 heat units) compared with general radiographic tubes (about 300,000 heat units). In general, the X-ray tube and generator generally must perform according to the same standards as radiographic units and are evaluated in a similar way. Factors such as filtration (half-value layer [HVL]), focal spot size, X-ray tube heat sensors, overload protection, kilovolt (peak) (kVp) accuracy, reproducibility, linearity, output waveforms, automatic exposure control (for spot film devices), and grid uniformity and alignment all should be tested at least every 6 months with the methods and test tools discussed in previous chapters.

Image Intensifiers

Components

Fluoroscopic systems must use an image intensifier, which brightens electronically the image obtained during fluoroscopy. The most common type of image intensifier in fluoroscopic systems is the tube-type image intensifier, which works by converting a low-intensity, full-size image to a high-intensity, minified image. This type of device was first developed in 1948 by Coltman, who used technology similar to an electron microscope (Fig. 7.1). A newer alternative to the tube-type image intensifier is the flat-panel sensor (detector) made up of an active matrix array very similar to digital radiographic systems, which are discussed in detail in Chapter 8. The essential parts of the tube-type image intensifier are the glass envelope, input phosphor, photocathode, electrostatic focusing lenses, anode, and output phosphor.

Glass envelope. A tube-type image intensifier is a vacuum tube that allows the free flow of electrons from one side of the device (photocathode) to the other (anode). The glass

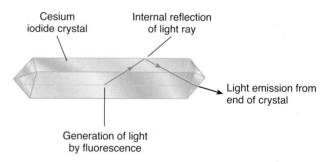

Fig. 7.2 Cesium iodide light pipe.

envelope is necessary to contain this powerful vacuum, which can experience as much as 1 ton of force from the outside air pressure pushing against it. Breakdown of vacuum integrity is the usual cause of the limited life of the image intensifier.

Input phosphor. On entry into the image intensifier, the X-rays strike the input phosphor, which absorbs them and converts their energy into visible light. The image intensifier ranges in diameter from 6 to 16 inches (15–40 cm) and is curved to maintain an equal distance between all points on the input and output phosphors. An input phosphor consists of either a glass or thin aluminum base (used in most newer input phosphors) with a coating of sodium-activated cesium iodide crystals placed in a layer 0.1- to 0.2-mm thick. The crystals form long, needlelike shapes that act as light pipes to emit light with minimal divergence (Fig. 7.2). The light emitted has a wavelength of about 4200 Å (420 nm), which places it in the blue portion of the color spectrum.

Photocathode. Light photons from the input phosphor immediately strike the photocathode, which is a thin layer of antimony and cesium compounds. The light photons release electrons from the photocathode through the process of photoemission.

Electrostatic focusing lenses. Electrostatic focusing lenses are positively charged metal plates that focus and accelerate the electrons as they travel toward the output phosphor.

Anode. The anode is a positively charged electrode that attracts the electrons toward the output phosphor. The potential difference between the anode and photocathode is 25–35 kV.

Output phosphor. Output phosphor is usually a piece of glass or aluminum about 1 inch (2.54 cm) in diameter and is coated with a thin layer (4–8 μm) of zinc cadmium sulfide (also known as *P20*). When electrons from the photocathode strike these crystals, light is emitted with wavelengths between 5000 and 6500 Å (500–650 nm), which places it in the yellow-green portion of the color spectrum. Because the light is placed in the approximate center of the visible light spectrum, video cameras (and the human eye) can detect this light easily.

Image Brightness

The image intensifier increases the brightness of the image by the following two processes:

1. The image from the larger input phosphor is condensed onto the smaller output phosphor. Because the image is emitted from a smaller area, it appears to be brighter. This increase in brightness is known as minification gain and is calculated with the following equation:

$$\text{Minification gain} = \frac{\text{Input diameter}^2}{\text{Output diameter}^2}$$

2. High voltage accelerates the electrons from the photocathode and their kinetic energy is increased, releasing many times more light photons from the output phosphor surface. This increase in brightness is known as the flux gain. At 25 kV, one electron incident on the output phosphor releases 50 light photons. The flux gain is then considered to be 50 times.

The total brightness gain is determined by multiplying the minification gain by the flux gain. Brightness gain may be referred to as the amount of brightness of an image-intensified image versus a nonimage-intensified fluoroscopic image. The brightness level of a fluoroscopic image is affected by milliamperes (mA), kVp, automatic brightness control, variable tube current, and variable pulse width, as shown in Box 7.1.

Multifield Image Intensifiers

The multifield image intensifier allows the fluoroscopic image to be magnified electronically by changing the voltage on the electrostatic focusing lenses, which decreases the amount of the input phosphor image sent to the output phosphor. The resulting image is then magnified (Fig. 7.3). Because the minification gain is decreased, the mA must be increased to maintain image brightness, which results in significantly increased entrance skin exposure. Another disadvantage is that the field of view is decreased. This type of image intensifier is used in digital fluoroscopic units and interventional, vascular, and cardiac studies.

The two basic types of multifield image intensifiers are dual focus and trifocus.

Dual focus. The dual-focus multifield image intensifier allows for a choice of two different fields of view to be used.

BOX 7.1 Factors Affecting the Brightness of Fluoroscopic Images

Milliamperes
An increase in the fluoroscopic X-ray tube mA multiplies the number of X-ray photons incident on the image intensifier, and therefore image brightness increases.

Kilovolts (Peak)
An increase in the fluoroscopic X-ray tube potential difference (i.e., kVp) multiplies the number of X-ray photons reaching the image intensifier, causing an increase in image brightness.

Patient Thickness and Tissue Density
An increase in patient thickness and tissue density reduces the number of X-ray photons reaching the image intensifier, thereby decreasing the image brightness.

Automatic Brightness Control or Automatic Brightness Stabilization
Automatic brightness control, or automatic brightness stabilization, allows the fluoroscopic unit to maintain the brightness level of the image automatically for variations in patient thickness and attenuation. This maintenance is accomplished by one of the following three methods, depending on the manufacturer:

- *Variable kilovolts (peak).* Variable kVp systems use a motor-driven autotransformer that varies the kVp in response to image brightness-sensing electrodes. These electrodes monitor the output phosphor directly or use a signal generated by a video camera. This method covers a wide range of patient thicknesses. However, it is slow, and the images may demonstrate quantum noise and low image contrast at high kVp values.
- *Variable tube current.* A variable tube current system varies the mA or tube current in response to image brightness-sensing electrodes, which requires a large-capacity X-ray generator.
- *Variable pulse width.* Using the variable pulse width method, the X-ray output is pulsed with a grid-controlled X-ray tube at a sequence rapid enough to avoid image flicker. A faster pulsing sequence is selected by the equipment to increase fluoroscopic image brightness and vice versa.

The most common dual-focus option is called the 9/6, which means the input phosphor can vary from a 9-inch diameter for a normal field of view to a 6-inch diameter for a magnified field of view (also called 23/15 for centimeter diameter measurement).

Trifocus. The trifocus option provides the user a choice of three input phosphor diameters, the most common of which is the 10/7/5 (in inches) or the 25/18/12 (in centimeters).

Image Intensifier Artifacts

The use of image intensifiers in fluoroscopic systems may lead to five basic types of artifacts: veiling glare, or flare; pincushion distortion; barrel distortion; vignetting; and S distortion.

Veiling glare, or flare. Veiling glare, or flare, is caused by light being reflected from the window of the output phosphor,

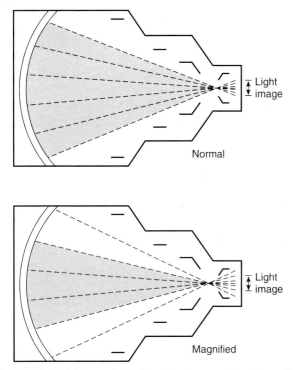

Fig. 7.3 Multifield image intensifier showing normal and magnification modes.

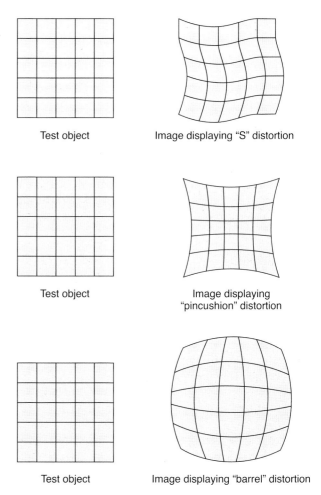

Fig. 7.4 S, pincushion, and barrel distortion.

which reduces image contrast. This artifact occurs most often when moving from one portion of a patient's anatomy to another (such as when imaging the chest and moving down to the abdominal area), causing a sudden increase in image brightness. Most manufacturers incorporate designs to reduce veiling glare to minimize this effect.

Pincushion distortion. **Pincushion distortion** is caused by projecting an image from a curved surface (input phosphor) onto a flat surface (output phosphor). This effect is similar to that of a carnival mirror that distorts appearance and is greater toward the lateral portions of the image. With pincushion distortion, magnification increases toward the periphery (Fig. 7.4).

Barrel distortion. Barrel distortion is similar to pincushion distortion and is caused, again, by projecting from a curved surface to a flat one (or vice versa), but magnification is reduced toward the periphery (also seen in Fig. 7.4).

Vignetting. **Vignetting** is a decrease in image brightness at the lateral portions of the image and is caused by a combination of pincushion distortion and the coupling of the television camera to the output phosphor.

S distortion. An **S distortion** artifact is a warping of the image along an S-shaped axis and is the result of strong magnetic fields changing the trajectory of the electrons moving across the image intensifier tube.

Image Monitoring Systems

Because the output phosphor is only 1 inch (2.54 cm) in diameter, the image projected is relatively small and therefore must be magnified and monitored by an additional system. The main methods used include mirror optics, closed-circuit television (CCTV) monitoring, cinefluorography, photofluorospot, film/screen spot devices, and digital image recorders.

Mirror Optics

Mirror optics is the oldest method of monitoring the image from an image intensifier. It uses a system of mirrors and lenses. The final image is projected onto a 6-in-diameter mirror mounted on the side of the image intensifier tower. The field of view is small, so only one person can view the image at a time. Image resolution of this system is 3–4 line pairs per millimeter (lp/mm). This method is rarely used today.

Closed-Circuit Television Monitoring

CCTV is the most common method for monitoring the fluoroscopic image. A television camera is focused onto the output phosphor and then displayed on a monitor. The components necessary for television monitoring are a television camera, linkage from the camera to the output phosphor, and a television monitor.

Television camera. The television camera converts visible light images into electronic signals. Four basic types of television cameras have been in use throughout the years: the **orthicon**, plumbicon, vidicon, and charge-coupled device (CCD).

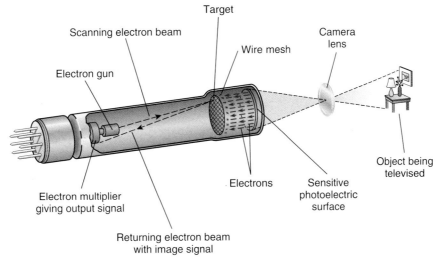

Fig. 7.5 Orthicon television camera tube.

Orthicon. The image-orthicon is the largest and most sensitive type of television camera, and it functions as both an image intensifier and a television pickup tube. Image quality is excellent and completely free of lag; however, it is expensive, is extremely sensitive to temperature changes, and requires a long warmup time (Fig. 7.5).

Plumbicon. The plumbicon camera uses lead oxide as the target phosphor and is often used in digital fluoroscopy because of its short lag time.

Vidicon. The vidicon camera is currently the most common type of video camera in fluoroscopic systems. Target material in the camera is antimony trisulfide, which has a relatively long lag time (helpful in GI studies) to help reduce image noise.

Charge-coupled device/complementary metallic oxide semiconductor. These are solid-state cameras that are not made up of a vacuum tube but rather, an array of millions of photosensors on a small circuit board. This forms an array of 100–1000 tiny (5–20-μm) photodiodes on a solid-state computer chip that form pixels to create the signal (Fig. 7.6). When light strikes these photodiodes, electrons are released in direct proportion to the amount of incident light. These electrons build up charges that form electronic pulses. These pulses then form the electronic video signal containing the image information. The advantages of a charge-coupled device (CCD) or complementary metallic oxide semiconductor (CMOS) are smaller size, less power consumption, lower price, longer life, virtually no lag, and less fragility. Both types of imagers convert light into electric charge and process it into electronic signals. In a CCD sensor, every pixel's charge is transferred through a very limited number of output nodes (often just one) to be converted to voltage, buffered, and sent off-chip as an analog signal. All of the pixel can be devoted to light capture, and the output's uniformity (a key factor in image quality) is high. It is also very sensitive to low levels of light, so fewer mA can be used on the patient (compared to the tube-type cameras). In a CMOS sensor, each pixel has its own charge-to-voltage conversion,

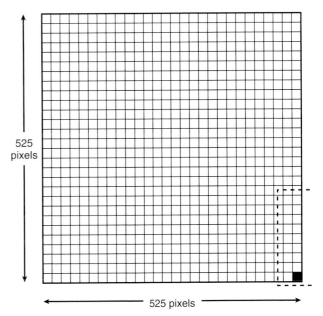

Fig. 7.6 Representation of a photodetector/pixel arrangement in a charge-coupled device.

and the sensor also includes amplifiers, noise-correction (high signal-to-noise ratio), and digitization circuits, so that the chip outputs digital bits. These other functions increase the design complexity and may reduce the area available for light capture (lower fill factor) and more electronic noise. However, they consume less power than a CCD chip. For these reasons, most newer units are being equipped with either CCD or CMOS cameras.

Linkage from the television camera to output phosphor. The television camera must be coupled, or linked, to the output phosphor so that image quality is maintained. To maintain image quality, one of two methods is used: fiber optics and lens coupling.

Fiber optics. Fiber optics linkage uses flexible glass or plastic fibers in which total internal reflection occurs (Fig. 7.7). This device is small, rugged, and relatively inexpensive but

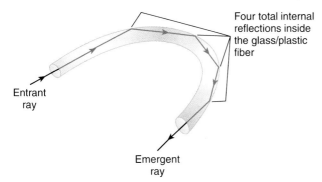

Fig. 7.7 Principle of fiber optics.

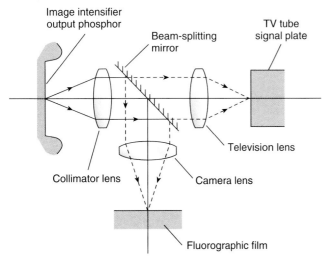

Fig. 7.8 Split mirror for monitoring fluoroscopic images.

cannot accommodate auxiliary units such as cine or spot film cameras.

Lens coupling. The lens coupling method uses a system of lenses and mirrors to split the image so auxiliary devices can view the image simultaneously with the television camera (Fig. 7.8).

Television monitor. The television monitor found on an older system uses a cathode ray tube (CRT) to display the fluoroscopic image. The CRT monitor uses the Electronics Industries Association's RS-170 standard for closed-circuit black-and-white television, which uses 525 lines per frame, with 30 separate frames appearing each second and an aspect ratio of 4:3. Standard monitors use a method called *interlaced horizontal scanning* to avoid flicker, which involves scanning the odd-numbered lines in the first half of the frame and the even-numbered lines during the second half rather than all 525 at once. This type of monitor can resolve between 2 and 2.5 lp/mm. Noninterlaced, or progressive, scan monitors (which scan all lines in order and have a frame rate of 60 frames/s) also are available and are used in most personal computer displays. These monitors are preferred in angiographic and interventional procedures because of their reduced flickering. High-resolution monitors with up to 1023 lines per frame are available and demonstrate 2.5–5 lp/mm. Newer fluoroscopic systems are now incorporating high-resolution flat-panel monitors in which a liquid crystal display

is used instead of a CRT monitor. These LCD monitors have aspect ratios of 16:9 or 21:9, with faster frame rates and greater contrast. The next chapter contains a more complete discussion of viewing monitors. As high-definition television systems have become more cost effective, they have rapidly replaced CRT monitors.

Cinefluorography

With the cinefluorography method, a motion picture camera is used to monitor the image from the output phosphor. This high-speed motion picture camera records the image of fast-moving objects, and it is ideal for cardiac catheterization studies (95% of all cine studies involve cardiac studies). The film used is either 16 mm or, most often, 35 mm (98% of all cine studies) black-and-white motion picture film. The larger size yields better image quality but requires a greater patient dose. The camera is capable of recording framing frequencies of 7.5, 15, 30, 60, and 120 frames/s, depending on the motion of the object. The greater the framing frequency, the greater the ability to minimize motion in the resulting image. However, it also results in an increased patient dose. The X-ray beam is pulsed with a grid-controlled X-ray tube to match the framing frequency. These systems have been replaced by fast-pulse fluoroscopic systems that record the image with a digital recording system for playback.

Photofluorospot, or Spot Film, Camera

The **photofluorospot**, or spot film, method uses a spot film camera that takes a static photograph of the fluoroscopic image with a lens coupling device. The lens has a longer focal length than that of cine cameras to cover a larger film format. These cameras use 70-, 90-, 100-, or 105-mm roll or cut film sizes. The larger the film format, the better the image quality, but the patient receives a greater dose. The patient dose with this method is less than that from film/screen spot filming. In addition, the cost of film and processing is less than that of film/screen spot filming. These systems have been replaced with digital recording systems.

Film/Screen Spot Film Devices

Film/screen spot film devices do not monitor the fluoroscopic image from the image intensifier; rather, they use a fluoroscopic X-ray tube to create a radiograph on a standard cassette. This cassette is usually kept in a lead-shielded compartment until the spot film device is activated. It is then placed into the X-ray beam path behind a grid, and a field format is selected (e.g., one on one, two on one) (Fig. 7.9). The fluoroscopic X-ray tube is then changed from approximately 3 mA to as much as 1000 mA, and the exposure is made and then controlled with an automatic exposure control system. The images created with this method have a greater contrast and spatial resolution than photofluorospot images. Spot film devices are preferred for most angiographic procedures, air contrast GI examinations, endoscopic retrograde cholangiopancreatography, arthrography, and sialography. These systems have been replaced with digital recording systems.

Cassette formats

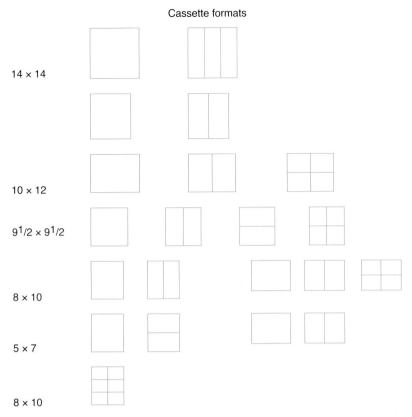

14 × 14

10 × 12

9½ × 9½

8 × 10

5 × 7

8 × 10

Fig. 7.9 Film/screen spot film formats.

Digital Image Recorders

Digital image recorders now are being used in many fluoroscopic systems to view fluoroscopic images at a later time. These systems store images using a magnetic or solid-state hard drive for later playback. These systems are discussed in Chapter 8.

QUALITY CONTROL OF FLUOROSCOPIC EQUIPMENT

The procedure for evaluating fluoroscopic systems involves much of the same processes as the evaluation of radiographic systems, with the components of visual inspection, environmental inspection, and performance testing.

Visual Inspection

A fluoroscopic system visual inspection should be performed at least every 6 months, using a checklist, by either a quality management technologist or a medical physicist. A sample checklist is included at the Evolve website. The following should be included in the checklist:

- *Fluoroscopic tower and table locks.* Operate all locks manually to verify function.
- *Power assist.* Activate the power assist. The tower should move smoothly over the tabletop.
- *Protective curtain.* Ensure that a protective curtain or drape is in place and moves freely so that it can be placed between the patient and any personnel in the fluoroscopic room. This curtain must contain at least a 0.25-mm lead equivalent, which should be verified on acceptance. Verification is

accomplished by exposing the lead curtain to 100-kVp X-rays and taking radiation measurements on either side. The reading behind the lead curtain should be about 50% of the input reading (because the HVL of lead at 100 kVp is 0.24 mm).

- *Bucky slot cover.* Move the Potter–Bucky diaphragm to the far end of the examination table. A metal cover should move in place and must attenuate to the equivalent of at least one-tenth-value layer or TVL (about 0.5 mm of lead). Radiation readings should be taken on either side of the cover, with the amount outside the cover being 10% of the input exposure, and should be verified on acceptance. Verify operation of the cover during each inspection.
- *Exposure switch.* Every fluoroscopic system exposure switch must be a dead man type of switch, which requires continuous pressure for activation, and should be verified on acceptance. Subsequent visual inspections should focus on sticking or malfunction of this switch.
- *Fluoroscopic timer.* A 5-min reset timer is required for monitoring the length of time the fluoroscopic X-ray tube is energized. An audible signal should sound at the end of 5 min. Timer accuracy can be verified with a stopwatch.
- *Lights/meter function.* All indicator lights and meters should function as specified by the manufacturer. A display of the fluoroscopic irradiation time at the fluoroscopist's working position is required for all fluoroscopic equipment manufactured after 2006. When the X-ray tube is activated, the fluoroscopic irradiation time in minutes and tenths of minutes shall be continuously displayed and updated at least once every 6 seconds. The fluoroscopic irradiation time

shall also be displayed within 6 seconds of termination of an exposure and remain displayed until reset. Means shall be provided to reset the display to zero prior to the beginning of a new examination or procedure.

- *Compression device, or spoon, observation.* The compression device, or spoon, should move easily and be free of any splatters of contrast media.
- *Park position interrupt.* When the tower is in the parked position, it should not be possible to energize the X-ray tube. Check the park position while wearing a lead apron and depressing the fluoroscopic exposure switch to determine whether the system is activated.
- *Primary protective barrier.* The entire cross-section of the useful beam should be intercepted by a primary protective barrier at all source-to-image distances (SIDs). The barrier is usually built into the tower assembly for units in which the image intensifier is above the X-ray table. **With the tower at the maximum SID and the shutters wide open, the exposure rate above the tower should not exceed 2 mR/h or 20 µGy air kerma (measured at 10 cm from any accessible surface of the fluoroscopic imaging assembly beyond the plane of the image receptor for every roentgen [R] or 10 mGy air kerma per minute measured at tabletop (1020.32 (a), 21 CFR Subchapter J)).** The effectiveness of the primary protective barrier can be evaluated by using a dosimeter with a homogenous phantom made of 15 cm of acrylic in place or with the shutters completely closed to protect the image intensifier. Moveable grids and compression devices should be removed from the useful beam during measurement.
- *Collimation shutters.* **In fluoroscopic mode, when the adjustable collimators are fully open, the primary beam should be restricted to the diameter of the input phosphor and must be accurate to within ±2% of the SID. For spot imaging, the edges of the X-ray field and corresponding image receptor edges must agree to within ±3% of the SID (1020.32 (b), 21 CFR Subchapter J).** For rectangular X-ray fields used with circular image receptors, the error alignment is determined along the length and width dimensions of the X-ray field that pass through the center of the visible area of the image receptor. Means must be provided to permit further limitation of the field. Beam-limiting devices manufactured after May 22, 1979, and incorporated in equipment with a variable SID and/or visible area of greater than 300 cm² should be provided with means for stepless adjustment of the X-ray field. Equipment with a fixed SID and a visible area of 300 cm² or less should be provided with either stepless adjustment of the X-ray field or with means to limit the X-ray field size further at the plane of the image receptor to 125 cm² or less. Stepless adjustment should, at the greatest SID, provide continuous field sizes from the maximum obtainable to a field size of 5 cm × 5 cm or less. In addition, the primary beam should be aligned to the center of the image intensifier to within 2% of the SID. This can be verified with a commercially available fluoroscopic beam alignment test tool that consists of ruler increments or a series of equally spaced holes and is placed on the face of the

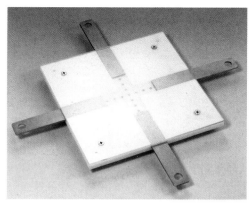

Fig. 7.10 Fluoroscopic beam alignment device. (Courtesy Nuclear Associates, Inc., Carle Place, New York.)

image intensifier (Fig. 7.10). When the image is observed, the ruler markings or holes should indicate the size of the input phosphor being irradiated. If this is not available, a phantom can be imaged under the fluoroscope with the shutters fully open. When viewing the image on the monitor, a shutter tangent must be seen at all edges of the monitor at both the lowest and highest SID positions. For spot image devices, the total misalignment of the edges of the X-ray field with the respective edges of the selected portion of the image receptor along the length or width dimensions of the X-ray field in the plane of the image receptor must not exceed 3% of the SID when adjusted for full coverage of the selected portion of the image receptor. The sum without regard to sign of the misalignment along any two orthogonal dimensions should not exceed 4% of the SID. It should be possible to adjust the X-ray field size in the plane of the image receptor to a size smaller than the selected portion of the image receptor. The minimum field size at the greatest SID should be greater than or equal to 5 cm × 5 cm. The center of the X-ray field in the plane of the image receptor should be aligned with the center of the selected portion of the image receptor to within 2% of the SID.

- *Monitor brightness.* Place a penetrometer on a homogenous phantom (6–10 inches of water in a plastic bucket, 15 cm of acrylic plastic [Lucite], or 1.5-inch-thick block of aluminum). The brightness and contrast controls on the monitor should be adjusted to show as many of the steps as possible.
- *Table angulation and motion.* The table should move freely to the upright position and stop at the appropriate spot. The table angle indicator and the actual table angle should coincide within 2 degrees.
- *Lead aprons and gloves.* Lead apparel should be exposed during remote fluoroscopy at 100 kVp, with the image observed on the television monitor for the presence of any cracks or irregularities. Otherwise, radiographs of the apron should be made to reduce operator exposure. This was discussed in detail in Chapter 5.

Environmental Inspection

Environmental inspections are essentially the same in fluoroscopic units as in radiographic units and should be performed

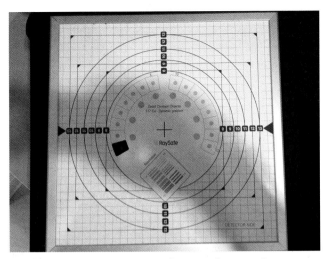

Fig. 7.11 Multifunction fluoroscopic test tool.

at least every 6 months. In general, these inspections are performed at the same time as the visual inspection of many of the items included in the checklist. The condition of high-tension cables and the mechanical condition of the image intensifier tower and table are especially important.

Performance Testing

As with radiographic units, performance testing of fluoroscopic units is critical to avoid variation in system performance. Many states have strict guidelines for fluoroscopic systems and mandate performance testing as a condition for granting the license to operate such equipment. Because of the potentially high patient dose in fluoroscopic procedures, these tests should be performed at least every 6 months (semiannually) or as indicated by state law. Specialized test tools are available for quality control testing of fluoroscopic systems (see Fig. 7.11). The fluoroscopic system should be tested in both the vertical and horizontal positions if the system is capable of operating in both positions.

Reproducibility of Exposure

PROCEDURE: REPRODUCIBILITY OF EXPOSURE

1. Place a homogenous phantom on the fluoroscopic tabletop and place a dosimeter between the phantom and the image intensifier input phosphor. Select the maximum mA and kVp available on the fluoroscopic unit.
2. Center the dosimeter probe to the center of the fluoroscopic X-ray beam. Depress the expose button for 10 seconds (use a stopwatch) and record the reading.
3. Clear the dosimeter and repeat this procedure twice.
4. Determine the milliroentgen-to-milliampere-second ratio for each 10-second exposure of the dosimeter. Compare the readings and calculate the reproducibility variance using the equation from Chapter 5. **The reproducibility variance must be less than 0.05 (5%)**. Reproducibility outside the accepted variance can result in fluctuations in image quality and patient dose, and is caused most likely by problems with the X-ray generator or fluoroscopic X-ray tube.

Focal Spot Size

PROCEDURE: FOCAL SPOT SIZE

1. Place any one of the focal spot test tools described in Chapter 5 on top of a homogenous phantom that is on the tabletop and centered to the fluoroscopic X-ray field. Set the fluoroscopic mA and kVp to the most commonly used settings.
2. Tape a nonscreen film to the bottom of the image intensifier tower and expose (you will probably need about 10 seconds of fluoroscopic exposure). If one is not available, use a high-resolution computed radiography cassette with preprocessing image data recognition set to fixed mode (computed radiography acts like a film/screen cassette) and print a hard copy using a dry laser printer.
3. After the film is processed, calculate the focal spot size according to the instructions with the test tool. Focal spot blooming should conform to the guidelines of the National Electrical Manufacturers Association discussed in Chapter 5.

Filtration Check

The fluoroscopic circuitry in the X-ray generator is different from the radiographic circuitry, so radiographic beam quality results do not apply to the fluoroscopy capabilities of the unit. For fluoroscopic systems with manual kilovolt control override, the preferred method for determining the HVL is to set the kilovolts and determine the HVL just as one would for a radiographic unit, measuring exposure rate instead of exposure. When a manual kilovolt setting is not available on the fluoroscopic system, the HVL will have to be measured in automatic exposure rate control (AERC) mode. To accomplish this, the field of view is minimized, and the exposure probe is placed as far away from the X-ray tube as possible. Several 1-mm sheets of aluminum are placed between the probe and the image intensifier. The sheets need to be big enough to span the minimized field of view and there needs to be enough of them to drive the kilovolts to at least 80 kVp. The exposure rate/air kerma is measured, and a single sheet of aluminum is removed from the stack behind the chamber and placed in front of the chamber midway between the X-ray tube and the probe. Again, the exposure rate/air kerma is measured and the next filter is moved, and so on. This procedure keeps the same amount of aluminum in the beam for each measurement while varying the filtration in front of the probe. The AERC should hold a constant mA and kilovolts. In practice, knowing the HVL without knowing the kilovolts is not that valuable, and so the kilovolts reported by the fluoroscopic kilovolts indicator on the system should be recorded. If the X-ray system does not have a kilovolts indicator, there is no value in determining the HVL other than to ensure compliance with accrediting body or state regulations.

PROCEDURE: FILTRATION CHECK

1. Use the aluminum plates and a dosimeter to measure the HVL, using the same procedure described in Chapter 5 for radiographic systems. The dosimeter probe should be placed in a

Continued

PROCEDURE: FILTRATION CHECK—cont'd

support stand that holds it halfway between the tabletop and the bottom of the image intensifier tower. Be sure to collimate to an area that is slightly smaller than the aluminum plates.

2. Because fluoroscopic kVp values are usually greater than those in radiography, the HVL should be determined with the most common kVp used for that unit. For example, if a particular fluoroscopic unit is used mostly for upper GI examinations at 100 kVp, then calculate the HVL for 100 kVp. Table 7.1 contains the HVL values for common fluoroscopic kVp. Filtration that is less than adequate increases the patient skin dose.

Kilovolt (Peak) Accuracy

In fluoroscopy, the kilovolts may be continuously changing as a result of the AERC. For most systems, there is very little need to know whether the kilovolts are accurate or not, since this knowledge will affect neither the image quality nor the dose to the patient in a direct sense. The easiest way to determine fluoroscopic kilovolts is to use a noninvasive kilovolt meter such as the one described in Chapter 7. The kilovolt meter is placed in the fluoroscopic beam and the kilovolts are read out. Kilovolts indicators should be accurate to ±5%.

PROCEDURE: KILOVOLT (PEAK) ACCURACY

1. The digital kVp meter is used as described in Chapter 5.
2. Place the kVp meter on the tabletop facing the direction of the X-ray tube and centered to the fluoroscopic X-ray field. Set the fluoroscopic kVp to 80.
3. Expose the kVp meter for 2 seconds and record the reading. Repeat two more times.
4. Repeat the first two steps for the 90-, 100-, 110-, and 120-kVp stations.
5. Average the three meter readings for each kVp station and compare this value with the value selected on the control panel.
6. Calculate the kVp variance using the following equation:

$$kVp\ variance = \frac{(kVp_{max} - kVp_{min})}{(kVp_{max} + kVp_{min})}$$

7. The kVp variance should be less than or equal to 0.05. **The measured kVp and the value indicated on the control should coincide within ±5%.**

TABLE 7.1 Half-Value Layer Valves for Common Fluoroscopic Kilovolts (Peak)

Fluoroscopic kVp	Minimum HVL (mm Al)
80	2.3
90	2.5
100	2.7
110	3
120	3.2
130	3.5
140	3.8
150	4.1

HVL, Half-value layer; *kVp*, kilovolt (peak).

Voltage Waveform

To evaluation the voltage waveform, attach an X-ray output detector to an oscilloscope or personal computer. The voltage waveform of the X-ray generator is displayed as discussed in Chapter 5.

Several pulse shapes are available for monitoring by the medical physicist. The kilovolts and radiation pulse shapes are the most convenient to acquire (mA pulses require invasive techniques). These, however, may be under software control during cine, rendering their evaluation difficult at best. The manufacturer's representative should be consulted concerning proper evaluation of pulse shapes. Minimally, these pulses should be checked for duration of the width and timing with the imaging chain. The pulse width, if excessive, can result in significant loss of image quality due to motion unsharpness. If the capacitive tail of the kilovolt waveform is excessively long, it may lengthen the effective pulse width. This not only further degrades image quality but also eliminates many of the dose-saving features of pulsed fluoroscopy. Pulse timing must be properly coordinated with the image recording system to ensure that no exposure is produced between frames. This minimizes patient dose and reduces image blur.

Milliampere Linearity

A dosimeter and stopwatch are used with a homogenous phantom in place.

PROCEDURE: MILLIAMPERE LINEARITY

1. With the dosimeter placed between the phantom and the image intensifier and centered to the fluoroscopic X-ray field, make a 10-second exposure at 0.5 mA.
2. Record the reading and calculate the milliroentgen/milliampere-second values.
3. Repeat at 1 mA and then 2 mA (or all other fluoroscopic mA stations available on your particular fluoroscopic unit).
4. Determine the milliroentgen/milliampere-second values for each mA station tested and then calculate the linearity variance using the following equation:

$$Linearity\ variance = \frac{(mR/mAs_{max} - mR/mAs_{min})}{(mR/mAs_{average})} \div 2$$

The linearity variance should be within 0.1 (10%).

X-ray Tube Heat Sensors

X-ray tube heat sensors can be tested with the same basic procedure used in Chapter 5, but with a stopwatch and a homogenous phantom to determine the exposure time.

PROCEDURE: X-RAY TUBE HEAT SENSORS

1. Calculate the heat units for a 30-second exposure at the maximum fluoroscopic kVp and mA, then compare them with the maximum tube limit stated in the manufacturer's specifications.

PROCEDURE: X-RAY TUBE HEAT SENSORS—cont'd

2. Now look at the light-emitting diode readout on the sensor to determine whether the values coincide. If necessary, continue fluoroscopy until 75% of the maximum is achieved to determine whether an alarm is activated. If the alarm is not activated, contact a service engineer.

Grid Uniformity and Alignment

The grid can become dented or positioned incorrectly in the system with clinical usage. If possible, the X-ray grid should be removed from the system and radiographed to see if any artifacts are present. It should also be tested for proper alignment and uniformity.

PROCEDURE: GRID UNIFORMITY AND ALIGNMENT

Follow the same procedure as discussed in Chapter 5 for grid uniformity, using a spot film for evaluation.
1. For grid alignment, tape the test tool to the bottom of the image intensifier and acquire an image with a homogenous phantom in place.
2. Determine alignment according to the test tool instructions.

Automatic Exposure Rate Control

The automatic exposure rate control (AERC) system should adjust the technical parameters (kVp, mA, and pulse width) automatically for changes in part thickness. A dosimeter and homogenous phantom of varying thickness should be in place.

PROCEDURE: AUTOMATIC EXPOSURE RATE CONTROL

1. Place the dosimeter between the phantom and the X-ray source, using a phantom of 7.5-cm-thick acrylic plastic (Lucite).
2. Expose for 10 seconds and record the reading.
3. Add another 7.5-cm thickness (15 cm total) and repeat. The dosimeter reading should be approximately double the 7.5-cm reading if the system is functioning properly.

Automatic Gain Control

Some fluoroscopic systems are equipped with automatic gain control to maintain image brightness. These systems vary the gain of the video system rather than adjust the technical factors.

PROCEDURE: AUTOMATIC GAIN CONTROL

1. Place a dosimeter under the 7.5-cm homogenous phantom and expose for 10 seconds while watching the monitor for image brightness.
2. Repeat the procedure for a 15-cm thickness. The radiation readings and the image brightness should be the same for both exposures.

Maximum Entrance Exposure Rate/Air Kerma

The maximum entrance exposure rate is the greatest possible exposure rate the fluoroscopic system can deliver to the patient. This rate is measured at the tabletop for fluoroscopic tubes mounted under the table or where the beam enters the patient for fluoroscopic tubes mounted above the tabletop (see Fig. 7.12). *The intensity of the X-ray beam at the tabletop should not exceed 10 R/min or 100 mGy/min air kerma rate for units equipped with* automatic brightness stabilization *(ABS) and 5 R/min or 50 mGy/min air kerma rate for units without ABS (1020.32(d), 21 CFR Subchapter J).*

The radiology departments in some states use a value known as air kerma rate (AKR), rather than exposure or intensity, to measure the amount of radiation entering the patient. Kerma is an acronym for kinetic energy released in matter, and it measures the amount of kinetic energy released into particles of matter (such as electrons created during Compton and photoelectric interactions) from exposure to X-rays. Kerma is measured in either rads or the International System of Units gray (Gy). Air kerma is the kinetic energy released per unit mass of air. An exposure of 1 R corresponds to an air kerma of about 8.8 mGy. For fluoroscopic systems, the air kerma rate is measured in air at the position where the center of the useful beam enters the patient (the probe position on the phantom of the Centers for Devices and Radiological Health [CDRH] is placed for air kerma measurement). According to standards of the US Food and Drug Administration (FDA), the air kerma rate for all fluoroscopic units should be less than 44 mGy/min or 5 rad/min and should be less than 88 mGy/min (10 rad/min) unless a high-level control is provided.

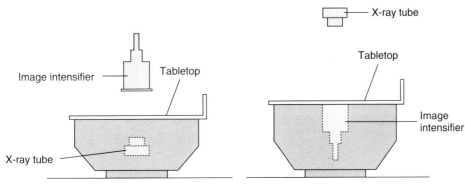

Fig. 7.12 Diagram of fluoroscopic units with the image intensifier mounted above or below the tabletop.

For photofluorographic spot film cameras, the entrance kerma to the image intensifier at maximum tube potential and mA should not be greater than 0.0003 cGy (0.3 rad) per exposure. This limits the entrance kerma to the patient to about 0.1 cGy (0.1 rad) per exposure. For cinefluorography, the entrance kerma to the image intensifier should not be more than 0.3 µGy (0.03 rad) per frame.

Magnification studies in which multifield image intensifiers (specially activated fluoroscopy) and high-level-control fluoroscopy (also known as *boost fluoroscopy*) must limit the maximum entrance exposure rate to 20 R/min (5.2 mC/kg) or 200 mGy/min air kerma rate when acquiring images without recording devices. High-level-control fluoroscopy is an operating mode for fluoroscopic equipment in which a greater exposure rate is produced to allow for visualization of smaller and lower-contrast objects that may not be seen during conventional fluoroscopy. The FDA and the Conference of Radiation Control Program Directors are investigating these studies, and possible limits may be forthcoming. These fluoroscopic units are required to have a separate exposure switch or pedal, and an audible sound must be emitted by the system when high-intensity fluoroscopy is delivered.

Fluoroscopic equipment manufactured on or after June 10, 2006, shall display at the fluoroscopist's working position the AKR and cumulative air kerma. The following requirements apply for each X-ray tube used during an examination or procedure:

1. When the X-ray tube is activated and the number of images produced per unit time is greater than six images per second, the AKR in miligrays per minute shall be continuously displayed and updated at least once every second.
2. The cumulative air kerma in units of mGy shall be displayed either within 5 seconds of termination of an exposure, or displayed continuously and updated at least once every 5 seconds.
3. The display of the AKR shall be clearly distinguishable from the display of the cumulative air kerma.
4. The AKR and cumulative air kerma shall represent the value for conditions of free-in-air irradiation at one of the following reference locations specified according to the type of fluoroscope. If the source is below the X-ray table, the AKR shall be measured at 1 cm above the tabletop or cradle. If the source is above the X-ray table, the AKR shall be measured at 30 cm above the tabletop, with the end of the beam limiting device or spacer positioned as closely as possible to the point of measurement.

PROCEDURE: MAXIMUM ENTRANCE EXPOSURE RATES

1. Place a dosimeter so that the maximum exposure rate or AKR is measured 1 cm above the tabletop or cradle, along with two 3-mm-thick lead sheets placed in front of the image intensifier. For units in which the image intensifier is under the table and the X-ray tube is over the table (Fig. 7.12), the dosimeter should be placed 30 cm above the tabletop.
2. Expose for 30 seconds using the maximum kVp and mA available.
3. Record the dosimeter reading in roentgens, coulombs per kilogram, or milligrays of air kerma, and multiply by two to obtain the roentgens per minute or milligray per minute (AKR) value. Compare with the previously mentioned limits.

Standard Entrance Exposure Rates

Accrediting agencies such as The Joint Commission and DNV-GL Healthcare require that standard or typical exposure rates be monitored because the maximum values do not represent typical use. For this information to be obtained, a dosimeter, along with a CDRH fluoroscopic phantom, is recommended by both the American College of Radiology and the AAPM (Fig. 7.13). This phantom contains a 7-inch acrylic block to simulate tissue equivalence, along with lead and copper attenuators for air kerma measurement. It also contains an optional high- and low-contrast test pattern (discussed in the next section).

For photofluorospot cameras, the entrance exposure should be monitored with a dosimeter and a homogenous phantom at an exposure that creates an optical density between 0.8 and 1.2 on the resulting film. The exposure should be in the range of 50–200 µR/image (13–52 nC/kg/image). For cine film exposures, the Inter-Society Commission for Heart Disease Resources recommends a minimum entrance exposure of 15 µR/frame (4 nC/kg/frame) for

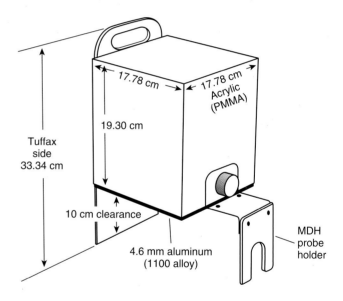

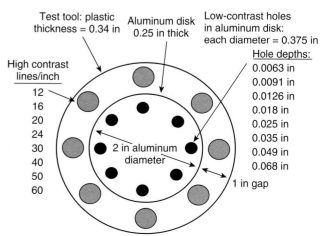

Fig. 7.13 Fluoroscopic phantom of the Centers for Devices and Radiological Health. (Courtesy Centers for Devices and Radiological Health, Rockville, Maryland.)

9-inch-diameter (23-cm-diameter) image intensifiers and 35 μR/frame (9 nC/kg/frame) with the 6-inch (15-cm) mode.

The standard entrance exposure rate should remain constant for a single room each time this test is performed (every 6 months). When different rooms are compared, any variation exceeding ±25% should be investigated.

High-Contrast Resolution

High-contrast resolution is the ability to resolve small, thin, black-and-white areas and is a measure of spatial resolution. A test tool for high-contrast resolution usually consists of copper mesh patterns with sizes of 16, 20, 24, 30, 35, 40, 50, and 60 holes per inch (Fig. 7.14).

An image intensifier with a 9-inch input phosphor should be able to resolve at least 20–24 holes per inch in the center of the image and 20 holes per inch at the edge when monitored with a CCTV system. With a 6-inch image intensifier, the center of the image should resolve a pattern of at least 30 holes per inch and at least 24 holes per inch at the edges. If a mirror optic system is present rather than a CCTV system, the 9-inch mode should image at least 40 holes per inch in the center and 30 holes per inch at the edges; 6-inch systems should resolve at least 40 holes per inch in the center and 35 holes per inch at the edges. Flat-panel image intensifiers should resolve at least 40 holes per inch throughout the entire field of view.

PROCEDURE: STANDARD ENTRANCE EXPOSURE RATES

1. Place the phantom on the tabletop for tower image intensifiers or at 30 cm above the tabletop for image intensifiers mounted under the tabletop (see Fig. 7.12). Be sure the dosimeter probe is placed in the appropriate slot on the phantom.

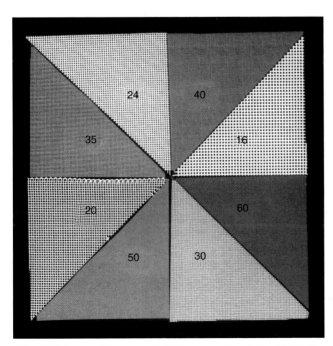

Fig. 7.14 Image of fluoroscopic high-contrast resolution test tool.

2. The exposure should be made at the standard kVp and mA levels for that unit for 30 seconds.
3. Record the reading in roentgens or millicoulombs per kilogram and multiply by two to determine the roentgen per minute or millicoulombs per kilogram per minute value. Exposure values should range from 1 to 3 R/min (0.3–0.5 mC/kg per minute) for typical use. Air kerma equivalent values are 8.7–26 mGy/min (0.87–2.6 rad/min). Grid exposures may be 1.5 to 2 times greater. With multifield image intensifiers, this procedure should be performed for each mode.

PROCEDURE: HIGH-CONTRAST RESOLUTION

1. Center and tape the test tool to the bottom of the image intensifier.
2. Set the kVp to the lowest possible setting.
3. Collimate the fluoroscopic X-ray beam to the size of the test tool and observe the image on the monitor.

The evaluation of high-contrast resolution of images created with spot image systems also can be performed with the same test tool, as follows:

PROCEDURE: HIGH-CONTRAST RESOLUTION OF SPOT IMAGE SYSTEM

1. Complete steps 1 and 2 in the previous list.
2. Obtain a spot image with the spot image device present in your fluoroscopic system (e.g., cassette spot film, photofluorospot, cine, or digital recorder).
3. Process the image and evaluate the image of the test tool from the hard copy obtained.

Spot images should demonstrate at least 40 holes per inch at the center and 30 holes per inch at the edge of the image. The Image Quality Test Object, which is a part of the CDRH fluoroscopic phantom, contains a high-contrast resolution test pattern that can be used with the listed procedures.

Low-Contrast Resolution

Low-contrast resolution is the ability to resolve relatively large objects that differ slightly in radiolucency from the surrounding area. Contrast resolution is determined by viewing a phantom containing various objects that span a range of subtle contrasts. The preferred phantom for determining fluoroscopic contrast resolution is the CDRH fluoroscopic phantom. A low-contrast resolution tool consists of two 1.9-cm-thick aluminum plates and a 0.8-mm aluminum sheet with two sets of holes of 1.5, 3.1, 4.7, and 6.3 mm (Fig. 7.15). The Image Quality Test Object, which is a part of the CDRH fluoroscopic phantom, contains a low-contrast resolution test pattern consisting of a series of 0.375-in-diameter holes in an aluminum disk. These holes range in depth from 0.0063 to 0.068 inches and should create a subtle shade of gray beneath each hole in the resulting image. If this is not available, other low-contrast phantoms such as those discussed in Chapter 3 can be substituted.

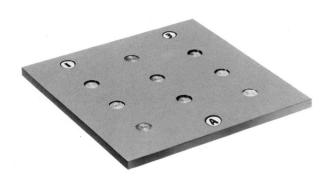

PROCEDURE: LOW-CONTRAST RESOLUTION

1. Place the low-contrast resolution test tool or CDRH fluoroscopic phantom between the focal spot and the image intensifier.
2. Expose at 100 kVp and observe the image on the monitor. With the low-contrast resolution test tool, the contrast between the holes and the surrounding area is 2%. All fluoroscopic systems should image the two largest holes clearly, and the third largest (3.1-mm) hole should just barely be visible. With the CDRH phantom, the three deepest holes should be visible. Better systems are able to visualize the smaller holes on the test tool or the shallower holes on the CDRH phantom.

Source–Skin Distance

The following are the minimum source–skin distances (SSDs) for fluoroscopic units established by the FDA (1020.31(i), 1020.32(g), 21 CFR Subchapter J):

Fixed or stationary units: 38 cm or 15 inches

Mobile units: 30 cm or 12 inches

Specialized units[1]: 20 cm or 8 inches

In units in which the fluoroscopic X-ray tube is above the tabletop, a tape measure is used to measure the SSD. For units in which the X-ray tube is under the table, two metal plates are used: one that is 4 inches long and another that is 2 inches long.

PROCEDURE: SOURCE–SKIN DISTANCE

1. Tape the 4-inch plate to the bottom of the image intensifier and place the 2-inch plate on the tabletop. Place a homogenous phantom of 15-cm acrylic plastic (Lucite) on top of the 2-inch plate to protect the image intensifier. The long axis of the two plates should be in the same direction, with both centered to the central ray of the X-ray beam.
2. During fluoroscopy, the height of the image intensifier should be adjusted until the outer edges of the plates coincide.

---

[1]Fluoroscopes intended for specific surgical application that would be prohibited at the source-skin distance.

Under these conditions, the distance between the tabletop and the 4-inch metal plate is equal to the target-to-tabletop distance (and therefore the SSD). An alternative is to use the similar triangle method discussed in Chapter 5. For mobile C-arm fluoroscopic units, a cone or spacer frame should be attached permanently to maintain a 12-inch or 30-cm SSD.

Distortion

Tape a wire mesh pattern (similar to that used for film/screen contact) to the bottom of the image intensifier and place a homogenous phantom on the X-ray table. During fluoroscopy, observe the image of the wire mesh for any signs of pincushion or S distortion (see Fig. 7.4). If any signs are present, consult a service engineer.

Image Lag

Image lag is defined as a continuation or persistence of the image, and it blurs objects as the image intensifier is moved over the patient. Tests should be completed to verify that the frame-to-frame persistence of the video does not result in unnecessary smearing of moving objects within the fluoroscopic image. This is most easily confirmed by using a commercially available plastic disc that spins at 30 rpm. The disc contains six different gauges of piano wire and lead shot. The lead shot moves at approximately 180 mm/s and provides a high-contrast object that can be used to measure image persistence. This phantom is used in conjunction with a large polypropylene container in which 15, 20, or 25 cm of water is placed to create clinical levels of contrast and noise. If this is not available, a metal washer with a ¼-inch (6-mm) hole (or lead diaphragm with a similar-size hole) in the center of a homogenous phantom can be substituted.

Image Noise

Most noise in fluoroscopic images results from either quantum mottle or electronic noise. To determine the specific nature of the noise, first observe the monitor with no fluoroscopic image. If noise is present, it is electronic in nature and a service engineer should be contacted to correct the problem, usually by reducing the gain of the video amplifier. After the noise is corrected, use the following procedure.

PROCEDURE: IMAGE LAG (METAL WASHER METHOD)

1. Place a metal washer with a ¼-inch (6-mm) hole (or lead diaphragm with a similar-size hole) in the center of a homogenous phantom.
2. Perform fluoroscopy on the phantom while moving the image intensifier back and forth; observe the image for lag. Some amount of lag is inherent in the system, with vidicon camera tubes demonstrating more than the other types of cameras. *The maximum amount of lag should be less than 10% for cardiac, vascular, and interventional studies because a 0.014-inch moving guide wire must be visualized. For GI studies, lag times up to 20% are acceptable.* If excessive lag is present, consult a service engineer to adjust the system or, possibly replace the camera.

1. Place a homogenous phantom on the fluoroscopic table and expose at the lowest possible mA and 80 kVp.
2. Increase the mA gradually to the maximum value. If the amount of noise decreases with increased mA, the noise is quantum mottle. To compensate, increase the mA until the noise is at an acceptable level.

Relative Conversion Factor

The relative conversion factor measures the amount of light produced by the output phosphor per unit of X-radiation incident on the input phosphor, which is measured with the following units:

$$\frac{\text{Candela/m}^2}{\text{mR/s}} \quad \text{or} \quad \frac{\text{Nit}}{\mu\text{C/kg/s}}$$

A dosimeter measures the amount of X-radiation at the entrance to the input phosphor and a photographic light meter measures the light emitted from the output phosphor, which should be measured at 80 kVp with the same fluoroscopic mA each time. Place a homogenous phantom in the beam path to protect the image intensifier. Record the value and compared it with all future values. Image intensifiers may deteriorate at a rate of 10% per year, which is reflected by the resulting values. When the values have degraded by more than 50% from the value at acceptance, consult a service engineer because image quality becomes poor and patient dose increases significantly.

Veiling Glare, or Flare

As mentioned previously, veiling glare, or flare, is defined as scattered or reflected light, usually within the linkage between the output phosphor and the television camera, which reduces image contrast. Two methods are used to evaluate for flare. The first involves a homogenous phantom and a small lead disk of 1–2 cm in diameter. Obtain a photofluorospot or cine film image, along with optical density values of the center of the disk area and the area outside the disk. Then use these optical density values to calculate the contrast modulation of the system with the following equation:

$$\text{Contrast modulation} = \frac{(\text{OD}_{max} - \text{OD}_{min})}{(\text{OD}_{max} + \text{OD}_{min})} \times 100$$

where OD_{max} is the optical density of the film outside the image of the lead disk and OD_{min} is the optical density in the center of the lead disk. This value should be at least 70% for most fluoroscopic applications.

Another method of measuring flare involves a video waveform monitor attached to the camera output video cable (accessed most easily by disconnecting it from the back of the television monitor). Use the same setup with the lead disk and homogenous phantom but do not take any spot films. Instead, image the disk during fluoroscopy and observe the voltage waveform pattern on the waveform monitor, which plots voltage versus time (Fig. 7.16). Compare the voltage measurements from the area behind the disk and outside the disk and use the following equation to calculate the contrast:

$$\text{Contrast\%} = \frac{1 - \text{Voltage behind lead strip}}{\text{Peak white voltage}} \times 100$$

Video signal levels should be within ±5% of those specified in the RS 170 standards. This procedure is described in detail elsewhere.[2]

Fluoroscopic Systems for Cardiac Catheterization and Interventional Procedures

Fluoroscopic systems used during cardiac catheterization and interventional procedures must demonstrate a type of resolution known as *temporal resolution*, which is the ability of the imaging system to display events in time (*temporal* refers to *time*) that are occurring close together as separate events. With these procedures, a physician guides various catheters and guide wires through blood vessels to a desired location. The fluoroscopic system must be able to capture the motion of these guide wires precisely (with minimal motion blur) so the physician can place them in the correct location at the correct time, which requires a high (fast) frame rate for the fluoroscopic system. The ability of these fluoroscopic systems to display clear images of moving guide wires is evaluated with a rotatable spoke test pattern (Fig. 7.17). This test object consists of six 5-inch-long steel wires of varying diameters (ranging in size from 0.005 to 0.022 inches) arranged at 30-degree intervals like spokes in a wheel. The wheel is attached to an electric

---

[2]Gray J, Winkler N, Stears J, et al. *Quality Control in Diagnostic Imaging.* University Park Press; 1982.

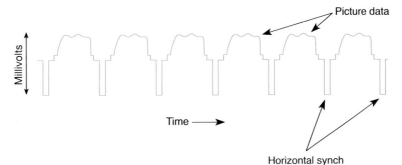

Fig. 7.16 Video waveforms.

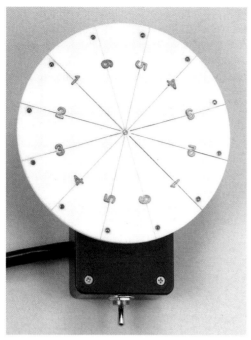

Fig. 7.17 Rotatable spoke test pattern. (Courtesy Nuclear Associates, Inc., Carle Place, New York.)

motor with a rotation speed of 30 rpm. The image of this moving pattern is displayed on the monitor, and the ability to visualize the moving wire is evaluated. These fluoroscopic systems should be able to visualize wire diameter, which is 0.013 inches or smaller, for optimum performance. If they do not visualize, a faster frame rate must be utilized. However, this will increase patient dose. The test pattern also should be visualized using cine cameras and digital recorders to ensure that these systems are delivering optimal image quality.

Video Monitor Performance

The final fluoroscopic image is usually displayed on a television monitor, although this is the weakest link in the imaging chain in terms of loss of resolution. Over time, monitors are subject to defocusing, which reduces the spatial resolution of the observed image. Newer computer monitors used for viewing digital images may also develop unique problems. These monitors contain video cards that "drive them" (allow them to display the digital information). Sometimes these cards generate enough heat to "pop" out of their slots, with a resulting loss of operation. A test pattern created by a multiformat test generator or downloaded from a computer is required for the evaluation of proper monitor performance. These test patterns vary according to the manufacturer of the pattern, but the most common pattern is that designed by the Society of Motion Picture and Television Engineers (SMPTE), in accordance with SMPTE Recommended Practice RP 133-1986, "Medical Diagnostic Imaging Test Pattern for Television Monitors and Hard Copy Recording Cameras" (Fig. 7.18). An alternative test pattern is the AAPM task group (TG) 18-quality control (QC) test pattern, created by the American Association of Physicists in Medicine. A more in-depth discussion of video monitors and their performance takes place in the next chapter.

PROCEDURE: VIDEO MONITOR PERFORMANCE

1. Remove the input cable from the television monitor and replace it with the output cable from the test pattern generator or computer.
2. After the image is displayed, evaluate resolution, geometry, contrast, aspect ratio, uniformity, brightness, and grayscale, and compare the results with the manufacturer's specifications. The 10% steps from the test pattern should be visible.

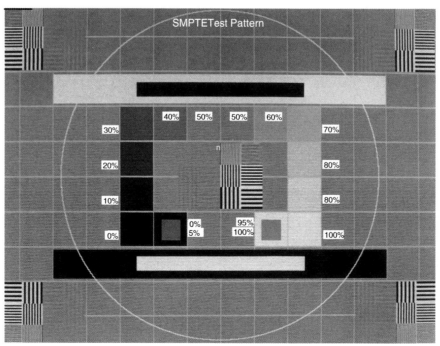

Fig. 7.18 Test pattern of the Society of Motion Picture and Television Engineers (SMPTE).

Standard fluoroscopic (analog black-and-white television) monitors should be monitored every 6 months with the previous procedure. Monitors used to display digital images (such as digital fluoroscopic or radiographic images) should be evaluated using the procedures described in the next chapter.

SUMMARY

Fluoroscopic examinations administer potentially high doses of X-radiation, particularly if the equipment is not functioning within accepted guidelines. For this risk to be minimized, quality control protocols for this equipment are essential for diagnostic radiology departments.

Refer to the Evolve website at https://evolve.elsevier.com for Student Experiments 7.1: Fluoroscopic Visual Inspection, 7.2: Fluoroscopic Exposure Levels, 7.3: Image Resolution of a Fluoroscopic System, 7.4: Fluoroscopic Image Noise, and 7.5: Fluoroscopic Automatic Brightness Control.

REVIEW QUESTIONS

1. Which of the following is not part of an image intensifier tube?
   a. Filament
   b. Photocathode
   c. Anode
   d. Output phosphor
2. Which material is most often used in the input phosphor of an image intensifier?
   a. Calcium tungsten
   b. Cesium iodide
   c. Zinc cadmium sulfide
   d. Lanthanum oxybromide
3. Which of the following terms best describes the increase in image brightness resulting from the difference in size between the input and output phosphors?
   a. Brightness gain
   b. Flux gain
   c. Minification gain
   d. Resolution gain
4. Which of the following increases the brightness of a fluoroscopic image: (1) an increase in kVp, (2) an increase in mA, or (3) an increase in pulse width?
   a. 1 and 2
   b. 2 and 3
   c. 1 and 3
   d. 1, 2, and 3
5. Which of the following is the main advantage of using a multifield image intensifier?
   a. The field of view is increased.
   b. The image brightness is increased.
   c. Magnification option is available.
   d. The patient dose is decreased.

6. Which of the following terms best describes the type of image intensifier artifact that results from projecting an image onto a flat surface?
   a. Veiling glare
   b. Pincushion distortion
   c. Vignetting
   d. S distortion
7. Which of the following is not a "tube" type of television camera?
   a. Orthicon
   b. Plumbicon
   c. Vidicon
   d. CCD
8. The primary beam should be restricted to the diameter of the input phosphor to within ±_____% of the source-to-image distance.
   a. 2
   b. 3
   c. 4
   d. 5
9. The video monitor of a fluoroscopic system should be evaluated with a test pattern created by which of the following organizations?
   a. The National Electrical Manufacturers Association
   b. The American College of Radiology
   c. The Society of Motion Picture and Television Engineers
   d. The American Society of Radiologic Technologists
10. The intensity of the X-ray beam at the tabletop should not exceed _____ R/min for units that are equipped with an automatic brightness stabilization system.
    a. 3
    b. 5
    c. 10
    d. 20

Digital Radiographic and Fluoroscopic Systems and Advanced Imaging Equipment

OBJECTIVES

At the completion of this chapter, the reader should be able to do the following:

- Describe the basic methods of obtaining digital radiographs
- State the advantages and disadvantages of digital radiography vs. analog radiography
- Discuss the quality control (QC) procedures for evaluating digital radiographic systems
- Describe the basic methods of obtaining digital fluoroscopic images
- Explain how digital subtraction angiography is performed
- Discuss the QC procedures for evaluating digital fluoroscopy

- Describe the basic principle of image production from dry laser printers and digital recorders, and discuss the QC procedures for each
- Describe the various types of electronic display devices and discuss the applicable QC procedures
- Explain the basic image informatics and archiving networks and discuss the applicable QC procedures
- Describe the basic QC process for special procedures equipment
- Explain the various methods for obtaining bone mineral density measurements

KEY TERMS

Active matrix array
Algorithm
Amorphous
Analog-to-digital converters
Application program interface (API)
Archive test
Artificial intelligence
Aspect ratio
Capture element
Collection element
Compression ratio

Computed radiography (CR)
Contrast balance
Contrast ratio
Cosine law
Coupling or conversion element
Daily tests
Deep learning
Detective quantum efficiency (DQE)
Deviation index (DI)
DICOM broker

DICOM Modality Worklist (DMWL)
Digital Imaging and Communications in Medicine (DICOM)
Digital fluoroscopy
Digital radiography
Digital subtraction angiography
Digital X-ray radiogrammetry
Direct-to-digital radiographic systems

In recent years, diagnostic imaging has undergone an explosion in technology with the advent of computerized imaging, magnetic resonance imaging (MRI), and digital archiving and retrieval systems. All of these technologies are now commonplace in diagnostic imaging departments and can be subject to variations with age and use; therefore quality control (QC) protocols should be in place to monitor for these variations so that they can be kept to a minimum.

DIGITAL RADIOGRAPHIC IMAGING SYSTEMS

Virtually all diagnostic imaging systems can be considered to have the following key components: image acquisition, image processing, and image display. Since the late 1890s, radiographic images were acquired by exposing a screen/film combination that required chemical processing and was displayed on a viewbox illuminator. In digital imaging, an image acquisition system obtains image data in the form of an electronic signal, which is processed electronically in a computer memory whereby the image exists as electronic values in a computer matrix (rather than as grains of silver on a sheet of polyester plastic) and displayed on an electronic display device (computer monitor). The computer matrix is made up of tiny squares called pixels (a contraction of the term *picture element*). The more pixels in a matrix, the smaller each pixel becomes, thereby increasing spatial resolution (Fig. 8.1). The production of digital radiographic images has virtually replaced this method of film/screen radiography. Creating radiographic images in a digital format has many advantages over the analog format (film/screen images), including:

- Reducing repeat images resulting from technique error (most overexposures and slight underexposure can be

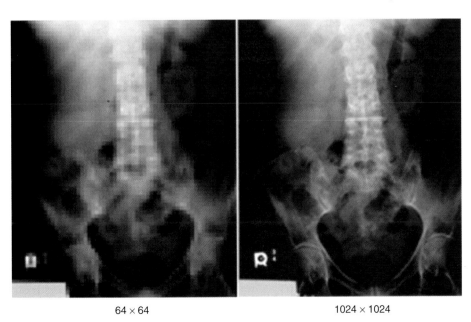

64 × 64   1024 × 1024

Fig. 8.1 Images showing the difference in spatial resolution as the size of the matrix increases.

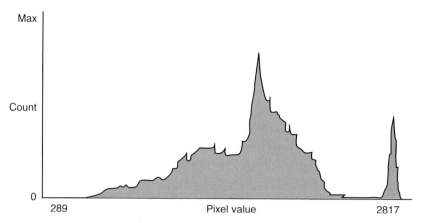

Fig. 8.2 A histogram from a digital radiographic system.

corrected with software and not have to be repeated, but gross underexposure may not)

- Simplifying the filing of images (they can be stored electronically rather than in hard copy)
- Reducing the number of lost images (digital images are stored electronically and can be retrieved as long as they have been correctly entered and saved in the computer system)
- Postprocessing of the image (spatial resolution and contrast can be enhanced by the computer software)
- Transmitting the electronic images (this allows for teleradiology, which is the sending of images over long distances for diagnosis and consultation)

The pathway for digital radiographic imaging consists of the following steps:

1. Image acquisition—Consists of an X-ray exposure to an image receptor
2. Image processing—A computer processes the electronic signal generated by the image receptor into an image made up of pixels using algorithms. An algorithm is a step-by-step procedure or mathematical process for solving a problem or accomplishing a specific task. Processing can occur in three steps:
   a. Preprocessing—Anything done to image data before they have been entered into the computer memory. This includes entering the patient's demographic information and selecting the exam and view to be performed.
   b. Processing—Manipulation of data as they are entered into the computer memory. This includes:
      - Data recognition—This is used to determine parameters such as the average value of a signal, which data are clinically useful, the orientation of the part(s) on the image receptor (IR), the number of projections present on the IR.
      - Pixel arrangement—Image data received from the image receptor are assigned to a specific pixel location in the image matrix.
      - Histogram analysis—A histogram is a graph of signal intensity values that corresponds to a spectrum of pixel values (Fig. 8.2). The x-axis has the pixel brightness value and is related to the amount of exposure to the image plate; the y-axis displays the number of pixels with that brightness value for each exposure. The computer generates a histogram from

the data in the scanned area and compares it with an existing histogram for the programmed body part. This histogram is selected by body part by the radiographer during preprocessing.

- Automatic rescaling (aka: auto ranging, normalization, histogram modification, or stretching)—If the exposure to the IR is outside the range from underexposure or overexposure, then the computer will correct the image by shifting or rescaling the histogram to the correct area. Overexposures of 500% and underexposures as low as 60% can be rescaled without losing image quality.
- LUT adjustment—A lookup table (LUT) is applied to the data that has the standard contrast for that examination to give the desired image contrast for display. The proper LUT will provide the proper gray scale, regardless of variations in kilovolt (peak) (kVp) and milliamperes (mA), resulting in consistent images (Fig. 8.3). The LUT is a histogram of

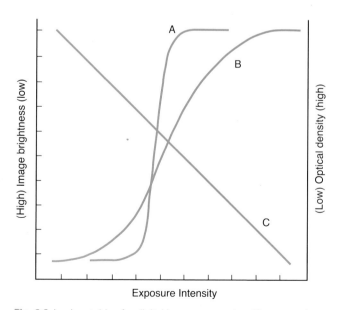

Fig. 8.3 Lookup tables for digital image processing. The curve shape defines the relationship between the intensity of exposure and image brightness (comparable to optical density in film images). (A) High-contrast curve. (B) Low-contrast (wide latitude) curve. (C) Linear response curve with a reversed gray scale.

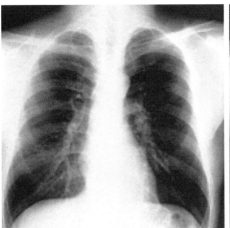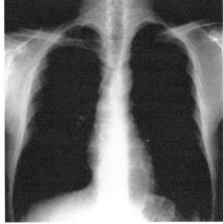

Fig. 8.4 Effect of contrast enhancement on a radiographic image.

luminance values (for image display) derived from the image receptor values (from image acquisition). There is a LUT for every anatomic part. The LUT is graphed by plotting the original values on the x-axis and the new values on the y-axis. Contrast can be increased or decreased by changing the slope of the graph. Brightness is increased or decreased by moving the line up or down the y-axis. In other words, it is a table that maps the image grayscale values into some visible output intensity on a monitor or printed film. This is comparable to adjusting the characteristic curve in film/screen imaging and can be used to enhance a particular portion of the image such as fractures that are difficult to visualize. Digital systems have a linear response that would result in a low-contrast image if it is applied without this step.

c. Postprocessing—Manipulation of data after they have been entered into the computer memory. Common postprocessing functions may include:

- Gradational enhancement (contrast); may also be known as G setting, contrast enhancement, contrast rescaling, contrast processing, tone scaling, or multiscale image contrast algorithm by various equipment manufacturers. Fig. 8.4 shows the effect of gradational enhancement on the radiographic image.
- Spatial frequency enhancement (recorded detail); may also be known as R setting, edge enhancement, unsharp masking, or frequency processing. This postprocessing function allows enhancement of spatial resolution at the expense of increased noise and artifacts. Fig. 8.5 shows the effect of contrast enhancement on the radiographic image.
- Histogram equalization eliminates black-and-white pixels that contribute little diagnostic information and expands the remaining image data to use the full dynamic range.
- Subtraction/addition option is used to remove bony structures or reduce the effect of scatter to increase image contrast.

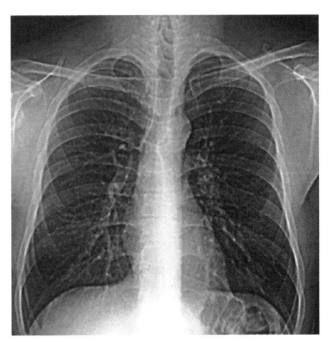

Fig. 8.5 Effect of edge enhancement on digital radiographic image.

- Image magnification electronically magnifies or zooms into specific areas.
- Image inversion allows the option of displaying either a negative (standard radiographic appearance) or a positive (a reverse image whereby the bones are black and air-filled areas are white) image.
- Statistical analysis is used for calculating surface areas and estimating volumes or changes in tissue density.
- Windowing is the manipulation of window width and level to adjust image brightness and contrast.
- Image annotation is the addition of text information such as view, position, time sequence, etc., to the image.
- Image flip allows images to be rotated horizontally or vertically.

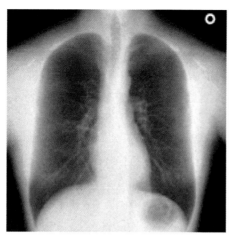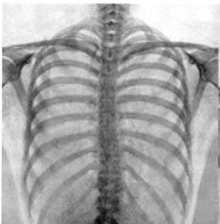

Fig. 8.6 Effect of energy subtraction on a chest examination. The image on the left has bony structures subtracted, whereas the image on the right shows soft tissue subtraction.

- Energy subtraction is based on subtracting projection radiographs obtained at two different photon energies. These are often used for chest radiography to diminish bony rib structures and better visualize lung and soft tissue. Fig. 8.6 shows the effect of energy subtraction on the radiographic image.
- Image stitching is the formation of a long body part image (such as a complete spine during a scoliosis study) from a series of overlapping subimages.
- Database functions are used for image storage and display, distribution to local network workstations, archive query, transfer to a picture archiving and communication system (PACS), and for printing hard-copy images.

3. Image display—Digital images are soft-copy images, so they must be viewed on a display monitor. These will be discussed later in this chapter.
4. Image analysis—The image is viewed to determine if proper image quality is present.
5. Image archiving—Images are stored in a PACS, to be discussed later in this chapter.

Currently, digital images can be acquired by using one of three methods: secondary capture, computed radiography (CR), or digital radiography (DR).

Secondary Capture

This method of creating digital images involves the initial creation of an analog image (on film) and then its conversion into a digital format. One method of accomplishing this conversion would involve taking a photograph of a film radiograph with a digital camera. This method has been used for years by diagnostic imaging educators to obtain digital images. However, there is considerable loss of resolution, even with a large matrix (>3 megapixel) camera. Therefore it may be acceptable for teaching files or professional meeting presentations but should never be used to make a diagnosis. More acceptable conversion of analog film images to digital format can be accomplished by a laser scanning digitizer or a

charge-coupled device (CCD) scanner. Common uses of secondary capture devices include:
- Film radiographs are archived into a picture archiving and communication system (PACS).
- Computer-aided diagnosis is a software program in which the computer can search for abnormalities in mammography and chest radiographs.
- Teleradiology is the process of sending digitized images to distant locations for interpretation and consultation.
- Duplicate images allow the original film-based radiograph to remain at the original clinical site while an electronic copy made by the digitizer can be burned onto a CD or DVD and given to the patient.

Laser Scanning Digitizer

The laser scanning digitizer is used to convert an existing radiographic image that is recorded on film into a digital format that can be stored and transmitted electronically (Fig. 8.7).

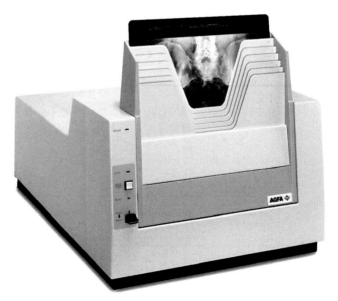

Fig. 8.7 Laser scanning digitizer. (Courtesy Agfa in Bushong SC. *Radiologic science for technologists*, 12th ed. Elsevier-Mosby; 2021.)

It is similar in function to a scanner used with a personal computer to scan photographic images into the computer data storage. The existing radiograph is placed in the digitizer, where it is scanned by a laser and then detected by photosensors on the other side. The analog electronic signals created by these photosensors are then sent through analog-to-digital converters (ADCs), which transform them into a digital electronic signal. Once the electronic signal is in digital form, it can enter into the computer memory for processing. The higher optical density areas of the film image attenuate a higher percentage of the laser light than the areas with a lower optical density. The differences in the amount of laser light transmitted through the various areas are used to convert the analog image information into a digital image. The shade values are then displayed on a computer monitor based on an LUT that indicates which shade of gray is associated with each value. Scanning takes about 25 seconds, depending on the scanning resolution. These systems currently have a resolution capability of about 5 megapixels. They have been around since about 1990 and are considered the gold standard for film digitization. As with the scanner for a personal computer, it is important to keep the scanning surface clean and free of any dirt or dust. Otherwise, artifacts that are not present in the original film image can appear in the digital version of the image.

Charge-Coupled Device Scanner

The CCD scanner is similar to a document copier or a scanner that you would use with your personal computer. Light is focused on a line on the film, which strikes a linear array CCD detector. When light strikes the CCD, it causes electrons to leave in a signal that is proportional to the amount of light transmitted through the film. This device is smaller and less expensive than the laser scanning digitizer, but it has poorer contrast resolution. It is also slower than laser scanning digitizers (up to 80 seconds per scan) and can have problems accurately reproducing extreme light and dark areas on the original film radiograph.

Computed Radiography

CR is a digital image acquisition and processing system for producing static radiographs. It was developed in 1981 by the Fuji Corporation, with the first clinical application in 1983. This system uses standard X-ray tubes and generators but requires specialized image receptors and processing. CR systems consist of the image receptors, an image reader device (IRD), computer, and a workstation.

Most CR image receptors resemble a traditional film/screen cassette but do not contain intensifying screens and film (some CR systems can be integrated into a bucky assembly or chest unit so that they are not visible and the technologist does not need to handle a cassette). The outside is made of carbon fiber and has a bar code that is scanned into a computer to link it with patient data in the Radiology Information System (RIS). Inside of the cassette is an imaging plate (IP) made of either metal or plastic that is coated on one side with photostimulable phosphors (PSPs) in a layer less than 1 mm thick. The phosphor material can be either barium fluorobromide (BaFbR:Eu^{2+}) doped with europium

(an activator or impurity) or cesium bromide (CsBr:Eu^{2+}) doped with europium. The cesium bromide phosphor yields better resolution because of light divergence as compared with barium fluorobromide. The K-edge of these materials is between 35 and 50 keV (lower than rare earth phosphors), making them more sensitive to scattered radiation.

When these crystals are exposed to X-rays, they are energized until they are exposed to light from a laser. This is known as photostimulated luminescence. The crystal electrons (after X-ray absorption) are trapped in empty lattice sites called F-centers. When laser light hits the F-centers, the trapped electrons are released, causing the emission of visible light (which is blue in color), which is then detected by photosensors and sent through ADCs and into the computer for processing. The standard plate has a relative speed of between 200 and 400, whereas the high-resolution plate is between 50 and 100 (comparable to film/screen systems). Once an IP is exposed to X-rays, a latent image is present and can remain on the IP for up to 24 hours but will gradually weaken through a process called *fading*. This fading process will occur exponentially over time. A typical IP will lose about 25% of its stored energy within 8 hours of exposure.

The exposed image receptor is placed into a slot in the front of an image reader device (IRD) (Fig. 8.8) that removes the plate from the cassette for processing. The plate is then stimulated

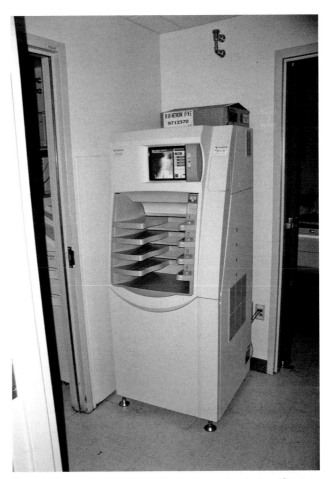

Fig. 8.8 The computed radiography image reader device. (Courtesy Advocate Good Samaritan Hospital, Downers Grove, Illinois.)

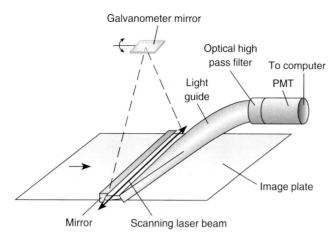

Fig. 8.9 Schematic diagram of a computed radiography reader system. *PMT*, Photomultiplier tube.

by a scanning helium–neon laser (emitting a red light with a wavelength of 633 nm) or a solid-state laser (670 nm), which causes the crystals to release blue-violet light (390–400 nm wavelength). The F-centers in the IP respond best to red light having a wavelength of about 600 nm. A rotating polygon or an oscillating mirror deflects the laser beam back and forth across the IP as it is moving. This is known as the "fast scan" mode. The light emitted by the PSPs is then detected by photosensors that convert the amount of light detected to an electronic signal value that is sent through an ADC and then to the computer for processing (Fig. 8.9). The IP must be moved at a constant, slow speed (known as slow scan) along the long axis of the IP. Any fluctuations in velocity can result in banding artifacts.

After the image is obtained from the IP, it is transferred to another part of the IRD, where a high-intensity sodium discharge lamp erases any residual image so that it can be reused. These plates are kept in a storage bin until needed, at which time they can be transferred back into the image receptor. Most current systems can process about 200 IPs per hour and take about 30–60 seconds to process. There are also X-ray tables and upright bucky units that contain multiple PSP plates and a reader in the unit so that no cassette handling is required. The units will move and process the IPs after each exposure, which allows the radiographer to view the images on a monitor in the control booth area.

Once the IRD has scanned the image plate, the signal from the photodetectors is sent to a computer for processing. A workstation console where the radiographer can perform both pre- and postprocessing functions is attached to this computer.

The image is usually created with a 2560 × 2048 matrix. Hard-copy images can be created with a dry laser printer.

Advantages of Computed Radiography vs. Film/Screen Radiography

CR has several advantages over conventional film/screen radiography including the following:

1. A lower patient dose is incurred as a result of the higher quantum detection efficiency (up to 50%) of the IP phosphors (in

TABLE 8.1 **Percentage Dose Reduction for Various Radiographic Examinations**

Examination	Decrease in Patient Dose (%)
Upper GI tract	5
Pelvis	12
Chest	14–20
IVP or IVU	50

GI, Gastrointestinal; *IVP*, intravenous pyelogram; *IVU*, intravenous urography.

some systems only). Table 8.1 lists the percentage dose reduction for various radiographic examinations. Some CR systems may require an increase in exposure of the IP, in which case the dose reduction would occur because of a lower repeat rate.

2. The repeat rate is lower because computer can correct pixel brightness and contrast if improper technical factors were used.

3. Higher-contrast resolution and wider-exposure latitude are possible than with radiographic film emulsion. These can be demonstrated with a sensitometric curve (Fig. 8.10). The response of the CR IP is linear over an X-ray exposure range of four orders of magnitude between 5 and 50 mR or 0.05–0.5 mGy air kerma. The film/screen combination is limited to about two orders of magnitude and a sigmoidal response. This means that at high and low exposures, the contrast is greatly reduced; a linear response exists only for about one order of magnitude in exposure.

4. No darkroom or film costs are incurred (unless hard-copy images are desired).

5. The images can be postprocessed to improve quality.

6. Image storage is easy through either hard copy or electronic storage.

7. Easy interface is possible with PACS.

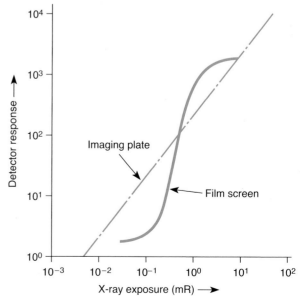

Fig. 8.10 Plot of system response of film/screen imaging system and digital radiographic imaging plate.

Disadvantages of Computed Radiography vs. Film/Screen Radiography

The disadvantages of CR include the following:

1. Capital costs are high for image receptors, CR reader units, and computer hardware and software.

2. Spatial resolution may be lower in older systems. Spatial resolution is controlled by the dimension of the crystals in the IP, the size of the laser beam in the CR reader unit, and the matrix size. Film/screen combinations can resolve more than 5 line pairs per millimeter (lp/mm) compared with 4–5 lp/mm for some CR systems. This can make visualization of linear fractures in bone difficult. CR systems with spatial frequencies of 10 lp/mm are available for mammographic imaging and are discussed in Chapter 9.

3. Collimation and centering of the part are critical for the computer to determine the proper pixel shade brightness (optical density) and contrast.

4. The patient could potentially be overexposed to radiation. With film/screen systems, the correct amount of radiation exposure is necessary to obtain an acceptable radiographic image. With CR systems, the computer can compensate overexposure of up to 500% above the necessary amount of milliampere-second (mAs), which can cause radiographers to routinely overexpose the patient to unnecessary radiation. The ALARA (as low as reasonably achievable) concept should be remembered to keep exposure as low as reasonably achievable. Various CR system manufacturers use a numeric system to monitor the amount of exposure to the IP (and therefore the patient). Unfortunately, these systems vary by manufacturer and are not standardized (unlike the relative system speed value that all radiographers can use with film/screen systems). For example, the Fuji CR system uses a value known as the sensitivity (or "S" value), which is inversely proportional to the amount of exposure reaching the IP. These values are calibrated so that an exposure of 1 mR (0.01 mGy air kerma) from an 80-kVp beam to a standard IP will yield an "S"-number of 200 in the semiautomatic mode. Therefore an exposure of 0.1 mR (0.1 μGy air kerma) to the same plate would yield an S-number of 2000, whereas 10 mR (0.1 mGy air kerma) would yield a value of 20. In the normal mode, cutting the exposure in half would double the S-number and vice versa. Proper exposure to IPs should produce S-values of between 150 and 250. An S-value of greater than 250 for nonbucky exposure or 400 for bucky exposure indicates underexposure, whereas a value of less than 100 would indicate overexposure. In comparison, Carestream Health (formerly known as Kodak) uses a value known as the exposure index (EI), which is directly proportional to the amount of radiation that strikes the IP. This index is the average pixel value calculated within the defined anatomic region. It is calibrated so that an exposure of 1 mR (0.01 mGy air kerma) from an 80-kVp beam on a standard plate would yield a value of 2000. Thus an exposure of 0.1 mR (0.1 μGy air kerma) results in an EI of 1000, whereas 10 mR (0.1 mGy air kerma) would produce a value of 3000. Doubling the exposure will cause an increase in the EI of 300, whereas cutting the exposure in half causes it to drop by 300. IPs should produce EI values between 1800 and 2200 when properly exposed. Agfa uses a value known as the log of the median exposure (log M). It is calibrated with a beam of 75 kVp for a 20-mR exposure, and the plate is scanned using a speed class setting of 100 to yield a log M value of 2.6. For a given speed class setting, the value of log M varies according to the log of the radiation dose to the IP. A doubling of the exposure should result in an increase in the value of log M by 0.301. The typical range of log M values is between 1.95 and 2.6. Regardless of the system manufacturer, it is important for the radiographer to keep these values within the manufacturer's specifications. An underexposed IP (less than 60% below the ideal exposure) can create an image that will demonstrate quantum mottle, even though the brightness level is acceptable. Overexposed IPs (greater than 200% above ideal exposure) can create images that may suffer from low contrast (even though most software can produce a diagnostic image with up to a 500% overexposure). When the plate receives greater than 500% overexposure, saturation occurs and the image remains black despite all postprocessing attempts to brighten it. Because there is greater latitude in being able to use postprocessing to fix an overexposed image than an underexposed image, many radiographers can have a tendency to overexpose an image plate. This has led to a condition known as dose creep, whereby patient dose for many exams is higher than ideal standards. Automatic exposure control systems can be calibrated to work with CR systems and should be used to ensure proper exposure of the image plate. An exposure technique chart that has been formulated for the individual CR system must also be present and used.

5. Image artifacts may occur with the use of grids. A moiré or zebra pattern artifact (discussed in the next chapter) can occur if the grid is stationary during the exposure, and the grid frequency and the scan frequency of the IRD are similar and oriented in the same direction (grid lines should run perpendicular to the plate reader's scan lines to avoid this problem). Using a grid frequency of greater than 60 lines per centimeter should eliminate this problem. These artifacts also can be caused by the sampling rate of the ADC in the reader unit having a rate that is too slow. Thus grid frequency should be about 85/inch (33–34/cm) for a 14-inch × 17-inch image receptor and 103/inch (40–43/cm) for a 10-inch × 12-inch image receptor. Because IPs are especially sensitive to scatter, grids should be used for all exposures greater than 80 kVp. The IPs are also very sensitive to background radiation (even more than film/screen systems). Most plates can respond to radiation exposures as low as 10 μR, whereas background radiation can vary between 40 and 80 μR/day in many areas. It is therefore recommended that the plates be erased daily if they have not been used to eliminate unwanted noise. They also will need to be routinely cleaned, just like intensifying screens in film/screen cassettes. The use of CR imaging equipment in the United States has decreased significantly

since reimbursement for images obtained with this method have been reduced by the federal government (and private insurers).

Digital Radiography

This method of creating digital radiographic images, also known as either digital radiography (DR) or *flat-panel* or *flat-plate* imaging, appeared in the late 1990s and is now the method of choice for creating digital radiographic images. They also have been referred to as direct-to-digital radiographic systems (DDRs). The main components of a DR system include the image receptor, computer and software (for image processing), and a workstation to display the image and carry out postprocessing functions.

This method originally involved the installation of a flat-panel image receptor in the bucky of a radiographic table or an upright bucky, whereas newer cassette-based DR systems have been introduced and have become the industry standard in hospitals and medical centers. This flat-panel image receptor creates an electronic signal in proportion to the amount of X-rays striking its surface and then sends this signal directly to a digital image processor. The flat-panel image receptor is a large-area (the size of conventional film/screen image receptors) integrated circuit called an active matrix array (AMA) that consists of millions of identical semiconductor elements deposited on a glass base (Fig. 8.11). These act as tiny radiation detectors (also called detector elements, DELs, or DEX-ELS) that convert X-ray energy into an electronic signal that can be processed by a computer.

The AMA is similar to a CCD/complementary metallic oxide semiconductor (CMOS) camera (used in digital

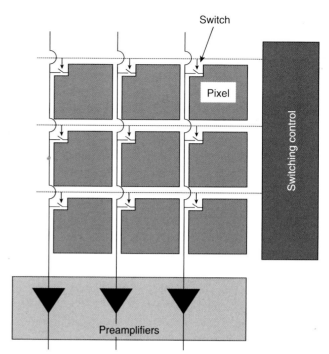

Fig. 8.12 Illustration of a section of the active matrix array showing the switch associated with each pixel.

cameras, digital video camcorders, and television cameras in fluoroscopic systems) but much larger in size. These flat-panel image receptors also can be used for fluoroscopic imaging as well as radiographic imaging. Each element in the AMA is known as a *pixel*. Each pixel of the array has a switch made from a thin-film transistor (TFT). These TFT switches are connected to switching control circuitry that allows all switches in a row of the array to be operated simultaneously (Fig. 8.12). For radiographic imaging, all of the TFT switches are kept in the "off" position during the X-ray exposure. Once the exposure is complete, the switches in the first row are turned on and the signal from each pixel is amplified, converted into digital form by an ADC, and then stored in the memory of the digital image processor. These switches are then turned off and the switches in the second row are turned on, then the third, and so on, until the image from the entire array is acquired. For fluoroscopic exposures, the array is scanned continuously. The AMA can get signal data immediately to the computer for processing, so the image will appear on the monitor quickly. Most AMAs are assembled using a process known as tiling, whereby several flat-panel detectors are joined to obtain one large image receptor. Care must be taken to make sure that the segments have equal response to radiation exposure or have good flat-fielding software that can compensate for any difference in performance between the various tiles. The main parts of an AMA are:

1. Capture element—This is the top portion of the AMA that will absorb the X-rays that exit the patient (much like the PSP in CR systems). This could be either a scintillator such as cesium iodide or gadolinium oxysulfide, or a photoconductor such as amorphous selenium in direct DR systems.

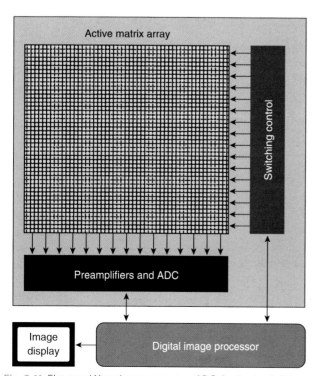

Fig. 8.11 Flat-panel X-ray image receptor. *ADC,* Analog-to-digital converter.

2. **Coupling or conversion element**—This will convert the X-ray–generated image data from the capture element into an electronic charge that will be transferred to a collection element. This is most often made up of a photodiode (made of amorphous silicon), or it can be fiber optics, lens coupling, or amorphous selenium (which will act as both the coupling and capture element).

3. **Collection element**—This is the bottom portion of the AMA and would collect the charge created by the coupling element and send it to through an ADC and on to the computer for processing. This can be made up of a CCD, CMOS, or a TFT array.

Two different types of flat-panel devices have been developed: indirect-conversion and direct-conversion image receptors.

Indirect-Conversion or Scintillator DR System

This type of system involves first converting X-ray energy into light energy and then converting that light energy into an electronic signal (hence the term *indirect* because the X-ray energy is not converted directly into an electric signal). These systems are available in two basic designs, a flat panel with a scintillator capture element and a TFT collection element, or a scintillator capture element with a CCD or CMOS collection element.

a. The flat panel with a scintillator and TFT system involves coupling the scintillator (usually cesium iodide or terbium-doped gadolinium dioxide sulfide) with amorphous silicon as the coupling element. The term *amorphous* means "without form." In this context, it means that silicon (which normally exists in a crystalline state) is in a noncrystalline state. Because the atomic number of silicon is 14, it will not absorb X-rays well. Therefore a scintillator consisting of a phosphor layer of cesium iodide or a rare earth intensifying screen composed of lanthanum and gadolinium oxysulfides (sometimes called Gadox) that emits light when struck by X-rays, is used. Cesium iodide requires about 10% less radiation than Gadox and has slightly better image quality, but DR image receptors using Gadox are about 20%–30% cheaper. This light then activates the amorphous silicon photodetectors (of which there are millions in the AMA). This interaction results in the creation of an electric signal that is stored by a TFT assembly until readout, at which time the signal is sent to the computer. A disadvantage to this design is decreased spatial resolution resulting from light divergence from the scintillator. These detectors are manufactured in columns to minimize this light diffusion and increase spatial resolution. The main advantage of this design is relatively low patient dose (about 20%–50% lower as compared with CR or film/screen image receptors, depending on the examination). The potential disadvantage of this design is decreased spatial resolution due to light divergence from the scintillator. To help prevent this loss of spatial resolution, the scintillator crystals are manufactured in needles or columns about 10–20 μm in diameter to minimize this light diffusion and increase spatial resolution.

b. The flat panel with scintillator and CCD or CMOS system couples (by lenses or fiber optics) a scintillator made of rare earth phosphors such as gadolinium oxysulfide ($Gd_2O_2S{:}Tb$) or cesium iodide to a CCD or CMOS device. Both CCD and CMOS devices will convert light into an electric charge and then process it into electronic signals. In a CCD sensor, every pixel's charge is transferred through a very limited number of output nodes to be converted into a voltage, buffered, and sent off from the chip as an analog signal. All of the pixel can be devoted to light capture, and the output signal's uniformity (a key factor in image quality) is high. It is also very sensitive to low levels of light, so fewer mAs can be used on the patient. In a CMOS sensor, each pixel has its own charge-to-voltage conversion, and the sensor often includes amplifiers, noise correction (to increase the signal to noise ratio), and digitization circuits so that the chip can output a digital signal. However, these other functions increase the design complexity and reduce the area available for light capture (lower fill factor) and increase electronic noise. With each pixel doing its own conversion, uniformity is lower. This results in fast, continuous readout at video rates, and is currently used in time delay and integration systems (also known as slit systems), whereby a slit camera and X-ray tube travel over the field of view.

Direct-Conversion or Photoconductor DR System

This type of system involves the use of the photoconducting material amorphous selenium rather than a scintillator as the capture element. The amorphous silicon used in indirect-conversion image receptors has an atomic number of 14, so X-rays do not interact to a significant degree unless thick amounts are used. Selenium has an atomic number of 34 and therefore interacts more readily with X-rays to create an electronic signal (so no scintillator is necessary). The electric charge produced after X-ray interaction is detected by an array of pixels that consists of an electrode and a capacitor, which store the charge until switched by a TFT. This yields better spatial resolution than the indirect systems, since no light divergence occurs. However, selenium is not good for high kVp exposures because of its relatively low K-edge (13 keV) and is used mainly for mammography. Photoconductors such as lead iodide and mercury iodide are being introduced to replace selenium for higher kVp studies.

The advantage of the direct-conversion method over the indirect-conversion method is that there is no spreading of light from the phosphor material (similar to the effect in conventional intensifying screens) and the loss of spatial resolution that occurs as a result. However, the phosphor used in the indirect-conversion system possesses a higher detective quantum efficiency (DQE) (see Chapter 3) and therefore results in a lower patient dose. The relatively low DQE of amorphous selenium also means that it is not quite suitable for higher kVp exposures because of its relatively low K-edge. Photoconductors such as lead iodide and mercury iodide are being introduced to replace selenium for higher kVp studies.

The spatial resolution of direct-conversion systems is determined primarily by the detector size (also known as aperture size) and the sampling pitch (which is the length of an array divided by the number of detectors along that length). For example, if there are 2000 detectors on a line that is 35 cm long, the sampling pitch is 175 µm (35 divided by 2000). The sampling pitch determines the limiting spatial resolution that is achievable by the digital imaging system in line pairs per millimeter. The limiting spatial resolution, also known as the **Nyquist frequency**, is equal to one-half of the sampling frequency. For example, if a DR image receptor contains 2 pixels in each millimeter, the maximum spatial frequency that can be resolved is 1 lp/mm since one pixel would display the black line and one pixel would be needed to display a white line. Systems currently available have pixels as small as 85 µm, which yield a spatial resolution of approximately 5 lp/mm (comparable to CR systems).

Another feature that can influence spatial resolution and patient dose with direct-conversion image receptors is the **fill factor.** The fill factor is the percentage of pixel area that is sensitive to the image signal (contains the X-ray detector). The fill factor for most current systems is approximately 80% because some of the pixel area must be devoted to electronic conductors and the TFT.

The computer that is purchased with a DR system should have a fast processor (at least an I-7, with an I-9 or newer preferred). The random-access memory of the computer should be at least 16–32 GB. Random-access memory gives applications a place to store and access data on a short-term basis. It stores the information your computer is actively using so that it can be accessed quickly. The hard drive should be a solid-state device that is swappable for future use. The software that comes with DR systems should also have certain characteristics such as:

- Open architecture design, which means that it should not cause conflicts with other programs
- Allow for web interface support
- Be intelligent and offer artificial intelligence (AI) tools that increase speed and precision, and contain productivity aids such as:
  - Positioning guides
  - Image communication tools, web viewers, email and Digital Imaging and Communications in Medicine (DICOM) compatibility
  - Technique/X-ray exposure setting assistance during image acquisition
  - Automated report generation for radiologists

The display monitor for DR images should have at least 1920 × 1080 pixels; have a contrast ratio of at least 1000:1, with 10,000:1 preferred; a minimum brightness of 300 nit, with 350–400 preferred; and should be touchscreen, with a glove hand version preferred.

Comparison of CR with DR

Both the CR and DR methods create digital images that have many advantages over the analog images created by film/screen radiography. But how do they compare with each other? Both methods produce spatial resolution that is comparable to that of film/screen systems (about 5 lp/mm). They also have superior contrast resolution compared with film/screen systems. Both systems provide image processing software to enhance the image. To make a better comparison of image quality among digital systems, many physicists recommend using a parameter known as DQE. DQE is a measure of the information transfer efficiency of a detector and is defined as the signal-to-noise ratio squared (SNR^2) coming out of a detector divided by the signal-to-noise ratio squared going into a detector (SNR^2_{out}/SNR^2_{in}). As with modulation transfer function values, DQE values will always range from 0 to 1. A DQE value of 1 would be a perfect detector because no information is lost between the detector input and detector output. Therefore the greater the DQE, the better the digital detector system at displaying image quality.

The advantage of DQE is that it is a measure of the combined effect of the noise and contrast performance of an imaging system expressed as a function of object detail. Greater DQE values will increase one's ability to view small, low-contrast objects (such as in mammography). The DQE of the cesium iodide with TFT indirect DR system is very high at diagnostic kVp values and when spatial resolution requirements are not too high. This is one of the reasons why it is the most common DR system used today. Direct DR systems have a higher DQE at lower kVp values or when higher spatial resolution is required. Any type of DR image receptor should have a DQE of at least 0.65 (65%) at 0 lp/mm.

The DR image receptor system's response to radiation exposure is linearly related to radiation dose, so image contrast does not change with the dose. Also, DR systems are not subject to saturation or a loss of contrast because of overexposure, meaning that overexposed images do not have to be repeated as they do with CR systems. In addition, exposures should not be repeated with DR systems because of brightness or contrast concerns. As with CR image receptor systems, DR systems cannot compensate for excessive noise caused by quantum mottle (caused by severe underexposure). As with CR systems, dose creep can also occur with DR systems. Numeric values to indicate proper exposure to the DR image receptor (similar to those used in CR systems) are used by the various manufacturers to help radiographers avoid dose creep. These can include dose area product or kerma area product, EI, and detector EI. In 2009, the International Electrotechnical Commission (IEC) and the American Association of Physicists in Medicine (AAPM) proposed an international standardization for exposure indicators used in digital radiographic systems as standard IEC 62494-1 and AAPM Task Group 116, which have been adopted by many equipment vendors. The values they proposed include the exposure index (EI), **target exposure index (EI$_t$),** and **deviation index (DI).**

1. EI is an index of exposure to the image receptor in a relevant region. It is derived from the image signal-to-noise ratio (SNR), which relates to the absorbed energy at the detector (not the patient) after each exposure. The value of the EI is linear with the amount of mAs used and will change exponentially with the kVp. The EI numbers are derived from an air kerma value of 10 µGy to the image

receptor, which will yield an EI number of 1000. If 20 μGy is received, the EI number would be 2000, and 5 μGy will yield an EI value of 500.

2. EI_t is the target reference exposure that is obtained when the image receptor is properly exposed and will differ for each body part and projection.

3. DI is obtained from the equation:

$$DI = 10 \times \log_{10}(EI/E_t)$$

This measures how far the actual EI value deviates from the projection-specific EI_t. These values most often range from −4 to +4, with a DI of 0 being optimal. The following table demonstrates various DI values.

DI	Exposure Factor	% Change
4	2.60	160
3	2.0	100
2	1.6	60
1	1.26	26
0	1.00	0
−1	0.80	−20
−2	0.60	−40
−3	0.50	−50
−4	0.40	−60

As with those of CR systems, these exposure indicators vary by manufacturer and no uniform set of values has been accepted by the industry. Various exposure indicators for a number of DR systems is listed in Table 8.2. Accepted values are specified by the manufacturer and techniques should be developed to ensure that radiographers adhere to these target values. The technique charts containing proper exposure parameters must be in place to ensure that the image receptor is exposed to enough radiation to avoid quantum mottle but minimize exposure to the patient (they are also part of the standard of care expected by The Joint Commission). They should also be formulated to function over a wide range of adult sizes and include a wide range of pediatric sizes.

In the past, the majority of DR systems have been built into the bucky assembly and were therefore confined to bucky use. However, there are now cassette-based DR systems that can be used in table and upright bucky assemblies or during mobile radiography. The image data can be downloaded from the cassette-based DR AMA via a cable or through a wireless connection that also can be used for non-bucky use. The DR systems have a higher capital cost than CR systems because of the intricacy of designing and constructing the AMA. The cost per room for DR systems that are built into the bucky assembly is approximately three to four times greater than CR systems, whereas cassette-based DR systems are closer in cost to a CR system (but with fewer image receptors). However, DR systems have a much shorter image acquisition time and are less labor intensive because the image receptor does not have to be entered into a reader unit. This also reduces examination time, which can increase patient satisfaction. It also can allow for more patients to be

TABLE 8.2 List of Digital Radiography Manufacturers (Selling in the United States)

Manufacturer	Web Address
Agfa HealthCare	https://www.agfahealthcare.com
Canon USA, Inc.	https://us.medical.canon
Carestream Health (formerly Kodak)	www.carestreamhealth.com
FujiFilm Medical Systems USA	https://www.healthcaresolutions.us.fujifilm.com
GE Healthcare	https://www.gehealthcare.com
iCRco Inc.	www.icro.com
IDC (Imaging Dynamics Company)	https://www.imagingdynamics.com
Konica Minolta Medical Imaging	https://www.medical.konicaminolta.us
Philips Medical Systems	https://www.usa.philips.com
Rayence Inc.	https://www.rayenceusa.com
Siemens Medical Solutions	https://www.siemens-healthineers.com/en-us
Swissray International	https://www.swissray.com
Thales Electron Devices	https://www.thalesgroup.com
Viztek	https://www.viztek.net

served in a given period, especially with high-volume examinations such as chest radiography. Indirect-conversion DR systems with cesium iodide phosphors have achieved US Food and Drug Administration approval for mammographic procedures (discussed in Chapter 9). For these reasons, DR systems have rapidly replaced CR systems, especially in larger hospitals and medical centers. A listing of manufacturers selling DR imaging equipment in the United States (complete as of the writing of this edition) can be found in Table 8.2. As mentioned in Chapter 2, reimbursement for images created with CR systems have been reduced by 7%–10% compared to those obtained with DR systems.

Potential DR Image Problems

1. Dropped pixels—Areas of no data (usually appearing as black dots or lines) caused by damage to the AMA

2. Electronic noise—Each detector element has a certain amount of electronic noise associated with it (also known as dark noise).

3. Incomplete charge transfer—Caused by the collection element not sufficiently sending all data to the computer for processing, resulting in incomplete image formation

4. Electronic memory artifact—Exposures are taken in too rapid a sequence, resulting in not enough time for each previous exposure to transfer the entire signal, creating an artifact known as "ghosting."

5. Uneven amplification—In large detector arrays, several amplifiers are used that can vary in gain from one to the next. To correct for differences in gain between detector elements (tiling), a process known as flat-fielding is used. Flat-fielding or equalization is a software correction that is performed to equalize the response of each pixel to a non-uniform X-ray beam.

6. Backscatter—Scattering through the back of the cassette that can either create noise in the image or may create an image of the internal circuitry found in the back of the cassette

7. High capital cost—DR image receptors are very expensive. Therefore they must be rugged to handle the workload during radiographic examinations. When purchasing DR image receptors, the manufacturer's specifications should indicate that they should be able to pass a drop test from a distance of at least 70 cm to 1 m and still function normally without any artifacts present. They should also have a moisture barrier rating with an International Protection Rating (IPX) score of 4 or higher. This means that it will offer protection from splashes of water in any direction for at least 5 min.

Quality Control of Digital Radiographic Imaging Systems

Because the image is created digitally, variation in system performance is less than with film/screen systems. However, digital imaging can create a host of new problems requiring a quality management program that must take into consideration the entire imaging chain (and the people involved within it). For example, a misidentified conventional film image can be fixed rather easily with an adhesive label containing the correct information taped over the incorrect information. With digital imaging, several copies of the image may have been created, archived, and transmitted electronically within a PACS, making correction more difficult. In addition, new versions of system software might cause changes in image quality when added to existing systems. Three levels of system performance for QC and system maintenance exist:

1. Routine—Performed by QC technologists
2. Full inspection—Performed by medical physicists and involves radiation measurements and noninvasive adjustments
3. System adjustment—Performed by vendor service personnel and involves hardware and software maintenance

Unfortunately, many different types of digital systems exist, and there is no standard QC process that can be used by all systems. This means that QC technologists must rely on the manufacturer's guidelines for specific QC procedures. However, some basic QC procedures are common to all systems:

- CR system inspection. The IP loading and unloading mechanisms in the CR reader unit must be cleaned and lubricated regularly (at least weekly). Care must be taken to avoid dirt or dust on the IPs to prevent artifacts on the final image, which can mimic pathologic conditions (Fig. 8.13). CR plates also can yellow over time, which can

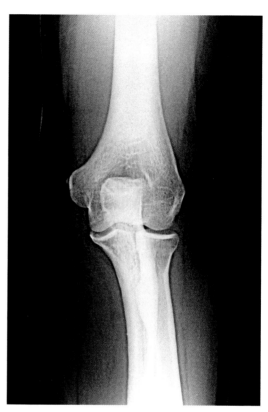

Fig. 8.13 Digital radiographic image with artifact caused by dirt on plate.

reduce their efficiency. It is important to use a dry cloth or a cleaning solution that is specified by the manufacturer and is not water based. The IPs also should be inspected for hairline cracks at least monthly because these cracks also can cause artifacts on the image that can mimic pathology. The IPs also should be erased daily to reduce image noise. They are especially sensitive to exposure from fluorescent lighting, so they should be stored in the IRD or erased before use.

- Laser scanning digitizers must be kept clean and free of dirt and debris, as previously mentioned.
- The image receptors used with DR systems also must be kept clean and free of dirt, debris, blood, contrast media, and other items. The internal batteries on wireless DR cassettes should be inspected to make sure that they are fully charged (most have a charge indicator on the cassette).
- Check the performance of the display monitors at least monthly, as recommended by the American College of Radiology (ACR). A high-resolution monitor is used for all types of digital radiographic systems to display the final image. These monitors are available with either a cathode-ray tube (CRT) display or a liquid crystal display (LCD) flat-panel display. Many radiologists are making their diagnoses according to the images from these monitors rather than hard-copy film images, and they may perform operations 24 hours a day, 7 days a week. The CRT monitors can defocus over time and lose image brightness and contrast. They are the weakest link in terms of the variability in the quality of digital image display. The LCD flat-panel

displays have a disadvantage of limited viewing angle (you have to look straight at them to see the image clearly). They also may require periodic replacement of their light source after approximately 30,000 hours of operation. However, LCD displays are subject to far less variability than CRT display monitors. Procedures for checking video monitor performance are discussed later in this chapter.

- Phantom image testing should be performed on all digital systems. Phantom images are obtained from special test tools that can either be supplied by the digital system manufacturer, or a multipurpose test phantom that can evaluate any digital system can be purchased. Phantom images are obtained as suggested by the manufacturer of the test phantom and various image parameters are evaluated both qualitatively and quantitatively. Box 8.1 summarizes the parameters that are most often evaluated during phantom image testing. If a phantom or test tool is unavailable, the following options may be used as an alternative for CR systems:
  - Uniformity—Expose the CR or DR image receptor to a uniform dose of radiation by using a 72-inch SID (to eliminate heel effect variation) and a technique of 80 kVp and enough mAs to produce about 100 µGy of radiation to the image receptor. Process the image receptor and examine the image for uniformity. One way to accomplish this is to print the image with a dry laser printer and take optical density readings across the surface of the image. These should be within a value of ±0.2 of each other. To evaluate uniformity of the soft image on the monitor, you can use the region of interest to check brightness at various points throughout the image. These should be within 10% of each other. Most digital systems use a preprocessing manipulation known as flat-fielding, which is a software correction that equalizes the response of each pixel to make the image more uniform. For DR systems, acceptance testing should determine the number and type of any bad pixels (flat-fielding software should correct for a few scattered nonfunctioning detectors in the AMA). QC routine performance evaluation testing should include a process to report any new bad pixels that may develop during use over time.
  - Spatial accuracy—The wire mesh test tool used for evaluating film/screen contact can be used to evaluate this parameter by placing it on a CR or DR image receptor and making an exposure at 72-inch SID, 60 kVp, and enough mAs to produce about 50 µGy to the image receptor. After processing, the image should appear uniform in brightness and resolution, with no geometric distortions. If any appear, inspect the CR plate or DR AMA for any defects. If these appear across multiple plates, the cause is probably the laser in the reader unit for a CR system.
  - Erasure test (CR systems)—Use a knee or other phantom and make an extreme overexposure. After processing, verify that the image has been completely erased from the plate.

- Laser function—A metal ruler can be imaged on a CR cassette using 80 kVp, 72-inch SID, and enough mAs to yield about 50 µGy to the IP. Be sure that the ruler is placed perpendicular to the laser scan lines. After processing the image, view it on the monitor and verify that the edges of the ruler appear as straight lines. If not, there is a problem with the laser in the reader unit and a service engineer should be called.
- Wireless transmission integrity (wireless DR systems)—An exposure of a phantom can be made on a wireless DR cassette and then viewed on the monitor to make sure that the wireless signal was received uncorrupted. It is important to ensure that no signal interference or corruption between different systems occurs when they are communicating on the same wireless network. There must also be appropriate signal encryption to maintain Health Insurance Portability and Accountability Act privacy standards. In addition, a loss prevention and image recovery procedure must be in place for images that have interrupted or corrupted transmission.

The AAPM suggests the following QC program for digital radiographic systems:

Acceptance tests are performed by a medical physicist. You may recall from Chapter 1 that acceptance testing is done on brand-new equipment or equipment that has undergone a major repair to make sure that it is performing at manufacturer's specification.

1. Erasure thoroughness (CR) or ghost imaging DR. For CR systems, erasure thoroughness evaluates the ability of the sodium discharge lamp in the reader unit of a CR system to completely erase previous data (especially those from extreme overexposure). If not completely erased, ghosting artifacts that can mimic disease processes can appear on subsequent images. Testing involves creating an image of a metal plate (such as the copper plate in the Leeds Test Kit) at extreme overexposure (about 50-mR exposure or 500 µGy air kerma to a CR image plate), processing the plate (including erasure), and then taking a second image of the same plate with about 1-mR (10 µGy air kerma) exposure. The image created by this second exposure of the IP is then analyzed for the presence of the previous image taken at 50 mR (500 µGy air kerma). DR systems do not have an erasure cycle, but the thin TFTs should release all of their charge created by one exposure before the next exposure occurs. If any residual charge still exists, a ghost image of the previous image will appear in the new image. The same procedure for CR systems can be used to verify that residual charges from a previous image is removed by the DR array.
2. Phantom image testing is discussed in Box 8.1, which includes specific phantom image data.
3. Exposure indicator calibration—Determines if manufacturer's indicator value is consistent with the amount of radiation to the IR. Testing involves exposing a digital dosimeter (or comparable radiation detection device) in a digital image receptor and making an exposure. The

BOX 8.1   Computed Radiography and Digital Radiography Phantom Image Testing

Both CR and DR systems are relatively new; federal QC standards that are uniform for all manufacturers have yet to be implemented. Each system manufacturer has QC protocols described in the operating manual provided to each user. Many equipment vendors as well as private organizations have developed evaluation phantoms for CR and DR systems such as the Boston Test Tool (see Fig. 8.14) or the Leeds Test Objects (see Fig. 8.15). The phantom image can evaluate the performance of the IRD and image plates (CR systems), detector array function (DR systems), workstations, hard copy printer, and the X-ray exposure room. Most manufacturers recommend that these phantom images be taken on acceptance and then at least once a month (can be performed by a QC technologist or medical physicist) or when problems are suspected. Information obtained from phantom image testing most often includes the following:

- Relative sensitivity test—Used to confirm that the CR reader system sensitivity calibration or DR system sensitivity is consistent with the baseline test. The sensitivity of a CR or DR system affects patient dose. This same test also can provide information on the X-ray generator output and consistency. A CR or DR system should display a consistent sensitivity index number when an image receptor with the same dose is digitized. Each CR or DR manufacturer should provide an acceptable standard deviation.
- Shading or uniformity test—Evaluates the uniformity of the image brightness (comparable to optical density in film/screen imaging) across the scanning width (CR) or the active matrix array of a DR system. The test pattern incorporates a fine mesh pattern (such as the Leeds MS4 Test Object in Fig. 8.16) that is viewed after processing. It also confirms the CR reader system's light guide position and optics. If a laser is not performing uniformly, low-contrast light and dark bands may appear running either horizontally or vertically. Nonuniformity may be caused by uneven pixel gain, dead pixels, tiling, etc. Areas of image should be uniform to within ±10%. Flat-fielding software can correct for nonuniformity.
- Contrast evaluation—Measures the contrast resolution capability of the image processor, workstation monitors, and hard-copy printers using a low-contrast resolution tool such as the Leeds TO 20 Test Object (see Fig. 8.17). Low-contrast

areas should be visible and should not change over time. The procedure involves taking image of a low-contrast resolution phantom at 75 kVp and mAs to produce 0.5 mR (0.005 mGy air kerma), 1.0 mR (0.01 mGy air kerma), and 5.0 mR (0.05 mGy air kerma). Contrast detail threshold should be proportionally lower at higher exposures.

- Spatial accuracy or sharpness test—The test phantom should contain a wire mesh pattern similar to one used to measure film/screen contact in analog image receptors. After processing, the image should appear uniform in brightness with no geometric distortions. Deviation should be less than 2%. It also will demonstrate whether the CR or DR system is presenting images with the correct geometric relationships.
- Laser jitter test—Evaluates the horizontal and vertical performance of the laser optic and transport systems of the CR reader and hard copy printer. Laser jitter should not exceed ±1 pixel.
- Image noise test—Evaluates the presence of dark noise (signal being present even though no radiation exposure occurred, caused mainly by electronic noise). The amount of noise present should not exceed a pixel value of 280.
- Accuracy of measurement tools—Ensures the accuracy of workstation measurement tools and hard copy printer software. The test object should produce geometric patterns of a known size, such as the Leeds M1 Test Object, which produces squares of exactly 20 mm (see Fig. 8.18). Any difference between the measured distance of an object and the actual distance of the object should be <2%.
- System linearity test—Measures CR reader system or DR system linearity. Linearity is also an important factor regarding patient dose. For example, if exposures of 0.1, 1.0, and 10 mR are digitized, the systems exposure guide indicator numbers should track linearly within 10% changes.
- Spatial resolution test—The test tool should incorporate a spatial frequency pattern in lp/mm. The spatial frequency in lp/mm should not vary over time. Procedure: Place three line-pair patterns, two in orthogonal directions and one at a 45-degree angle. After processing, determine the maximum discernable spatial frequency in each direction. The spatial frequency divided by the Nyquist frequency should be >0.9.

CR, Computed radiography; *DR,* digital radiography; *IRD,* image reader device; *QC,* quality control.

exposure in milliroentgen or micrograys is recorded from the dosimeter and the exposure indicator is obtained from the workstation monitor. As an example, if a digital system utilizes the IEC's EI exposure indicator system, a 5-μGy exposure to the image receptor should show an EI value of 500. Variation between stated value and actual value should be <10%.

4. System linearity test—This test measures the uniformity of the detector system exposed to varying amounts of radiation (3 powers of 10 difference). The test involves exposing an IR to approximately 0.1 mR (1 μGy air kerma), 1.0 mR (0.01 mGy air kerma), and 10.0 mR (0.1 mGy air kerma). A semilog plot of pixel value vs. exposure on a linear-log plot should result in a straight line. System linearity should not vary by more than 10%.

5. System uniformity test—This test measures the uniformity of the detector response when exposed to the same dose. Procedure: Expose three different CR plates or DR detectors to the same dose with 10 mR (0.1 mGy air kerma) of exposure at 80 kVp. After processing, the pixel value standard deviation for all three should be determined (usually displayed with pixel brightness value) from over 80 % of the image area and compared. The pixel value standard deviation should be <400.

Daily tests are performed by a technologist.

1. As part of the general inspection, inspect CR or DR cassettes for cleanliness (surfaces should be free of dirt and debris to avoid image artifacts or processing problems in the IRD) and bar code labels (make sure that they are clean and free of any surface dirt), and check that hinges and

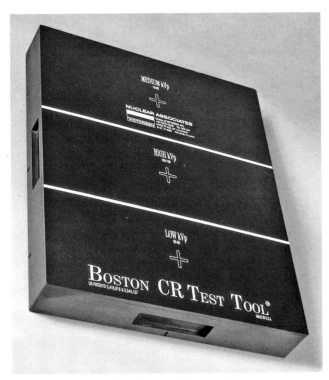

Fig. 8.14 Boston CR Test Tool.

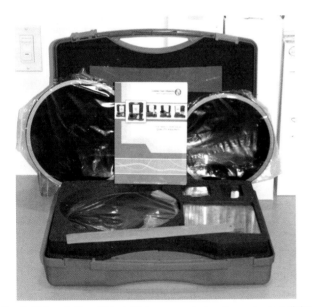

Fig. 8.15 Leeds Test Object Kit for computed radiography and digital radiography.

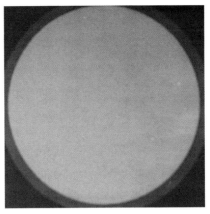

Fig. 8.16 Image of Leeds TO.MS4 mesh Test Object for uniformity, blurring, and stitching artifact evaluation.

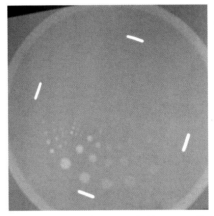

Fig. 8.17 Image of Leeds TO.20 threshold contrast Test Object.

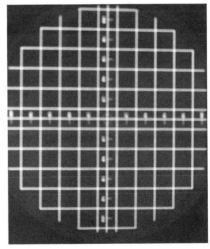

Fig. 8.18 Image of Leeds TO.M1 geometry Test Object.

latches are in good condition. Also make sure that IRD removes IPs smoothly and easily and that they are read and replaced in the cassette properly. Once these tasks are completed, a system walkthrough should be performed to verify general equipment operation and network transmission. For wireless DR cassettes, their internal batteries must be kept fully charged when not in use.

2. Check the laser printer to make sure it is functioning properly to obtain hard copy images. If paper printers are used, make sure that they are working properly.

3. Erase all CR image plates before use.

4. Verify that the CR reader unit and workstations are communicating properly with each other. Also make sure that the bar code readers are working properly. For DR cassettes, make sure that image data are transmitted from the cassette to the central processing unit of the imaging system. This is accomplished via a cable connection or wireless connection. Loose cable or a dead battery in a wireless

cassette can cause a lack of connection, as can interference in a wireless network.

5. Perform processor QC if a laser camera is used for obtaining hard copy images.

Weekly tests are performed by a technologist.

1. Verify monitor calibration (CRT only).
2. Test phantom images by performing phantom image analysis as suggested by the manufacturer, and compare with previous images and look for any variation.
3. Clean and inspect all image receptors.
   - CR—Clean and inspect all CR cassettes.
   - DR—Clean and inspect DR cassettes. For DR image receptors that are contained in a bucky or chest unit, inspect that top surface of the AMA area for dirt and scratches. Also inspect any visible cables leading to the DR image receptor for any cracks in the insulation or plastic connectors or any exposed or bare wires.
4. Clean the air intake ports on the CR system IRD. This will prevent damage to the IRD and minimize artifacts that may be caused by dirt on the reader mirrors or on the lens of the scanning laser.
5. Clean the computer keyboard and mouse according to the manufacturer's guidelines. This will prolong the life of the computer components and also reduce the transmission of illness among the department staff.
6. Clean the screen of CRT monitors according to the manufacturer's guidelines. CRT monitors attract dirt and dust due to electrostatic attraction. In addition, many monitors utilize touchscreen technology, which can cause dirt to build up quickly. LCD monitors are less likely to attract dirt and debris but should still be inspected. Care must be taken in cleaning LCD screens, as it is easy to damage the plastic face and the LCD crystals underneath the face. Closely follow manufacturer's guidelines.

Monthly tests are performed by a technologist.

1. Film processor maintenance is necessary only if the laser camera is used instead of a dry laser printer for hard copies.
2. Inspect and clean all image receptors.
   - CR—Remove the image plates from each cassette and clean them according to manufacturer's specifications. Generally, a lint-free cloth (photographic lens cloth) or a camel-hair brush should be used to gently wipe any loose debris from the image plate. Most manufacturers have a special cleaning solution that can be used for IPs that have any dirt that is more difficult to remove. IPs that can no longer be cleaned effectively will have to be replaced. Because the PSP material contains some barium, they cannot be disposed of in the standard trash and must be disposed of according to Environmental Protection Agency regulations. A licensed disposal company should be contacted to properly dispose of these IPs, and the proper paperwork must be kept on file.
   - DR—Clean and inspect DR cassettes. For DR image receptors that are contained in a bucky or chest unit,

inspect that top surface of the AMA area for dirt and scratches. Also inspect any visible cables leading to the DR image receptor for any cracks in the insulation or plastic connectors or any exposed or bare wires. A thorough cleaning of the DR image receptor should be performed by a qualified service technician and scheduled accordingly.

3. Perform a repeat analysis and review the data to correct any ongoing issues. A repeat or reject analysis looks at images that were not acceptable diagnostically and determines why they occurred to minimize the chance of recurrence in the future. This generally involves looking at these images and using a repeat analysis form to classify the rejects according to cause. This procedure is discussed in detail in Chapter 10. Repeat rates should be within 1%–3%. A review of various literature revealed that repeated image rates hovered around 10% in screen-film departments, with approximately 45% of images repeated owing to exposure errors, which have been greatly reduced in digital imaging. Rejected image rates in digital departments have been reported to range from 4% to 8%. Therefore the AAPM recommends that 8% be used as a target for overall rejected image rate, and 10% as a threshold for investigation and possible corrective action. As mentioned previously, this rate should be adjusted to reflect the operator's clinical practice. Repeated image rates in pediatric imaging departments have been reported to be approximately 3%–5%. The task group recommends that a target of 5% be used in pediatric imaging and 7% as a threshold for investigation and possible corrective action.
4. Service logs of digital equipment should be reviewed to see if a specific problem is reccurring. If so, possible solutions should be explored to minimize downtime.

Semiannual/annual tests are performed by a medical physicist.

1. X-ray generator testing involves testing the X-ray generator, tube, and accessories according to the procedures discussed in Chapter 5. This type of testing is done to make sure that any errors discovered are caused by the digital imaging components and not by the X-ray generator.
2. Evaluate image quality by reviewing actual patient images as well as phantom images. Phantom images should be obtained and analyzed in both automatic and nonautomatic modes.
3. Image processing evaluations are conducted to make sure that all of the preprocessing (histogram analysis, LUT, etc.) and postprocessing functions are operating properly.
4. Repeat acceptance tests to reestablish baseline values.
5. Review patient exposure trends, repeat analysis data, QC records, and service history.
6. Evaluate exposure indicator accuracy using a dosimeter to record exposure to image receptors.
7. Determine the necessity for system adjustment by vendor service personnel.

A summary of these tests is listed in Box 8.2.

BOX 8.2   Summary of QC Tests for CR and DR Systems

Acceptance Tests—Performed by Medical Physicist
1. Erasure thoroughness (CR systems)
2. Phantom imaging testing (CR and DR)

Daily Tests—Performed by Technologist
1. General inspection of cassettes and viewing monitors (CR and DR)
2. Laser printer (if applicable)
3. Erasure thoroughness (CR)
4. Workstation communication with IRD (CR systems) or DR cassettes
5. Processor QC (laser cameras only)

Weekly Tests—Performed by Technologist
1. Verify monitor calibration (CRT monitors only)
2. Phantom image testing (CR and DR)
3. Clean and inspect all image receptors (CR and DR)
4. Clean air intake ports on IRD (CR) and CPU (CR and DR)
5. Clean computer keyboard and mouse (CR and DR)
6. Clean monitor screen (CR and DR)

Monthly Tests—Performed by Technologist
1. Film processor maintenance (laser cameras only)
2. Clean and inspect all image receptors (CR and DR)
3. Perform repeat analysis (CR and DR)
4. Service log review (CR and DR)

Semiannual/Annual Tests—Performed by Medical Physicist
1. X-ray generator testing (CR an DR)
2. Image quality evaluation (CR and DR)
3. Image processing evaluation (CR and DR)
4. Repeat acceptance tests to reestablish baseline values (CR and DR)
5. Review patient exposure trends, repeat analysis data, QC records, and service history (CR and DR)
6. Evaluate exposure indicator accuracy (CR and DR)
7. Determine necessity for system adjustment by service personnel (CR and DR)

CR, Computed radiography; *DR*, digital radiography; *IRD*, image reader device; *QC*, quality control.

Digital Fluoroscopy

Digital fluoroscopy (DF), or computerized fluoroscopy, was developed during the 1970s at the University of Wisconsin and the University of Arizona. The concept involves taking the fluoroscopic image (whether from the television camera or a flat-panel system), digitizing the electronic signal carrying the image information, and sending this digital signal into a computer for real-time processing. Advantages of digital fluoroscopy include *last frame–hold, road mapping, digital temporal filtering, image enhancement,* and *image restoration.*

Last Frame–Hold

One of the many advantages of digital fluoroscopy includes a *last frame–hold* feature that allows the last image in the computer memory to be displayed on the monitor, even though the X-ray beam is off.

Road Mapping

Another advantage is a feature known as *road mapping,* which can permit an image to be captured and displayed on a monitor, whereas a second monitor shows a real-time image. Road mapping also can be used to record an image with contrast material that can then be overlaid onto a live fluoroscopic image.

Digital Temporal Filtering

Still another advantage is a feature known as *digital temporal filtering* (also known as *frame averaging*), which can add together different image pixel values and then average the values during display of successive images. This process is used to reduce the effect of random noise (quantum mottle) but does cause a noticeable increase in image lag because of a lower image frame rate.

Image Enhancement

The computer allows image improvement or image enhancement of structures of interest in the image through various means. The image contrast can be manipulated by controlling window width, and the image brightness can be manipulated by controlling window level. Window width selects the width of the band of values in the digital signal, which can be represented as gray tones in the image. This provides a means of compressing or expanding image contrast. The window level selects the level of the displayed band of values within the complete range. This allows for the manipulation of the pixel brightness in different parts of the image to optimize image quality.

Image Restoration

The computer allows image restoration to correct for distortion and vignetting that may occur in the image intensifier.

Currently, two methods are used for performing DF: with an analog image intensifier tube or with a flat-panel or flat-plate image receptor.

Image Intensifier Tube Digital Fluoroscopy Systems

Standard fluoroscopic units feed the image from the television camera (which is focused onto the output phosphor of an image intensifier tube) directly to the monitor for immediate viewing. In this method of DF, the analog signal from the camera is first sent through an ADC and then through a microprocessor circuit that processes the image (Fig. 8.19).

Flat-Panel Digital Fluoroscopy Systems

This method of DF uses similar flat-panel image receptors such as those in direct-conversion radiographic systems. This flat-panel image receptor replaces the image intensifier and television camera combination and feeds the image information directly into an image processor, which is essentially the same as that used in DF, with an image intensifier tube. The rows of pixels in the AMA are switched continuously, rather than in sequential rows (used in DR radiographic systems). This allows continuous updating of the image to obtain a real-time image.

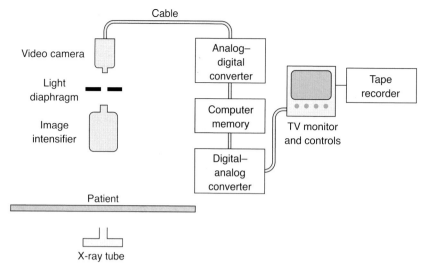

Fig. 8.19 Block diagram of digital fluoroscopic system.

The digitally generated image can be displayed on the monitor either with monochrome grayscale images, in which each pixel produces a certain gray tone (most common), or with bistable images, in which the pixel is either black or white, with no intermediate gray tones. This is generally used in radionuclide imaging. The monitor can use several scan modes for image display, including continuous fluoroscopy mode, pulsed interlaced scan mode, pulsed progressive scan mode, and slow scan mode.

Continuous Fluoroscopy Mode

A standard 525-line monitor is used with continuous fluoroscopy at a low mA value (<5 mA). With this lower mA value, quantum mottle and low SNR ratio are problems; therefore the computer uses as many as 20–30 separate frames to produce a single image.

Pulsed Interlaced Scan Mode

In the pulsed interlaced scan mode, the X-ray tube delivers radiation in short, high-intensity pulses at about one per second. This reduces quantum mottle and increases resolution and SNR ratio. This pulsed mode also can reduce patient dose and is more commonly used than continuous fluoroscopy.

Pulsed Progressive Scan Mode

In the pulsed progressive scan mode, the X-ray beam is pulsed, but the monitor scans the lines in natural order rather than in an interlaced manner. This reduces image flicker and improves resolution but requires a 1023-line monitor.

Slow Scan Mode

In slow scan mode, 7.5, 1050-line frames are scanned per second, which doubles image resolution.

All modes have freeze-frame and last-image recall options that allow the image to remain on the monitor even though no fluoroscopy is currently taking place. This function reduces patient dose.

Digital Subtraction Angiography

The main application for DF systems is for digital subtraction angiography (DSA). This involves removing or subtracting background structures from an image so that only contrast media–filled structures remain (Fig. 8.20). Before DSA, radiographs were taken before the administration of contrast media. Because a standard radiograph is a photographic negative, a positive of this image, called a *mask image,* is then created. When a second radiograph is taken with contrast media present (again, a photographic negative), it is combined with the mask image to create the subtraction image. This method is time consuming and cumbersome. DSA involves imaging the patient before the arrival of contrast media; the computer stores the image as the mask. When the image with the contrast media is created, the computer stores it in a separate area

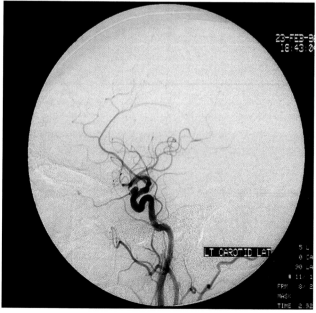

Fig. 8.20 Image obtained during digital subtraction angiography.

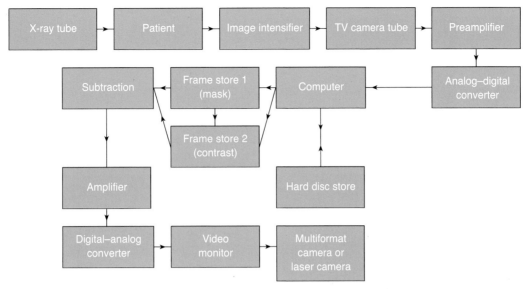

Fig. 8.21 Block diagram of digital subtraction angiography.

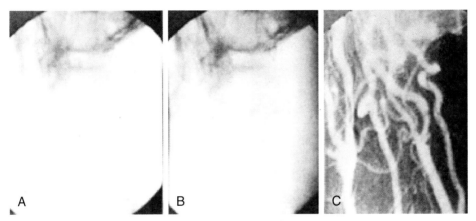

Fig. 8.22 Images demonstrating temporal subtraction. (A and B) subtraction; (C) original image.

and then combines it with the mask to create the subtracted image. Fig. 8.21 shows a block diagram of this process.

The advantages of DSA over the film method include wider exposure latitude, computerized enhancement of image contrast (contrast differences of <1% can be visualized), and quick image acquisition. The main disadvantages are small field of view (because it is limited by the input phosphor size) and lower spatial resolution (because of pixel size and the limitation of the monitor). A laser camera should be used to create hard copy images. DSA is of several types, including temporal mask subtraction, time-interval difference subtraction, and dual-energy subtraction.

Temporal Mask Subtraction

Temporal mask subtraction is the standard type of DSA described earlier, in which the computer uses a noncontrast mask with the contrast media image to create the subtracted image. Patient motion must be avoided between the two images, or image noise and degradation result (Fig. 8.22).

Time-Interval Difference Subtraction

In the process of time-interval difference subtraction, a series of images is obtained at equally spaced times after injection

of contrast media. Each image is subtracted from the next to form new subtraction images. This helps identify certain pathologic conditions in the vasculature that inhibit the flow of contrast media over time (Fig. 8.23).

Dual-Energy Subtraction

In dual-energy subtraction, two different qualities (energies) of X-ray beam are used, one at just below 33 keV and one at just above this value. This is because the K-edge of iodine is at 33 keV, so the images created at each different energy level are compared by the computer to create the subtracted image.

QC of Digital Fluoroscopy Units

The nondigital functions of DF units should be checked with the use of the conventional fluoroscopic methods described in Chapter 7. Once these have been evaluated and are performing within specified parameters, then the DF functions should be checked on acceptance and then every 6 months or when service is performed on the system. This requires a phantom that conforms to the recommendations found in Report No. 15 by the AAPM Digital Radiography/Fluorography Task Group of the Diagnostic Imaging Committee (Fig. 8.24). The

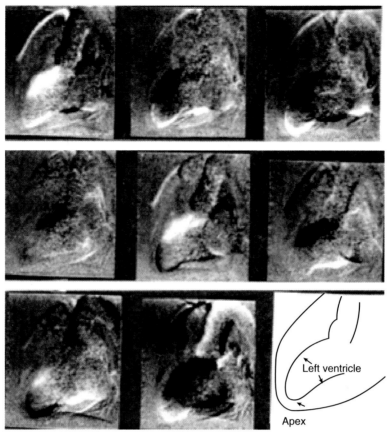

Fig. 8.23 Images showing the effect of time-interval difference subtraction process.

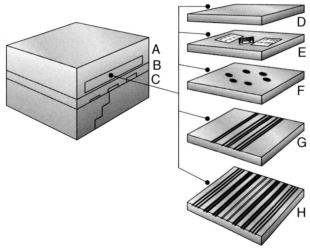

Fig. 8.24 Digital subtraction angiography phantom. (A) Slot block; (B) bone block; (C) step wedge; (D) block insert; (E) high-contrast resolution pattern insert; (F) linearity insert; (G) low-contrast artery insert; (H) low-contrast iodine line pair insert. (Courtesy Nuclear Associates, Carle Place, New York.)

phantom evaluates the variables of high- and low-contrast resolution, spatial resolution, subtraction effectiveness, image uniformity, amplifier dynamic range, registration (to detect any changes in pixel position between the test image and the mask image), and linearity. Linearity in this context refers to changes in iodine content (measured in milligrams per square centimeter) within a specific area, which should change the pixel shade or tone accordingly. For example, if an image is obtained of two iodine-filled vessels, one with an iodine content of 1 mg/cm^2 and the other 2 mg/cm^2, then the shade or tone of the pixel should differ by a factor of 2. Some phantoms also have components that simulate blood vessels and aneurysms of various sizes.

ELECTRONIC DISPLAY DEVICES

All digital diagnostic imaging modalities must display the final image on some type of electronic display device such as a television or computer monitor. This is sometimes referred to as "soft-copy" viewing (as opposed to hard-copy viewing, such as a film image on a conventional viewbox). The obvious advantage of soft-copy viewing is the ability to postprocess the image while viewing. However, disadvantages include limited luminance range; poor resolution; reflection of ambient light; veiling glare (a light-spreading phenomenon caused by internal light scattering; light leakage; or electron backscattering, causing a degradation of image contrast); and degradation over time. Oftentimes, these devices can be the weakest link in the imaging chain in terms of image resolution. This means that the quality of the display device can have a direct bearing on the quality of the image and therefore the accuracy of the diagnosis obtained from this image. Flat-panel LCD and plasma monitors are much less likely to suffer from the above disadvantages. All electronic display devices must

TABLE 8.3   List of Primary Display Monitor Manufacturers (Selling in the United States)

Manufacturer	Web Address
Barco	https://www.barco.com
Canvys, a division of Richardson Electronics	https://www.canvys.com
Double Black Imaging	https://www.doubleblackimaging.com
Eizo	https://www.eizo.com
NDSsi	https://www.ndssi.com
NEC Display Solutions of America, Inc.	https://www.necdisplay.com
Sony Medical	https://http://pro.sony.com
U.S. Electronics, Inc.	https://www.us-electronics.com
Wide USA Corp.	https://www.widecorp.com

conform to the Digital Imaging and Communications in Medicine (DICOM) Grayscale Standard Display Function (GSDF) standard, which specifies a function that relates pixel values to displayed luminance levels.

The ACR and the Food and Drug Administration classify electronic display devices as being either primary (also known as diagnostic) or secondary (also known as clinical). Primary or diagnostic display devices are those that will be used for the interpretation of diagnostic images by radiologists and other providers. The recommended matrix size for primary display devices used to view radiographic images is 2048 × 2560 (5 megapixels). The active pixel size is about 0.15 mm. A list of manufacturers selling primary display devices can be found in Table 8.3. Secondary or clinical display systems are those used for viewing diagnostic images for purposes other than for providing medical interpretation (such as operators' console monitors and QC workstations, PACS workstations, and workstations used by general medical staff). Secondary matrix sizes can range from 1024 × 1280 (1.3 megapixels) to 1200 × 1600 (2 megapixels). The active pixel size is about 0.3 mm. Monitors for viewing digital mammographic images have a matrix size of 4096 × 6144 with an active pixel size of 40–50 μm. This is necessary for proper display of spatial resolution but can cost up to $40,000. Care must be taken when viewing an image of a certain matrix size to a display device of another size because information can be lost from the image. Interpolation refers to the mapping of an image of one matrix size to a display of another size. For example, if an image created in a computer with a matrix size of 2 k × 2 k is displayed on a 1 k × 1 k monitor, 4 pixels from the original image will have to be mapped to each single pixel in the monitor, causing a loss of image data. Another factor that determines how much detail can be presented by a viewing monitor is the pixel pitch, which is the distance between the pixels on the screen. The smaller the pixel pitch of a display, the better the spatial resolution. Pixel pitch may be also be called dot pitch, aperture grill pitch, or slot pitch, depending on the manufacturer. Still another important characteristic of

an electronic display device is a value known as the aspect ratio. This is the ratio of the width of the display to the height of the display. Most standard CRT computer monitors have an aspect ratio of 4:3, whereas flat-screen LCD and plasma monitors have a ratio of 16:9. Primary display monitors for viewing radiographic images are generally 5-megapixel displays and have an aspect ratio of 5:4. The software settings of the computer controlling the display device must be adjusted to match the aspect ratio of the monitor or geometric distortions will occur in the image. Another important monitor characteristic is the refresh rate (also known as the frame rate or vertical scan frequency) of the monitor. This refers to how many times each second that the monitor rewrites or updates the image on the display. A refresh rate that is too low can cause a flickering effect that can cause eye strain and fatigue for the viewer. The refresh rate for viewing monitors can range from 55 to 150 Hz (in this context, a Hertz refers to a frame per second). A minimum refresh rate of 70 Hz is recommended for primary class CRT displays. LCD and plasma displays take longer to switch from one image to the next, so less flicker is visible.

In the past, high-resolution monochrome (black-and-white) CRTs have been the most common displays for viewing digital radiographic and fluoroscopic images. Currently, flat-panel active matrix LCDs have become the display devices of choice, as their capital cost continues to decline. CRT displays are rarely manufactured or sold today because of the previously mentioned disadvantages, as well as the fact that they require special disposal procedures because many contain mercury. Flat-panel plasma displays are beginning to appear as image display devices. Fig. 8.25 shows the various classifications of electronic display devices.

Cathode-Ray Tube Displays

The CRT has been around since the late 1870s (the Crooke's tube that Roentgen was experimenting with when he discovered X-rays was a CRT, as is the fluoroscopic image intensifier tube) and is still used today for both image display as well as television camera tubes to acquire the initial image. The basic components (Fig. 8.26) include a cathode (which will release electrons through thermionic emission); control grids; accelerating electrodes; electrostatic focusing lenses (to accelerate and focus the electrons toward the front screen); deflection coils (to move the electron beam back and forth and up and down to create scan lines and pixels); an anode (to attract the electrons from the cathode); and the front screen (which is a glass plate coated with crystals that will emit light when struck by the electron beam). An antireflection layer is placed on the faceplate of the screen to reduce ambient light reflection and veiling glare. Veiling glare is light scattering in display devices, which induces a diffuse luminance that veils the intended image. The addition of this diffuse secondary component has the overall effect of reducing contrast in a manner similar to contrast reduction from scattered X-rays in radiography. This contrast reduction is most severe in the dark regions of the primary image.

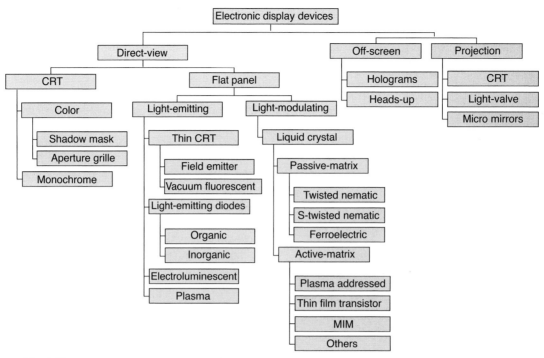

Fig. 8.25 Block diagram showing various classifications of electronic display devices. *CRT*, Cathode-ray tube; *MIM*, *MIN Software Inc.* (Courtesy Badano, Chakraborty, Samei et al. Assessment of display performance for medical imaging systems. Draft report of the American Association of Physicists in Medicine (AAPM) Task Group 18, Version 10.0, August 2004.)

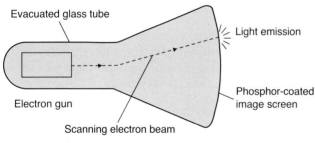

Fig. 8.26 Basic components of a cathode-ray tube display device.

Phosphor materials that are used in the screens are designated by a P-number system created by the U.S. Electronics Industry Association. A higher P-number indicates that it will create a greater degree of luminance for a given amount of current in the electron beam (i.e., a P45 phosphor will emit more light for a given tube current than a P11). Currently, P4, P45, and P104 phosphors have all been used successfully in high-resolution monitors used in diagnostic imaging. The P45 phosphor is the most commonly used because it is more stable than the others at high beam currents, exhibits a slower loss of efficiency from aging, and has less noise. Monochrome monitors produce a luminance level of 300–500 nit, as compared with 2000 (general radiography) to 3500 (mammographic) nit for film images on a viewbox. To obtain a higher brightness level with a CRT, a larger beam current would be necessary; however, this would tend to increase the size of the beam and therefore reduce spatial resolution, as well as reduce the life of the tube. The advantages and disadvantages of cathode ray tube monitors are:

Advantages:
- High contrast ratio (over 15,000:1)
- Excellent viewing angle
- Can be used or stored in both extreme hot and cold temperature conditions

Disadvantages:
- Large size and weight
- Prone to geometric distortions
- High power consumption (2–10 times that of an identically sized LCD monitor)
- Large amount of heat emitted during operation
- Can suffer screen burn
- Produces flicker at refresh rates lower than 85 Hz
- Sensitive to magnetic interference
- Image edges are slightly diffuse (blurred) compared to other monitors
- Glass envelopes contain toxic lead and barium as X-ray shielding.
- Phosphors can contain cadmium (toxic substance), which prohibits their disposal in landfills or by incineration.

Liquid Crystal Displays

Flat-panel LCDs have become the most popular display devices used in diagnostic imaging, much as they are with home desktop computers (laptop computers have used LCDs from the beginning). LCDs consist of a large array of liquid crystal cells (each of which will represent a single pixel in the image), polarizer filters, and a backlight (usually a light-emitting diode in newer monitors) (Fig. 8.27). The liquid crystals will change their molecular orientation when an electrical field is applied to them. This in turn will change the light transmission capability of the liquid crystal,

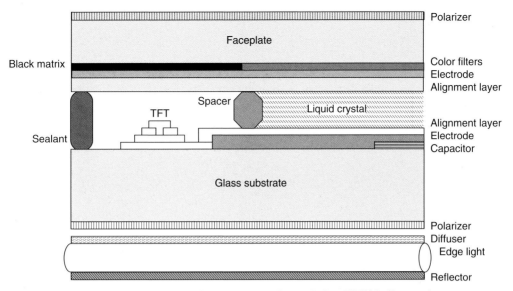

Fig. 8.27 Basic components of a liquid crystal display device. *TFT*, Thin-film transistor.

thereby causing more or less light to be transmitted through it, thus controlling the brightness value of the pixel. Filter materials are added for color displays. LCDs have many advantages over CRT monitors in that they do not defocus over time because no electron beam is used to create the image, they have better grayscale definition than CRTs, and they better reduce the effect of ambient light on image contrast. LCDs also produce a higher level of luminance than CRTs (up to 2100 nit). They also give the appearance of greater resolution and contrast because of the light emission being emitted perpendicular to the faceplate (caused by the passage of light through the polarizing filters). This also leads to a significant disadvantage in that they have a limited viewing angle (usually 40 degrees either side of a line that is perpendicular to the center of the faceplate). This is known as angular dependence of viewing. LCDs used for diagnostic imaging should have at least an 80 degree or higher viewing angle in the horizontal direction and 50 degrees in the vertical direction. CRT monitors have a curved face and therefore a wider viewing angle. The complete list of advantages and disadvantages is as follows:

Advantages:
- They are very compact and lightweight.
- They do not defocus over time because no electron beam is used to create the image.
- They have better grayscale definition than CRTs.
- They use less electricity (lower operating cost).
- Very little heat is emitted during operation.
- They are not affected by magnetic fields.
- There is little or no flicker.
- They better reduce the effect of ambient light on image contrast (greater contrast resolution).
- LCDs also produce a higher level of luminance than CRTs (up to 700 nit) and less noise.
- They give the appearance of greater resolution and contrast due to the light emission being emitted perpendicular to the faceplate (caused by the passage of light through the polarizing filters), as well as having lower black levels (minimum luminance).

Disadvantages:
- They have a limited viewing angle (usually 40 degrees either side of a line that is perpendicular to the center of the faceplate). This is known as angular dependence and is governed by the cosine law, which states that when a monitor is viewed straight on, the luminous intensity is at its maximum. When a monitor is viewed from an angle, the contrast and the luminous intensity are reduced. LCDs used for diagnostic imaging should have at least an 80-degree or higher viewing angle in the horizontal direction and 50 degrees in the vertical direction.
- They are subject to dead pixels, which are dark specks in white images that do not change location when a different white image is displayed.

Plasma Displays

Flat-panel plasma displays consist of an active matrix of tiny fluorescent bulbs that will emit light from each pixel location. An advantage of this type of display device is that they are thinner than LCD panels but have a higher luminance output than CRT or LCD displays and a wide angle of viewing capability. However, they are much more expensive than LCD monitors and have a shorter life span.

QC of Electronic Display Devices

Because electronic display devices are responsible for image display in all digital imaging, it is imperative that they be evaluated for optimum performance on a regular basis. Many groups have published guidelines for QC procedures, including the National Electronics Manufacturer's Association, the Society of Motion Picture and Television Engineers (SMPTE), the DICOM group, and the AAPM, as well as the various manufacturers of these devices. As of the writing of this edition, no one set of recommendations has been endorsed by the medical community. Medical physicists and radiologists should be consulted for setting the performance standards at facilities until universal standards are adopted.

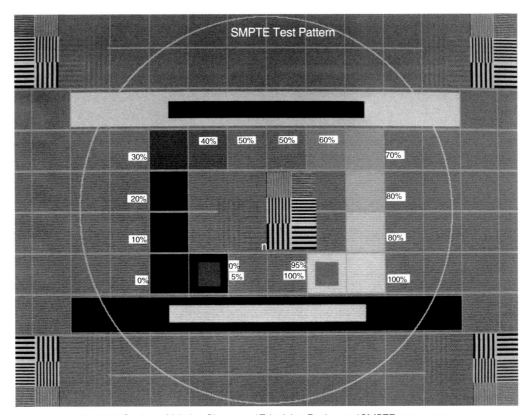

Fig. 8.28 Society of Motion Picture and Television Engineers (*SMPTE*) test pattern.

Virtually all display device manufacturers recommend that they be operated between 0 and 40°C with a relative humidity range of between 10% and 70% (to avoid condensation). LCD monitors are especially sensitive to changes in temperature. The ACR recommends evaluating performance at least monthly. The AAPM is more rigorous in its recommendations, suggesting evaluation on acceptance, daily, monthly/quarterly, and annually. Acceptance and annual evaluation should be performed by a physicist, whereas daily and monthly/quarterly evaluation can be performed by either a physicist or a trained QC technologist. Daily QC should take less than 1 min to complete and involves imaging either an SMPTE test pattern (Fig. 8.28) or the AAPM TG18-QC (Fig. 8.29) test pattern. Parameters to evaluate during daily QC include the following:

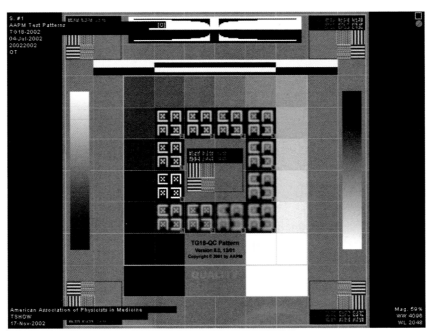

Fig. 8.29 American Association of Physicists in Medicine TG-18 QC test pattern. (Courtesy Badano, Chakraborty, Samei et al. Assessment of display performance for medical imaging systems. Draft report of the American Association of Physicists in Medicine (AAPM) Task Group 18, Version 10.0, August 2004.)

1. Turn on the monitor and execute the normal boot-up procedure. Allow CRT monitors to warm up for 30 min. Set the display window width/level to the manufacturer-specified values for the test pattern. Do not set these values by eye, as this will invalidate the results of this procedure.

2. Cleanliness of front screen—Clean the front screen using manufacturer's guidelines if dirty. Be especially careful in cleaning flat-panel LCD monitors, as they usually have a softer plastic front.

3. Geometric distortion—Involves verification that all lines and borders in the pattern are visible, and straight and centered within the active area of the display device.

4. General image quality and appearance—Involves evaluating the overall appearance of the pattern for any nonuniformities or artifacts such as dropped pixels (dark specks in white or light gray images that do not change location when a different image is displayed).

5. Luminance—Involves verification that all 16 luminance patches are distinctly visible from adjacent patches. It is especially important that the 5% patch can be distinguished in the 0%/5%patch and that the 95% patch can be distinguished in the 95%/100% patch.

6. Resolution—Involves verification that all letters and numbers within the pattern are visible.

7. Ambient light—Measure illuminance in the area where primary reading (diagnosis) will take place and make sure that it does not exceed 4.5 foot-candles (50 lux).

Monthly or quarterly inspections should take about 20 min, and the following procedure should be used:

PROCEDURE: DISPLAY MONITORS

Monthly/Quarterly

1. Turn on the monitor and execute the normal boot-up procedure. Allow CRT monitors to warm up for 30 min.
2. Inspect the front screen of the monitor for cleanliness. If dirty, clean using the manufacturer's instructions.
3. Determine whether specular reflection of light sources (e.g., lights, other monitors, viewboxes, windows) are present on the monitor from a normal viewing direction. Reduce or eliminate if possible.
4. Assess the following image quality parameters while viewing the appropriate SMPTE or AAPM-TG 18 test pattern:
   a. Maximum luminance (luminance response)—**Luminance response** refers to the relationship between displayed luminance (luminance values obtained during testing) and the input values of a standardized display system (test pattern brightness). Use a photometer (some PACS monitors have internal photometers) and AAPM TG18-LN test patterns (Figs. 8.30–8.32) to measure luminance at the center of the monitor. Primary display monitors (those used by providers to diagnose images) should have a maximum luminance of at least 170 nit (50 foot-lamberts), whereas secondary display monitors (those used by technologists) should have a maximum luminance of at least 100 nit (30 foot-lamberts). These luminance values should not vary by more than 10% from values that were previously obtained. Also, workstations with multiple monitors should not vary by more than 10%. The monitor brightness control can be readjusted if the luminance is not within limits. If a photometer is not available, luminance response can be evaluated visually using the TG18-CT test pattern (Fig. 8.33). This pattern should be evaluated for visibility of the central half-moon targets and the four low-contrast objects at the corners of each of 16 different luminance regions. The pattern should be evaluated from a distance of approximately 30 cm. The low-contrast targets in all 16 regions should be visible (a common failure is not being able to see the targets in one or two of the dark regions). In addition, the bit depth resolution of the display (the maximum number of gray scales that can be displayed simultaneously) should be evaluated using the TG18-MP test pattern (Fig. 8.34). The relative location of contouring bands and any luminance levels should not be further than the distance between the 8-bit markers (long markers). No contrast reversal (bright areas appearing dark and dark areas appearing bright) should be visible.
   b. **Contrast ratio**—This is determined by taking the luminance readings from the center of the TG18-LN01 pattern (L_{min}) and the TG18-LN18 pattern (L_{max}). A photometer is used to measure the luminance of the minimum black level (L_{min}) and the maximum white level (L_{max}) displayed on the monitor. The contrast ratio is the ratio of the maximum white level (L_{max}) to the minimum black level (L_{min}), or L_{max}/L_{min}, and should be greater than 250 (most will be at least 600 or greater) for primary monitors and greater than 100 for secondary monitors. As a comparison, this corresponds to optical density values in film screen imaging of between 0.1 and 2.5, which is where most diagnostically useful structures would typically be found.
   c. Luminance uniformity—Luminance uniformity refers to the uniformity of the brightness across the entire screen by comparing the luminance values at the center of the screen to those at the edges of the screen. Nonuniformity refers to the maximum variation in luminance across the display area when a uniform pattern is displayed. This is a common characteristic in CRT displays, with the luminance typically decreasing from the center to the edges and corners of the display because of differences in the path length and beam landing angle of the electron beam (because the glass front is curved). This effect is less pronounced in LCD displays but must still be evaluated. Use the photometer to measure the luminance of the TG18-UNL10 (relatively dark image) and TG18-UNL80 (relatively bright image) test patterns (Figs 8.35 and 8.36) in the center of the display, as well each of the four corners. The five luminance readings from each of the same test pattern should be within 20% of each other. If not, the monitor controls can be adjusted, or a physicist or biomedical engineer should be consulted. If a photometer is not available, luminance nonuniformity can be evaluated visually using the TG18-UN10 and TG18-UN80 test patterns. When viewing, each pattern should be free of gross nonuniformities from the center to the edges. No luminance variations with dimensions on the order of 1 cm or larger should be observed.
   d. Workstation monitor uniformity—This value is determined by using the TG18-LN 18 pattern on each workstation monitor and measuring the brightness in the center of the monitor with a photometer. The center measurement of each monitor on a workstation should not vary by more than 10%. In addition, these values should remain consistent each time the test is performed.

Continued

PROCEDURE: DISPLAY MONITORS—cont'd

e. Luminance dependencies—Luminance dependencies refer to the luminance response mentioned above, but it is how this value is dependent on the viewing angle between the observer and the center of the display. Luminance or angular dependence is how bright the image appears from each viewing angle between the observer and the center of the display. Ideally, luminance and viewing angle should be independent of each other. However, this can vary considerably depending on the type of monitor used. Flat-panel LCD monitors tend to suffer severe variation due to viewing angle changes, even suffering from contrast reversal (light areas appearing dark and dark areas appearing bright). Angular response can be evaluated using the TG18-CT test pattern (see Fig. 8.33). Begin by viewing the pattern straight-on and determine the visibility of the half-moon targets. Then move to the right and left of center to see when or whether the patterns disappear (they probably will not with CRT or plasma displays but will with LCD displays). Any viewing angle limits should be clearly labeled on the front of the monitor, and these limits should not change from one test to the next. The change in image brightness with the viewing angle follows the cosine law, which states that the luminous intensity and image contrast with an LCD monitor will be greatest when the observer is viewing perpendicular to the center of the monitor and both will decrease as the viewing angle increases.

f. Spatial or geometric distortion—View the large squares of the SMPTE or AAPM TG18-QC pattern throughout the image using a viewing distance of 30 cm. They should appear as perfect squares over the entire screen and should show no pincushion or barrel distortion. A flexible ruler can be used to measure the width and height of each square. This should be done in each quadrant as well as at the center of the image. The difference between expected and measured lengths within the pattern should not exceed 2% for primary class displays or 5% for secondary class displays. Monitor controls can be adjusted if they are beyond these limits. Also make sure that there are no magnetic fields present, as these can cause geometric distortions in CRT monitors.

g. Spatial resolution—View high-contrast boundaries (such as white text on a dark background) and verify that they are well defined. Adjust monitor controls if they are not visible. A more detailed test involves assessing the appearance of the Cx patterns in either the TG18-QC or TG18-CX (Fig. 8.37) test patterns. Examine the displayed Cx patterns at the center and at the four corners of the image using a magnifying glass. Note any differences in the visibility of the test patterns between the horizontal and vertical lines (they should all be the same whether they are in the center or at the edges). CRT displays may show less resolution at the edges than at the center.

h. Low-contrast resolution—Verify that the 5% contrast patches are visible in both the 100% video (white) and 0% video (black) squares from either the SMPTE or the AAPM TG18-QC test pattern. In addition, verify that the proper contrast balance is available within the image. The contrast balance evaluates the contrast visible near the very black levels and the very white levels of the image. For this evaluation, display the SMPTE or AAPM TG18QC test pattern and look for the 5% and 95% squares. The perceived contrast difference between the 0% and 5% (darkest) squares should be the same as the perceived contrast between the 100% and 95% (whitest) squares.

i. Grayscale uniformity—Verify that the gray background of the SMPTE or AAPM TG18-QC pattern is uniformly gray across the entire display. The AAPM TG 18 PQC test pattern (Fig. 8.38) may also be used.

j. Display artifacts—Verify that the display does not contain streaks, lines, or dark/light patches. Also look for any small black dots, which indicate nonfunctioning (dropped) pixels.

k. Display reflection—Verify that all light coming from the display surface has been generated by the display device only and does not contain any reflected light. Generally, reflection from the face of the display comes in two basic forms: specular and diffuse. Specular reflection produces a mirror image of the light source creating it, and diffuse reflection produces a more uniform luminance on the display, with no detectable patterns of the source creating it. These reflections can be very common with CRT monitors but rarely occur with LCD monitors. Antireflective coatings on the faceplate of the display and reduction of ambient light in the viewing area should reduce these reflections. With the display in the power-save mode or turned off, observe the display with the ambient light at normal levels at a distance of about 30–60 cm and a viewing angle of ±15 degrees. Look for the presence of specularly reflected light sources or illuminated objects. Reflections from white laboratory coats and other bright clothing are common sources of specular reflection. If present, reduce ambient light levels. To test for diffuse reflection, observe the low-contrast patterns in the TG18-AD test pattern (Fig. 8.39) in both near-total darkness and in normal ambient lighting. The low-contrast patterns should appear the same whether viewed in total darkness or normal light conditions. If the patterns are not visible in normal light conditions, ambient light must be reduced, as this is causing a reduction in contrast within the image.

PROCEDURE: DISPLAY MONITORS

Annual

1. Turn on the monitor and execute the normal boot-up procedure. Allow CRT monitors to warm up for 30 min.
2. Inspect the front screen of the monitor for cleanliness. If dirty, clean using the manufacturer's instructions.
3. Determine whether specular reflection of light sources (e.g., lights, other monitors, viewboxes, windows) are present on the monitor from a normal viewing direction. Reduce or eliminate if possible.
4. Assess the following image quality parameters while viewing the appropriate SMPTE or AAPM-TG 18 test pattern:
   a. Luminance response—Luminance response refers to the relationship between displayed luminance (luminance values obtained during testing) and the input values of a standardized display system (test pattern brightness). Use a photometer (some PACS monitors have internal photometers) and AAPM TG18-LN test patterns (Figs. 8.30–8.32) to measure luminance at the center of the monitor. Primary display monitors (those used by providers to diagnose images) should have a maximum luminance of

PROCEDURE: DISPLAY MONITORS—cont'd

at least 170 nit (50 foot-lamberts), whereas secondary display monitors (those used by technologists) should have a maximum luminance of at least 100 nit (30 foot-lamberts). These luminance values should not vary by more than 10% from values that were previously obtained. Also, workstations with multiple monitors should not vary by more than 10%. The monitor brightness control can be readjusted if the luminance is not within limits. If a photometer is not available, luminance response can be evaluated visually using the TG18-CT test pattern (Fig. 8.33). This pattern should be evaluated for visibility of the central half-moon targets and the four low-contrast objects at the corners of each of 16 different luminance regions. The pattern should be evaluated from a distance of approximately 30 cm. The low-contrast targets in all 16 regions should be visible (a common failure is not being able to see the targets in one or two of the dark regions). In addition, the bit depth resolution of the display (the maximum number of gray scales that can be displayed simultaneously) should be evaluated using the TG18-MP test pattern (Fig. 8.34). The relative location of contouring bands and any luminance levels should not be further than the distance between the 8-bit markers (long markers). No contrast reversal (bright areas appearing dark and dark areas appearing bright) should be visible.

b. Contrast ratio—This is determined by taking the luminance readings from the center of the TG18-LN01 pattern (Lmin) and the TG18-LN18 pattern (Lmax). A photometer is used to measure the luminance of the minimum black level (L_{min}) and the maximum white level (L_{max}) displayed on the monitor. The contrast ratio is the ratio of the maximum white level (L_{max}) to the minimum black level (L_{min}), or L_{max}/L_{min} and should be greater than 250 (most will be at least 600 or greater) for primary monitors and greater than 100 for secondary monitors. As a comparison, this corresponds to optical density values in film screen imaging of between 0.1 and 2.5, which is where most diagnostically useful structures would typically be found.

c. Luminance uniformity—Luminance uniformity refers to the uniformity of the brightness across the entire screen by comparing the luminance values at the center of the screen to those at the edges of the screen. Nonuniformity refers to the maximum variation in luminance across the display area when a uniform pattern is displayed. This is a common characteristic in CRT displays, with the luminance typically decreasing from the center to the edges and corners of the display because of differences in the path length and beam landing angle of the electron beam (because the glass front is curved). This effect is less pronounced in LCD displayed but must still be evaluated. Use the photometer to measure the luminance of the TG18-UNL10 (relatively dark image) and TG18-UNL80 (relatively bright image) test patterns (Figs. 8.35 and 8.36) in the center of the display, as well each of the four corners. The five luminance readings from each of the same test pattern should be within 20% of each other. If not, the monitor controls can be adjusted or a physicist or biomedical engineer should be consulted. If a photometer is not available, luminance nonuniformity can be evaluated visually using the TG18-UN10 and TG18-UN80 test patterns. When viewing, each pattern should be free of gross nonuniformities from the center to the edges. No luminance variations with dimensions on the order of 1 cm or larger should be observed.

d. Workstation monitor uniformity—This value is determined by using the TG18-LN 18 pattern on each workstation monitor and measuring the brightness in the center of the monitor with a photometer. The center measurement of each monitor on a workstation should not vary by more than 10%. In addition these values should remain consistent each time the test is performed.

e. Luminance dependencies—Luminance dependencies refer to the luminance response mentioned above, but it is how this value is dependent on the viewing angle between the observer and the center of the display. Angular dependence is how bright the image appears from each viewing angle between the observer and the center of the display. Ideally, luminance and viewing angle should be independent of each other. However, this can vary considerably depending on the type of monitor used. Flat-panel LCD monitors tend to suffer severe variation due to viewing angle changes, even suffering from contrast reversal (light areas appearing dark and dark areas appearing bright). Angular response can be evaluated using the TG18-CT test pattern (see Fig. 8.33). Begin by viewing the pattern straight-on and determine the visibility of the half-moon targets. Then move to the right and left of center to see when or whether the patterns disappear (they probably will not with CRT or plasma displays but will with LCD displays). Any viewing angle limits should be clearly labeled on the front of the monitor, and these limits should not change from one test to the next. The change in image brightness with the viewing angle follows the cosine law, which states that the luminous intensity and image contrast with an LCD monitor will be greatest when the observer is viewing perpendicular to the center of the monitor and both will decrease as the viewing angle increases.

f. Spatial or geometric distortion—View the large squares of the SMPTE or AAPM TG18-QC pattern throughout the image using a viewing distance of 30 cm. They should appear as perfect squares over the entire screen and should show no pincushion or barrel distortion. A flexible ruler can be used to measure the width and height of each square. This should be done in each quadrant, as well as at the center of the image. The difference between expected and measured lengths within the pattern should not exceed 2% for primary class displays or 5% for secondary class displays. Monitor controls can be adjusted if they are beyond these limits. Also make sure that there are no magnetic fields present, as these can cause geometric distortions in CRT monitors.

g. Spatial resolution—View high-contrast boundaries (such as white text on a dark background) and verify that they are well defined. Adjust monitor controls if they are not visible. A more detailed test involves assessing the appearance of the CX patterns in either the TG18-QC or TG18-CX (Fig. 8.37) test patterns. Examine the displayed CX patterns at the center and at the four corners of the image using a magnifying glass. Note any differences in the visibility of the test patterns between the horizontal and vertical lines (they should all be the same whether they are in the center or at the edges). CRT displays may show less resolution at the edges than at the center.

h. Low-contrast resolution—Verify that the 5% contrast patches are visible in both the 100% video (white) and 0% video (black) squares from either the SMPTE or the AAPM TG18-QC test pattern. In addition verify that the proper contrast balance is

Continued

PROCEDURE: DISPLAY MONITORS—cont'd

available within the image. The contrast balance evaluates the contrast visible near the very black levels and the very white levels of the image. For this evaluation, display the SMPTE or AAPM TG18QC test pattern and look for the 5% and 95% squares. The perceived contrast difference between the 0% and 5% (darkest) squares should be the same as the perceived contrast between the 100% and 95% (whitest) squares.

i. Grayscale uniformity—Verify that the gray background of the SMPTE or AAPM TG18-QC pattern is uniformly gray across the entire display. The AAPM TG 18 PQC test pattern (Fig. 8.38) may also be used.

j. Display artifacts—Verify that the display does not contain streaks, lines, or dark/light patches. Also look for any small black dots, which indicate nonfunctioning (dropped) pixels.

k. Display reflection—Verify that all light coming from the display surface has been generated by the display device only and does not contain any reflected light. Generally, reflection from the face of the display comes in two basic forms: specular and diffuse. Specular reflection produces a mirror image of the light source creating it, while diffuse reflection produces a more uniform luminance on the display with no detectable patterns of the source creating it. These reflections can be very common with CRT monitors but rarely occur with LCD monitors. Antireflective coatings on the faceplate of the display, and reduction of ambient light in the viewing area should reduce these reflections. With the display in the power-save mode or turned off, observe the display with the ambient light at normal levels at a distance of about 30–60 cm and a viewing angle of ±15 degrees. Look for the presence of specularly reflected light sources or illuminated objects. Reflections from white laboratory coats and other bright clothing are common sources of specular reflection. If present, reduce ambient light levels. To test for diffuse reflection, observe the low-contrast patterns in the TG18-AD test pattern (Fig. 8.39) in both near total darkness and in normal ambient lighting. The low-contrast patterns should appear the same whether viewed in total darkness or normal light conditions. If the patterns are not visible in normal light conditions, ambient light must be reduced as this is causing a reduction in contrast within the image.

l. Display noise—Display noise is evaluated using the TG18-AFC test pattern. The test image is divided into four quadrants. Each quadrant is divided into 48 squares, with each square having a low-contrast dots in random positions within the squares. The contrast-size values for the target dots are a constant in each quadrant, but the values are different for each quadrant. The image is viewed at a distance of 30 cm at the normal ambient lighting conditions in which the workstation will be used. On a calibrated monitor used for primary diagnosis, the evaluator should be able to determine the location of all of the dots in three out of the four quadrants. On other calibrated monitors, the evaluator should be able to determine the location of the dots in two out of the four quadrants.

m. **Display chromaticity**—In LCD monitors, the color tint of grayscale monitors can be affected by the spectrum of the backlight and by the viewing angle. Grayscale monitors used for primary diagnosis on multimonitor workstations should be matched for tint at the factory and sold and installed in matched sets to avoid perceivable differences in the tint of monitors on the same workstation. To perform this test, display the TG18-UN80 test pattern (Fig. 8.40) on the grayscale monitors. Note any perceivable differences in the relative color uniformity across the display area of each monitor and between the monitors on the same workstation. The observer must be looking straight on at the monitor to reliably perform this test. Angled viewing will result in an invalid test.

A checklist for documentation of this procedure is provided on the accompanying Evolve website.

Annual inspections should only be performed by a medical physicist using the procedures described by the AAPM Task Group 18. The procedures are extensive and beyond the scope of this book but can be downloaded from the following website: https://www.aapm.org.

The monthly/quarterly and annual tests are summarized in Box 8.3.

PROCEDURE: DRY LASER PRINTER

1. A multiformat test generator should be used to create either an SMPTE, TG18-QC, or a TG18-PQC test pattern.
2. Display the SMPTE test pattern on the filming console. Set the display window width/level to the manufacturer-specified values for the SMPTE pattern.
3. Film the SMPTE pattern. Use six-on-one format and capture the pattern in all six frames.
4. A densitometer should be used to record the following areas of the hard-copy SMPTE film:
   40% patch: This value determines the level of the middensity or speed indicator, which should be approximately 1.15 ± 0.15.
   10% and 70% patches: The optical densities of these two regions are subtracted from each other to yield the contrast indicator, which should be approximately 1.2 ± 0.15.
   90% patch: This value is just above the base + fog and should be about ±0.15 of 0.30.
5. Plot these optical densities in the appropriate places on the laser film QC chart. Circle any points that fall outside the control limit.

SMPTE Patch	Optical Density	Control Limits
0%	3.00	±0.15
10%	2.20	±0.15
40%	1.15	±0.15
90%	0.30	±0.15

6. Put the film on a viewbox and inspect it for streaks, uneven densities, and other artifacts.
7. If optical densities fall outside of control limit or if artifacts are found, corrective action should be taken.

Dry Laser Printers

Most imaging departments have replaced multiformat cameras and laser cameras with dry laser printers to produce hard copies of digital images. These devices were introduced in 1996 and

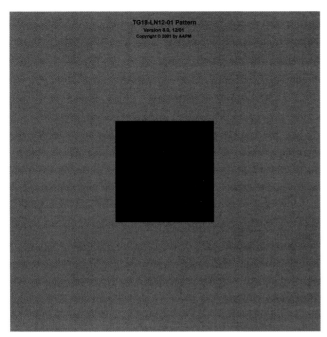

Fig. 8.30 American Association of Physicists in Medicine TG18-LN01 test pattern.

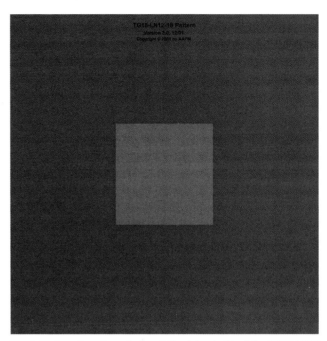

Fig. 8.32 American Association of Physicists in Medicine TG18-LN18 test pattern.

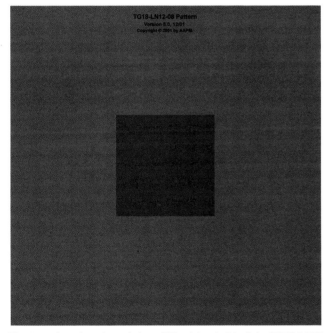

Fig. 8.31 American Association of Physicists in Medicine TG18-LN08 test pattern.

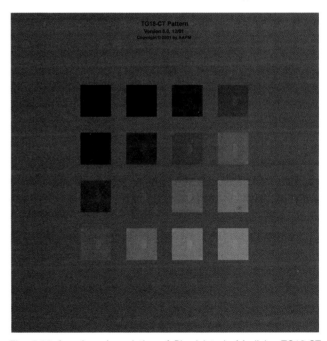

Fig. 8.33 American Association of Physicists in Medicine TG18-CT test pattern.

require specialized film (photothermographic) that uses silver behenate rather than silver halide to produce the image, and is processed thermally rather than with liquid developer and fixer. Silver behenate is a crystalline long-chain silver carboxylate $(AgC_{22}H_{43}O_2)$ that has been used in X-ray diffraction as well as microfilms for many years. The silver metal image formation is based on the heat-induced reduction of the silver behenate. The film is exposed with a scanning laser, much the same as with a laser camera. After laser exposure, the film is heated to a temperature of 120°C for 24 seconds to process the image (Fig. 8.41).

After the image has been recorded and the film ejected from the machine, it is still in the process of image development. The room illumination or light emanating from a viewbox illuminator can cause slight changes in the optical density. This can cause traces of overlapped films or transferred images to appear temporarily, but they disappear when those films are left under normal light conditions. The images recorded on these films can experience an increase in optical density over time if stored at temperatures above 30°C; however, because the images originally existed in digital form,

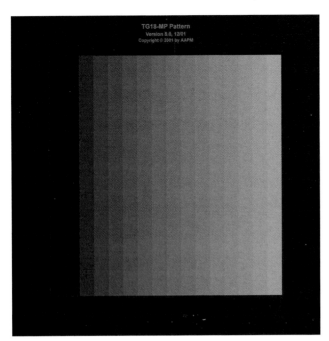

Fig. 8.34 American Association of Physicists in Medicine TG18-MP test pattern.

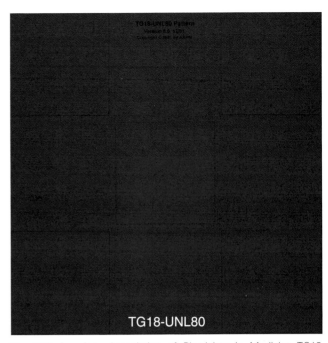

Fig. 8.36 American Association of Physicists in Medicine TG18-UNL80 test pattern.

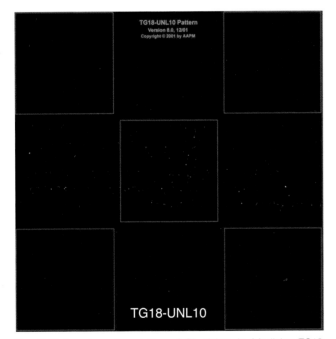

Fig. 8.35 American Association of Physicists in Medicine TG18-UNL10 test pattern.

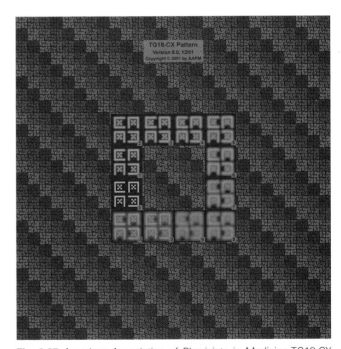

Fig. 8.37 American Association of Physicists in Medicine TG18-CX test pattern.

they can be recalled in soft form (if stored properly) and then reprinted in hard copy at the desired future date.

For QC, dry laser printers can be evaluated by imaging a test pattern (usually an SMPTE or internal). Documentation of dry laser printer QC can be done with the control chart found in Box 8.4. Many models of dry laser printers have a built-in test pattern generator programmed into the unit that can be printed and evaluated according to the manufacturer's guidelines (Fig. 8.42). This usually involves the creation of a characteristic curve from this pattern and comparing it with those obtained on previous days. If this option is unavailable on a particular system, an external test pattern generator can be used and the procedure for evaluation of the laser camera followed.

DIGITAL RECORDERS

Digital image recorders (also known as *digital photospot imaging*) have replaced videotape and videodisc recorders, as well as

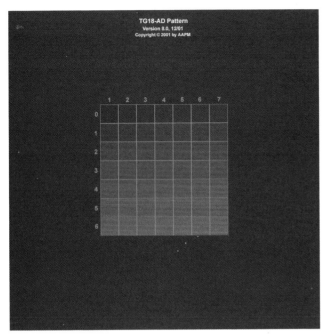

Fig. 8.38 American Association of Physicists in Medicine TG18-PQC test pattern.

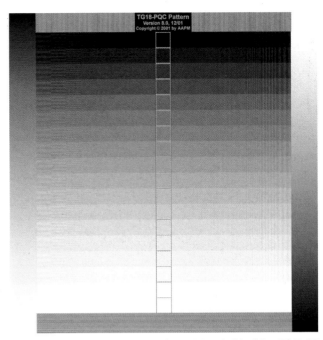

Fig. 8.39 American Association of Physicists in Medicine TG18-AD test pattern.

spot film and photospot imaging in many newer applications. These systems will obtain static spot images by having a short exposure of the image intensifier made with a high mA while the real-time video is inactivated. Instead, the fluoroscopic television camera will send the signal through an ADC and then into a computer memory for later retrieval and processing. The images are usually 1024 × 1024 pixels, although some newer systems have 2048 × 2048 pixels. These units store the image in a digital form through computer hardware and software until needed. They are essentially computer hard drives. The image can then be recalled onto a video monitor, or hard copies may be generated with a laser camera or dry laser printer. Images can be stored on computer disks. Digital image recorders also allow images to be enhanced or manipulated for better visualization of anatomic structures, but currently they record only a few frames in their memory circuits.

QC of Digital Recorders

Digital recorders should be evaluated on acceptance and then at least every 6 months.

PROCEDURE: DIGITAL RECORDER

1. A multiformat test generator that creates an SMPTE or TG18-QC test pattern should be used for evaluation of these units (they are usually built into the software of these systems for easy access and display).
2. When the test pattern image is recorded and evaluated, the image should display all of the 10% patches and distortion should be minimal. The contrast or gray scale on the recorded image should be the same as on the original image.

A regular preventive maintenance program should be in place to ensure that the internal components are cleaned and evaluated. Digital recorders have fewer moving parts and are not

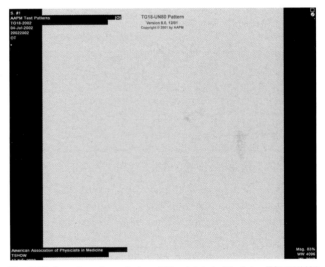

Fig. 8.40 American Association of Physicists in Medicine TG18 UN80 test pattern.

subject to as much variation as analog units. The SMPTE test pattern can be used to evaluate the performance of these units in the same way as with analog units. Digital units generally perform correctly or not at all because of the solid-state nature of the equipment.

DIAGNOSTIC IMAGING INFORMATICS

With digital imaging becoming the dominant acquisition mode for diagnostic imaging, the storage of these images into a central computer system for retrieval at a later date has become an essential component of imaging departments. This reduces the space required for film storage in analog

BOX 8.3   Summary of Viewing Monitor QC

Test Parameter	Variance Allowed (If Applicable)	Test Parameter	Variance Allowed (If Applicable)
Monthly/quarterly		Maximum luminance	>170 nit for primary and >100 nit for secondary
Monitor cleanliness	Front screen should be clean	Contrast ratio	>250
Specular reflection	Reduce or eliminate	Display noise	Primary—dots visible in 3 of 4 quadrants
Maximum luminance	>170 nit for primary and >100 nit for secondary		Secondary—dots visible in 2 of 4 quadrants
Contrast ratio	>250	Luminance uniformity	±20%
Luminance uniformity	±20%	Workstation monitor uniformity	Luminance values of each monitor should not vary by more than 10%
Workstation monitor uniformity	Luminance values of each monitor should not vary by more than 10%	Luminance dependency	Image should be visible with viewing angle of at least 40 degrees from center
Luminance dependency	Image should be visible with viewing angle of at least 40 degrees from center	Spatial or geometric distortion	±2% for primary and ±5% for secondary
Spatial or geometric distortion	±2% for primary and ±5% for secondary	Spatial resolution	Should not change from acceptance test
Spatial resolution	Should not change from acceptance test	Low-contrast resolution	5% and 95% patches must be visible
Low-contrast resolution	5% and 95% patches must be visible	Grayscale uniformity	Should be uniform across entire display
Grayscale uniformity	Should be uniform across entire display	Veiling glare	Glare ratio (GR) ≥400 for primary and ≥150 for secondary
Display artifacts	None should be visible	Chromaticity	No perceivable differences should be observed
Display reflection	Reduce or eliminate if possible		
Annual			
Monitor cleanliness	Front screen should be clean		
Specular reflection	Reduce or eliminate		

QC, Quality control.

departments and increases the speed and accuracy of retrieval. Computer systems allow remote access of patient images and other pertinent information from within the hospital itself and from providers' offices and clinics several miles away, and even around the world as a result of satellite transmission of digital data. Digital images can be easily downloaded into these systems from their original units. Conventional film images (which are analog in nature) must be converted to digital data by means of film digitization scanners that are similar to scanners used with personal computers to enter pictures or data (discussed earlier in this chapter). Most scanners use a CCD digitizer or a laser to scan the image and convert it to digital form. The resolution created by these scanners is usually less than the original film image because the pixel size used is larger than the silver grains found in the film.

The most common system for storing and retrieving digital images is the PACS, which stores digital images and allows access from remote locations. If you are not familiar with computer terminology, you may wish to familiarize yourself with these terms in Box 8.5 before proceeding any further. Most PACS systems use the DICOM network protocol, which is a system of computer software standards that allows different

digital imaging programs to understand one another. For example, a digital radiographic system, a digital fluoroscopic system, CT scanners, and MRI scanners in a healthcare organization can all share the same PACS, even though they are different systems and may have been made by different manufacturers. The ACR and the National Electrical Manufacturers Association formed a committee to develop a standard network protocol for digital imaging and communications (DICOM) in 1983. DICOM version 3.0 is the current standard developed by this committee and has become the de facto global standard. As the field of digital imaging continues to evolve, the DICOM-3 standard is subject to continuous revision, with supplements issued by the committee at various times. Instead of using the version number, the standard is often version numbered using the release year, such as "the 2017 version of DICOM," which is currently being used. PACS and modalities vendors each publish a DICOM conformance statement that defines their data elements and protocols. Most imaging modalities have a DICOM Modality Worklist (DMWL) that can interface with the PACS. The minimum DMWL data elements include:

- Patient name
- Patient ID

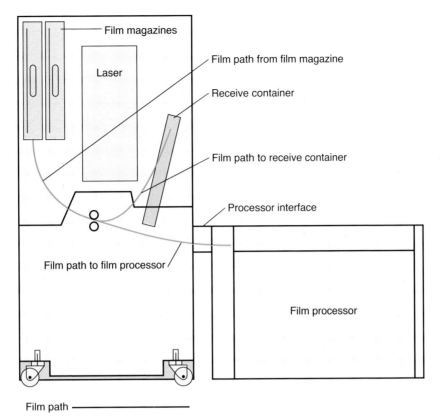

Fig. 8.41 Schematic diagram of a laser camera.

- Accession number
- Patient's date of birth
- Patient's gender
- Exam requested
- Modality type

One of the most important functions of the DICOM protocol is the DICOM Grayscale Standard Display Function (GSDF), which specifies a standardized display function that would convert digital pixel values to luminance values for consistent display of grayscale images on different devices and monitors, and that these values that are displayed are perceived as being equal by human viewers. It also ensures that images display similar contrast whether on display monitors or printed media such as those created by a dry laser printer.

PACS systems contain four main components: image acquisition, image display and interpretation, image storage and retrieval, and a communications network. A list of PACS vendors can be found in Table 8.4.

1. Image acquisition is achieved by downloading the image from a particular modality such as CR, DR, MR, CT, nuclear medicine, sonography, or from a film digitizer.
2. Image display and interpretation are the workstations for viewing images. Each workstation in the system is called a node or a client.
3. Image storage and retrieval is controlled by an archive server (known as a workflow manager). It is composed of a database server or image manager, short-term storage, long-term archive, and redundant or disaster recovery archive that is maintained separately from the long-term archive. The servers for these three levels of storage can be housed within the healthcare organization or by an outside provider. Disaster recovery servers are most often located at a different location for safety purposes.
4. The communications network allows images to be transmitted to remote workstations. The networks can be a local area network (LAN), a wide area network (WAN), or a virtual private network. A LAN is a network confined to one facility and usually connected by cable, optical fiber, or a wireless system. A WAN includes remote facilities and uses telecommunication devices such as the Internet. *Teleradiology* is the term given when images are transmitted over a WAN from one location to another for the purposes of interpretation and consultation. A virtual private network is constructed using public telecommunication like a WAN but uses encryption software and other security measures such as username and password login to gain entry into the network (much like an online banking system). This allows providers to view images on laptop computers, smartphones, and so on.

Traditionally, healthcare institutions have had a RIS and an HIS. RISs contain patient imaging history and scheduling information but do not store images. HISs contain the patient's electronic medical record systems that contain data such as patient admission, diagnostics, treatment, discharge and billing information, and employee information and pharmaceutical and equipment supply data but again, do not store images. The federal government and private insurance companies prefer to use EHRs to reduce the file space required

BOX 8.4   Laser Film Printer Control Chart (May be Reproduced for Use)

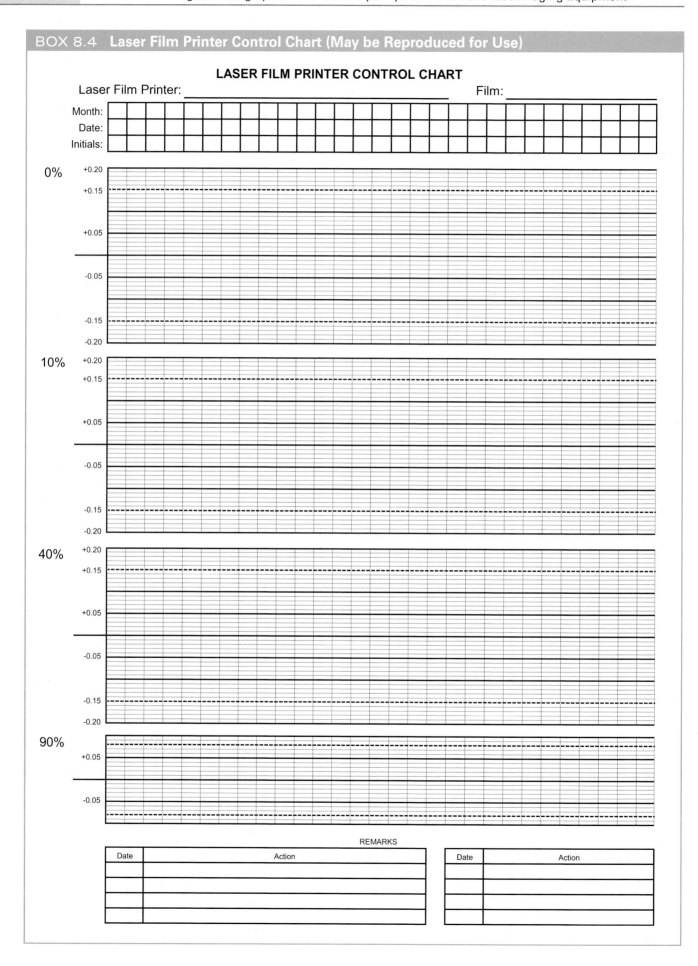

LASER FILM PRINTER CONTROL CHART

| Density step 0 |
| Density step 1 |
| Density step 2 |
| Density step 3 |
| Density step 4 |
| Density step 5 |
| Density step 6 |
| Density step 7 |
| Density step 8 |
| Density step 9 |
| Density step 10 |
| Density step 11 |
| Density step 12 |
| Density step 13 |
| Density step 14 |
| Density step 15 |
| Density step 16 |
| Density step 17 |
| Density step 18 |
| Density step 19 |
| Density step 20 |
| Density step 21 |
| Density step 22 |
| Density step 23 |
| Density step 24 |
| Density step 25 |
| Density step 26 |
| Density step 27 |
| Density step 28 |
| Density step 29 |
| Density step 30 |
| Density step 31 |

Fig. 8.42 Demonstration of step test pattern for evaluation of dry laser printer.

to store paper records (the American Recovery and Reinvestment Act of 2009 and the Patient Protection and Affordable Care Act of 2010 have enacted penalties in the form of decreased Medicare and Medicaid reimbursement for providers and healthcare organizations who do not use EHRs). The Centers for Medicare & Medicaid Services (https://www.CMS.gov) has an EHR Incentive Program that provides financial incentives for the "meaningful use" of certified EHR technology to improve patient care. To receive this payment, healthcare providers must demonstrate that they are "meaningfully using" their EHRs by meeting thresholds for a number of objectives. The CMS has also established the objectives for "meaningful use" that eligible professionals, eligible hospitals, and critical access hospitals must meet to receive these incentive payments. A problem with developing EHRs is that the DICOM-3 standard used for transmission of images is not designed for transmission of other patient data such as laboratory reports. The current standard for transmission of medical record data is the Health Level 7 (HL7) standard, developed by the Healthcare Information and Management Systems Society. Most HL7 programs use the Minimal Lower Layer Protocol. Both the HIS and RIS vendors will publish an HL7 conformance statement that will define to the data element level; information that can be shared between systems. The Radiological Society of North America has formed a joint committee with the Healthcare Information and Management Systems Society that has completed work to integrate

the DICOM-3 and HL7 standards to allow for a universal format for PACS and EHRs. This is known as the Integrating Healthcare Enterprise (IHE) the latest information can be found on its web site at https://www.ihe.net. Most PACS utilize a DICOM broker that changes the format between the HL7 information in the EHR and the DICOM information in PACS. The most relevant IHE integration profile for diagnostic imaging departments is the *Scheduled Workflow Integration Profile*. This profile establishes the continuity and integrity of basic departmental imaging data. It specifies a number of transactions that maintain the consistency of patient and ordering information as well as providing the scheduling and imaging acquisition procedure steps. This profile also makes it possible to determine whether images and other evidence objects associated with a particular performed procedure step have been stored (archived) and are available to enable subsequent workflow steps, such as reporting. It may also provide central coordination of the completion of processing and reporting steps as well as notification of appointments to the provider or department that placed the order.

Another important IHE profile is the Radiation Exposure Monitoring (REM) Integration Profile. This integration profile specifies how details of radiation exposure resulting from imaging procedures are exchanged among the imaging systems, local dose information management systems, and cross-institutional systems such as dose registries. The data flow in the profile is intended to facilitate recording individual procedure dose information, collecting dose data related to specific patients, and performing population analysis. The profile addresses dose reporting for imaging procedures performed on CT and projection X-ray systems, including mammography. It does not currently address procedures such as nuclear medicine (PET or SPECT), radiotherapy, or implanted seeds.

Other concerns with the digital transmission of image data are the privacy and security of the information. Health Insurance Portability and Accountability Act required that security standards for electronic transactions of patient information be implemented by October 2002 (October 2003 for small health plans) and are now in place. Similar legislation has been created by the European Community (EC Data Protection Directive 95/46/EC) and in Japan (HPB 517). To help integrate images into EHRs, most PACS incorporate remote viewing technology that uses application program interface (API) to integrate into the system. APIs specify how certain software components should interact with other software components. This allows access to imaging information securely on a variety of web-enabled devices such as personal computers, tablets, and mobile devices.

A main concern for instituting the PACS is the amount of computer hardware and data storage required. A current digital chest series (posteroanterior and lateral) requires about 20 Mb of digital storage space, while a digital screening mammogram can range from 32–220 Mb, so a typical diagnostic imaging department could generate enough

BOX 8.5   Computer and PACS Terminology

1. Informatics—The body of ideas, devices, and processes related to handling multiple types of information
2. Platform—A particular configuration of informatics devices and processes
3. Biomedical informatics—The platforms that are used for medical purposes
4. Bandwidth—Defines the maximum amount of information that can be transferred over a data channel per unit time, and measured in units of megabits per second or gigabits per second
5. Server—A computer that manages resources for other computers, servers, and network devices. There may be one server that provides storage for files, one that manages the print functions, and another that provides Internet access for the network.
6. Workflow—How a process is done, step by step. In radiology, it refers to how we complete an examination from order entry to transcribed report. Workflow in digital departments is greatly increased when compared with a film/screen department.
7. Network—System that allows two or more computer to exchange information
8. Network interface—The connection between two computers or parts of computers; also known as a network adapter, and consists mainly of electronic circuitry
9. Network interface card—Connects each computer to a network (also known as a network adapter)
10. Network address—A unique number that identifies each interface between a node and a network
11. Disaster recovery plan—Periodic back-up of archived files.
12. Router—A computer system that connects and directs information from one network to another by selecting the best available pathway
13. Network protocols—The codes and conventions under which a network operates; they are the guidelines by which two different computer devices communicate with each other. Examples include:
    * Simple mail transfer protocol (SMTP)—Used for e-mail
    * Hypertext transfer protocol (HTTP)—Used for transferring and viewing web pages
14. RIS—Contains patient imaging history, scheduling information and the radiologists report
15. Hospital information system (HIS)—Tracks patient admission, diagnostics, treatment, discharge, and billing information, as well as employee information, pharmaceutical, and equipment supply data
16. Electronic (or enterprise) medical record or electronic healthcare (or health) record (EHR)—electronic version of an individual's collection of medical documents
17. Universal resource locator (URL)—A string of characters used to obtain a service from another computer on the Internet. The first part of the URL specifies the protocol (http, etc.) the second part is the host name of the computer from which the resource is requested, and the third part specifies the location of the file on the destination computer.
18. Baud rate—Describes the rate of information transfer in a network in bits per second. A baud rate of 56,000 corresponds to 56,000 bits per second. Computers linked using an Ethernet connection (10 Mbps) transmit a chest X-ray (10 MB) in about 1 min. Fast Ethernet (100 Mbps) transmits the chest X-ray in less than 10 seconds, and gigabit Ethernet (1,000 Mbps) in less than 1 second.

image data to require a total memory of 20 terabytes (20 trillion bytes) or more. Another problem is the network capacity because most hospital-based PACS systems must share the LAN and its bandwidth with the rest of the healthcare organization, which can slow the speed of image transmission. The large data sets can benefit from image compression, which reduces the size of data files by removing and encoding redundant information. Compression allows faster retrieval of images from the PACS system, reduces bandwidth and physical space cost, and allows for more efficient use of teleradiology. When discussing compression, a term known as compression ratio is often used. Compression ratio is the ratio of the size of the original file to the compressed image file. For example, a compression ratio of 2:1 would correspond to a compressed image with one-half the file size of the original. There are two basic types of compression that can be used for diagnostic images:

A. Lossless compression (also known as recoverable compression) is completely reversible with compression up to five times (or a compression ratio of 5:1). This does not compromise image quality. Disadvantages of lossless compression include:
   * It takes time to encode and decode.
   * It brings only modest savings in terms of size.
   * Both ends have to support it during transmission.
   * Future software needs to be able to read it.

B. Lossy (or nonrecoverable) compression is not reversible and can introduce some degree of data loss but can compress data size from 5 to 50 times. It achieves higher compression ratios but introduces some degree of data loss. This means that less disk space is used in the archive servers, which lowers bandwidth requirements. It also can enable teleradiology from areas where only slow Internet connections are available. Disadvantages of lossy compression include:
   * Loss of image data
   * Does not archive the image that was originally used for diagnosis so may pose legal questions
   * Should not be used for primary interpretation
   * May not be good for portable media
   * Forbidden in some applications such as mammography

A widely used lossy compression standard is JPEG (Joint Photographic Export Group), which breaks the digital image into 8 × 8 pixel blocks and then compresses these blocks. Compression also can exaggerate original image errors and archival image errors. A new storage protocol called the storage area network is being introduced to PACS systems

TABLE 8.4 Picture Archiving and Communication System Vendors (Selling in the United States)

Agfa HealthCare	https://www.agfahealthcare.com
AMD Technologies	https://www.amd.com
Avreo Inc.	https://www.avreo.com
Brit Systems	https://www.brit.com
Candelis, Inc.	https://www.candelis.com
Carestream Health	www.carestream.com
Cerner Corp.	https://www.cerner.com
CoActiv Medical	https://www.coactiv.com
DR Systems	https://www.dominator.com
Fujifilm Medical Systems USA Inc.	https://www.fujifilmusa.com
GE Healthcare	https://www.gehealthcare.com
iCRco	www.icrco.com
Image Information Systems Ltd	https://www.image-systems.biz
Imsi Med	https://www.imsimed.com
Infinitt	https://www.infinitt.com
Intelerad	https://www.intelerad.com
Intuitive Imaging	https://www.intuitiveimaging.com
McKesson	https://www.mckesson.com
Medweb	https://www.medweb.com
Merative	https://www.merative.com
NovaRad Corp.	https://www.novarad.net
PACSPlus	https://www.pacsplus.com
Philips Healthcare	https://www.healthcare.philips.com
Radlink	https://www.radlink.com
Radsource	https://www.radsource.us
RamSoft	https://www.ramsoft.net
ScImage	https://www.scimage.com
Sectra	https://www.sectra.com
Siemens Healthcare	www.smed.com
Viztek	http://viztek.net
Voyager Imaging	https://www.intellirad.com

that can transfer large data files much more quickly. Storage area networks use fiber channels, which can carry five times more bandwidth than the more commonly used small computer system interface. Because this is a considerable amount of hardware to maintain, many healthcare organizations have turned to application software providers, which are sometimes referred to as cloud storage systems. These are independent storage contractors outside of the healthcare organization who maintain the hardware and software necessary for a successful archiving system. A list of Cloud-based PACS vendors can be found in Table 8.5.

Because archiving systems are digital, variation in system performance is relatively rare. However, a QC mechanism should be in place to guarantee optimum performance (see procedure box). PACS systems that use a wireless transmission communication network must have additional procedures to ensure that the signal is encrypted to protect patient privacy, to prevent signal interference and corruption from other systems using the same network, and have a strategy for loss prevention and image recovery if the wireless signal is interrupted during transmission of data. A disaster recovery plan must also be in place to ensure that images are not lost from the system (usually in the form of periodic backup archiving of images in the system). Documentation of other characteristics such as system down-time and system training for department employees also should be included in quality control/quality management (QC/QM) programs. This can be accomplished through the use of a log noting the details (e.g., name, dates, reason for problem, what was done to fix the problem).

For imaging departments that are transferring analog (film/screen) images into a PACS system using film digitization scanners, these devices should be kept clean and free of dust or debris to avoid artifacts on the downloaded images.

PROCEDURE: PACS QUALITY CONTROL

1. An image of an SMPTE test pattern, AAPM TG18-QC, AAPM TG18-BR (also known as a Briggs test pattern) (Fig. 8.43) or a special PACS test pattern (see Fig. 8.44) consisting of horizontal, vertical, and diagonal lines should be digitized and displayed on the monitor. If one is not available, a phantom image can be created. Register this pattern as a test patient and verify that the patient data are available in the RIS.
2. The test pattern image should be captured, transmitted, archived, retrieved, and displayed by the PACS system, and compared with the original image for any changes in quality. This should be performed at least weekly.
3. Image resolution should conform to the manufacturer's specifications. This test should be performed at least monthly to test the overall operation of the system under conditions that simulate the normal operation of the system. No change should be observed from one month to the next.
4. Compression recall should be evaluated quarterly by saving the following versions of the test patterns mentioned in step one of this procedure: (a) no compression, (b) lossless compression (usually a 2:1 ratio), and (c) lossy compression (if used by your department). Examine the images of the test patterns in each of the above versions and determine whether any information, image quality, or significant spatial resolution has been lost.
5. A thread test should be performed upon acceptance and then monthly. A **thread test** evaluates how the PACS passes data from module to module to ensure that they link up appropriately. They utilize clinical scenarios to evaluate the information from acquisition to display, printing, reporting and archive. Steps in a thread test include:
   - Register test patient in the HIS and verify that the patient appears in the RIS.
   - Enter a test order for an examination on the test patient in the RIS. Verify that the patient and examination appear in the modality's workstation DICOM worklist.

Continued

PROCEDURE: PACS QUALITY CONTROL—cont'd

- Select the test patient and test order from the modality's workstation and verify that the data elements map correctly into the workstations fields. Acquire an image using a phantom.
- After the image appears on the workstation monitor, send it to the PACS. The test patient and completed image(s) should appear on the radiologist's "to be read" worklist. There should be an indication on the radiologist's PACS desktop that a dictation system is ready to receive the radiologist's dictation. Enter a test dictation and notify the transcriptionist that the dictation is present. The transcriptionist should select the test patient/test exam from the transcription system's worklist. Once this is complete, verify that the preliminary report is available with images in the PACS.
- Verify that the completed report is available at a clinical workstation along with the images.
- Have the vendor or system administrator log into each archival location to verify that the test patient's examination and report are available.

6. An **archive test** should be performed to test each server in the archive. This test consists of the following steps:
   - Process and acquire an examination on a test patient at a modality workstation in the normal manner and send it to the PACS.
   - Log into a diagnostic (radiologist's) workstation and verify that the examination is on the "exams pending" interpretation worklist. Display the examination and save specific annotations and window width/level settings to several images in the examination. Check and record the file size of the examination and the number of images.
   - At the PACS administrator workstation, access the short-term storage server and verify that the examination on the test patient is present. Check and record the file size of the examination and the number of images.
   - Access the long-term archive and verify that the examination on the test patient is present. Check and record the file size of the examination and the number of images. If image compression is utilized, verify that the compression ratio utilized reduced the file size by the appropriate amount (i.e., a 2:1 compression ratio should reduce the file size by one-half).
   - Access the disaster recovery archive and verify that the test examination on the test patient is present. Some PACS may only archive to this system at specific times, so you may have to wait to verify until this time.
   - Go to the HIS/RIS and change the test patient's middle name. Verify that the name change on the test patient migrates through all of the systems so that the short-term storage, long-term archive, and disaster recovery have updated the test patient's name.
   - Have the PACS administrator delete or "age" the test examination from the short-term storage. Verify that the test examination is no longer on the short-term storage worklist and verify that it is in the long-term archive. Then go to a PACS workstation, select the test patient, and retrieve the test examination from the long-term storage. Verify that the window width/level settings saved to the examination are present.

7. Perform a disaster recovery archive test (may not be possible with certain system architecture). Steps for this test include:
   - Remove the disaster recovery archive connection to the long-term storage. Have the PACS administrator delete the test examination from the archive test procedure discussed previously from the short-term storage and long-term archive.
   - Verify that the test examination is no longer available in the short-term storage or long-term archive worklist.
   - Reconnect the disaster recovery archive and long-term archive.
   - Go to a PACS workstation, select the test patient, and retrieve the examination. Verify that the annotations and window width/level settings are present.

8. Perform a workstation functionality test to ensure each function is available. Steps for this test include:
   - Verify that the user is presented with a worklist/patient list and that the worklist is configurable according to the vendor's specifications.
   - Verify that the following are available for the user:
     a. Move the cursor across multiple monitors and verify that it moves across all screens of the workstation.
     b. Verify that window width/level are available in both single-image and multiple-image examinations.
     c. Verify that the digital magnifying glass is able to move/roam throughout the image, increase or decrease the zoom, inverse video, and that window width/level functions are available inside the window.
     d. Verify that the horizontal flip, vertical flip, and sequential 90-degree rotation of an image is available.
     e. Verify that inverse video is available.
     f. Verify that image roam and zoom functions are available.
     g. Verify that pixel brightness values can be obtained.
     h. Verify text annotation, image identification, undo last keystroke, save, view full image header information, stack, cine, and multiplanar reformatting is available and functioning.
   - Verify that the measurement software is available in both metric and English units by measuring an object of known size.
   - Verify that the workstation supports angle measurements.
   - Verify that the workstation supports perimeter measurement of objects.
   - Verify that a user can define and save image display protocols.
   - Verify that the display protocol allows a user to define image presentation order and number of images on a screen.
   - Verify that the display protocol can be modality specific.

9. Laser printers, which are used to make hard-copy images from a PACS system, and electronic display devices (both primary and secondary) should be evaluated as previously discussed.

10. Evaluate workstation monitors using the procedures previously covered in this chapter.

11. Perform display monitor evaluation using the procedures previously discussed in this chapter.

12. Additional testing specified by the system's manufacturer should be performed.

TABLE 8.5 Cloud Storage Systems for Picture Archiving and Communication System

Accelerad	https://www.accelerad.com
Brit Systems	https://www.brit.com
Candelis, Inc.	https://www.candelis.com
Carestream Health	www.carestream.com
CoActiv Medical	https://www.coactiv.com
Dell Inc.	https://www.dell.com
Intelerad	https://www.intelerad.com
Etiam Corp.	www.etiam.com
Hyland Software Inc.	https://www.hyland.com/en/healthcare
Infinitt North America	https://www.infinitt.com
Integrated Modular Systems Inc.	https://www.imsimed.com
Iron Mountain	https://www.ironmountain.com
Kjaya Medical	https://www.kjayamedical.com
Medweb	https://www.medweb.com
Merge Healthcare	https://www.merge.com
MIM Software	https://www.mimsoftware.com
ScImage, Inc.	https://www.scimage.com
Shina Systems	https://www.shina-sys.com
Siemens Healthcare	www.smed.com
TeraRecon	https://www.terarecon.com
Viztek	http://viztek.net

ARTIFICIAL INTELLIGENCE

A relatively new trend in diagnostic imaging is the use of artificial intelligence (AI) to help increase both quality and efficiency in diagnostic imaging departments. AI refers to a field of computer science dedicated to the creation of systems performing tasks that usually require human intelligence, branching off into different techniques. Two subsets of AI are machine learning and deep learning. Machine learning is a subset of AI that includes all those approaches that allow computers to learn from data without being explicitly programmed and has been extensively applied to medical imaging. It utilizes algorithms that improve as they are exposed to more data. Deep learning methods belong to representation-learning methods with multiple levels of representation, which process raw data to perform classification or detection tasks. They are made up of artificial neural networks structured in multiple layers to decode imaging raw data. Currently, AI systems have four basic applications in diagnostic imaging departments: computer-aided diagnosis, imaging optimization, workflow improvement, and analytics reporting.

Computer-aided diagnosis is the use of a computer-generated output as an assisting tool for a clinician to make a diagnosis. As an early form of AI, computer-aided diagnosis systems have been used extensively within radiology for many years. The most common applications are for detection of breast cancer on mammography and of pulmonary nodules on chest CT and radiographs.

Image optimization includes processing features for images of optimal quality while reducing quality errors and minimizing dose. It provides better image quality by lowering noise and lowering radiation dose without loss of image quality. This is especially important in neonatal and pediatric imaging, where imaging at the lowest possible dose is critical.

Workflow improvement automate manual tasks and workflow steps to streamline processes, support technologist productivity, save time and money, and enhance patient care. It can involve automated equipment positioning, and patient pose verification optimizes efficiency for radiographers and speed workflow. Many systems also utilize automated technique selection that can improve image consistency and support radiation dose control. There are also systems that provide improved infection control through task automation capabilities, removing the radiographer from direct contact with potentially infectious patients.

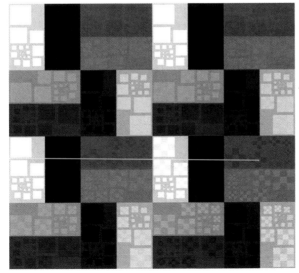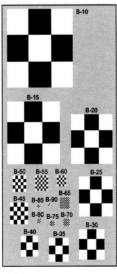

Fig. 8.43 American Association of Physicists in Medicine TG18-BR Briggs test pattern.

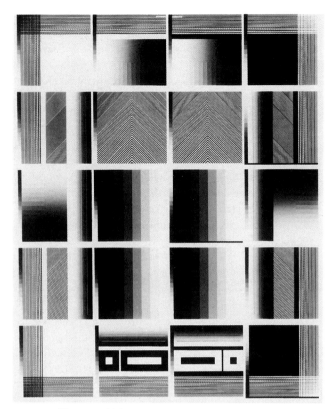

Fig. 8.44 Picture archiving and communication system test pattern. (Courtesy Nuclear Associates, Carle Place, New York.)

Analysis reporting can provide a centralized information management tool for tracking key performance metrics of technologists and imaging equipment. It can deliver continuous performance feedback, allowing managers to analyze results, ensure optimal workflow, implement cost control, and develop improvement plans, all to enhance patient care. As of the writing of this edition, QC of AI systems is the responsibility of the manufacturers and vendors of this equipment, and no government standards have yet been developed.

MISCELLANEOUS SPECIAL PROCEDURES EQUIPMENT

Many diagnostic imaging departments contain a so-called special procedures laboratory, or area in which angiographic, cardiac, and interventional procedures are performed. These types of procedures require additional equipment that is not normally found in standard radiographic and fluoroscopic suites, including pressure injectors for administration of contrast media, image receptors, electrocardiographic units, physiologic monitors, and recorders. Proper functioning of this equipment is critical to a successful procedure and patient well-being; therefore proper QC testing should be performed at least semiannually. However, this equipment varies greatly, and there are currently no uniform national protocols for QC testing. The operating manual for the equipment supplied by the manufacturer should be consulted for this testing, or a procedure should be developed by a medical physicist and the service representative for the equipment. One of the most important pieces of equipment is the pressure injector.

PRESSURE INJECTORS

Pressure injectors are used to administer contrast media into vascular or lymphatic vessels during many diagnostic procedures. Variables such as injected volume and injection flow rate (usually in mL/unit time) should be tested so that what is selected on the programmer is exactly what is administered to the patient. This usually involves the selection of a specific catheter and contrast media (usually the type most commonly used by the facility) and the injector's administration of the material into a beaker or other graduated container. The volume in this container can then be compared with the control panel for variation. This procedure also can be timed with a stopwatch so that the administration time can be compared with the value set on the unit.

The Pressuire Selection of pressure injectors should also be evaluated on a regular basis. This is the maximum pressure allowed to build up in the syringe and not the patient. Depending on the modality, pressures can be set anywhere from 50 pounds per square inch (PSI) to 1200 PSI.

The pause and hold functions also need to be assessed on a regular basis. The pause function will stop the entire injection process for a predetermined amount of time. A hold function will stop the entire injection process until the operator manually resumes the injection.

BONE DENSITOMETRY SYSTEMS

The ability to obtain accurate measurements of bone mineral density can help identify patients with osteoporosis and other atrophic diseases of the bone and minimize their risks for the development of painful and debilitating fractures. Various methods for the measurement of bone mineral density have been developed and marketed.

Single-Photon Absorptiometry

This method of measuring bone mineral density was first described in the early 1960s and uses a radioactive source and a detector (most often a sodium iodide scintillation detector). The radioactive source is most often iodine-125 (^{125}I), which emits a gamma ray with an energy of 35 keV. Because this is a relatively low-energy photon, bone measurement is most often performed in small, distal areas of the body, such as the distal forearm or lateral calcaneus. Radiation measurements are performed with and without the anatomic structure in the path of the gamma ray beam. Because of the difference in the radiation readings, the degree of attenuation of the beam allows for estimation of bone mineral density (i.e., a greater bone mineral density absorbs more of the radiation beam). The accuracy rate for this method approaches 98% if performed correctly. Because ^{125}I has a half-life of about 60 days, periodic replacement and recalibration of the equipment are required. This method is rarely used in clinical practice because of the cost of replacement and disposal of radioactive waste.

Single-Energy X-ray Absorptiometry

Single-energy X-ray absorptiometry is similar to single-photon absorptiometry (SPA), except that an X-ray source replaces the radioactive source. This eliminates the replacement cost of the radioactive material. The X-ray beam is heavily filtered so that it is monoenergetic. The amount of X-ray attenuation is used to estimate the bone mineral density.

Dual-Photon Absorptiometry

This method of bone mineral density measurement was introduced in the early 1970s. As with SPA, dual-photon absorptiometry (DPA) uses a radioactive source, but two different energy photons are released. The most common source is gadolinium-153, which emits gamma ray photons with energies of 44 and 100 keV. The higher energies allow for bone density measurement of thicker areas of the body, including lumbar and thoracic vertebrae. Using photons with two separate energies also allows the DPA technique to withdraw the absorption by soft tissues, which results in a more accurate measurement of bone mineral density than that obtainable with SPA or single-energy X-ray absorptiometry. The detector assembly also could be made larger and be scanned back and forth over the patient to create an image similar to a nuclear medicine scan. As with SPA, DPA uses a radioactive source with a finite half-life; periodic replacement is required. Because of this, DPA has been abandoned in most clinical sites in favor of dual-energy X-ray absorptiometry (DEXA).

Dual-Energy X-ray Absorptiometry

DEXA was introduced clinically in 1987. The premise is similar to that of DPA, except that an X-ray tube is used as the source of radiation rather than a radioactive source. As its name implies, X-rays with two separate energies are used to obtain the bone density data. Obtaining these different energies depends on the manufacturer; they can be obtained by either varying the amount of filtration in the X-ray beam or varying the X-ray generator output (kilovolts [peak]). Early versions of the unit emitted a single pencil beam of radiation and required 5 min or more to scan an area of interest. More advanced systems use a fan-shaped beam with an array of detectors, which drops scan time to as little as 5 seconds. Models are available for either peripheral scanning, known as *peripheral DEXA units* (distal extremities), or central body scanning (vertebra or hip). Both types of units have precision error rates of only 1%–2%. In addition to bone mineral density measurements of virtually any body part, DEXA scanners also allow for measurement of the total body calcium content and body composition (with a whole body scan). The DEXA scanners also are programmed to include a value known as the T-score, which is a comparison with the young adult peak bone mass. It is determined by the number of standard deviations above or below the mean bone mineral density for a healthy 30-year-old adult. The diagnosis of normal, osteopenia, or osteoporosis can be made with the T-score, according to criteria developed by the World Health Organization. T-scores indicate differences between a patient's bone mass

TABLE 8.6 **World Health Organization Definitions of Bone Density Levels**	
Category	**T Score**
Normal	−1 to +1 (bone density is within 1 SD of young adult mean)
Osteopenia	−1 to −2.5 (bone density is between 1 and 2.5 SD below the young adult mean)
Osteoporosis	−2.5 or lower (bone density is 2.5 SD or more below the young adult mean)
Established osteoporosis	−2.5 or lower with one or more osteoporosis-related fractures (bone density is more than 2.5 SD below the young adult mean, and there have been one or more osteoporotic fractures)

SD, Standard deviation.
Courtesy World Health Organization.

density and that of the healthy young adult and are measured in units called standard deviations that were discussed in Chapter 2. A T-score of 0 means that the bone mass density is equal to the normal amount for a healthy young adult. Table 8.6 contains the World Health Organization criteria using T-score standard deviations.

Quantitative Computed Tomography

Quantitative computed tomography uses a CT scanner with the patient placed in the gantry in the supine position. However, a phantom containing reference densities is placed under the patient that allows the computer in the CT scanner to compare the Hounsfield units (mathematical numbers indicating the mass density of the particular structure in the patient) of the vertebral bodies with the values in the phantom to obtain bone density information. This method results in relatively accurate bone density information (especially in the measurement of highly metabolically active trabecular bone in the spine), but the units are relatively large and considerably more expensive than DEXA scanners.

Quantitative Ultrasound

This method of obtaining bone density information has been performed since the mid-1960s. This method uses ultrasound with a relatively low frequency range (200–600 kHz) and measures the amount of attenuation of the ultrasound beam by a portion of bone (most often the calcaneus). Because normal bone generally attenuates more of the ultrasound beam than osteoporotic bone does, the approximate bone mineral density can be calculated. The precision error for measurement of these units is not as good as that of DEXA scanners. However, they are relatively low in cost and small in size, and they do not expose the patient to ionizing radiation. Their main application is their use as a screening tool in providers' offices, with a follow-up DEXA scan for patients who may have osteoporosis.

Digital X-ray Radiogrammetry

Digital X-ray radiogrammetry is a relatively new method of estimating bone density whereby an X-ray image of the hand is obtained and analyzed by computer software. For film-based images, a digitizer is used to scan the image into the computer. Images obtained with CR and DR can be called up from a PACS for analysis. The digital X-ray radiogrammetry technology is based on a radiogrammetry and texture analysis and is insensitive to the relevant variations affecting the quality of the X-ray image. The term "radiogrammetry" is the measure of distances on the image, and the computer software calculates bone volume based on measurements of the cortical bone thickness, bone width, and texture analysis. Texture analysis provides information on the microstructure of the bone, specifically the fraction of holes in the cortical bone. Specific regions of interest are automatically selected by the computer software to minimize error.

QC of Bone Densitometry Equipment

Currently, DEXA scanning is the primary method of evaluating bone mineral density, followed by quantitative ultrasound and quantitative computed tomography. Regardless of the equipment that is being used, careful QC procedures are required to ensure accurate bone mineral density measurements. Because of the variety of equipment in use, no uniform set of QC guidelines is in place for these systems. Technologists who perform these studies have to rely on the QC procedures specified by the manufacturer. These most often involve daily phantom scans, those either supplied by the manufacturer or commercially available from various vendors (Fig. 8.45). The accepted

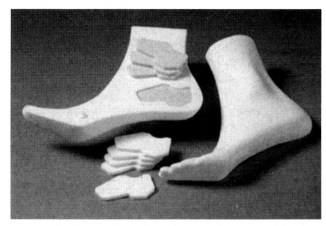

Fig. 8.45 Dual-energy X-ray absorptiometry phantom used for determining the accuracy of bone density measurements.

densities of the phantoms are then compared with what is obtained on the equipment during the phantom scan to determine whether the equipment is performing properly. The values from these daily scans should fall to within ±1.5% of the accepted value (±2.5% for peripheral DEXA systems). The daily values also should be plotted on a control chart with the 1.5% value used as the upper and lower limit. Some manufacturers will provide two phantoms for QC purposes, one for testing the mechanical operation and calibration of the system and the other to mimic bone density to detect a shift in bone mineral density values. Many equipment manufacturers have installed automated QC hardware and software to monitor performance (they will even create a control chart for documentation).

SUMMARY

Advanced imaging systems are commonplace in most diagnostic imaging departments. A current trend in diagnostic imaging is an emphasis toward digital imaging and away from conventional film images to reduce department costs. This should increase the use of these devices in the future; therefore proper QC protocols must be in place to ensure that this equipment is operating within accepted guidelines.

Refer to the Evolve Website at https://evolve.elsevier.com for Student Experiments 8.1: Digital Image Display Monitor Evaluation and 8.2: Computed Radiography (CR) Quality Control.

REVIEW QUESTIONS

1. Which of the following would not be a part of a direct capture AMA?
   a. Scintillator
   b. Capture element
   c. Conversion element
   d. Collection element
2. Which of the following is an advantage of digital radiographic systems vs. analog radiography?
   a. Lower patient dose
   b. Higher-contrast resolution
   c. Edge enhancement
   d. All of the above
3. A quality control test for digital radiographic image receptors is to check for dark noise. What is the reason for this test?
   a. To determine the minimum exposure required for a satisfactory image
   b. To assess the accuracy of the exposure indicator value
   c. To assess the level of detector noise in the system
   d. To evaluate the monitor's calibration
4. Which of the following identifies the fluoroscopic scan mode by which the X-ray tube delivers radiation in short, high-intensity pulses?
   a. Continuous fluoroscopic mode
   b. Pulsed interlaced scan mode
   c. Slow scan mode
   d. All of the above

5. When evaluating low-contrast resolution in digital viewing monitors, which patches of the SMPTE or AAPM TG18-QC test pattern must be visible?
   a. 0% and 100%
   b. 30% and 70%
   c. 5% and 95%
   d. 10% and 80%

6. Types of DSA include (1) temporal mask subtraction, (2) time-interval difference subtraction, and (3) dual-energy subtraction.
   a. 1 and 2
   b. 2 and 3
   c. 1 and 3
   d. 1, 2, and 3

7. In direct capture DR systems, remnant radiation is converted into an electric signal by:
   a. PSP crystals
   b. Amorphous selenium
   c. Cesium iodide
   d. Amorphous silicon

8. Which of the following should be a part of initial acceptance testing of a digital radiographic system?
   a. Evaluation of image uniformity
   b. Presence of dropped pixels
   c. Accuracy of exposure indicator
   d. All of the above

9. A flat panel image receptor is exposed with nothing between the X-ray tube and image receptor. Five images are acquired at five different mAs values. The pixel readings with a certain region of interest are compared to determine the relationship between the X-ray output to the pixel brightness values. What quality control test is being performed?
   a. System sensitivity
   b. System linearity
   c. System repeatability
   d. System uniformity

10. Luminance response evaluation of a digital display device would require which of the following?
    a. Charge-coupled device
    b. Densitometer
    c. Sensitometer
    d. Photometer

9

Mammographic Quality Standards

OBJECTIVES

At the completion of this chapter, the reader should be able to do the following:

- Explain the difference between dedicated mammography equipment and conventional equipment
- Describe the composition of the X-ray tube target in mammographic equipment
- Discuss the advantages of compression during mammographic procedures
- Describe the image receptor systems currently used in mammography
- Indicate the quality control tasks relating to the radiologist and the medical physicist
- Describe the quality control duties of the mammographer on a daily, weekly, quarterly, and semiannual basis
- Describe the various components of a Food and Drug Administration/Mammography Quality Standards Act inspection

KEY TERMS

Adverse event
Annotations and measurements
Beryllium window
Compression
Consumer
Digital breast tomosynthesis

Emission spectrum
Grayscale processing
Image inversion
Magnification
Mammography Quality
    Standards Act

Postprocessing
Serious adverse event
Serious complaint
Target composition
Tissue equalization
Workflow

Mammography is soft tissue radiography of the breast. It requires different equipment and techniques from conventional radiography because of the close similarities among anatomic structures (low subject contrast). Low kilovolt (peak) (kVp) in the 20- to 30-kVp range must be deployed to maximize the amount of photoelectric effect and to enhance differential absorption, which will increase subject contrast. The low contrast of the images makes it very difficult to see early signs of breast cancer, such as microcalcifications. The radiologist must have sufficient contrast and resolution available in the image to visualize microcalcifications as small as 0.1–0.3 mm, and other parenchymal structures. The side effect of using lower-kVp exposure factors is correspondingly higher milliampere-second (mAs) values, which increase the total radiation dose to the patient. The American College of Radiology (ACR) recommends the average glandular dose for a 4.2-cm thick breast should be less than 300 mrad (3 mGy) per view for image receptors used with a grid. If no grid is used, the average glandular dose should be less than 100 mrad (1 mGy) per view. Because the glandular tissue of the breast is inherently radiosensitive, care must be taken to minimize radiation exposure through dedicated equipment and quality control (QC) procedures.

DEDICATED MAMMOGRAPHIC EQUIPMENT

X-ray Generator

The X-ray generators used in mammographic studies must be dedicated solely to mammographic imaging (Fig. 9.1) per the Mammography Quality Standards Act (MQSA). All current mammographic imagers are high-frequency X-ray generators (see Chapter 5) that are smaller in size and less expensive than earlier single- and three-phase mammographic units. High-frequency X-ray generators also provide exceptional exposure reproducibility, which is essential for consistent image quality. The power ratings of mammography generators vary between 3 and 10 kW.

The kVp range available on most units is between 20 kVp and 35 kVp, and typical X-ray tube currents are about 80–200 mA. The advantage of using low kVp is that it produces high subject contrast. The breast is made up exclusively of soft tissue (glandular, fibers and fat), that has a very low subject contrast, so the lower-kVp values will help to increase both subject contrast and visibility of detail. Exposure times are approximately 1 second but can be as long as 4 seconds for dense or thick breasts, or for those with implants. For a normal compressed breast (4.5 cm), a typical X-ray tube voltage is 28 kVp with a milliampere–exposure time combination of about 120 mAs. All systems must be equipped with an automatic exposure control (AEC) system that consists of two to three sensors to regulate the pixel brightness of the

resulting image. Each system should provide an AEC mode that is operable in all combinations of equipment configuration provided (for example, grid, nongrid, magnification, nonmagnification, and various target–filter combinations). The positioning or selection of the detector permits flexibility in the placement of the detector under the target tissue. The size and available positions of the detector must be clearly indicated at the X-ray input surface of the breast compression paddle. The system also must provide a means for the operator to vary the selected signal-to-noise ratio (SNR)/pixel brightness from the normal (zero) setting. The X-ray tube/image receptor assembly must be capable of being fixed in any position and not undergo any unintended motion or fail in the event of power interruption. The backup mAs for grid techniques must be set no higher than 600 mAs, and for nongrid and magnification techniques, 300 mAs.

X-ray Tube

Modern mammographic X-ray units use rotating anode X-ray tubes just as conventional radiographic units do. However, some significant differences exist, including the X-ray tube window, target composition, focal spot size, and source-to-image distance (SID) and target angle.

X-ray Tube Window

X-ray tubes used in conventional radiographic, fluoroscopic, and computed tomographic units incorporate a window made primarily of glass (which is essentially silicon with an atomic number of 14). Because relatively high-kVp exposure factors are used in these studies, absorption of lower-energy X-rays in the window material is acceptable and actually desired. Mammographic X-ray tubes use a thinner glass window or a beryllium window (atomic number of 4), which is less likely to absorb the low-kVp X-rays used in mammographic procedures. The inherent filtration of the beryllium is about 0.1 mm aluminum (Al) equivalent, compared with 0.5-mm Al equivalent for standard radiographic tubes.

Target Composition

Conventional radiographic X-ray tubes use a target composition of a tungsten–rhenium alloy. A mixture of X-rays produced by both bremsstrahlung (the slowing down of the projectile electron, causing a wide range of X-ray energies) and characteristic radiation (X-rays created by electron transitions between orbits resulting in specific or discrete energies) exists in the X-ray beam created with these X-ray tubes. This effect can be demonstrated with an X-ray emission spectrum graph (Fig. 9.2). This wide band of energies may be desirable in conventional radiography but is not desirable in mammography because of the low subject contrast. Factors affecting the X-ray emission spectrum graph include milliamperes, kVp, added filtration, target material, and voltage waveform/ripple.

Milliamperes. The factor of milliamperes changes the amplitude of the curve (height of the y-axis) but not the shape of the curve (Fig. 9.3).

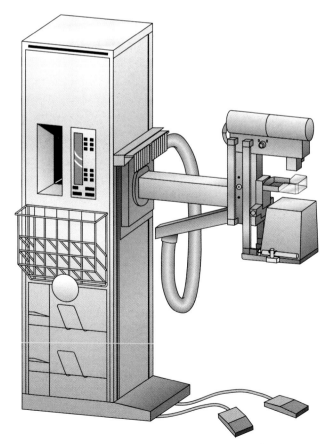

Fig. 9.1 Dedicated mammographic unit.

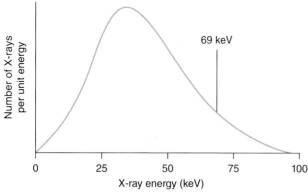

Fig. 9.2 Emission spectrum for tungsten-rhenium target. *keV*, Kiloelectron volt.

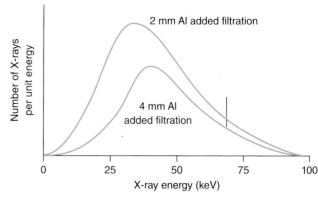

Fig. 9.5 Effect of added filtration on emission spectrum. *Al*, Aluminum; *keV*, kiloelectron volt.

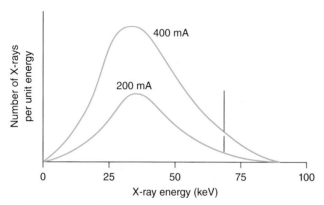

Fig. 9.3 Effect of milliamperes on emission spectrum. *keV*, Kiloelectron volt; *mA*, milliampere.

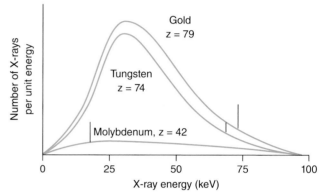

Fig. 9.6 Effect of target material on emission spectrum. *keV*, Kiloelectron volt; *z*, atomic number.

Kilovolts (peak). The factor of kVp changes both the amplitude and the position of the spectrum curve. An increase in kVp shifts the spectrum to the right, indicating greater energy values (Fig. 9.4).

Added filtration. Because filtration affects X-ray quality, the effect on the X-ray emission spectrum is similar to that of kVp. If filtration is increased, the amplitude decreases and the spectrum shifts slightly to the right (Fig. 9.5).

Target material. The amplitude and shape of the emission spectrum graph vary with any changes in the atomic number of the target material. If the atomic number increases,

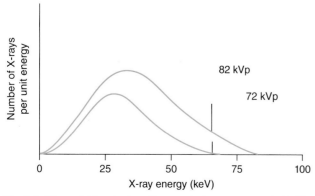

Fig. 9.4 Effect of kilovolts (peak) on emission spectrum. *keV*, Kiloelectron volt; *kVp*, kilovolt (peak).

the continuous portion of the spectrum (bremsstrahlung) increases slightly in amplitude, especially to the high-energy side, whereas the discrete portion of the spectrum (characteristic X-rays) shifts to the right (Fig. 9.6). The target materials used in mammographic X-ray tubes include tungsten, molybdenum, rhodium, or a combination of them.

Tungsten (atomic number 74). Tungsten produces a wide band of X-ray energies, including some that are not useful in mammographic imaging. The emission spectrum is then shaped with filters made of aluminum, molybdenum, or rhodium.

Molybdenum (atomic number 42). The lower atomic number reduces the number of bremsstrahlung X-rays significantly, so virtually all the X-rays exiting the X-ray tube housing are characteristic X-rays of 17.9 kiloelectron volts (keV) and 19.5 keV (well within the K-edge of the image receptor being used). A 30–50-μm molybdenum filter is added to eliminate any additional bremsstrahlung X-rays (which improves subject contrast). This target material is commonly used for normal or fatty breast composition.

Rhodium (atomic number 45). Rhodium creates an emission spectrum similar to that of molybdenum. The characteristic X-rays have an energy of 20.2 keV and 22.7 keV (slightly greater than molybdenum, making it better for more dense breast tissue), and more bremsstrahlung X-rays are created. A 50-μm rhodium filter is used.

Molybdenum–Rhodium–Tungsten alloy. Molybdenum–rhodium–tungsten alloy target material exhibits a mixed-emission

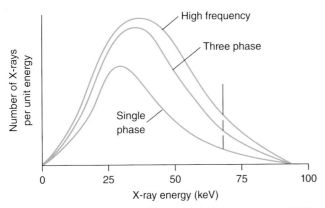

Fig. 9.7 Effect of voltage waveform on emission spectrum. *keV,* Kilo-electron volt.

spectrum with characteristics of each element. With the selection of an aluminum, rhodium, or molybdenum filter, the emission spectrum can be shaped to fit the image receptor used. When more than one target material is available with the mammographic unit, the system must indicate, before exposure, the preselected target material.

Voltage waveform/ripple. High-frequency X-ray generators create X-rays with a greater average energy (quality) and in greater numbers (quantity) than single-phase X-ray generators; therefore the amplitude and relative position of the spectrum are different. With high-frequency generators, the increasing amplitude and the right-shifting spectrum indicate greater average energy (Fig. 9.7).

Focal Spot Size

The spatial resolution required in mammographic images is greater than that of conventional radiography because of the need to demonstrate microcalcifications, which is accomplished with a small focal spot ranging from 0.1 mm (for magnification studies) to 0.3 mm (for routine images). When more than one focal spot is available on the unit, the system must indicate, before exposure, which focal spot is selected. Some manufacturers tilt the X-ray tube toward the cathode side (about 25 degrees), which reduces the effective focal spot size even more. Most mammographic X-ray tubes use a circular focal spot rather than the rectangular focal spots found in conventional radiographic X-ray tubes. Circular focal spots provide better geometric sharpness but have a lower heat capacity because of less surface area of the anode under bombardment by the projectile electrons. Mammographic X-ray tubes often utilize the heel effect (increase in radiation toward the cathode side of the X-ray field) by placing the cathode side of the tube toward the chest wall (not all units allow for rotation of the X-ray tube). However, because geometric "unsharpness" is also greater toward the cathode side of the X-ray field, any suspicious areas near the chest wall are often reimaged with the anode side closer to the chest wall.

Source-to-Image Distance and Target Angle

The SID used in dedicated mammographic units ranges from 50–80 cm, with 65 cm being typical. Because of this relatively short SID, a larger target angle is necessary for mammographic X-ray tubes (angles of 22–24 degrees compared with 7–13 degrees for standard radiographic X-ray tubes) to create an X-ray field size large enough to cover the image receptor.

Compression

All modern mammographic units must be equipped with a compression device, usually made of radiolucent plastic. The amount of X-ray transmission through these devices is about 80% at 30 kVp. The function of these devices is to compress the breast tissue gently with a force of between 25 lb and 45 lb (111 N and 200 N). An automatic adjust-and-release mechanism is found on most systems. Each mammographic system must provide (1) an initial power-driven compression activated by hands-free controls operable from both sides of the patient and (2) fine adjustment compression controls operable from both sides of the patient. The chest wall edge of the compression paddle should be straight and parallel to the edge of the image receptor. The advantages of breast compression are shown in Box 9.1. The principal disadvantage of compression is patient discomfort.

Mammographic systems also must be equipped with various-size compression paddles that match the sizes of all full-field image receptors provided for the system. The compression paddle should be flat and parallel to the breast support table and should not deflect from parallel by more than 1 cm at any point on the surface of the compression paddle when compression is applied.

Grids

The presence of scattered radiation in a diagnostic image always reduces or lowers image contrast. Because mammographic images have an inherently low subject contrast, it is imperative that scattered radiation be reduced as much as possible. Carbon fiber–interspaced grids are often used to reduce scattered radiation (and therefore help to increase image contrast). The grid ratios range from 3:1–5:1, and the grid frequency can range from 30–50 lines/cm. The mammographic grids also are focused to the X-ray source and move during the exposure to eliminate grid lines. Uniformity of construction and motion is paramount for proper image quality. A new type of crosshatch grid, called the *high transmission cellular* (HTC) *grid,* has been developed for mammographic systems. Crosshatch grids are superior at removing scattered radiation (compared with focused or parallel linear grids) but require significantly greater mAs exposure because of increased

---

BOX 9.1   Advantages of Breast Compression

1. Because of the part's immobilization, motion blur is reduced.
2. Part thickness is more uniform, which manifests as more uniform optical densities in the final image.
3. Bringing all object structures closer to the image receptor reduces geometric "unsharpness" and improves spatial resolution.
4. Because the part is thinner, patient dose and scattered radiation are reduced.

absorption of primary radiation. For alleviation of this problem, the HTC mammographic grid uses copper as the grid strip material (compared with lead in conventional grids) and air as the interspace material. The grid ratio of the HTC mammographic grid is 3.8:1. Systems with film/screen image receptors should be equipped with moving grids matched to all image receptor sizes provided. Systems used for magnification procedures should be capable of operating with the grid removed from between the X-ray source and the image receptor. Some studies have suggested that a grid can be omitted from mammographic examinations performed with full-field digital mammography (FFDM) for breasts less than 5 cm thick when compressed to decrease patient dose because postprocessing of the digital images can maintain contrast despite the lack of a grid. Virtual grid software programs are also available to remove scatter without having a physical grid in place.

Image Receptors

In the past, most mammographic examinations that have been performed have used film/screen combinations as the primary image receptor. Full-field digital and computed radiographic (CR) mammographic systems have replaced film/screen image receptors in many facilities. Regardless of the image receptor used, exposure to the patient should be kept as low as reasonably achievable. The use of an AEC system and having a working technique chart available (Fig. 9.8) helps obtain precise techniques.

CR and digital radiographic (DR) systems have been common imaging systems for conventional radiography. However, early versions of these systems tended to have less spatial resolution than film/screen imaging systems and a greater capital cost, which slowed their application into mammographic imaging. On January 28, 2000, the Food and Drug Administration (FDA) approved the Senographe 2000D FFDM system for marketing and immediate use in facilities certified for film/screen imaging systems according to the Mammography Quality Standards Act (MQSA). As of the writing of this edition, several additional digital mammographic systems have been approved by the FDA, along with digital breast tomosynthesis (DBT).

The spatial resolution for 2D mammography systems must be ≥4.0 line pairs per millimeter (lp/mm) for contact mode and 6.0 lp/mm for magnification mode. For DBT systems, spatial resolution must be ≥2.0 lp/mm for contact mode. The images may be read directly from the monitor (soft copy review) or from hard copy images created by a dry laser printer. These hard copy images provide better contrast resolution and better visibility of detail than images from traditional film/screen mammography. The dry laser printer, with a maximum density (D_{max}) of 3.5 or greater, a base + fog level of less than 0.25, and 16-bit images with at least 12-bit gray levels, is recommended for printing hard copy digital mammographic images. They should support true-size printing, and images should be justified so that the chest wall is printed as close to the edge of the film as possible by the printer. In addition, film artifacts are virtually eliminated. The Digital Mammographic Imaging Screening Trial, which was sponsored by the National Cancer Institute and coordinated by the ACR Imaging Network, demonstrated that digital mammographic systems are as effective as analog systems as a screening tool. For some women (such as those with dense breasts), digital mammography (DM) is more effective than film/screen in finding cancer.

A major advantage of digital imaging is postprocessing of the image, which can improve lesion visibility in underexposed or overexposed regions. Postprocessing is a manipulation of the image data in the memory of the computer before the image is displayed on a monitor. Postprocessing functions available with FFDM and CR systems may include the following:

1. Tissue equalization—Image processing that compensates for varying breast tissue densities so the entire breast (from the chest wall to the skin line) can be visualized in a single image
2. Magnification—Electronic digital zoom with software manipulation that can reduce the need to take additional magnification views, as with film/screen mammography
3. Image inversion—Conversion of a negative image (standard radiographic image) to a positive image (meaning a reverse of the negative image, where white areas on the negative image are black on the positive image and vice versa)
4. Grayscale processing—Manipulation of grayscale values displayed in the image, including windowing (or window width), which controls image contrast, and leveling (or window level), which controls image brightness (comparable with optical density) (OD in film/screen imaging), allowing for increased contrast resolution
5. Annotations and measurements—Software manipulation allowing electronic annotation on the image and electronic measurement tools for calculating sizes and volumes

Improved workflow (the number of patients imaged per hour) is another advantage of FFDM and CR mammography over the older film/screen mammography. A report published by the London-based Center for Evidence-based Purchasing looked at an average of 16,000 screening mammograms per year between 2002 and 2006 and found the following times to produce four mammographic images:

Film/screen: 3.5–6.5 min
CR: 2.5–4 min
FFDM: 1.3–4.7 min

Another advantage of digital systems is the use of scanning software known as *computer-aided detection* or *artificial intelligence* to help radiologists locate suspicious areas in the images. Initial studies have shown this type of software has sensitivities as much as 90%, so they can help increase the accuracy of mammographic diagnoses. Patient dose in DM is the same or less (up to 50% less in some studies) than that obtained with film/screen systems. Fewer recalls for additional imaging with DM also contribute to lower patient dose.

Patient convenience/satisfaction also is considered an advantage for DM because less time is required to perform mammographic procedures, especially with FFDM. This procedure is shorter because the image is available in less than a minute with digital systems, compared with 3.5–6.5 min with film/screen mammography.

Mammography Technique Chart

Image Mode *(2D, 2D w/Add-on DBT, DBT)* _____

Facility Name _____   **MAP ID-Unit#** *(00000-00)* _____ - _____

Mfr & Model _____   Room ID _____

Survey Date _____

Screening/Diagnostic Digital Mammography

Compressed Breast Thickness	50% Fatty - 50% Dense Breast		
	AEC Mode	Target/Filter	kVp
< 3 cm			
3 to 5 cm			
5 to 7 cm			
> 7 cm			

Implant Displaced Mammography Views (Manual Technique)

Breast Size	Target/Filter	kVp	mAs
Small			
Medium			
Large			

ACR DM Phantom Technique (Weekly QC)

	Digital Mammography	DBT	2D w/DBT Fixture
AEC mode			
Paddle size (IR Size)			
Paddle type (reg or flex)			
View/selected image type			
Slice or Slab # (DBT only)			
Compression force			
AEC cell position *(if avail)*			
Target/filter *(if app)*			
kVp *(if app)*			
Density setting *(if app)*			

Fig. 9.8 Technique chart for mammographic imaging with an automatic exposure control system.

A new application of DM is digital breast tomosynthesis or DBT (also known as 3D mammography), which requires multiple images from many angles to generate tomographic slices that can eliminate overlapping structures. This process combines digital image capture and processing with simple tube/detector motion. FFDM image receptors are required for DRT systems because they provide rapid readout. This requires about 10 static exposures at slightly different central ray angles through the region of interest. Depending on the system, either a continuous sweep or stop-and-shoot motion of the tube can be utilized.

Each exam requires a specific sweep angle that can range from 10 to 50 degrees. Larger sweep angles provide better separation of structures and resolution but suffer more elongation. Postacquisition image processing permits reconstruction of any desired plane through the exposed area. Postacquisition software can also modify blur, image brightness, contrast, and resolution. Playback of the sequence of slices is via a cine loop, similar to that used in computed tomographic scanning. These images can be used ultimately with three-dimensional visualization software to create three-dimensional images of breast structure. The main benefits of DBT are:

- Greater accuracy for earlier and easier detection. 3D mammography has been shown to improve breast cancer detection by 27%–50%.
- Fewer callbacks. 3D mammography has been shown to lower recall rates by 17%–40%.

The Centers for Medicare and Medicaid Services has enacted a policy to facilitate access to these examinations by covering beneficiaries for tomosynthesis and urges private payers to do the same. As of the writing of this edition, the FDA has approved the following DBT systems:

- GE Senographe Pristina with DBT option—March 3, 2017
- Fujifilm ASPIRE Cristalle with DBT option—January 10, 2017
- Siemens MAMMOMAT Inspiration with DBT option—April 21, 2015
- GE SenoClaire DBT system—August 26, 2014
- Hologic Selenia Dimensions DBT system—February 11, 2011

An emerging application of DM is dual-energy subtraction imaging (similar to the type being used in chest imaging), which can enhance certain structures by subtracting background structures from the region of interest.

The main disadvantage of digital systems are greater capital cost for the equipment (currently about three to five times the cost of a film/screen system), greater maintenance costs, and greater adjunct costs (such as 5-megapixel primary viewing monitors that can cost up to $40,000 and last about 2 years). Because reimbursement of mammographic services by private insurance companies and the federal government (Medicare, Medicaid) is relatively low, it has been difficult for healthcare organizations to recover their investment in these systems. Technological issues also pose problems, such as file storage issues (the file size of digital mammograms may be as large as 200 MB) and remote viewing (person accessing the image also must have a 5-megapixel high-resolution monitor to be able to diagnose the image). Therefore picture archiving and communication systems must be able to store as much as 40 GB of image data per month just for mammographic images and must have a 5-megapixel monitor available to view the images for diagnosis, increasing both the cost and operational difficulties of these systems. For picture archiving and communication systems to transmit digital mammographic images, lossless compression capability is essential. Magnification studies may also be of concern in DM. Film/screen mammography uses geometric magnification, such as increased object-to-image distance (OID) and/or decreased SID, to obtain magnification studies. Digital systems can use electronic magnification, which usually increases pixel size to magnify the image. This results in less exposure to the patient and a shorter examination time but greatly decreases the spatial resolution compared with those studies using geometric magnification.

Magnification Mammography

Magnification studies are common during mammographic procedures to investigate small microcalcifications or lesions that may appear ambiguous at normal size. They are requested when the visibility of detail in small structures or microcalcifications needs to be enhanced, and as many as 10% of patients require additional magnification views. According to the FDA, mammographic systems used to perform noninterventional, problem-solving procedures should have radiographic magnification capability available for use by the operator. These systems should provide, at a minimum, at least one magnification value within the range of 1.4–2. This magnification factor is determined by the ratio of the image size compared with the object size or by the ratio of SID to source-to-object distance. Magnification of the image is achieved by increasing the OID, which reduces the source-to-object distance (typically 35 cm in magnification studies). Because this increase also reduces image sharpness, it is essential that the effective focal spot size for magnification studies not exceed 0.1 mm. However, the small focal spot can only tolerate low tube currents (25 mA), which can result in long exposure times of several seconds. The air gap created by the increased OID normally eliminates the need for a grid, thereby reducing the required mAs.

Stereotactic Localization

Stereotactic localization is a method that has been developed to perform core needle biopsies using mammographic imaging. As with the old process of stereoradiography, two views of the breast are acquired, with the central ray at a different angle for each view (usually within 15 degrees of normal). Images of the lesion shift by an amount depending on lesion depth, which permits a 3D localization of the lesion. A biopsy needle gun is positioned at the correct location and then fired to obtain a core sample of the tissue. This type of biopsy is quick, accurate, and less invasive than other methods, with less scarring of the breast tissue. Full-field digital systems are better suited than film/screen systems for this technique because image acquisition is faster (no film processing is required), and the computer software can align the two images for optimum visualization.

MAMMOGRAPHIC QUALITY ASSURANCE

The importance of mammography to an early diagnosis of breast cancer has been well demonstrated. Breast cancer can be detected by means of mammograms as early as 2 years before a lump can be felt during a manual examination. For breast cancer detection to be accomplished successfully, the images must be of the highest quality and the interpreting physician must be highly trained. This means a detailed quality management program must be in place to minimize any variations, which are even more detrimental to image quality in mammography because of the low subject contrast.

MQSA and the Mammography Quality Standards Reauthorization Act

Before 1992, quality standards for mammography were the responsibility of individual state agencies. The ACR began a voluntary Mammography Accreditation Program in 1987 that required specific QC and quality assurance procedures for equipment and personnel. Approximately 30% of facilities that initially applied for ACR accreditation failed on their first attempt. Because so few facilities sought and obtained ACR accreditation voluntarily, concern of mammographic image quality prompted the US Senate Committee on Labor and Human Resources to hold hearings on breast cancer in 1992. This committee discovered many problems with mammographic procedures in the United States, including poor-quality equipment, a lack of quality assurance procedures, poorly trained interpreting physicians, and no consistent oversight or facility inspections. These discoveries led to the enactment of Public Law 102-539 (the MQSA), which passed on October 27, 1992. This law required all facilities (except for those of the Department of Veterans Affairs) to be accredited by an approved accrediting body and certified by the Secretary of Health and Human Services to provide mammography services legally after October 1, 1994. The Secretary of Health and Human Services delegated the authority to approve accreditation bodies and to certify facilities to the FDA. Certification of facilities can be through the FDA or by the states of Illinois, Iowa, or South Carolina. These state agencies use the same certification requirements as the FDA. The MQSA has been superseded by the Mammography Quality Standards Reauthorization Act (MQSRA) of 1998. As part of the new law, final FDA regulations regarding mammographic procedures became effective on April 28, 1999, replacing interim regulations that were used during the original law. In 2002, the amended final regulations were published with new subparts that included addressing alternatives such as digital mammographic systems. The final regulations emphasize performance objectives rather than specify the behavior and manner of compliance.

The main provisions of MQSA and MQSRA include the following:

- Accreditation of mammography facilities by private, nonprofit organizations (such as the ACR) or state agencies that have met the standards established by the FDA (including Illinois, Iowa, and Texas) and have been approved by the FDA
- An annual mammography facility physics survey, consultation, and evaluation performed by a qualified medical physicist
- Annual inspection of mammographic facilities performed by FDA–certified federal and state inspectors
- Establishment of initial and continuing qualification standards for interpreting physicians, radiologic technologists, medical physicists, and mammographic facility inspectors
- Specification of boards or organizations eligible to certify the adequacy of training and experience of mammography personnel
- Establishment of quality standards for mammographic equipment and practices, including quality assurance and QC programs
- Establishment of infection control policies and procedures for cleaning and disinfecting mammographic equipment after contact with blood or other potentially infectious materials

- Standards governing the final assessment of findings in the evaluation of mammographic provision in the final report of overall final assessment findings, classified as one of the following categories:
  1. Negative—nothing on which to comment (if the interpreting physician is aware of clinical findings or symptoms, despite the negative assessment, these should be explained)
  2. Benign—also a negative assessment
  3. Probably benign—findings have a high probability of being benign
  4. Suspicious—findings without all the characteristic morphology of breast cancer but indicating a definite probability of being malignant
  5. Highly suggestive of malignancy—findings have a high probability of being malignant
  6. Incomplete/additional imaging evaluation needed—assigned in cases in which no final assessment category can be determined because of an incomplete workup; reasons for a nonassessment must be stated by the interpreting physician
- Communication of mammography results to the patient. Each facility should send each patient a summary of the mammography report written in lay terms within 30 days of the mammographic examination. If assessments are "suspicious" or "highly suggestive of malignancy," the facility should make reasonable attempts to ensure the results are communicated to the patient as soon as possible.
- Record keeping. Each facility that performs mammograms should maintain mammographic images and reports in a permanent medical record of the patient for a period of not less than 5 years, or not less than 10 years if no additional mammograms of the patient are performed at the facility, or a longer period of time if mandated by state or local law. This storage may be in either digital data or hardcopy films. Each facility should, on request or on behalf of the patient, transfer permanently or temporarily the original mammograms (hardcopy films) and copies of the patient's reports to a medical institution or to a physician or healthcare provider of the patient, or to the patient directly.
- Specific regulations for accrediting bodies
- General facility provisions—such as requirements for the content and terminology in the mammography report, specific guidelines for mammography reports, definition of the responsibilities of facility personnel, review of mammography medical outcomes data every 12 months, and standards for examinees with breast implants—and the requirement of facilities to develop a system for collecting and resolving serious complaints
- Personnel regulations for interpreting physicians, medical physicists, and mammographers. Facilities should maintain records to document the qualifications of all personnel who worked at the facility as interpreting physicians, radiologic technologists, or medical physicists. These records must be

available for review for MQSA inspectors. Records of personnel no longer employed by the facility should not be discarded until the next annual inspection has been completed and the FDA has determined that the facility is in compliance with MQSA personnel requirements.

Quality Control Responsibilities

The MQSA designates specific responsibilities for various members of the diagnostic imaging department.

Radiologist (Interpreting Physician)

The primary responsibility for mammography QC is the lead interpreting physician or radiologist. Minimum qualifications include a license to practice medicine and certification by the American Board of Radiology, the American Osteopathic Board of Radiology, or the Royal College of Physicians and Surgeons of Canada, and at least 3 months of documented full-time training in the interpretation of mammograms. The physician or radiologist also must continue to read and interpret 960 mammographic examinations for 24 months and obtain at least 15 category I continuing education units (CEUs) in mammography during a 36-month period. These individuals also have the responsibility of following up with any patient who has a positive diagnosis.

Medical Physicist

Medical physicists are responsible for the QC evaluation of the mammographic equipment. They must have a license or state approval or be certified by an FDA-approved accrediting body. Their continuing experience must be maintained by surveying at least two mammographic facilities and at least six mammographic units in a 24-month period and obtain at least 15 continuing medical education/continuing education unit (CME/CEUs) in mammography during a 36-month period.

The FDA mandates that, at least once a year, each facility must undergo mammographic equipment evaluation (MEE), which must be performed by a medical physicist, and the following QC tests must be performed: AEC; kVp accuracy and reproducibility; focal spot condition; beam quality and half-value layer (HVL); breast entrance air kerma and AEC reproducibility; dosimetry; X-ray field/light field, image receptor, and compression paddle alignment; uniformity of screen speed, system artifacts, radiation output, decompression, QC tests for other modalities, viewbox illuminators and viewing conditions, comparison of test results with action limits, and additional evaluations.

Automatic exposure control. The AEC must be capable of maintaining proper image receptor exposure in digital systems when the thickness of a homogenous material is varied over a range of 2–6 cm and the kVp is varied appropriately for such thickness over the kVp range used clinically in the facility (in contact mode only). If this requirement cannot be met, a technique chart should be developed showing appropriate techniques (kVp and SNR control settings) for different breast thicknesses and compositions. The ACR Mammographic Accreditation programs mandates that the medical physicist performs an annual test to assess the performance of the AEC function and to verify consistency in

detector signal-to-noise level for a range of breast thickness. For the initial MEE and annual inspection, the SNR must be ≥40.0 for 4.0 cm in contact mode and must be within ±15% of MEE over the clinically used phantom thickness and imaging modes.

Kilovolt (Peak) accuracy and reproducibility. The kVp must be accurate within ±5% of the indicated or selected kVp at the lowest clinical kVp level that can be measured by a kVp test device, the most commonly used clinical kVp, and the highest available clinical kVp level. The coefficient of variation of reproducibility of the kVp must be equal to or less than 0.02 (test at the most common kVp used clinically).

Focal spot condition. According to MQSA regulations, facilities must evaluate focal spot condition only by determining the system spatial resolution. These are performed for all target materials, focal spots, and image receptors used clinically. They should be performed for both contact mode (using the most commonly used SID) and magnification mode (using the SID giving a magnification factor of 1.5). The system resolution requirement is that the image receptor used in the facility should provide a minimum resolution of 11 lp/mm when a high-contrast resolution bar test pattern is oriented with the bars perpendicular to the anode-cathode axis, and a minimum of 13 lp/mm when the bars are parallel to the axis. The bar pattern should be placed 4.5 cm above the breast support surface, centered with respect to the chest wall edge of the image receptor, and positioned with its edge within 1 cm of the chest wall edge of the image receptor. When focal spot dimensions are measured, standards of the National Electrical Manufacturers Association apply (Table 9.1).

Beam quality and half-value layer. At a given kVp setting in the mammographic kilovoltage range (below 50 kVp), the HVL determined with the compression paddle in place must be equal to or greater than the values in the table from the FDA regulations listed in Table 9.2.

Breast entrance air kerma and automatic exposure control reproducibility. Each AEC detector or cell must be tested and should produce the same air kerma reading at the same console settings. The coefficient of variation must not exceed 0.05.

Dosimetry. The average glandular dose delivered during a single craniocaudal view of an FDA-accepted phantom (Fig. 9.9A) simulating a standard breast must not exceed

TABLE 9.1 Standards of the National Electrical Manufacturers Association for Focal Spot Tolerance Limits

Nominal Focal Spot Size (mm)	Maximum Measured Dimensions	
	Width (mm)	Length (mm)
0.1	0.15	0.15
0.15	0.23	0.23
0.2	0.3	0.3
0.3	0.45	0.65
0.4	0.6	0.85
0.6	0.9	1.3

TABLE 9.2 Values for Minimum Acceptable HVL X-ray Tube Voltage (kVp) and Minimum HVL

Designed Operating Range (kVp)	Measured Operating Voltage (kVp)	Minimum HVL (mm Al)
>50	20	0.2
	25	0.25
	30	0.3

Al, Aluminum; *HVL*, half-value layer; *kVp*, kilovolt (peak).

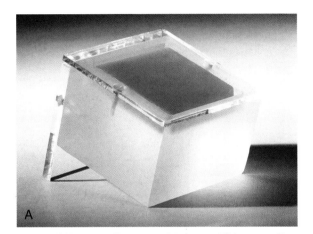

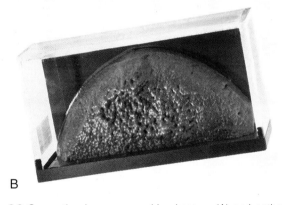

Fig. 9.9 Conventional mammographic phantom (A) and anthropomorphic (lifelike) phantom (B). (Courtesy Nuclear Associates, Inc., Carle Place, New York.)

3 mGy (0.3 rad) per exposure. The dose must be determined for all image receptors, targets, and filters for a standard breast.

X-ray field/light field, image receptor, and compression paddle alignment. All systems must have beam-limiting devices that allow the entire chest wall edge of the X-ray field to extend to the chest wall edge of the image receptor and to provide a means to ensure the X-ray field does not extend beyond any edge of the image receptor by more than 2% of the SID. If a light field that passes through the X-ray beam limitation device is provided, it must be aligned with the X-ray field so the total of any misalignment of the edges of the light field and the X-ray field along either the length or the width of the visually defined field at the plane of the breast support surface does not exceed 2% of the SID. The chest wall edge of the compression paddle must not extend beyond the chest wall edge of the image receptor by more than 1% of the SID when tested with the compression paddle placed above the breast support surface at a distance equivalent to standard breast thickness. The shadow of the vertical edge of the compression paddle should not be visible on the image. Testing is to be performed on all combinations of collimators, image receptor sizes, targets, and focal spots clinically used for full-field imaging in the contact mode.

System artifacts. System artifacts must be evaluated with a high-grade, defect-free sheet of homogenous material large enough to cover the mammography image receptor and should be performed for all cassette sizes used in the facility with a grid appropriate for the cassette being tested. System artifacts also must be evaluated for all available focal spot sizes and target filter combinations used clinically.

Radiation output. The system must be capable of producing a minimum output of 7 mGy air kerma/s (800 mR/s) when operating at 28 kVp in standard mammography (molybdenum per molybdenum) mode at any SID where the system is designed to operate and when measured by a detector with its center located 4.5 cm above the breast support surface with the compression paddle in place between the source and the detector. The system must be capable of maintaining the required minimum radiation output averaged over a 3-second period. Instruments used by medical physicists in their annual survey to measure the air kerma or air kerma rate from a mammographic unit should be calibrated at least once every 2 years and each time the instrument is repaired. The instrument calibration must be traceable to a national standard (either by the National Institute of Standards and Technology or by a laboratory that participates in and has met the National Institute of Standards and Technology's proficiency test requirements) and calibrated with an accuracy of ±6% (95% confidence level) in the mammographic energy range.

Decompression. If the system is equipped with a provision for automatic decompression after completion of an exposure or interruption of power to the system, the system must be tested to confirm it provides (1) an override capability to allow maintenance of compression, (2) a continuous display of the override status, and (3) a manual emergency compression release that can be activated in the event of power or automatic release failure.

Viewbox illuminators and viewing conditions. Viewbox illuminators and viewing conditions are not listed by the FDA in 21 Code of Federal Regulations Part 900 as an annual duty but are recommended by the ACR in its 1999 edition of the *Mammography Quality Control Manual.* The acrylic plastic (Plexiglas) illuminator fronts should be clean and free of any loose dirt, marks from grease pens, or scratches. The viewbox luminance, color temperature, and ambient light conditions (room luminance) should be measured with the equipment and procedures outlined in Chapter 4. The luminance from the center of the illuminator should be at least 3000 nit, and the room luminance (ambient light), should be 50 lux or less. Fluorescent bulbs should be replaced at least every 2 years. The MQSA specifies that facilities must make available to the interpreting physicians special lights for film illumination (hot lights) capable of producing light levels greater than those provided by the viewbox. Facilities also must ensure that film masking devices that can limit the illuminated area to a region equal to or smaller than the exposed portion of the film are available to all physicians interpreting for the facility.

Comparison of test results with action limits. After completion of the annual QC tests, the facility should compare the test results with the corresponding specified action limits or, for digital modalities, with the manufacturer's recommended action limits. If the test results fall outside the action limits, the source of the problem should be identified, and corrective actions taken (1) before any additional examinations are performed or any films processed with a component of the mammography system that failed any tests of dosimetry or QC tests for digital systems and (2) within 30 days for all other tests.

Additional evaluations. Additional evaluations of mammography units or image processors must be conducted whenever a new unit or processor is installed, when a unit or processor is disassembled and reassembled at the same time or at a new location, or when major components of a mammography unit or processor equipment are changed or repaired. All problems must be corrected before new or changed equipment is put into service for examinations or film processing. The MEE should be performed by a medical physicist or by an individual who is supervised directly by a medical physicist. Major repairs would include the following:

- AEC replacement, thickness compensation internal[1] adjustment, AEC sensor replacement, AEC circuit board replacement
- Bucky replacement if the AEC system is also replaced
- Collimation system, including collimator replacement and collimator reassembly with blade replacement
- Filter replacement
- X-ray unit kVp, milliampere, or time internal adjustments, high-voltage generator replacement, X-ray tube replacement, installation, reassembly
- Software changes and upgrades for digital mammographic systems

The ACR medical physicist's tests for DM systems are summarized below:

Test	Minimum Frequency	Corrective Action Timeframe
MEE MQSA requirements	MEE	Before clinical use
ACR DM phantom image quality	MEE and annual	Before clinical use
DBT z resolution	MEE and annual	Within 30 days
Spatial resolution	MEE and annual	Within 30 days
DBT volume coverage	MEE and annual	Before clinical use
Automatic exposure control system performance	MEE and annual	Within 30 days
Average glandular dose	MEE and annual	Before clinical use

Test	Minimum Frequency	Corrective Action Timeframe
Unit checklist	MEE and annual	Critical: before clinical use; less critical: within 30 days
Computed radiography (if applicable)	MEE and annual	Before clinical use
Acquisition workstation monitor QC	MEE and annual	Within 30 days; before clinical use for severe defects
Radiologist workstation monitor QC	MEE and annual	Within 30 days; before clinical use for severe defects
Film printer QC (if applicable)	MEE and annual	Before clinical use
Evaluation of site's technologist QC program	MEE and annual	Within 30 days
Evaluation of display device technologist QC program	MEE and annual	Within 30 days
Beam quality (half-value layer) assessment	MEE or troubleshooting	MEE—before clinical use; Troubleshooting—within 30 days
kVp accuracy and reproducibility	MEE or troubleshooting	MEE—before clinical use; Troubleshooting—within 30 days
Collimation assessment	MEE or troubleshooting	MEE—before clinical use; Troubleshooting—within 30 days
Ghost image evaluation	troubleshooting	Before clinical use
Viewbox luminance	troubleshooting	NA

ACR DM, American College of Radiology digital mammography; *DBT*, digital breast tomosynthesis; *kVp*, kilovolt (peak); *MEE*, mammography equipment evaluation; *MQSA*, Mammography Quality Standards Act; *NA*, not applicable; *QC*, quality control.

Mammography equipment evaluation. The ACR Mammography Accreditation program requires the medical physicist to perform a MEE upon initial accreditation and then annually thereafter. If new mammography equipment or image output devices (review workstations) were obtained, disassembled, and then reassembled (either at the same or a new location), or a major component was changed or repaired since the previous inspection, a new MEE is required. This is to conform to MQSA Requirements for Equipment [FDA Rule Sec. 900.12 (b)] and only applies to MEE. The ACR form is found in Fig. 9.10.

ACR phantom image quality. The medical physicist will use an ACR DM phantom (Fig. 9.11) to determine score for fibers, specks, and masses, as well as assess SNR, contrast-to-noise ratio (CNR) and distance measurement accuracy of the software system. ACR DM phantom image must be free of clinically

1. Mammography Equipment Evaluation (MEE)

Facility Name ....

Mfr & Model ....

MAP ID-Unit# *(00000-00)* .... - ....

Room ID ....

Survey Date ....

MQSA Requirements for Equipment [FDA Rule Sec. 900.12 (b)] - only applies to MEE

Feature	FDA Rule	Requirement	Meets? Yes/No/NA
Motion of tube-image receptor	3(i)	The assembly shall be capable of being fixed in any position where it is designed to operate. Once fixed in any such position, it shall not undergo unintended motion.	
	3(ii)	This mechanism shall not fail in the event of power interruption.	
Image receptor sizes	4(iii)	Systems used for magnification procedures shall be capable of operation with the grid removed from between the source and image receptor.	
Light fields	5	For any mammography system with a light beam that passes through the X-ray beam-limiting device, the light shall provide an average illumination of not less than 160 lux (15 ft-candles) at 100 cm or the maximum source-image receptor distance (SID), whichever is less.	
Magnification	6(i)	Systems used to perform noninterventional problem-solving procedures shall have radiographic magnification capability available for use by the operator.	
	6(ii)	Systems used for magnification procedures shall provide, at a minimum, at least one magnification value within the range of 1.4 to 2.0.	
Focal spot selection	7(i)	When more than one focal spot is provided, the system shall indicate, prior to exposure, which focal spot is selected.	
	7(ii)	When more than one target material is provided, the system shall indicate, prior to exposure, the preselected target material.	
	7(iii)	When the target material and/or focal spot is selected by a system algorithm that is based on the exposure or on a test exposure, the system shall display, after the exposure, the target material and/or focal spot actually used during the exposure.	
Application of compression	8(i)(A)	Each system shall provide an initial power-driven compression activated by hands-free controls operable from both sides of the patient.	
	8(i)(B)	Each system shall provide fine adjustment compression controls operable from both sides of the patient.	
Compression paddle	8(ii)(A)	Systems shall be equipped with different sized compression paddles that match the sizes of all full-field image receptors provided for the system.	
	8(ii)(B)	Compression paddle shall be flat and parallel to the breast support table and shall not deflect from parallel by more than 1.0 cm at any point on the surface of the compression paddle when compression is applied.	
	8(ii)(C)	Equipment intended by the manufacturer's design to not be flat and parallel to the breast support table during compression shall meet the manufacturer's design specifications and maintenance requirements.	
	8(ii)(D)	Chest wall edge of the compression paddle shall be straight and parallel to the edge of the image receptor.	
	8(ii)(E)	Chest wall edge may be bent upward to allow for patient comfort but shall not appear on the image.	
Technique factor selection and display	9(i)	Manual selection of mAs or at least one of its component parts (mA and/or time) shall be available.	
	9(ii)	The technique factors (kVp and either mA and seconds or mAs) to be used during an exposure shall be indicated before the exposure begins, except when AEC is used, in which case the technique factors that are set prior to the exposure shall be indicated.	
	9(iii)	Following AEC mode use, the system shall indicate the actual kVp and mAs (or mA and time) used during the exposure.	
Lighting**	14	The facility shall make special lights for film illumination, i.e., hot-lights, capable of producing light levels greater than that provided by the view box, available to the interpreting physicians.	
Film masking devices**	15	Film masking devices that can limit the illuminated area to a region equal to or smaller than the exposed portion of the film are available to all interpreting physicians interpreting for the facility.	
Beam quality assessment	*	Must meet the specifications of FDA's Performance Standards for Ionizing Radiatiion Emitting Products (Part 1020.30)	
kVp accuracy &	*	The mean kVp must not differ from the nominal by more than + 5% of the nominal kVp.	
	*	The coefficient of variation must be ≤0.02.	
Collimation assessment	*	If sum of left plus right edge deviations or anterior plus chest edge deviations exceeds 2% of SID, seek service adjustment.	
	*	If X-ray field exceeds image receptor at any side by more than + 2% of SID or if X-ray field falls within image receptor on the chest wall side, seek service adjustment.	
	*	If chest-wall edge of compression paddle is within the image receptor or projects beyond the chest-wall edge of the image receptor by more than 1% of SID, seek service correction.	
		Overall Pass/Fail	

* ACR adoption for MEEs of pertinent sections in FDA Rule 900.12(e)(5) that apply to annual testing of screen-film only
** NA is acceptable if 1) no hard copy interpretations are made, 2) no hard copy comparisons are made or 3) for new units at existing facilities if these were previously evaluated and have not changed

Fig. 9.10 American College of Radiology medical physicist Mammography Equipment Evaluation (MEE) checklist.

MEDICAL PHYSICIST'S MAMMOGRAPHY QC TEST SUMMARY
Preliminary Results

Site		Survey Date	
		Room ID	
X-Ray Unit Manufacturer		Model	

Medical Physicist's QC Tests

Pass/Fail

	ACR Guides	MQSA Regs

1. Mammographic Unit Assembly Evaluation
2. Collimation Assessment
3. Evaluation of Focal Spot Performance
4. Automatic Exposure Control (AEC) System Performance
5. Uniformity of Screen Speed
6. Artifact Evaluation
7. **Phantom Image Quality Evaluation****
8. kVp Accuracy and Reproducibility
9. Beam Quality (Half-Value Layer) Assessment
10. **Breast Entrance Exposure, Average Glandular Dose,****
    AEC Reproducibility, and
    Radiation Output Rate
11. Viewbox Luminance and Room Illuminance

**If any of the starred MQSA tests fail (Phantom Image Quality and Average Glandular Dose), corrective action must be taken <u>before any further exams are performed</u>. Failure of any other MQSA-mandated tests requires corrective action within 30 days of the test date.

Recommendations for Corrective Actions

Evaluation of Site's Technologist QC Program

	ACR Guides	MQSA Regs

1. Darkroom cleanliness (daily)
2. Processor QC - performed, records maintained, action taken when needed (daily)
3. Screen cleaning (weekly)
4. Mammo phantom imaging - performed, records maintained, action taken as needed (weekly)
5. Darkroom fog (semiannually)
6. Film-screen contact test (semiannually)
7. Compression pressure monitored (semiannually)
8. Repeat analysis - performed, records maintained, reviewed by radiologist (quarterly)
9. Viewboxes and viewing conditions (weekly)
10. Analysis of fixer retention (quarterly)
11. Visual checklist (monthly)

Specific Comments

This is only a preliminary list of findings. A full and final report will be mailed to you shortly. Please call me if you have any questions about this summary.

Signature	_____
Physicist's Name	_____
Phone Number	_____

Fig. 9.11 American College of Radiology Medical Physicist's Mammography QC Test Summary.

Medical Physicist's ACR DM QC Test Summary

Facility Name _____   MAP ID-Unit# _____ - _____
Address _____

Room ID _____
Report Date _____
Survey Date _____

X-Ray Unit Manufacturer _____   **Model** _____

Control Panel Serial # _____   **Manufacture Date** _____   **Installation Date** _____

DM Unit Type: ☐ Digital radiography (DR)   ☐ Computed radiography (CR)   ☐ Digital Breast Tomosynthesis (DBT)

Unit Use: ☐ Diagnostic and screening mammography   ☐ Diagnostic only   ☐ Screening only

Survey Type: ☐ Mammography equipment evaluation (MEE) - Full   ☐ MEE - Partial   ☐ Annual survey

Equipment Tested: ☐ DM unit   ☐ AW monitor   ☐ RW monitor   ☐ Viewbox   ☐ Printer   Other: _____

Oversight Level: ☐ Medical physicist on-site   ☐ Medical physicist oversight

Quality Control Manual Used for Survey and Facility QC: *2018 ACR Digital Mammography QC Manual (with 2D and DBT QC)*

Medical Physicist _____   Signature _____

QC Test Results

Test	2D**	2D Add-on DBT	DBT	CA
		Pass/Fail*		
Medical Physicist Tests				
1. Mammography Equipment Evaluation - MQSA Reqs				
2. ACR DM Phantom Image Quality				
3. DBT Z Resolution				
4. Spatial Resolution				
5. DBT Volume Coverage				
6. Automatic Exposure Control System Performance				
7. Average Glandular Dose				
8. Unit Checklist				
9. Computed Radiography *(if applicable)*				
10. Acquisition Workstation Monitor QC				
11. Radiologist Workstation Monitor QC				
12. Film Printer QC *(if applicable)*				
13. Evaluation of Site's Technologist QC Program				
14. Evaluation of Display Device Technologist QC Program				
15. Manufacturer Calibrations *(if applicable)*				
16. Collimation Assessment				
MEE/Troubleshooting - Beam Quality (HVL) Assessment				
MEE/Troubleshooting - kVp Accuracy and Reproducibility				
Troubleshooting - Ghost Image Evaluation				
Troubleshooting - Viewbox Luminance				
Technologist QC Evaluation	Date reviewed if after new unit MEE:			
1. ACR DM Phantom Image Quality				
2. Computed Radiography Cassette Erasure *(if applicable)*				
3. Compression Thickness Indicator				
4. Visual Checklist				
5. Acquisition Workstation Monitor QC				
6. Radiologist Workstation Monitor QC				
7. Film Printer QC *(if applicable)*				
8. Viewbox Cleanliness *(if applicable)*				
9. Facility QC Review				
10. Compression Force				
11. Manufacturer Calibration *(if applicable)*				
Optional - Repeat Analysis				

Your Phantom Results - 2D
Fiber (≥ 2.0) ☐
Speck grp (≥ 3.0) ☐
Mass (≥ 2.0) ☐
AGD (≤ 3.0 mGy) ☐

Your Phantom Results - DBT
Fiber (≥ 2.0) ☐
Speck grp (≥ 3.0) ☐
Mass (≥ 2.0) ☐
AGD (≤ 3.0 mGy) ☐

* "Pass" means all components of test passes; "Fail" means any or all components fail; if "CA" checked, see Corrective Action Summary
** or DBT aquistition only

Fig. 9.12 American College of Radiology Medical Physicist's ACR DM QC Test Summary.

Continued

significant artifacts. The fiber score must be ≥2.0; speck group score must be ≥3.0; mass score must be ≥2.0. For 2D only, the MEE and annual: SNR must be ≥ 40.0 and the CNR ≥ 2.0. For annual inspection, the CNR must be ≥ 85% of MEE. For distance measurement accuracy, the measured wax insert distance must be 70.0 ± 14.0 mm. The ACR Medical Physicist form for evaluating phantom image quality is found in Fig. 9.12).

Digital breast tomosynthesis z resolution. In traditional DBT image reconstructions, serious artifacts can be found along the depth direction (z direction), resulting in the blurring of lesion edges in the off-focus planes parallel to the detector. The medical physicist will use an image of an ACR DM phantom to graph the z-axis point spread and determine the full width at half maximum value. During

Medical Physicist's ACR DM QC Test Summary *(cont)*

Facility Name _____

Mfr & Model _____

MAP ID-Unit# *(00000-00)* _____ - _____

Room ID _____

Survey Date _____

Corrective Action Summary*

Note: This is only a summary page, the Corrective Action Log Form may contain further details.

Required/ Recommended	Time Frame	Description	Utilize Corrective Action Log Form	Date Completed	Initials

Fig. 9.12, cont'd

the annual survey, the full width at half maximum must be within ±30% of the baseline (MEE) value. The ACR form is found in Fig. 9.13.

Spatial resolution. The ACR Spatial Resolution evaluation is performed to evaluate both the condition of the X-ray tube focal spot as well as the capability of the image receptor system to deliver sharp images. Testing involves using a line pair/mm resolution pattern. For 2D systems, the spatial resolution must be ≥4.0 lp/mm for contact mode and 6.0 lp/mm for magnification mode. For DBT, spatial resolution must be ≥2.0 lp/mm for contact mode. The ACR form for documenting spatial resolution evaluation is shown in Fig. 9.14.

DBT volume coverage. This test is performed to ensure that the entire imaged object is included in the reconstructed image with minimal distortion. The procedure involves placing aluminum sheets on top and bottom of the DM phantom diagonally across the chest wall. On the resulting image, both sheets must be focused in volume. The ACR form is shown in Fig. 9.15.

Automatic exposure control system performance. This test measures how well the AEC system compensates radiation output for changes in phantom thickness as well as to determine any changes in SNR. For MEE and annual inspections, the SNR must be ≥40.0 for 4.0 cm in contact mode. Also,

DBT Z Resolution

Facility Name _____   MAP ID-Unit# *(00000-00)* _____ - _____
Mfr & Model _____   Room ID _____
Survey Date _____

| **Procedure** | Equipment: DBT image from ACR DM Phantom Image Quality test   MEE Date: _____ |
| | MEE Baseline FWHM: |

Slice #	Relative Slice Location	Center Speck	12:00 Speck	2:00 Speck	5:00 Speck	7:00 Speck	10:00 Speck	Ave Max Signal	Mean Background Signal
	Maximum Speck Signal								
	−3								
	−2								
	−1								
	0								
	1								
	2								
	3								

Half Max Location	
0.00	
0.00	Rising edge
0.00	
0.00	
0.00	Falling edge
0.00	

For Chart		
Loc	Val	FWHM
−3		0.00	0.50
−2		0.00	0.50
−1		
0		
1		
2		
3		

Z-Axis Point Spread

Fraction of Speck Intensity
0.6
0.5
0.4
0.3
0.2
0.1
0.0
−4 −3 −2 −1 0 1 2 3 4
Slice Position

Z-Res Diff (Ave Max - Background Mean)	Δ Z-Res Diff relative to DBT Slice 0
Current FWHM	0.00 mm
MEE Baseline FWHM	mm
% Change (Current vs MEE)	
Overall Pass/Fail	

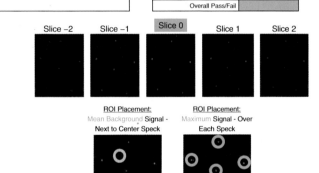

Slice −2   Slice −1   **Slice 0**   Slice 1   Slice 2

ROI Placement:
Mean Background Signal - Next to Center Speck

ROI Placement:
Maximum Signal - Over Each Speck

| **Action Limits** | Required: Annual Survey: FWHM must be within ±30% of the baseline (MEE) value. MEE: No action limit. |
| | Timeframe: Failures must be corrected within 30 days. |

Fig. 9.13   American College of Radiology DBT z Resolution form.

during the annual inspection, the SNR must be within ±15% of MEE over the clinically used phantom thickness and imaging modes. The ACR form to evaluate AEC performance for 2D systems is found in Fig. 9.16 and in Fig. 9.17 for DBT systems.

Average glandular dose. This is evaluated to ensure that the average glandular dose does not exceed the 3 mGy/view limit stated in MQSA. The test is performed with the ACR DM phantom and a dosimeter. The average glandular dose for a single craniocaudal view of the ACR DM phantom in either 2D or DBT mode must not exceed 3.0 mGy. The ACR form is found in Fig. 9.18.

Unit checklist. The checklist is used to document a visual inspection of the mammographic unit by the medical physicist to ensure the unit is mechanically safe as well as safe for the mammographer in terms of occupational dose reduction. All items, both critical and noncritical, must pass. The form for this procedure is found in Fig. 9.19.

Computed radiography (if applicable). For facilities that may be using CR image receptors, ACR requires testing of image plate consistency, artifact evaluation, CR reader performance, and SNR. The mAs required for each image receptor must be within ±10% of average mAs. The SNR for each image receptor must be within ±15% of average SNR, and the image must be free of clinically significant artifacts. For CR reader performance, a Tsquare phantom is used. The edges of the T should appear smooth and sharp. If they are not, and appear jagged or nonsmooth, then this could indicate a problem with the CR reader performance. The ACR forms for image plate consistency and artifact evaluation is shown in Fig. 9.20, while the form to evaluate CR reader scanner performance is shown in Fig. 9.21.

Acquisition workstation monitor quality control. The monitor used by the mammographer to view the acquired image is inspected by the medical physicist as part of the annual

Spatial Resolution

Facility Name _____ MAP ID-Unit# *(00000-00)* _____ - _____

Mfr & Model _____ Room ID _____

Survey Date _____

Procedure	Equipment:	ACR DM Phantom, line-pair test tool		Phantom Setup:	
	Place ACR DM Phantom reversed on breast support (wax insert away from chest edge)			Paddle size (IR size):	
	Place bar pattern on top of phantom and under paddle at ~45°			Paddle type (reg or flex):	
	Lightly compress paddle to touch bar pattern				
	Acquire "raw" images using manual mode closest to ACR DM Phantom technique				

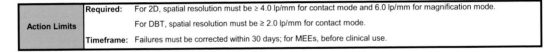

		Image Mode (2D, 2D w/Add-on DBT, DBT)				Mag Mode 2D
Setup Techniques	Mag factor		Contact			
	Target/filter					
	kVp					
	mAs					
Spatial Resolution Score	Line-pair score					
	Overall Pass/Fail					

Action Limits	Required:	For 2D, spatial resolution must be ≥ 4.0 lp/mm for contact mode and 6.0 lp/mm for magnification mode.
		For DBT, spatial resolution must be ≥ 2.0 lp/mm for contact mode.
	Timeframe:	Failures must be corrected within 30 days; for MEEs, before clinical use.

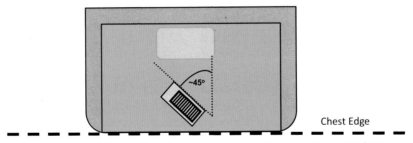

Fig. 9.14 American College of Radiology medical physicist's Spatial Resolution form.

inspection, using the form shown in Fig. 9.22. A photometer, along with Society of Motion Picture and Television Engineers (SMPTE) and/or American Association of Physicists in Medicine (AAPM) Task Group (TG) 18 test patterns, will be utilized. Any identified screen blemish that could interfere with clinical information must be removed. Test pattern image quality must pass all visual tests. L_{min} must be within ±30% of manufacturer specifications (or, if not available ≤1.5 cd/m²). L_{max} must be within ±10% of manufacturer specifications (or, if not available ≥150 cd/m²). Luminance uniformity must be ≤30%. Grayscale display function measured contrast response must be within ±10% of targeted contrast response. Any manufacturer's automated tests must pass manufacturer specifications. Any significant monitor cleanliness defects found during the inspection must be corrected before clinical use, while all other required tests must be corrected within 30 days.

Radiologist workstation monitor quality control. The radiologist's primary viewing monitor will also be inspected during the medical physicist's annual inspection. This is especially important since the final diagnosis from the mammographic images will be obtained from this device. A photometer, SMPTE and/or AAPM test patterns, and an ACR DM phantom will be utilized. Any identified monitor blemish that could interfere with clinical information must be removed. The ACR DM phantom image must be free of clinically significant artifacts. The fiber score must be ≥2.0; speck group score must be ≥3.0; mass score must be ≥2.0. The measured distance of wax insert must be 70.0 ±14.0 mm. The test pattern image quality must pass all visual tests. L_{min} must be within ±30% of manufacturer specifications (or, if not available ≤1.5 cd/m²). L_{max} must be within ±10% of manufacturer specifications (or, if not available ≥420 cd/m²). Luminance uniformity must be ≤30%; luminance

DBT Volume Coverage

Facility Name		MAP ID-Unit# *(00000-00)*	-
Mfr & Model		Room ID	
		Survey Date	

	Equipment: ACR DM Phantom, 2 sheets of 0.1 mm Al	**Phantom Setup:**
Procedure	Place ACR DM Phantom on breast support in the usual position	Paddle size (IR size):
	Place Al sheets on top and bottom of DM phantom, diagonally across chest wall	Paddle type (reg or flex):
	Acquire DBT image of phantom	
	View reconstructed image and verify that both Al sheets are in focus within the volume	

		Contact Mode
Setup Techniques	Mag factor	Contact
	Target/filter	
	kVp	
	mAs	
Results (Yes/No /NA)	Lower Al sheet in focus within the volume	
	Upper Al sheet in focus within the volume	
	Overall Pass/Fail	

| **Action Limits** | **Required:** Both sheets must be focused in volume |
| | **Timeframe:** Failures must be corrected before clinical use. |

Fig. 9.15 American College of Radiology medical physicist's DBT Volume Coverage form.

matching must be ≤20%. The grayscale display function measured contrast response must be within ±10% of targeted contrast response. Any manufacturer's automated tests must pass manufacturer specifications. Ambient light conditions should be appropriate for mammography, with a maximum of 45 lux recommended. The phantom must pass and significant monitor cleanliness defects must be corrected before clinical use; all other required tests must be corrected within 30 days. The ACR form to document this procedure is shown in Fig. 9.22.

Film printer quality control (if applicable). For mammography departments that print hard copies of mammographic images, the film printer will be evaluated during the medical physicist's annual inspection. An image from the ACR DM phantom will be printed from the workstation/computer typically used to print clinical films. The phantom image will be scored, and optical density values will be measured with a densitometer. The ACR DM phantom image must be free of clinically significant artifacts. The fiber score must be ≥2.0; speck group score must be ≥3.0; mass score must be ≥2.0. The background OD must be ≥1.6 (1.7–2.2 is recommended, and approximately 2.0 is optimal). The contrast (cavity OD – background OD) must be ≥0.1. The D_{max} must be ≥3.1 (≥3.5 is recommended). The measured distance of wax insert must be 70.0 ± 14.0 mm. Any failures of required items must be corrected before printing of clinical images. The ACR documentation form is shown in Fig. 9.23.

Evaluation of site's technologist quality control program. The ACR requires that the technologist QC program be evaluated by the medical physicist during the annual inspection. MQSA

regulations [FDA Rule 900.12(d)(1)(iii)] specify that "each facility shall have the services of a medical physicist available to survey mammography equipment and oversee the equipment-related quality assurance practices of the facility." Completion of this Evaluation of Display Device Technologist QC Program form documents that this oversight has been conducted. For the overall evaluation to pass, (a) there must be no significant missing data, (b) the tests must be analyzed without gross errors, and (c) appropriate corrective action for failures must be taken (and documented). Any failures must be corrected within 30 days. The ACR documentation form is shown in Fig. 9.24.

Evaluation of display device technologist QC program. Like the site's technologist QC program, the technologist's display device QC program must also be evaluated. MQSA regulations [FDA Rule 900.12(d)(1)(iii)] specify that "each facility shall have the services of a medical physicist available to survey mammography equipment and oversee the equipment-related quality assurance practices of the facility. " Completion of this Evaluation of Display Device Technologist QC Program form documents that this oversight has been conducted. For the overall evaluation to pass, (a) there must be no significant missing data, (b) the tests must be analyzed without gross errors, and (c) appropriate corrective action for failures must be taken (and documented). Any failures must be corrected within 30 days. The ACR documentation form is shown in Fig. 9.25.

Manufacturer calibrations (if applicable). Some manufacturers of FFDM units require periodic calibration. If so, the medical physicist will follow the manufacturer's instructions and document any calibrations made. Units must pass

Automatic Exposure Control System Performance (2D)

Image Mode *(2D, 2D w/Add-on DBT, DBT)* _____

Facility Name _____	MAP ID-Unit# *(00000-00)* _____ - _____
Mfr & Model _____	Room ID _____
	Survey Date _____

Procedure	Equipment: 2, 4, 6, 8 cm of BR-12, BR-50 or acrylic	Phantom Setup:	Paddle size (IR Size): _____
	Install small paddle (reg or flex) (Use large if small not available)		Paddle type (reg or flex): _____
	Use regular or flex paddle used for most clinical imaging		AEC cell position (if avail): _____
	Set thickness at actual thickness of phantom (2, 4, or 6 cm)		Mag setting: _____
	Acquire images using clinical techniques		Mfr DC offset, if app: _____
	SNR data must be obtained from raw image		Other settings: _____
	Magnification stand, if used clinically for 2D		

AEC Thickness Tracking

Mode	Thick-ness (cm)	Setup Techniques		Resultant Techniques				Signal and Noise Measurements			
		AEC Mode	Density setting	Target/Filter	kVp	mAs	Other	Mean Bkgd Signal	Std Dev of Bkgd	DC Offset (if app)	SNR
Contact	2										
Contact	4										
Contact	6										
Contact	8										
Mag*	4										

*2D only

$$SNR = \frac{(Mean\ Bkgd\ Signal - DC\ offset)}{Std\ Dev\ of\ Bkgd}$$

Analysis

Mode	Thick-ness (cm)	SNR	MEE and Annual		Annual			
			Lowest Limit for SNR*	Pass/Fail	MEE SNR	Lower Limit	Upper Limit	SNR within ±15% of MEE (P/F)
Contact	2							
Contact	4		40.0					
Contact	6							
Contact	8							
Mag*	4							

*2D only   **Overall Pass/Fail**

Action Limits	Required:	MEE and Annual: SNR must be ≥ 40.0 for 4.0 cm in contact mode.
		Annual: SNR must be within ±15% of MEE over the clinically used phantom thickness and imaging modes.
	Timeframe:	Failures must be corrected within 30 days; for MEEs, before clinical use.

Fig. 9.16 American College of Radiology medical physicist's Automatic Exposure Control System Performance (2D).

all manufacturer's calibrations to pass overall, and any failures must be corrected before clinical use. The ACR documentation form is shown in Fig. 9.26.

Collimation assessment. MQSA requires that the collimators on all mammographic units be inspected by a medical physicist on an annual basis, so this is included in the ACR program. If the sum of left plus right edge deviations or anterior plus chest edge deviations exceeds 2% of SID, seek service adjustment. If the X-ray field exceeds image receptor at any side by more than +2% of SID or if X-ray field falls within image receptor on the chest wall side, seek service adjustment. If the chest wall edge

of compression paddle is within the image receptor or projects beyond the chest wall edge of the image receptor by more than 1% of SID, seek service correction. Any failures must be corrected within 30 days: for MEEs, before clinical use. The ACR documentation form is shown in Fig. 9.27.

Mammography equipment evaluation/troubleshooting— beam quality (half-value layer) assessment. Since MQSA requires evaluation of beam quality, the ACR will require assessment during the initial MEE and then for troubleshooting any potential problems during the annual inspection. This will be evaluated using 0.1-mm aluminum sheets and a

Automatic Exposure Control System Performance (DBT)

Image Mode *(2D, 2D w/Add-on DBT, DBT)* _____

Facility Name _____   MAP ID-Unit# *(00000-00)* _____ - _____

Mfr & Model _____   Room ID _____

Survey Date _____

| Procedure | Equipment: 2, 4, 6, 8 cm of BR-12, BR-50 or acrylic
 Install small paddle (reg or flex) (Use large if small not available)
 Use regular or flex paddle used for most clinical imaging
 Set thickness at actual thickness of phantom (2, 4, or 6 cm)
 Acquire images using clinical techniques
 SNR data must be obtained from raw image
 Magnification stand, if used clinically for 2D | Phantom Setup: | Paddle size (IR Size): _____
 Paddle type (reg or flex): _____
 AEC cell position (if avail): _____
 Mag setting: _____
 Mfr DC offset, if app: _____
 Other settings: _____ |

AEC Thickness Tracking

Mode	Thick-ness (cm)	Setup Techniques		Resultant Techniques				Signal and Noise Measurements			
		AEC Mode	Density setting	Target/ Filter	kVp	mAs	Other	Mean Bkgd Signal	Std Dev of Bkgd	DC Offset (if app)	SNR
Contact	2										
Contact	4										
Contact	6										
Contact	8										
Mag*	4										

*2D only

$$SNR = \frac{(Mean\ Bkgd\ Signal - DC\ offset)}{Std\ Dev\ of\ Bkgd}$$

Analysis

Mode	Thick-ness (cm)	SNR	MEE and Annual		Annual			
			Lowest Limit for SNR*	Pass/Fail	MEE SNR	Lower Limit	Upper Limit	SNR within ±15% of MEE (P/F)
Contact	2							
Contact	4							
Contact	6							
Contact	8							
Mag*	4							

*2D only   **Overall Pass/Fail**

Action Limits	Required:	MEE and Annual: SNR must be ≥ 40.0 for 4.0 cm in contact mode. Annual: SNR must be within ±15% of MEE over the clinically used phantom thickness and imaging modes.
	Timeframe:	Failures must be corrected within 30 days; for MEEs, before clinical use.

Fig. 9.17 American College of Radiology medical physicist's Automatic Exposure Control System Performance (DBT).

dosimeter. At least one measurement for each available target-filter combination used for 2D and DBT (as applicable) will be made. The HVL must meet the specifications of FDA's Performance Standards for Ionizing Radiation Emitting Products (Part 1020.30) as discussed earlier in this chapter. Any failures must be corrected before clinical use. The ACR documentation form is shown in Fig. 9.28.

Mammography equipment evaluation/troubleshooting—kilovolt (peak) accuracy and reproducibility. Like beam quality (HVL), MQSA requires evaluation of kVp accuracy and reproducibility. Therefore it is included in the ACR

program during the initial MEE and for troubleshooting during annual inspections. The mean kVp must not differ from the nominal kVp by more than ±5% of the nominal kVp. The coefficient of variation must be ≤0.02. Any failures must be corrected within 30 days: for MEEs, before clinical use. The ACR documentation form is shown in Fig. 9.29.

Troubleshooting—ghost image evaluation. FFDM systems can have ghost images (image data from a previous image occurring in a new image), so ACR does have a troubleshooting procedure that the medical physicist can perform during the annual inspection. The ghosting index obtained must be

Average Glandular Dose

Facility Name _____ MAP ID-Unit# *(00000-00)* _____ - _____
Mfr & Model _____ Room ID _____
ACR DM Phantom Mfr & S/N _____ Survey Date _____

Procedure	Equipment:	Dosimeter	Dosimetry system:	
		ACR DM Phantom	Calibration date:	
	Use the technique from the ACR DM Phantom image page.		Correction factor, if app:	
	Measure mR/mAs or total exposure for dose calculation(s).		SID (cm):	
	Make exposure measurements at 4.2 cm			

		Imaging Mode (2D, 2D w/Add-on DBT, DBT)					
Technique Factors Resulting From ACR DM Phantom Acquisition	ACR DM Phantom equivalent breast thickness (cm)	4.2					
	ACR DM Phantom material	Acrylic					
	AEC mode						
	Target/filter						
	kVp						
	mAs						
Exposure Data (at skin surface)	Measured HVL (mm Al)						
	mAs setting for manual exposure measurement						
	Exposure #1 (mR)						
	Exposure #2 (mR)						
	Exposure #3 (mR)						
	Average exposure (mR)						
	Exposure/mAs at skin entrance (mR/mAs)						
	Total exposure (mR)						
AGD Calculation D = Kgcs	Average entrance exposure - K (mR)						
	g-factor x c-factor x (8.76 mGy/R)						
	s-factor						
	Computed AGD (mGy)						
AGD Result	**Pass/Fail**						
Indicated vs. Calculated AGD *(if avail)*	Unit-indicated AGD from DM Phantom image (mGy)						
	% Difference						
	Indicated within ±25% of measured?						

Action Limits	**Required:**	AGD for a single cranio-caudal view of the ACR DM Phantom in either 2D or DBT mode must not exceed 3.0 mGy.
	Recommended:	If available, unit-indicated AGD should be within ±25% of calculated AGD.
	Timeframe:	Doses > 3 mGy must be corrected before clinical use; failures of the unit-indicated AGD must be corrected within 30 days.

Fig. 9.18 American College of Radiology medical physicist's Average Glandular Dose form.

within 0 ± 0.3, and any failures must be corrected before clinical use. The ACR documentation form is shown in Fig. 9.30.

Troubleshooting—viewbox luminance. For departments that utilize viewboxes for viewing hard-copy mammographic images, MQSA (and therefore the ACR) requires that their performance be evaluated during annual inspections. Mammography viewboxes should be capable of a luminance of 3000 cd/m², be uniform, be clean, and have functioning masks. If these are not met, corrective action should be taken. The ACR documentation form is shown in Fig. 9.31.

Radiologic Technologist (Mammographer)

Technologists who perform mammograms must have at least 40 hours of training in mammography while under the supervision of a qualified instructor and must be licensed by the individual state or certified by an approved agency (such as the American Registry of Radiologic Technologists) to verify competency in radiography. The hours of documented training should include but are not necessarily limited to the following:

- Training in breast anatomy, physiology, positioning, compression, quality assurance/QC techniques, and imaging of patients with breast implants
- The performance of a minimum of 25 examinations while under the direct supervision of a qualified individual
- At least 8 hours of training in each mammography modality (such as DBT) to be used by the technologist in performing mammographic examinations

A continuing experience requirement for technologists dictates they must perform a minimum of 200 mammographic examinations during a 24-month period. Technologists also

Unit Checklist

Facility Name		MAP ID-Unit# *(00000-00)*	-
Mfr & Model		Room ID	
		Survey Date	

Procedure	**Equipment:** None Inspect the unit and evaluate the functionality according to the checklist below

Item	Yes/No/NA
1. **Free-standing unit is mechanically stable.***	
2. All moving parts move smoothly, without obstructions to motion.	
3. **All locks and detents work properly.***	
4. **Image receptor holder assembly is free from vibrations.***	
5. Image receptor slides smoothly into holder assembly (if applicable).	
6. **Image receptor is held securely by assembly in any orientation (if applicable).***	
7. **Patient or operator is not exposed to sharp or rough edges, or other hazards.***	
8. **Paddles are all intact with no cracks or sharp edges.***	
9. Mammography area is clean and free from significant dust and debris that may cause artifacts.	
10. **Operator protected during exposure by adequate radiation shielding.***	
11. All indicators working properly.	
12. **Autodecompression can be overridden to maintain compression (and status displayed).***	
13. **Manual emergency compression release can be activated in the event of a power failure.***	
14. Is the audible exposure indicator at an appropriate volume level?	
15. **DBT assembly moves as designed through its range of motion.***	
16. Operator technique charts are current and posted.	
17. Other:	
18. Other:	
19. Other:	
20. Other:	
Overall Pass/Fail	

Action Limits	**Required:**	All items, both critical (*) and noncritical, must pass.
	Timeframe:	Failures of critical items (*) must be corrected before clinical use; less critical items must be corrected within 30 days.

Fig. 9.19 American College of Radiology medical physicist's mammography Unit Checklist.

should obtain 15 CEUs in mammography every 36 months or as individual state guidelines dictate. QC duties are specified for technologists for film/screen, CR, and FFDM systems at daily, weekly, monthly, quarterly, and semiannual intervals.

Digital Mammography Systems

The technologist duties for DM systems for ACR accreditation are summarized in the chart below:

Digital QC Test	Minimum Frequency	Corrective Action Timeframe
ACR digital mammography phantom image quality	Weekly	Before clinical use
CR cassette erasure (if applicable)	Weekly	Before clinical use
Compression thickness indicator	Monthly	Within 30 days
Visual checklist	Monthly	Critical: before clinical use; less critical: within 30 days
Acquisition workstation monitor QC	Monthly	Within 30 days; before clinical use for severe defects
Radiologist workstation monitor QC	Monthly	Within 30 days; before clinical use for severe defects

Continued

Digital QC Test	Minimum Frequency	Corrective Action Timeframe
Film printer QC (if applicable)	Monthly	Before clinical use
Viewbox cleanliness (if applicable)	Monthly	Before clinical use
Facility QC review	Quarterly	Not applicable
Compression force	Semiannual	Before clinical use
Manufacturer detector calibration (if applicable)	Manufacturer recommendation	Before clinical use
Optional—repeat analysis	As needed	Within 30 days after analysis
Optional—system QC for radiologist	As needed	Within 30 days; before clinical use for severe artifacts
Optional—radiologist image quality feedback	As needed	Not applicable

ACR, American College of Radiology; *CR,* computed radiography; *QC,* quality control.

Daily duties. As with film/screen systems, mammographers may have daily responsibilities for DM systems, depending on the system manufacturer. The manufacturer's QC manual and the medical physicist should be consulted for the exact procedure to perform these duties. The ACR does not specify any required daily duties.

Weekly duties. The weekly duties performed by mammographers under the ACR accreditation program for digital mammographic systems include ACR DM phantom image quality testing and CR cassette erasure (CR systems only). The manufacturers' QC manuals and a medical physicist should be consulted for the exact procedure to perform these duties.

For the ACR DM phantom image quality test, the ACR DM phantom is imaged by the technologist and scored using the table below:

	Full point	Half point
Fibers	≥8 mm long	≥5 and <8 mm long
Specks	4–6 specks	2–3 specks
Masses	≥¾ border	≥½ and <¾ border

(Scoring)

The ACR technique and procedure form for performing this analysis is shown in Fig. 9.32. During analysis of the image, the ACR DM phantom image must be free of clinically significant artifacts. The fiber score must be ≥2.0; speck group score must be ≥3.0, and the mass score must be ≥2.0. Any unsatisfactory items must be corrected before clinical use. The ACR form to document the results of this test is shown in Fig. 9.32.

If CR systems are used, the ACR requires evaluation that adequate plate erasure is accomplished as part of the weekly technologist duties. Each cassette should successfully pass the CR cassette erasure process. Any failing cassettes must be corrected before clinical use. The ACR form to document the results of this test is shown in Fig. 9.33.

Monthly duties. The ACR accreditation program specifies monthly QC duties to be performed by the technologist. These will include compression thickness indicator, visual checklist, acquisition workstation and radiologist workstation monitor QC, film printer QC (if applicable), and viewbox cleanliness (if applicable).

For evaluation of the compression thickness indicator, the indicator must be accurate to within ±0.5 cm (±5 mm) of the actual thickness. Any failures must be corrected within 30 days. The ACR form to document this procedure is shown in Fig. 9.34.

The visual inspection is performed with the ACR Visual Inspection Form (Fig. 9.35). All items, both critical* and noncritical, must pass. Any failures of critical items (*) must be corrected before clinical use; less critical items must be corrected within 30 days.

The ACR requires the mammography technologist to evaluate both the acquisition workstation monitor as well as the radiologist's workstation monitor. For the acquisition workstation, the SMPTE or AAPM TG 18 test pattern is imaged and any identified screen blemish that could interfere with clinical information must be removed. The test pattern image quality must pass all visual tests. Any manufacturer's automated tests, if available, must pass manufacturer specifications. Significant monitor cleanliness defects must be corrected before clinical use; all other required tests must be corrected within 30 days. The ACR form to document this procedure is shown in Fig. 9.36. For the radiologist's workstation monitor, the test patterns as well as an image of the ACR DM test phantom will be imaged and analyzed. Any identified monitor blemish that could interfere with clinical information must be removed. The ACR DM phantom image must be free of clinically significant artifacts. The fiber score must be ≥2.0; speck group score must be ≥3.0; mass score must be ≥2.0. Test pattern image quality must pass all visual tests. Manufacturer's automated tests, if available, must pass manufacturer specifications. The phantom must pass, and significant monitor cleanliness defects must be corrected before clinical use; all other tests must be corrected within 30 days. The ACR form to document his procedure is shown in Fig. 9.37.

For mammography departments that utilize dry laser printers to print hard copies of digital images, the ACR does require that they be inspected monthly by the technologist. The hard-copy image is then analyzed to ensure that the hard copies meet image quality standards. The ACR DM phantom image must be free of clinically significant artifacts. The fiber score must be ≥2.0; speck group score must be ≥3.0; mass score must be ≥2.0. The background OD must be ≥1.6 (1.7–2.2 is recommended, while approximately 2.0 is optimal). The contrast (cavity OD – background OD) must be ≥0.1. The D_{max} must be ≥3.1 (≥3.5 is recommended). The ACR documentation form is found in Fig. 9.38.

If viewboxes are used to view mammographic images, the ACR mandates that a monthly inspection takes place. The procedure involves cleaning the viewbox surfaces and ensure that all marks have been removed. The technologist must

Computed Radiography *(if applicable)*

Facility Name	MAP ID-Unit# *(00000-00)*
Mfr & Model	CR Room
CR Reader Mfr & Model	Survey Date
CR Serial Number	Medical Physicist
CR Date of Manufacture	Signature

Inter-Plate Consistency & Artifact Evaluation

Procedure	Equipment: ACR DM Phantom	AEC mode:	AEC detector position:
	ACR DM Phantom on breast support plate with associated paddle.		Target/filter:
	Auto-Time, Set kV to ACR DM Phantom kV, cell position 2 if available.		kVp:

Small Cassettes

Cassette ID	mAs Evaluation		SNR Evaluation *(if available)*				Artifact Pass/Fail	Overall Pass/Fail
	mAs	P/F	Signal	Std Dev	SNR	P/F		
1								
2								
3								
4								
5								
6								
7								
8								

	Allowable			Allowable
Minimum mAs:		Minimum SNR:		
Mean mAs:		Mean SNR:		
Maximum mAs:		Maximum SNR:		

Small Cassettes

Cassette ID	mAs Evaluation		SNR Evaluation *(if available)*				Artifact Pass/Fail	Overall Pass/Fail
	mAs	P/F	Signal	Std Dev	SNR	P/F		
1								
2								
3								
4								
5								
6								
7								
8								

	Allowable			Allowable
Minimum mAs:		Minimum SNR:		
Mean mAs:		Mean SNR:		
Maximum mAs:		Maximum SNR:		

Action Limits	Required:	mAs must be within ±10% of average mAs.
		SNR must be within ±15% of average SNR.
		Must be free of clinically significant artifacts.
	Timeframe:	Failures must be corrected before clinical use.

Fig. 9.20 American College of Radiology medical physicist's computed radiography interplate consistency and artifact evaluation.

Continued

then visually inspect the viewboxes for uniformity of luminance and ensure that masking equipment is functioning. The ACR documentation form is found in Fig. 9.39.

Quarterly duties. The ACR requires a quarterly facility QC review by the technologist. This includes a review of any medical physicist's survey results, review of all technologist QC results, review and verification of any corrective action that has been taken if any unsatisfactory results were obtained,

review of the technique chart in each mammography room, review that all infection control protocols have been followed, review of QC for any offsite acquisition workstation monitors and film printers, a discussion of any past and future service or service upgrades, a discussion of any past of future state and/or MQSA inspections, and a discussion of any past and future ACR accreditation issues. The ACR checklist for the quarterly QC review is shown in Fig. 9.40.

Computed Radiography *(cont)*

Facility Name _____   MAP ID-Unit# *(00000-00)* _____ - _____

Mfr & Model _____   Room ID _____

Survey Date _____

CR Reader Scanner Performance

Procedure	**Equipment:** 2 thin metal rulers (or equivalent). Place rulers in the shape of a T on a cassette which is placed on top of the breast support. Expose at extremely low manual technique (~25 kVp, 4 mAs).

	Pass/Fail
Parallel to Chest Wall	
Perpendicular to Chest Wall	

Action Limits	**Recommendation:** The edges of the "T" should appear smooth and sharp. If they are not, and appear jagged or nonsmooth, then this could indicate a problem with the CR reader performance.

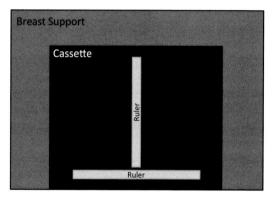

Fig. 9.20, cont'd

Semiannual duties. The technologist's semiannual duties for digital systems include compression force measurement using a scale. This is to ensure that the force is at least 25 lbs (111 N) but no more than 45 lbs (200 N). Failures must be corrected before further examinations are performed. The ACR form to document compression force is shown in Fig. 9.41.

Manufacturer's detector calibration. If applicable, digital mammographic units must pass the manufacturer's prescribed periodic calibration test. Failures must be corrected before further examinations are performed. The ACR checklist for the manufacturer's detector calibration is shown in Fig. 9.42.

As-needed quality control testing. The ACR lists three QC tests that are to be performed as needed. These include a Repeat Analysis, System QC for the Radiologist, and Radiologist Image Quality Feedback. The ACR forms for these tests are found in Figs. 9.43 through 9.45.

After completion of the required QC tests, the facility should compare the test results with the corresponding specified action limits or, for digital modalities, with the manufacturer's recommended action limits. If the test results fall outside the action limits, the source of the problem must be identified and corrective actions taken (1) before any

additional examinations are performed with a component of the mammographic system that failed any tests phantom image tests or compression device performance and (2) with 30 days for all other tests.

Table 9.3 summarizes the responsibilities for the radiologist, radiographer, and medical physicist.

Inspection by the Food and Drug Administration

As a result of the MQSA, only FDA-certified (or those certified by the states of Illinois, Iowa, South Carolina, and Texas) facilities may conduct mammography legally. To maintain its certified status, the following must be done for each facility:

- Have an annual survey performed by a qualified medical physicist
- Undergo periodic audits or clinical image reviews by the accrediting body
- Undergo annual inspection by an FDA-certified inspector (or those certified by the states of Illinois, Iowa, South Carolina, and Texas)
- Pay an inspection fee or reinspection fee if necessary
- Correct any deficiencies found during the inspections

The FDA-MQSA inspection covers equipment performance, technologist and physicist QC tests, medical audit and outcome analysis records, medical records (mammography

Acquisition Workstation (AW) Monitor QC

Facility Name _____   MAP ID-Unit# *(00000-00)* _____ - _____

Mfr & Model _____   Room ID _____

Medical Physicist _____   Survey Date _____

Signature _____

Procedure	
Equipment: Luminance meter	
Note: Some of these QC tests may or may not be possible to perform depending on the monitor QC capabilities	
Test Pattern Image Quality: Use TG18-QC, SMPTE or other relevant pattern (if available)	
Luminance Check: TG18 LN8-01 & LN8-18 test patterns, or others that provide measure of L_{min} & L_{max} (if available)	

Monitor manufacturer:	**Model:**	
	Monitor serial number	
	Monitor date of manufacture	
Monitor Condition	Significant findings P/F	
Test Pattern Image Quality *(if available)*	Test pattern centered appropriately?	
	0%-5% contrast boxes visible?	
	95%-100% contrast boxes visible?	
	Alphanumerics sharp and legible?	
	3 "Quality Control" patches visible (TG18)?	
	Line-pair images distinct (center)?	
	Line-pair images distinct (corners)?	
	Grayscale ramps smooth *(if avail)* ?	
	Test pattern P/F	
Luminance Check *(if available)*	Measured Luminance minimum (cd/m²)	
	Mfr recommendation for L_{min} *(if avail)*	
	L_{min} meets mfr recommendation ±30%?	
	Measured Luminance maximum (cd/m²)	
	Mfr recommendation for L_{max} *(if avail)*	
	L_{max} meets mfr recommendation ±10%?	
	Luminance check P/F	
DICOM GSDF	W/in ±10% of targeted contrast response P/F *(if avail)*	
Mfr Automated Test	Most recent set of mfr automated tests P/F	
	Overall Pass/Fail	

Significant findings indicated on figure below

Luminance Uniformity

Center	
Upper Left	
Upper Right	
Lower Left	
Lower Right	
Max	
Min	
% Diff	
P/F	

Action Limits	**Required:**	Any identified screen blemish that could interfere with clinical information must be removed.
		Test pattern image quality must pass all visual tests.
		L_{min} must be within ±30% of mfr specifications (or, if not available ≤ 1.5 cd/m²).
		L_{max} must be within ±10% of mfr specifications (or, if not available ≥ 150 cd/m²). Luminance uniformity must be ≤ 30%
		GSDF measured contrast response must be within ±10% of targeted contrast response.
		Mfr's automated tests must pass mfr specifications (if 1 test fails, indicate "F").
	Timeframe:	Significant monitor cleanliness defects must be corrected before clinical use; all other required tests must be corrected within 30 days.

Fig. 9.21 American College of Radiology medical physicist's Acquisition Workstation (AW) Monitor QC form.

reports and images), and personnel qualification records. Completing an inspection of a facility with a single mammographic unit takes approximately 6 hours.

Equipment Performance

For equipment performance, the inspector assesses the following:
- Collimation system (X-ray field/image receptor and image receptor/compression device alignment)
- Entrance skin exposure and exposure reproducibility
- Beam quality (HVL)
- Phantom image quality (including phantom scoring)

Records

The records the inspector asks to review include the following:
- Records for the previous 12 months for the technologist's QC tests/tasks mentioned previously

Radiologist Workstation (RW) Monitor QC

Facility Name _____ MAP ID-Unit# *(00000-00)* _____ - ___

Workstation ID _____ Survey Date _____

Medical Physicist _____ Signature _____

Procedure	**Equipment:** ACR DM Phantom Image, luminance meter **Note:** Some of these QC tests may or may not be possible to perform depending on the monitor QC capabilities ACR DM Phantom: use phantom acquired from any DM within facility network, preferably one MP has acquired Test Pattern Image Quality: Use TG18-QC, SMPTE or other relevant pattern Luminance: TG18 LN8-01, LN8-18 & TG18 UNL80 test patterns or other relevant test patterns

Monitor manufacturer:	Model:	Left*	Right*
	Monitor serial number		
	Monitor date of manufacture		
Ambient Light	Are ambient light conditions adequate for DM?		
Monitor Condition	Significant findings P/F		
ACR DM Phantom Evaluation	Artifacts P/F		
	Fiber score		
	Speck group score		
	Mass score		
	Phantom P/F		
Distance Measurement	Parallel to A-C axis (mm)		
	Meas = 70.0 ±14.0 mm (P/F)		
Test Pattern Image Quality	Test pattern centered appropriately?		
	0%-5% contrast boxes visible?		
	95%-100% contrast boxes visible?		
	Alphanumerics sharp and legible?		
	3 "Quality Control" patches visible (TG18)?		
	Line-pair images distinct (center)?		
	Line-pair images distinct (corners)?		
	Grayscale ramps smooth?		
	Test pattern P/F		
Luminance Check	Measured Luminance minimum (cd/m^2)		
	Mfr recommendation for L$_{min}$ *(if avail)*		
	L$_{min}$ meets mfr recommendation ±30%?		
	Measured Luminance maximum (cd/m^2)		
	Mfr recommendation for L$_{max}$ *(if avail)*		
	L$_{max}$ meets mfr recommendation ±10%?		
	Luminance check P/F		
DICOM GSDF *(if avail)*	W/in ±10% of targeted contrast response P/F		
Mfr Automated Test	Most recent set of mfr automated tests P/F		
	Overall Pass/Fail		

Significant findings indicated on figures below

Left and right monitors; complete additional forms if more than 2 monitors used

Luminance Uniformity

Monitor	Left	Right
Center		
Upper L		
Upper R		
Lower L		
Lower R		
Max		
Min		
% Diff		
P/F		

Luminance Matching

P/F	

Action Limits	**Required:** Any identified monitor blemish that could interfere with clinical information must be removed. ACR DM Phantom image must be free of clinically significant artifacts. Fiber score must be ≥ 2.0; speck group score must be ≥ 3.0; mass score must be ≥ 2.0. Measured distance of wax insert must be 70.0 ±14.0 mm. Test pattern image quality must pass all visual tests. L$_{min}$ must be within ±30% of mfr specifications (or, if not available ≤ 1.5 cd/m^2). L$_{max}$ must be within ±10% of mfr specifications (or, if not available ≥ 420 cd/m^2). Luminance uniformity must be ≤30%; luminance matching must be ≤ 20%. GSDF measured contrast response must be within ±10% of targeted contrast response. Mfr's automated tests must pass mfr specifications (if 1 test fails, indicate "F"). **Recommended:** Ambient light conditions should be appropriate for mammography; max of 45 lux is recommended. **Timeframe:** Phantom must pass and significant monitor cleanliness defects must be corrected before clinical use; all other required tests must be corrected within 30 days.

Fig. 9.22 American College of Radiology medical physicist's Radiologist's Workstation (RW) Monitor QC form.

- Phantom images and charting for the previous 12 months
- The annual medical physicist's report for each X-ray unit
- QA/QC documentation forms
- The latest version of all QC manuals for digital equipment
- Personnel orientation program for technologists
- Procedures for equipment use and maintenance
- Mammographic technique charts, including information pertinent to optimizing mammographic quality, such as positioning and compression
- Radiation safety policy and responsibilities

Film Printer QC *(if applicable)*

Facility Name		MAP ID-Unit# *(00000-00)*	-
Printer ID		Survey Date	
Medical Physicist		Signature	

Procedure	**Applicability:** If film printer is used clinically for mammography (i.e., for interpretation and to provide images to referring physicians and patients)
	Equipment: Densitometer
	Print an ACR DM Phantom image acquired from any DM unit within facility network, preferably one MP has just acquired.
	Do not change window/level settings from acquired image prior to printing.
	Print the phantom image from the workstation/computer typically used to print clinical films.
	Dmax should be measured either at extreme left or right edge of film or at extreme non-chest wall edge.

Film Printer Manufacturer		Film Printer Serial Number	
Film Printer Model		Film Printer Date of Manufacture	
Workstation for printing		DM ID or workstation ID	

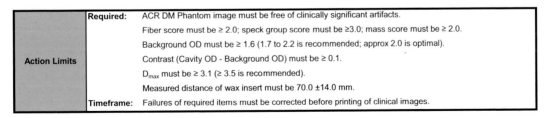

		Film size		
ACR DM Phantom		Artifacts P/F		
		Fiber score		
		Speck group score		
		Mass score		
		Phantom P/F		
Background		Bkgd OD *(Outside cavity)*		
		Bkgd OD ≥ 1.6 (P/F)		
Contrast		Cavity OD		
		Bkgd OD *(use value from above)*		
		Contrast = Cavity OD - Bkgd OD		
		Contrast ≥ 0.1 (P/F)		
D_{max}		D_{max} OD		
		D_{max} OD ≥ 3.1 (P/F)		
	Distance Measurement	Parallel to A-C axis (mm)		
		Meas = 70.0 ±14.0 mm (P/F)		
		Overall Pass/Fail		

Action Limits	**Required:**	ACR DM Phantom image must be free of clinically significant artifacts.
		Fiber score must be ≥ 2.0; speck group score must be ≥3.0; mass score must be ≥ 2.0.
		Background OD must be ≥ 1.6 (1.7 to 2.2 is recommended; approx 2.0 is optimal).
		Contrast (Cavity OD - Background OD) must be ≥ 0.1.
		D_{max} must be ≥ 3.1 (≥ 3.5 is recommended).
		Measured distance of wax insert must be 70.0 ±14.0 mm.
	Timeframe:	Failures of required items must be corrected before printing of clinical images.

Fig. 9.23 American College of Radiology medical physicist's Film Printer QC form.

In addition, the inspector:
- Determines whether all QC tests listed in the manuals have been conducted
- Determines whether all monitor and printer QC tests for digital equipment have been performed per the manufacturer's manual
- Determines whether timely corrective actions have been taken for any tests that have failed

- Examines the medical audit and outcomes analysis—a system designed to track positive mammograms and a process to correlate findings with surgical biopsy results. Analyses of these outcome data are made individually and collectively for all interpreting physicians at the facility. The ACR recommends that facilities use the Breast Imaging Reporting and Data System, or BI-RADS, final assessment codes and terminology for reporting and tracking

Evaluation of Site's Technologist QC Program

Facility Name _____ MAP ID-Unit# *(00000-00)* _____ - _____

Mfr & Model _____ Room ID _____

Survey Date _____

Radiologic Technologist's Quality Control Tests	Frequency	Test Performed, Analyzed & Documented	Missing Data	Incorrect Scoring or Calculations	Missing Corrective Action Documentation	Other	Comments
1. ACR DM Phantom Image Quality	Weekly						
			Tech Score		MP Score		
Medical physicist comparison on scores of latest phantom image:	Fiber						
	Speck group						
	Mass						
	Artifacts						
2. CR Cassette Erasure *(if app)*	Weekly						
3. Comp Thickness Indicator	Monthly						
4. Visual Checklist	Monthly						
5. AW Monitor QC	Monthly						
9. Facility QC Review	Quarterly						
10. Compression Force	Semiannual						
11. Mfr Calibrations *(if app)*							
Optional - Repeat Analysis	As Needed						
Optional - System QC for Radiologist	NA						
Optional - Radiologist IQ Feedback	NA						
Corrective Action Log documentation adequate?							

Overall Pass/Fail for Performance of Technologist QC Program ▢

Additional Comments: _____

_____

_____

_____

_____

Action Limits	Required:	MQSA regulations [FDA Rule 900.12(d)(1)(iii) specify that "each facility shall have the services of a medical physicist available to survey mammography equipment and oversee the equipment-related quality assurance practices of the facility." Completion of this "Evaluation of Site's Technologist QC Program" form documents that this oversight has been conducted. In order for the overall evaluation to pass, there must be a) no significant missing data, b) the tests must be analyzed without gross errors, and c) appropriate corrective action for failures must be taken (and documented). See test procedures for more information.
	Timeframe:	Failures must be corrected within 30 days.

Fig. 9.24 American College of Radiology medical physicist's Evaluation of Site's Technologist QC Program form.

of mammography outcomes. The BI-RADS categories are shown below:

Breast Imaging Reporting and Database System

Category	Assessment	Followup
0	Need additional imaging evaluation	Additional imaging needed before a category can be assigned
1	Negative	Continue regular screening mammograms
2	Benign (noncancerous) finding	Continue regular screening mammograms
3	Probably benign	Receive a 6-month followup mammogram
4	Suspicious abnormality	May require biopsy
5	Highly suggestive of malignancy (cancer)	Requires biopsy
6	Known biopsy-proven malignancy (cancer)	Biopsy confirms presence of cancer before treatment begins

Evaluation of Display Device Technologist QC Program

Facility Name _____   MAP ID-Unit# *(00000-00)* _____ - _____

Medical Physicist _____   Display Device Location _____

Signature _____   Survey Date _____

Display Device ID & Room	Display Device Description (RW, Printer, Viewbox)	Test Performed, Analyzed & Documented Incorrectly	Missing Data	Incorrect Scoring or Calculations	Missing Corrective Action Documentation	Mfr Automated Tests (if Applicable)	Other	Comments	P/F
Example: Mammography reading room	RW	✓	✓	✓	✓			Discussed with manager	P
Corrective Action Log documentation adequate?									

Overall Pass/Fail for Performance of Display Device Technologist QC Program _____

Additional Comments: _____

_____

_____

_____

_____

_____

_____

_____

_____

_____

_____

Action Limits	Required:	MQSA regulations [FDA Rule 900.12(d)(1)(iii) specify that "each facility shall have the services of a medical physicist available to survey mammography equipment and oversee the equipment-related quality assurance practices of the facility. " Completion of this "Evaluation of Site's Technologist QC Program" form documents that this oversight has been conducted. In order for the overall evaluation to pass, there must be a) no significant missing data, b) the tests must be analyzed without gross errors, and c) appropriate corrective action for failures must be taken (and documented). See test procedures for more information.
	Timeframe:	Failures must be corrected within 30 days.

Fig. 9.25 American College of Radiology medical physicist's Evaluation of Display Device Technologist QC Program form.

In addition, any cases of breast cancer among women who underwent imaging at the facility who subsequently become known to the facility should prompt the facility to initiate followup on surgical or pathologic results and review of the mammograms taken before the diagnosis of a malignancy.

- Examine permanent records, including the actual clinical images and mammography reports of the interpreting physician. Clinical images are evaluated based on the following parameters: positioning, compression, exposure level, sharpness, contrast, noise, artifacts, and examination identification. In digital departments, facilities must keep, in retrievable form, the original, raw mammographic image as well as the lossless compressed data or hard-copy films that duplicate the softcopy interpretive quality.

Manufacturer Calibrations *(if applicable)*

Facility Name _____   MAP ID-Unit# *(00000-00)* _____ - _____

Mfr & Model _____   Room ID _____

Survey Date _____

Procedure	Follow manufacturer's instructions.
	Notes: _____
	_____

	Name of Calibration	Detector	
Results (P/F)	2D		
	2D w/Add-on DBT Device		
	DBT		
	Overall Pass/Fail		

Action Limits	Required:	Unit must pass all manufacturer's calibrations to pass overall.
	Timeframe:	Failures must be corrected before clinical use.

Fig. 9.26 American College of Radiology medical physicist's Manufacturer's Calibrations form.

- Examine the infection control policy. Facilities that perform mammographic procedures must establish and comply with a system that specifies procedures to be followed by the facility for cleaning and disinfecting mammography equipment after contact with blood or other potentially infectious materials. This system must specify the methods for documenting facility compliance with infection control procedures. The procedures should comply with all applicable federal, state, and local regulations that pertain to infection control; with the manufacturer's recommended procedures for the cleaning and disinfection of the mammographic equipment used in the facility; or, if adequate manufacturer's recommendations are unavailable, with generally accepted guidance for infection control until such recommendations become available.
- Examine the consumer complaint mechanism. Each facility performing mammograms must establish a written and documented system for collecting and resolving consumer complaints. It also must maintain a record of each serious complaint received by the facility for at least 3 years from the date the complaint was received. The FDA defines a serious complaint as a report of a serious adverse event—an event that compromises clinical outcomes significantly or one for which a facility fails to take appropriate corrective action in a timely manner. Examples of serious adverse events include poor image quality, missed cancers, the use of personnel who do not meet FDA qualifications, or failure to send the mammography reports or lay summaries within 30 days. The facility also must provide the consumer with adequate directions for filing serious complaints with the facility's accreditation body if the facility is unable to resolve a serious complaint to the consumer's satisfaction. Each facility also is required to report unresolved serious complaints to the accreditation body in a manner and time frame specified by the accrediting body. An example of an acceptable system for collecting and documenting consumer complaints is described as follows.

PROCEDURE: CONSUMER COMPLAINT

1. The facility designates a facility contact person with whom consumers, the accreditation body, and the FDA can interact regarding serious consumer complaints. The contact person and other health professionals at the facility develop a clear understanding of the definitions of *consumer*, *adverse event*, *serious adverse event*, and *serious complaint*, so all parties are knowledgeable of the requirements of the consumer requirements of the consumer complaint mechanism (Box 9.2).

2. If the facility cannot resolve a complaint to the consumer's satisfaction, the facility provides the consumer with directions for filing serious complaints with the facility's accrediting body. These directions are to be provided in writing. The facility may want to post a sign to explain how to file

PROCEDURE: CONSUMER COMPLAINT—cont'd

complaints. In this case, the facility may use messages such as, "We care about our patients. If you have comments or concerns, please direct them to (the name of the person in the facility who is responsible for handling complaints)." The name and address of the accrediting body, listed on the facility's certificate, is also provided. The facility is required by law to post the certificate prominently in the facility.

3. The facility keeps documentation of the complaint on file for a period of 3 years from the date the complaint was received. The facility may develop a form to record, at a minimum, the following items concerning "serious complaints": the name, address, and telephone number of the person making the complaint; date of the complaint; date the serious adverse event occurred; precise description of the serious adverse event (including the names of the individuals involved); the manner of the complaint's resolution; and the date of the complaint's resolution. This record can be either handwritten or computerized, depending on the facility's preference.

4. The facility acknowledges the consumer's complaint, investigates the complaint, makes every effort to resolve the complaint, and responds to the individual filing the complaint within a reasonable time frame (these steps are usually accomplished within 30 days).

5. The facility ensures the complaint and any information about the complaint or its followup are shared only with those needed to resolve the complaint. In addition, the facility designs its complaint procedures to be responsive to the particular needs of the patients it serves. Patients or their representatives may complain in person or in writing.

6. The facility reports unresolved serious complaints to its accrediting body in a manner and time frame specified by the body. The facility may want to contact its accrediting body about this requirement. For easy reference, facilities may want to keep a separate listing of unresolved serious complaints, with the date of referral; summary; and date of response, if any, from the accrediting body. (This is in addition to the record described in step 3.)

BOX 9.2   Definitions by the Food and Drug Administration

1. **Consumer**—An individual who chooses to comment or complain in reference to a mammographic examination, including the patient or representative of the patient (for example, a family member or referring physician)

2. **Adverse event**—An undesirable experience associated with mammographic activities within the scope of the Mammography Quality Standards Reauthorization Act; adverse events include but are not limited to poor image quality, the failure to send mammographic reports to the referring physician within 30 days or to the self-referred patient in a timely manner, or the use of unqualified personnel (those who do not meet the applicable requirements of 21 Code of Federal Regulations Part 900, Section 12[a])

3. **Serious adverse event**—An adverse event that may compromise clinical outcomes significantly or an adverse event for which a facility fails to take appropriate corrective action in a timely manner

4. **Serious complaint**—A report of a serious adverse event

Courtesy Code of Federal Regulations.

Inspection Report

After the inspection, a report summarizing the inspection findings is sent to the institution. The findings belong to one of the following categories.

Level 1. A level 1 finding is a deviation from MQSA standards that may seriously compromise the quality of mammographic services offered by a facility. For example, a level 1 finding for the phantom image test exists when the score is less than three fibers, less than two speck groups, or less than two masses, or if the raw score is less than six. A level 1 finding also is issued if the interpreting physician is not certified by a board, has not had the initial (2 or 3 months) training in mammography, or has never had a valid license to practice medicine. A warning letter is sent if a level 1 finding exists to allow the facility to correct the problem before any enforcement action is implemented.

Level 2. A level 2 finding is not as serious a deviation from MQSA standards as a level 1 finding, but it still may compromise the quality of a facility's mammographic program and should be corrected as soon as possible. Facilities with these findings are rated "acceptable," but they must submit an acceptable corrective action plan to the FDA.

Level 3. A level 3 finding is a minor deviation from MQSA standards. Facilities with a level 3 finding are rated "satisfactory" but should institute policies and procedures to correct these conditions.

No findings. A report of no findings shows the facility has met all requirements of the MQSA.

Collimation Assessment

Image Mode *(2D, 2D w/Add-on DBT, DBT)* _____

Facility Name _____   **MAP ID-Unit#** *(00000-00)* _____ - _____

Mfr & Model _____   **Room ID** _____

    Survey Date _____

Procedure	**Equipment:** Coins, film, electronic collimation test tool(s), etc.
	Eqpt used: _____ **kVp:** _____ **mAs:** _____

		Largest Detector Size Available	Small Detector Size (CR only)
Technique	Target material		
	Collimator size (cm)		
	SID (mm)		
Deviation Between X-ray Field and Light Field	Left edge deviation (mm)		
	Right edge deviation (mm)		
	Sum of left and right edge deviations		
	Sum as % of SID		
	Anterior edge deviation (mm)		
	Chest edge deviation (mm)		
	Sum of anterior and chest edge deviations		
	Sum as % of SID		
	Pass/Fail		

		Largest Detector Size Available	Small Detector Size (CR only)
Deviation Between X-ray Field and Edges of the Image Receptor	Left edge deviation		
	% of SID (retain sign)		
	Right edge deviation		
	% of SID (retain sign)		
	Anterior edge deviation		
	% of SID (retain sign)		
	Chest edge deviation		
	% of SID (retain sign)		
	Pass/Fail		

Alignment of Chest-Wall Edges of Compression Paddle and IR	Difference between paddle edge and film		
	Difference as % of SID		
	Pass/Fail		

Overall Pass/Fail [ ]

Action Limits	**Required:**	If sum of left plus right edge deviations or anterior plus chest edge deviations exceeds 2% of SID, seek service adjustment.
		If X-ray field exceeds image receptor at any side by more than +2% of SID or if X-ray field falls within image receptor on the chest wall side, seek service adjustment.
		If chest-wall edge of compression paddle is within the image receptor or projects beyond the chest-wall edge of the image receptor by more than 1% of SID, seek service correction.
	Timeframe:	Failures must be corrected within 30 days; for MEEs, before clinical use.

Fig. 9.27 American College of Radiology medical physicist's Collimation Assessment form.

MEE or Troubleshooting
Beam Quality (Half-Value Layer) Assessment

Facility Name _____   **MAP ID-Unit#** *(00000-00)* _____ - _____

Mfr & Model _____   **Room ID** _____

                                              Survey Date _____

Procedure	**Equipment:** Dosimeter, 0.1 mm Al sheets, lead sheet	Dosimetry system: _____
	Cover the detector with lead sheet or apron	Calibration date: _____
	Make at least 1 measurement for each available target-filter combination used for 2D and DBT (as applicable)	

		Target/Filter 1		Target/Filter 2		Target/Filter 3		Target/Filter 4		Target/Filter 5		Target/Filter 6	
Target/filter													
Nominal kVp setting													
mAs													
		**Exposure Measurements**											
		mm AL	X (mR)	mm AL	X (mR)	mm AL	X (mR)	mm AL	X (mR)	mm AL	X (mR)	mm AL	X (mR)
No Aluminum	E_0	0		0		0		0		0		0	
Al Thickness (mm) t_a	E_a												
Al Thickness (mm) t_b	E_b												
Calculated or measured HVL (mm Al)													
Minimum allowed HVL													
Overall Pass/Fail													

$$HVL = \frac{t_b \ln[2E_a/E_0] - t_a \ln[2E_b/E_0]}{\ln[E_a/E_b]}$$

Action Limits	**Required:** The HVL must meet the specifications of FDA's Performance Standards for Ionizing Radiation Emitting Products (Part 1020.30) as shown below.
	Timeframe: All failures must be corrected before clinical use.

FDA X-ray Tube Voltage (kilovolt peak) and Minimum HVL		
Designed Operating Range (kV)	Measured Operating Voltage (kV)	Minimum HVL (mm of Al)
Below 50	20	0.2
	25	0.25
	30	0.3

Fig. 9.28 American College of Radiology medical physicist's MEE or Troubleshooting Beam Quality (Half-Value Layer) Assessment form.

MEE or Troubleshooting
kVp Accuracy and Reproducibility

Facility Name _____   MAP ID-Unit# *(00000-00)* _____ - _____

Mfr & Model _____   Room ID _____

Survey Date _____

kVp Accuracy and Reproducibility

Procedure	**Equipment:** kVp meter, lead sheet
	Cover the <u>entire detector</u> with lead sheet, a lead apron or other device.
	Remove the paddle.

kVp meter _____   Setting _____

Calibration Date: _____

		Low Clinical kVp*	ACR DM Phantom Clinical kVp (2D)	ACR DM Phantom Clinical kVp (DBT)	High Clinical kVp*
Technique	Nominal kVp setting				
	Target/filter				
	Focal spot				
	mAs				
Data	Measured kVp value 1				
	Measured kVp value 2				
	Measured kVp value 3				
Analysis	Mean kVp				
	Standard deviation (SD)				
	Mean kVp - nominal kVp				
	0.05 x nominal kVp				
	% error				
	% error P/F				
	Coefficient of variation (CV)				
	CV P/F				
Overall Pass/Fail					

* The low and high kVps may be either those used for 2D or DBT imaging, whichever are lowest or highest

Action Limits	**Required:**	Mean kVp must not differ from the nominal by more than ±5% of the nominal kVp.
		Coefficient of variation must be ≤ 0.02.
	Timeframe:	Failures must be corrected within 30 days; for MEEs, before clinical use.

Fig. 9.29 American College of Radiology medical physicist's MEE or Troubleshooting kVp Accuracy and Reproducibility form.

Troubleshooting
Ghost Image Evaluation

	Image Mode	2D
Facility Name	**MAP ID-Unit#** *(00000-00)*	-
Mfr & Model	**Room ID**	
	Survey Date	

Procedure	**Equipment:** ACR DM Phantom, 0.1 mm Al sheet (10 cm x 10 cm)	**Phantom Setup**	
	Largest image receptor size	**Paddle Size** *(IR size)* :	
	Clinical paddle (reg or flex)	**Paddle Type** *(reg or flex)* :	
	Apply 5 daN or 12 lbs comp force	**Exposure Mode:**	
		Compression Force:	12 lbs or 5 daN
	Position ACR DM Phantom with wax insert opposite from chest wall edge.	**AEC Cell Position** *(if avail)* :	
	AEC cell position to position "3".	**Density Setting:**	
	Use clinical (AEC) technique for both images		
	Image 1: Position phantom like Setup Image #1 (edge extends 1" beyond midline).		
	Image 2: Position phantom like Setup Image #2 with Al placed on top.		
	Signal data must be obtained from raw image		

			Image 1	Image 2
Resulting Techniques from Image Acquisition		Target/filter		
		kVp		
		mAs		
Ghosting Analysis *(see images below)*		S_1		
		S_2		
		S_3		
		Ghosting Index		
		Overall Pass/Fail		

$$\text{Ghosting Index} = \frac{(S_3 - S_2)}{(S_1 - S_2)}$$

Action Limits	**Required:** The ghosting index must be within 0±0.3.
	Timeframe: Failures must be corrected before clinical use.

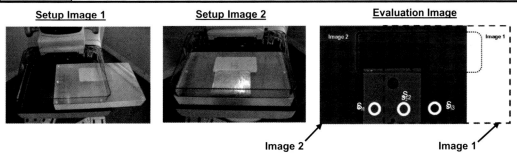

Setup Image 1	**Setup Image 2**	**Evaluation Image**

Image 2   **Image 1**

Fig. 9.30 American College of Radiology medical physicist's Troubleshooting Ghost Imaging Evaluation form.

Troubleshooting
Viewbox Luminance

Facility Name _____ **MAP ID-Unit#** *(00000-00)* _____ - _____

Medical Physicist _____ **Viewbox Location** _____

Signature _____ **Survey Date** _____

Procedure	**Equipment:** Luminance meter Measure luminance for all viewboxes, record the luminance value for the viewbox with the lowest luminance. Note: Only check a deficiency if it is significant and could impact interpretation; if the observation is not significant, just make a note in comments

Viewbox Designation	Measurements Viewbox Luminance (cd/m²)	Significant Deficiencies					Pass/Fail
		Dirt and Marks	Color Difference	Luminance Difference	Non-Uniformity	Functioning Masks Missing	
1.							
2.							
3.							
4.							
5.							
6.							
7.							
8.							
9.							
10.							
				Tech QC Review for Viewbox Luminance			
				Overall Pass/Fail			

Comments: _____
_____
_____
_____
_____
_____

Action Limits	**Recommended:** Mammography viewboxes should be capable of a luminance of 3,000 cd/m², be uniform, clean and have functioning masks; if these are not met, corrective action should be taken.

Fig. 9.31 American College of Radiology medical physicist's Troubleshooting Viewbox Luminance evaluation form.

ACR DM Phantom Image Quality   *Weekly*

Image Mode *(2D, 2D w/Add-on DBT, DBT)* _____

Facility _____   **Room ID** _____

MAP ID-Unit# *(00000-00)* _____ - ____ **Unit Mfr & Model** _____

		Year					
		Date *(month & day)*					
		Tech Initials					
Resulting Techniques		Image receptor size					
		View or selected image					
		Slice or slab # *(DBT only)*					
		AEC mode					
		Target/filter					
		kVp					
		mAs					
ACR DM Phantom		Artifacts P/F					
		Fiber score					
		Speck group score					
		Mass score					
Overall Pass/Fail							

P = Pass   F = Fail

Analyses:

Scoring		Full Point	Half Point
	Fibers	≥ 8 mm long	≥ 5 and < 8 mm long
	Specks	4 - 6 specks	2 - 3 specks
	Masses	≥ ¾ border	≥ ½ & < ¾ border

Action Limits	**Required:**	ACR DM Phantom image must be free of clinically significant artifacts.
		Fiber score must be ≥ 2.0; speck group score must be ≥ 3.0; mass score must be ≥ 2.0.
	Timeframe:	Required items must be corrected before clinical use.

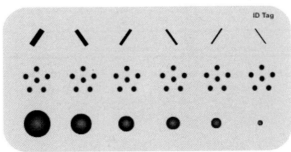

Fig. 9.32 American College of Radiology radiologic technologist's DM Phantom Image Quality form.

Computed Radiography (CR) Cassette Erasure   *Weekly*

(if applicable)   **Image Mode**   2D

Facility _____   **CR Room** _____

MAP ID-Unit# *(00000-00)* _____ - _____   **CR Reader Mfr & Model** _____

Year																								
Month	Jan				Feb				Mar				Apr				May				Jun			
Date																								
Tech Initials																								

Month	Jul				Aug				Sep				Oct				Nov				Dec			
Date																								
Tech Initials																								

Date and initial each test - | date |
                                 | initial |

Action Taken on Cassette *(include date & cassette #)* :

_____

_____

_____

_____

_____

_____

_____

_____

_____

_____

_____

_____

_____

_____

_____

Action Limits	Required:	Each cassette should successfully pass the CR cassette erasure process
	Timeframe:	Failing cassettes must be corrected before clinical use.

Fig. 9.33 American College of Radiology radiologic technologist Computed Radiography (CR) Cassette Erasure test form.

Compression Thickness Indicator   *Monthly*

Image Mode *(2D, 2D w/Add-on DBT, DBT)* _____

Facility _____   **Room ID** _____

MAP ID-Unit# *(00000-00)* _____ - _____   **Unit Mfr & Model** _____

		Jan	Feb	Mar	Apr	May	Jun	Jul	Aug	Sep	Oct	Nov	Dec
Year													
Month		Jan	Feb	Mar	Apr	May	Jun	Jul	Aug	Sep	Oct	Nov	Dec
Date													
Tech Initials													
Description of compression thickness indicator phantom													
Actual thickness of phantom		☐ cm	☐ mm	Select dot or check from dropdown, or type capital "P"	isplayed on the indicator)								
Indicated thickness													
Difference between indicated and actual thicknesses (Indicated - Actual)													
Overall Pass/Fail													

P = Pass   F = Fail

Action Limits	**Required:**	Compression thickness indicator ***must*** be accurate to within ±0.5 cm (±5 mm) of the actual thickness.
	Timeframe:	Failures ***must*** be corrected within 30 days.

Fig. 9.34 American College of Radiology Radiologic Technologist Compression Thickness Indicator test form.

Visual Checklist

Monthly

Image Mode *(2D, 2D w/Add-on DBT, DBT, All)* _____

Facility _____ **Room ID** _____

MAP ID-Unit# *(00000-00)* _____ - _____ **Unit Mfr & Model** _____

Procedure	Inspect the unit and evaluate the functionality according to the checklist below.

		Jan	Feb	Mar	Apr	May	Jun	Jul	Aug	Sep	Oct	Nov	Dec
Year													
Month		Jan	Feb	Mar	Apr	May	Jun	Jul	Aug	Sep	Oct	Nov	Dec
Date													
Tech Initials													
Room Cleanliness	Mag stands and paddles free from dust												
	Room and countertops free from dust												
	Cleaning solution available*												
X-Ray Unit	Indicators working												
	Locks *(all)* *****												
	Collimator light working												
	Are cables safely positioned												
	Smoothness of C-arm motion												
	Smoothness of compression paddle												
	Paddles/face shields not cracked*												
	Breast support not cracked*												
CR *(if app)*	**Cassette holder and lock** *(small and large)* *****												
	Condition of imaging plates and cassettes*												
Scanning Detector System *(if app)*													
DBT *(if app)*	**DBT assembly moves as designed***												
Other													

P = Pass   F = Fail   NA = Not Applicable

Action Limits	Required:	All items, both critical (*) and noncritical, must pass.
	Timeframe:	Failures of critical items (*) must be corrected before clinical use; less critical items must be corrected within 30 days.

Fig. 9.35 American College of Radiology radiologic technologist Visual Inspection checklist.

Acquisition Workstation (AW) Monitor QC   *Monthly*

Image Mode *(2D, DBT)* _____

Facility _____   **Room ID** _____

MAP ID-Unit# *(00000-00)* _____ - _____

		Jan	Feb	Mar	Apr	May	Jun	Jul	Aug	Sep	Oct	Nov	Dec
Year													
Month		Jan	Feb	Mar	Apr	May	Jun	Jul	Aug	Sep	Oct	Nov	Dec
Date													
Tech Initials													
Monitor Condition P/F *(significant findings)*													
Test Pattern Image Quality *(if available)*	0%-5% contrast boxes visible?												
	95%-100% contrast boxes visible?												
	Line-pair images distinct (center)?												
	Line-pair images distinct (corners)?												
	Test pattern P/F												
Monthly Check - Mfr Automated Test P/F *(if avail)*													
Overall Pass/Fail													

P = Pass   F = Fail

Action Limits	**Required:**	Any identified screen blemish that could interfere with clinical information must be removed.
		Test pattern image quality must pass all visual tests.
		Manufacturer's automated tests, if available, must pass mfr specifications (if 1 test fails, indicate F).
	Timeframe:	Significant monitor cleanliness defects must be corrected before clinical use; all other required tests must be corrected within 30 days.

Fig. 9.36 American College of Radiology radiologic technologist Acquisition Workstation (AW) Monitor QC Form.

Radiologist Workstation (RW) Monitor QC

Monthly

RW Location and ID

MAP ID# (00000) _____   **Monitor Mfr** _____   **Model** _____   **SN: Right** _____   **Left** _____

		Jan		Feb		Mar		Apr		May		Jun		Jul		Aug		Sep		Oct		Nov		Dec	
Year																									
Month		Jan		Feb		Mar		Apr		May		Jun		Jul		Aug		Sep		Oct		Nov		Dec	
Date																									
Tech Initials																									
Monitor		R*	L*	R	L	R	L	R	L	R	L	R	L	R	L	R	L	R	L	R	L	R	L	R	L
Monitor Condition P/F *(significant findings)*																									
ACR DM Phantom	Artifacts P/F																								
	Fiber score																								
	Speck group score																								
	Mass score																								
	Phantom P/F																								
Test Pattern Image Quality	0%-5% contrast boxes visible																								
	95%-100% contrast																								
	Line-pair images distinct (center)																								
	Line-pair images distinct (corners)																								
	Test pattern P/F																								
Monthly Check - Mfr Automated Test P/F *(if avail)*																									
Overall Pass/Fail																									

P = Pass   F = Fail

Action Limits	**Required:**	Any identified monitor blemish that could interfere with clinical information must be removed.	* R and L - right and left monitors; if only 1 monitor, use "R" column
		ACR DM Phantom image must be free of clinically significant artifacts.	
		Fiber score must be ≥ 2.0; speck group score must be ≥ 3.0; mass score must be ≥ 2.0.	
		Test pattern image quality must pass all visual tests.	
		Manufacturer's automated tests, if available, must pass mfr specifications (if 1 test fails, indicate F).	
	Timeframe:	Phantom must pass and significant monitor cleanliness defects must be corrected before clinical use; all other tests must be corrected within 30 days.	

Fig. 9.37 American College of Radiology radiologic technologist Radiologist Workstation (RW) Monitor QC form.

Film Printer QC *(if applicable)* *Monthly*

Film Printer Location and ID _____

Film Printer and Model _____

Workstation for printing _____ **Film size** _____

Procedure	**Applicability:** If film printer is used clinically for mammography (i.e., for interpretation and to provide images to referring physicians and patients) **Equipment:** Densitometer Print an ACR DM Phantom image acquired from any DM unit within facility network. Do not change window/level settings from acquired image prior to printing. Print the phantom image from the workstation/computer typically used to print clinical films. Dmax should be measured either at extreme left or right edge of film or at extreme non-chest wall edge.

		Jan	Feb	Mar	Apr	May	Jun	Jul	Aug	Sep	Oct	Nov	Dec
	Year												
	Month												
	Date												
	Tech Initials												
ACR DM Phantom	Artifacts P/F												
	Fiber score												
	Speck group score												
	Mass score												
	Phantom P/F												
Back-ground	Bkgd OD (Outside cavity)												
	Bkgd OD ≥ 1.6 (P/F)												
Contrast	Cavity OD												
	Bkgd OD (use value from above)												
	Contrast = Cavity OD - Bkgd OD												
	Contrast ≥ 0.1 (P/F)												
D_{max}	D_{max} OD												
	D_{max} OD ≥ 3.1 (P/F)												
	Overall Pass/Fail												

P = Pass   F = Fail

Action Limits	**Required:**	The ACR DM Phantom image must be free of clinically significant artifacts. Fiber score must be ≥ 2.0; speck group score must be ≥ 3.0; mass score must be ≥ 2.0. Background OD must be ≥ 1.6 (1.7 to 2.2 is recommended; approx 2.0 is optimal). Contrast (Cavity OD - Background OD) must be ≥ 0.1. D_{max} must be ≥ 3.1 (≥ 3.5 is recommended).
	Timeframe:	Failures of required items must be corrected before printing clinical images.

Fig. 9.38 American College of Radiology radiologic technologist Film Printer QC form.

Viewbox Cleanliness *(if applicable)*   *Monthly*

Viewbox Location and ID _____

Procedure	**Required Equipment:** Viewbox manufacturer-recommended cleaner; soft paper or cotton towels Clean viewbox surfaces and assure all marks have been removed. Visually inspect the viewboxes for uniformity of luminance and assure masking equipment is functioning.

	Year												
Month		Jan	Feb	Mar	Apr	May	Jun	Jul	Aug	Sep	Oct	Nov	Dec
Date													
Tech Initials													
Viewbox Designation													

P = Pass   F = Fail

Action Limits	**Required:**	Viewboxes must be clean and free of marks and uniform in brightness.
	Timeframe:	Failures must be corrected before clinical images are viewed on the viewbox.

Fig. 9.39 American College of Radiology radiologic technologist Viewbox Cleanliness form.

Facility QC Review   *Quarterly*

Image Mode *(2D, 2D w/Add-on DBT, DBT)* _____

Facility _____   **Date of QC Mtg** _____

Reviewed ☐

1. Review Medical Physics Surveys and Results

	Room 1	Room 2	Room 3	Room 4	Room 5
Room ID					
Date of last Medical Physicist (MP) survey					
MP DM QC Test Summary reviewed by radiologist?					
All MP corrective actions completed?					
ACR DM Phantom Average Glandular Dose (mGy)					
Fiber Score					
Speck Score					
Mass Score					

2. Review Tech QC   ☐

Test	Frequency	Summary Comments from Last Quarter	
1. ACR DM Phantom Image Quality	Weekly	_____	☐

		Room 1	Room 2	Room 3	Room 4	Room 5
Scores of most recent phantom image:	Date					
	Fiber score					
	Speck group score					
	Mass score					

Test	Frequency	Summary Comments	Reviewed
2. CR Cassette Erasure *(if app)*	Weekly	_____	☐
3. Compression Thickness Indicator	Monthly	_____	☐
4. Visual Checklist	Monthly	_____	☐
5. AW Monitor QC	Monthly	_____	☐
6. RW Monitor QC	Monthly	_____	☐
7. Film Printer QC	Monthly	_____	☐
8. Viewbox Cleanliness *(if app)*	Monthly	_____	☐
9. Facility QC Review	Quarterly	_____	☐
10. Compression Force	Semiannual	_____	☐
11. Manufacturer Calibrations *(if app)*		_____	☐
Optional - Repeat Analysis	As Needed	% Repeats [_____] _____	☐

3. Review and verify completion of all "Corrective Action"   ☐

4. Technique Chart review for each room (see MP report for recommendations) - (Annually)   ☐

5. Infection Control procedures followed   ☐

6. Offsite RW(s) & Film Printer(s) QC reviewed _____   ☐

7. Past and future service or service upgrades discussed *(if app)*   ☐

8. Past and future State and/or MQSA inspections discussed *(if app)*   ☐

9. Past and future ACR Accreditation issues discussed *(if app)*   ☐

Fig. 9.40 American College of Radiology radiologic technologist Facility QC Review form.

Continued

Facility QC Review *(cont)* *Quarterly*

Facility _____   **Date of QC Mtg** _____

Follow-up
Confirmed
(If App.)

10. Notable findings during QC meeting

_____   _____
_____   _____
_____   _____
_____   _____
_____   _____
_____   _____
_____   _____
_____   _____

11. Items for quality improvement from QC Meeting

_____   _____
_____   _____
_____   _____
_____   _____
_____   _____
_____   _____
_____   _____
_____   _____

12. Other QC Notes

_____   _____
_____   _____
_____   _____
_____   _____
_____   _____
_____   _____

Overall Pass/Fail [____]

_____   _____   _____
Lead Interpreting Radiologist   Facility Manager (If App)   QC Technologist
signature   *signature*   *signature*

Action Limit:	Required:	Lead interpreting radiologist and facility manager must review QC quarterly.
		The test passes if meeting held.
	Recommended:	Technologist and lead interpreting radiologist should review technique charts at least annually for each DM system.
	Timeframe:	Not applicable.

Fig. 9.40, cont'd

Compression Force   *Semiannual*

Image Mode *(2D, 2D w/Add-on DBT, DBT)* _____

Facility _____   **Room ID** _____

Unit Mfr & Model _____   **MAP ID-Unit#** *(00000-00)* _____ - _____

Procedure	**Required Equipment:** Bathroom scale; towels Place towel on detector, place bathroom scale on towel with dial or read-out positioned for reading. Place another towel on top of scale. Using manual fine-adjustment mode, activate compression until at least 25 pounds reached. Read and record the compression force. Using initial power-drive mode, activate compression until it stops automatically. Read and record the compression force. Check that force is maintained. **Note:** Ensure the scale used produces accurate readings as pressure is increased.

	Year				
	Date *(month & day)*				
	Tech Initials				
		Compression Force	**Units**	**Compression Force**	**Units**
Manual fine-adjustment compression force					
Force is at least 25 lbs (11.1 daN) P/F					
Initial power-drive compression force					
Force is at least 25 lbs (11.1 daN) but no more than 45 lbs (20.0 daN) P/F					
Compression remains at least 25 lbs (11.1 daN) throughout typical exposure P/F					
Overall Pass/Fail					

Enter number where appropriate.   **P = Pass   F = Fail**

Legend: lbs = pounds

daN = decanewton

Action Limit	**Required:**	Manual fine-adjustment compression force must be least 25 lbs (11.1 daN).
		Initial power-drive compression force must be at least 25 lbs (11.1 daN) but no greater than 45 lbs (20 daN).
		Compression remains at least 25 lbs (11.1 daN) throughout typical exposure.
	Timeframe:	Failures must be corrected before further examinations are performed.

Fig. 9.41 American College of Radiology radiologic technologist Compression Force form.

Manufacturer Calibrations *(if applicable)*

Image Mode *(2D, 2D w/Add-on DBT, DBT)* _____

Facility _____ _____ **Room ID** _____

MAP ID-Unit# *(00000-00)* _____ - _____ **Unit Mfr & Model** _____

Manufacturer Procedure	Frequency: _____
	Frequency: Per manufacturer recommendations (if app).
	Note: See medical physicist and manufacturer for instructions (if any).

Year					
Date *(month & day)*					
Tech Initials					
Name of Calibration					

P = Pass   F = Fail

Action Limits	Required:	Unit must pass manufacturer's prescribed periodic calibrations.
	Timeframe:	Failures must be corrected before further examinations are performed.

Fig. 9.42 American College of Radiology radiologic technologist Manufacturer Calibrations form.

Optional - Repeat Analysis - Summary Form   *As Needed*

Facility _____   **Year** _____

MAP ID *(00000)* _____

Procedure	Required Equipment: All repeated mammograms and means to count and sort them
	Record the ***total number of exposures*** for the collection period (month or quarter).
	Record the ***total number of repeat exposures*** for that time period.
	Calculate by hand, or use formulas in spreadsheet, to calculate repeat rate.
	Note: Some units may automatically calculate % Repeats. If so, enter this number into "% Repeats".

	Monthly Analysis				Quarterly Analysis			
	Total # of Exposures	# of Repeat Exposures	% Repeats	Pass or Fail	Total # of Exposures	# of Repeat Exposures	% Repeats	Pass or Fail
Jan								
Feb								
Mar								
Apr								
May								
Jun								
Jul								
Aug								
Sep								
Oct								
Nov								
Dec								

% Repeats = (# of Repeat Exposures / Total # of Exposures) * 100   P = Pass   F = Fail

Action Limits	Recommended:	If repeat rate changes from the previously determined rate by more than 2.0% of the total images included in the analysis, the reason(s) for the change must be determined.
	Timeframe:	Failures must be corrected within 30 days after analysis.

Fig. 9.43 American College of Radiology radiologic technologist Optional—Repeat Analysis—Summary form.

Optional - System QC for Radiologist
(For Quality Improvement)

As Needed

Facility _____

MAP ID-Unit# *(00000-00)* _____ - _____

Procedure	This test is to be performed or supervised by the lead interpreting radiologist. The technologist should deliver this form to the radiologist, ensure correct completion, follow-up on any failures, and place the form into QC notebook. This test can be performed on the same workstation for multiple DM or CR units. **Example:** A radiologist can sit at one workstation and view the images for all the DM and/or CR units within a facility. The radiologist does not need to evaluate every monitor at every workstation.

Objective   This test is for the Radiologist to perform an evaluation of the entire mammographic imaging chain with the focus being primarily on the detector and secondarily on the monitors. This test is not intended to evaluate technologist issues such as positioning, compression, etc.

Procedure for Radiologist

Step 1: Complete the demographics:

Room ID _____

DM or CR Unit Mfr & Model _____

Monitor ID _____

Radiologist Name _____

Date of Evaluation _____

Step 2. Pull up the recent mammographic study from the above listed DM unit and record ID & Study Date.

Image ID: _____

Study Date: _____

Step 3. Place the same MLO image on each monitor.

Left Monitor   Right Monitor

		Yes	No
Step 4. Evaluate the images for artifacts and check the appropriate boxes.	Comparing the monitors (or sides), do the background areas (outside of breast) appear different (darker or lighter, etc.)?	☐	☐
	Is there a difference in contrast between monitors/sides?	☐	☐
	Does the image contain excessive noise (not patient motion)?	☐	☐
For examples and more detailed descriptions, please see the Guide on Identifying Artifacts.	Do you see ghosting?	☐	☐
	Do you see "bad pixels" (singular or clusters) (white or black)?	☐	☐
	Do you see white dots that could be from excessive dust?	☐	☐
	Do you see any _image_ distortion (not architectural distortion)?	☐	☐
	Do you see gridlines?	☐	☐
	Do you see artifacts that could be due to image processing?	☐	☐
Step 5. If necessary, document any failures on the "Corrective Action Log" form and ensure items are resolved.	Do you see "line artifacts" (single or multiple pixels that form lines extending across image - horizontally or vertically)?	☐	☐
	Are there any other artifacts that are present and clinically significant (impeding interpretation)?	☐	☐

Action Limits	**Recommended:**	If any box is checked "Yes", then seek service.
	Timeframe:	If an image quality problem or artifact impedes clinical interpretation, seek service before further imaging or interpretations are performed.
		If the artifact does not impede clinical interpretation, seek service within 30 days.

Fig. 9.44 American College of Radiology radiologic technologist Optional-System QC for Radiologist form.

Optional - Radiologist Image Quality Feedback   *As Needed*
(For Quality Improvement)

Radiologist's Name _____

Date _____

Procedure	This report is to be completed by the Interpreting Radiologist when asked to interpret sub-optimal cases requiring the patient to be called back. The form may also be used to provide feedback on excellent quality. The radiologists should complete this form as needed for each case. A system should be in place for analyzing feedback and taking measures for improvement as necessary.

Objective   For the Radiologist to provide routine feedback to the technologists and manager on the quality of images.

Patient Identifier: _____

Technologist's Name: _____

Date of Exam: _____

Overall Assessment

☐ Excellent   ☐ Good   ☐ Needs improvement, but do not repeat   ☐ Sub-Optimal, and should be repeated

Image Evaluation

	RCC	LCC	RMLO	LMLO	Other View	Other View
Positioning						
Missing tissue						
Laterally						
Posteriorly						
Medially						
Inferiorly						
Nipple not in profile						
Skin fold						
Pectoralis not down to PNL						
Tissue droopy (camel nose)						
Narrow/concave pectoralis						
Inframammary fold						
Not open						
Not shown						
Centering not correct						
Technical Issues						
Not enough compression						
Exposure Too Low (Excessive Noise)						
Exposure Too High (Image Saturation)						
Patient Motion						
Artifacts						
Incorrect Patient ID						
Other						

Additional Images Needed for Complete Breast Evaluation

Requested views   ☐ RCC   ☐ LCC   ☐ RMLO   ☐ LMLO   ☐ Other View _____

Action Limits	Recommended:	Patients should be called back for additional images if the quality is suboptimal according to the interpreting radiologist's request.
	Timeframe:	Not applicable.

Fig. 9.45 American College of Radiology radiologic technologist Optional-Radiologist Image Quality Feedback form.

TABLE 9.3   Summary of Responsibilities for Mammography

Radiologist	Medical Physicist	Radiographer
Ensures the quality control program is implemented	Ensures proper functioning of mammographic equipment	Performs phantom image quality testing and CR cassette erasure weekly
Ensures the technical staff has adequate mammographic training and maintains continuing education	Performs yearly mammographic equipment evaluation	Performs monthly visual checklist, acquisition, and radiologist workstation monitor QC, film printer and viewbox cleanliness (if applicable)
Identifies primary quality control		Performs a quarterly facility QC review
Ensures technologist and medical physicist qualifications and performance of assigned duties		Performs a semiannual compression force evaluation
Reviews technologist and medical physicist test results		Performs any manufacturer calibration (if applicable)
Ensures procedures in infection control, quality control, radiation safety, and patient followup are maintained and updated		Performs repeat analysis, system QC for the radiologist, and radiologist image quality feedback analysis as needed

CR, Computed radiography; *QC*, quality control.

SUMMARY

QC and quality assurance of mammographic equipment and procedures are mandatory for compliance with the MQSA. Proper documentation of these procedures is essential for a facility to remain accredited to perform mammographic procedures.

Refer to the Evolve Website at https://evolve.elsevier.com for Student Experiment 11.1: Daily Mammographic Quality Control and 9.2: Phantom Image and Visual Inspection.

REVIEW QUESTIONS

1. What kVp range should be used during film/screen mammography?
   a. 15–20
   b. 20–28
   c. 30–40
   d. 40–50
2. Which of the following value ranges is the correct focal spot size for most mammographic X-ray tubes?
   a. 0.1–0.6 mm
   b. 0.6–1 mm
   c. 1–1.5 mm
   d. 1.5–2.5 mm
3. Which type of filter material should be used with a molybdenum target X-ray tube?
   a. Aluminum
   b. Copper
   c. Rhodium
   d. Molybdenum
4. Which of the following does not change the shape of the X-ray emission spectrum?
   a. Milliampere
   b. kVp
   c. Exposure time
   d. Target material
5. What is the usual range of force for mammographic system compression devices?
   a. 5–20 lb
   b. 15–30 lb
   c. 25–45 lb
   d. 45–60 lb
6. Severe defects found during acquisition workstation monitor QC must be corrected:
   a. Before clinical use
   b. Within 1 week
   c. Within 30 days
   d. By the next annual physics inspection

7. The light field/X-ray field alignment for mammographic units must be accurate to within ±____% of the source-to-image distance.
   a. 2
   b. 3
   c. 4
   d. 5

8. For ACR accreditation, which of the following tasks must the QC mammographer perform weekly for digital mammographic units?
   a. Compression force
   b. Acquisition workstation monitor QC
   c. Facility QC review
   d. Repeat analysis

9. When using the new ACR mammography phantom during phantom image analysis of digital mammographic systems, what is the minimum number of fibers that must be visible?
   a. 1
   b. 2
   c. 3
   d. 4

10. For ACR accreditation of mammographic facilities, how often must mammography technologists perform compression thickness indicator analysis?
    a. Daily
    b. Weekly
    c. Monthly
    d. Yearly

Quality Control in Computed Tomography

Lorrie Kelley*

OBJECTIVES

At the completion of this chapter, the reader should be able to do the following:

- Differentiate between high-contrast and low-contrast resolution
- Describe how basic quality control tests for computed tomography are conducted
- Describe the selection factors for quality control measurements
- Identify the parameters under the technologist's control that influence noise and spatial resolution

KEY TERMS

Acceptance testing
Action or control limit
Computed tomography dose index
  (CTDI)
Contrast scale
Control console

Gantry
High-contrast spatial resolution
Linearity
Low-contrast resolution
Mean CT number
Noise

Phantoms
Region of interest
Standard deviations
Volume computed tomography dose
  index (CTDIvol)

The goal of any quality control (QC) program is to ensure that the imaging equipment is producing the best possible image quality with a minimal radiation dose to the patient. The image quality in computed tomography (CT) can be difficult to maintain because of the complex nature of image acquisition and display. A contemporary CT system is composed of numerous electronic parts and computers that generate and process huge amounts of data. Because of the system's complexity, a quality assurance program is essential to ensure optimal system performance and image quality with the least amount of radiation dose to the patient. Quality assurance programs in CT are designed to provide certain performance parameters that allow for comparisons between two scanners and help determine whether a newly installed unit meets the specifications set by the vendor. A CT quality assurance program is conducted by a qualified team of medical physicists and radiologic technologists.

ACCEPTANCE TESTING

Typically, the installation of most CT units is immediately followed by extensive acceptance testing by qualified medical physicists. The purpose of the acceptance tests is to ensure that the equipment is performing according to the manufacturer's specifications before it is released for clinical use. Acceptance testing consists of measuring radiologic and electromechanical performance, analyzing image performance, and evaluating the system components. The results of the acceptance tests are used to identify system components that may need only slight adjustments and defective parts that should be replaced. At the end of the acceptance testing, scans are taken of standard objects so that their images, CT numbers, and standard deviations can be recorded as a baseline for future measurements of the system's performance.

---

*The author and publisher wish to acknowledge the previous edition's contributor.

ROUTINE TESTING

To provide more consistency in the performance measurements of CT scanners, federal performance standards state that the vendors of CT systems manufactured after September 1985 are required to supply the following: instructions for performing QC tests, a schedule for testing, allowable variations for the indicated parameters, a method to store and record the quality assurance data, and dose information in the form of a CT dose index. In addition each vendor is required to supply phantoms capable of testing the following parameters: contrast scale, noise, slice thickness, spatial resolution capabilities for both high-contrast and low-contrast objects, and the mean CT number for water or other reference material. Many routine QC tests can be performed by a CT technologist. In most instances, vendors specify the test conditions for evaluating their system's performance; therefore specific procedures for evaluating a system's performance may vary among manufacturers. Also, there is some disagreement among manufacturers about the proper monitoring frequency for high-contrast and low-contrast resolution, alignment, contrast scale, and slice thickness. Until standards for monitoring frequency can be agreed on, it is best to follow those recommended by the manufacturer. QC testing must also be completed after major repairs and before the first clinical scan after the repair. Major repairs include replacement or repair of any of the following subsystem components: X-ray tube, generator, collimator assembly, or X-ray detectors.

The performance of CT scanners is evaluated with a phantom as a test object. The phantoms that are supplied by the manufacturer can vary among vendors because of the differing requirements for performance evaluations and QC testing. However, a typical phantom used to assess the performance of a CT system is a multisectioned phantom, which enables the separate evaluation of different parameters (Figs. 10.1 and 10.2). In general, a phantom is constructed from plastic cylinders, with each section filled with water or other test objects to measure specific parameter performance. Some phantoms are designed so that numerous parameters can be evaluated with a single scan. The American College of Radiology (ACR) CT accreditation phantom is a solid phantom containing four modules and is constructed primarily from a water-equivalent material. Each module is 4 cm in depth and 20 cm in diameter. There are external alignment markings scribed and painted white (to reflect alignment lights) on each module to allow centering of the phantom in the axial (z-axis, cranial/caudal), coronal (y-axis, anterior/posterior), and sagittal (x-axis, left/right) directions. There are also "HEAD," "FOOT," and "TOP" markings on the phantom to assist with positioning. Module 1 (Fig. 10.2C) is used to assess positioning and alignment, CT number accuracy, and slice thickness. Module 2 (Fig. 10.2B) is used to assess low-contrast resolution. Module 3 (Fig. 10.2D) consists of a uniform, tissue-equivalent material to assess CT number uniformity. Module 4 (Fig. 10.2A) is used to assess high-contrast (spatial) resolution.

CT has undergone significant technologic advancements in recent years, resulting in new clinical applications and changes in clinical protocols in numerous CT departments across the United States. In 2002, in an effort to establish a reasonable standard of image quality, the ACR approved the implementation of the CT Accreditation Program. This program was designed to evaluate the primary determinants of clinical image quality, including the qualifications of the

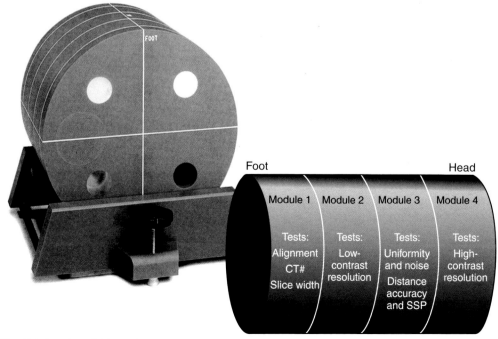

Fig. 10.1 American College of Radiology CT Accreditation Phantom. (From Bushong S. *Radiologic science for technologists,* 11th ed. Mosby; 2017.)

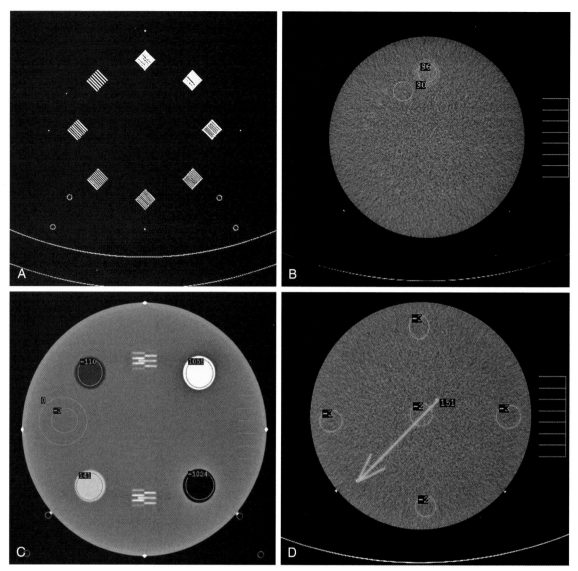

Fig. 10.2 Images of the four modules found in the American College of Radiology CT Accreditation Phantom: (A) Module 4; (B) Module 2; (C) Module 1; (D) Module 3. (From Bushong S. *Radiologic science for technologists,* 11th ed. Mosby; 2017.)

radiologists, medical physicists, and technologists; equipment performance; effectiveness of QC tests and measures; and clinical image quality and examination protocols. The ACR CT Accreditation Committee developed a specially designed CT phantom, along with test protocols for use in the accreditation process and for establishing quality assurance programs for clinical CT scanners. The multisectioned ACR CT accreditation phantom was designed to examine a wide variety of scanner parameters, including positioning accuracy, CT number accuracy, slice thickness, low-contrast resolution, high-contrast resolution, image uniformity and noise, distance measurement accuracy, section sensitivity profiles, and image artifacts. In the summer of 2008, Congress passed the Medicare Improvements for Patients and Providers Act of 2008, which mandates that any nonhospital institution performing advanced diagnostic services (such as CT) must be accredited by a Centers for Medicare & Medicaid Services–designated accrediting organization

to receive federal funding (Medicare reimbursement). As of the writing of this edition, Centers for Medicare & Medicaid Services have approved three national accreditation organizations: the ACR, the Intersocietal Accreditation Commission, and The Joint Commission. This rule affects providers of magnetic resonance imaging, CT, positron emission tomography, and nuclear medicine imaging services for Medicare beneficiaries on an outpatient basis. The accreditation applies only to the suppliers of the images and not to the physician's interpretation of the image. Therefore accreditation programs are becoming mandatory for CT departments to succeed.

All QC tests described in this chapter should be performed according to the following three basic tenets of QC:
- The QC tests should be performed on a regular basis.
- All QC test measurements should be documented with the data form provided by the manufacturer (Fig. 10.3) or accrediting agency.

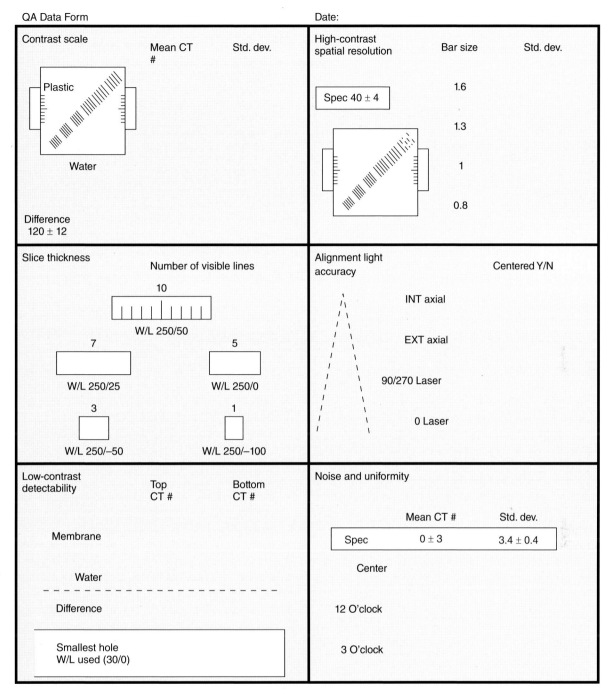

Fig. 10.3 Sample quality assurance data form.

- The QC test should indicate whether the tested parameter is within specified guidelines known as action or control limits.

The material in this chapter follows the procedures recommended by the ACR, but the Intersocietal Accreditation Commission and The Joint Commission require similar procedures. To maintain ACR CT accreditation status, the ACR states that a QC program must be implemented under the direction of a qualified medical physicist. The medical physicist is responsible for the annual performance evaluations of each CT unit as well as the establishment of a continuous QC program for implementation by a qualified CT technologist. The medical physicist will determine the frequency that each test must be performed on the basis of the facility and CT usage. The ACR recommends that a continuous QC program include but not be limited to evaluations of the following: alignment light accuracy, slice thickness, image quality, high-contrast resolution, low-contrast resolution, image uniformity, noise, artifact evaluation, CT number accuracy, and display devices.

The methodology of most of the following QC tests uses the ACR CT Accreditation Phantom and testing criteria, but the same tests can be performed with phantoms supplied by the CT system's vendor. When using a vendor-supplied phantom, test measures should be compared with the limits specified by the vendor or during acceptance testing.

The ACR CT Accreditation Phantom is a solid phantom constructed primarily from a water-equivalent material. It consists of four contiguous modules, each 4 cm in width and 20 cm in diameter. Various test objects are embedded within the phantom to measure the various image quality parameters of a QC program.

Before starting any QC tests, it is important to complete a tube warmup and daily system calibrations recommended by the manufacturer to optimize image quality.

ALIGNMENT LIGHT ACCURACY

Internal and external laser lights are used extensively for patient positioning and alignment. Accurate laser light performance is critical during stereotactic and interventional procedures.

Measurements to determine laser light accuracy can be made with the manufacturer's specific phantoms or a piece of covered, unexposed X-ray film.

After the X-ray film has been processed, the two sets of holes represent the internal and external light fields and the two dark bands from radiation exposure represent the radiation field. To measure the accuracy of the laser lights, one should check to see whether the dark bands of exposure fall directly over the associated holes (Fig. 10.4). For optimal performance, the light field should coincide with the radiation field to within 2 mm.

An alternative method to measure laser light accuracy is to scan the phantom and place a grid over the resultant image. The grid should line up accurately with the lines on the phantom.

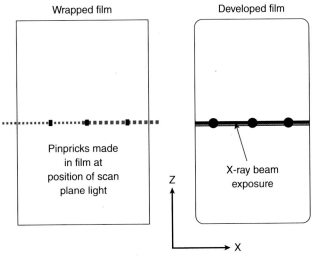

Fig. 10.4 Technique for assessing laser light accuracy. (Courtesy ImPACT, a Medical Devices Agency Evaluation Group, London, UK.)

PROCEDURE: ALIGNMENT LIGHT ACCURACY

1. Tape the unexposed X-ray film securely to the computed tomography table.
2. To measure the accuracy of the internal laser lights, turn on the internal laser lights and poke two or three small holes through the wrapper and X-ray film at the exact location of the light field. The holes should be located near the right and left edges and the center of the film.
3. Perform a scan through the location specified by the internal laser lights.
4. To measure the accuracy of the external laser lights, turn on the external laser lights and poke two small holes through either edge of the film at the exact location of the external light field.
5. Advance the table so that it is in position to scan, and perform a scan at that location.

Image Quality

High-Contrast (Spatial) Resolution

High-contrast spatial resolution is described as the minimum distance between two objects that allows them to be seen as separate and distinct. The parameters that influence the high-contrast spatial resolution of a CT scanner include the following:

1. Scanner design (focal spot size, detector size and spacing, magnification)
2. Image reconstruction (pixel size, reconstruction algorithm, slice thickness)
3. Sampling (number of rays per projection and number of projections)
4. Image display capabilities (display matrix)

The ACR CT Accreditation Phantom's Module 4 (Fig. 10.2A) is used to evaluate high-contrast spatial resolution. It contains 8-bar-resolution patterns, which represent spatial frequencies corresponding to 4, 5, 6, 7, 8, 9, 10, and 12 line pairs per centimeter (lp/cm), each fitting into a 15-mm × 15-mm square region.

PROCEDURE: HIGH-CONTRAST RESOLUTION

1. Scan Module 4 with adult abdomen and high-resolution chest protocols, making sure to use the appropriate reconstruction algorithm.
2. Display the images with a window width of 100 and window level ≈1100.
3. Record the bar pattern for which the bars and spaces are distinctly visualized for both images.

American College of Radiology Acceptance Criteria
- The adult abdomen and high-resolution chest protocols must be used.
- Window width = 100.
- Window level ≈1100.
- The 5-lp/cm bar pattern must be clearly resolved for adult abdomen protocol.
- The 6-lp/cm bar pattern must be clearly resolved for adult high-resolution chest protocol.

The limiting high-contrast spatial resolution of a CT scanner is measured in line pairs per centimeter. Even though many modern scanners have the ability to resolve holes as small as 0.3 mm, the spatial resolution of CT scanners is still lower than that of conventional radiography. The results of this test can be compared with the baseline measurement of the scanner collected during optimal system performance or with the manufacturer's specifications. Comparative measurements over time provide an index of the performance reproducibility of the CT system.

Low-Contrast Resolution

Low-contrast resolution refers to the capability of the CT system to demonstrate subtle differences in tissue densities from one region of anatomy to another. Compared with conventional radiography, CT provides superior low-contrast resolution. Typically, contrast resolution is expressed in one of two ways: the smallest diameter of an object with a specific contrast that can be detected or the smallest difference in X-ray attenuation that can be discriminated for an object of a specific diameter.

A phantom consisting of test objects such as holes drilled into plastic is used for this test (Module 2 of ACR Phantom). The rows of holes should be of varying sizes and filled with a liquid that has a CT number different from the CT number for the plastic by approximately 0.6%. The ACR CT Accreditation Phantom uses Module 2 (Fig. 10.5) to assess low-contrast resolution. It consists of a series of cylinders of varying diameters with a 0.6% Hounsfield unit (HU) difference from the background material, which has a CT number of approximately 90 HU. Four cylinders exist for each of the following diameters: 2, 3, 4, 5, and 6 mm. The space between each cylinder is equal to the diameter of the cylinder. An additional 25-mm cylinder is used to verify the contrast between the cylinders and the background material.

1. View the best image located in Module 2 for all submitted protocols using a window width = 100 and a window level = 100. Note that there are four cylinders for each of following diameters: 2, 3, 4, 5, and 6 mm (Fig. 10.6).
2. Place a region of interest (ROI) (≈100 mm²) over the large (25-mm diameter) cylinder and between the large cylinder and the 6-mm cylinders.
3. Record the mean signal in the ROI inside the 25-mm rod (A), the mean signal in the ROI outside the 25-mm rod over the background material (B), and the standard deviation (SD) from the ROI outside the 25-mm rod for your records. Use the following formula to calculate the contrast-to-noise ratio (CNR):

$$CNR = |A - B|/SD$$

4. Use the absolute value of the difference—that is, do not take into consideration whether the CNR is a positive or negative number. The CNR must be greater than 1.0 for the adult head and adult abdomen protocols. The CNR must be greater than 0.4 for the pediatric abdomen protocol and greater than 0.7 for the pediatric head protocol. In addition, all four of the 6-mm cylinders must be clearly visible.

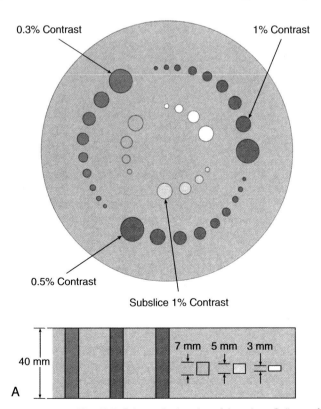

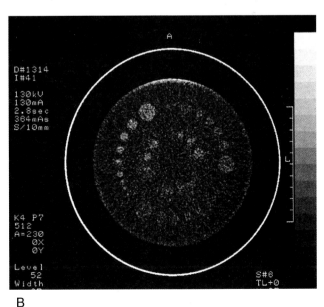

Fig. 10.5 Schematic drawing of American College of Radiology CT Phantom Module 2 (A) and its image (B). This test object is designed especially for multislice helical CT. (From Bushong S. *Radiologic science for technologists,* 11th ed. Mosby; 2017.)

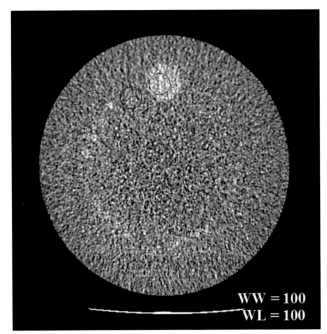

Fig. 10.6 Test image of Module 2 during low-contrast resolution evaluation. *WL*, Window length; *WW*, window width.

The primary factor limiting low-contrast resolution in CT is image noise caused by quantum mottle. As noise increases in an image, the edge definition of anatomic borders and subtle differences in attenuation between tissues decrease.

Image Uniformity

Uniformity refers to the ability of the CT scanner to yield the same CT number regardless of the location of the ROI within a homogenous object.

A simple 20-cm water phantom can be used to measure noise and uniformity in CT. Module 3 of the ACR CT Accreditation Phantom is used to assess image uniformity. Module 3 consists of a uniform, tissue-equivalent material with two small ball bearings placed at known distances within the material for optional measurements of in-plane distance (Fig. 10.2D).

PROCEDURE: IMAGE UNIFORMITY

1. Scan Module 3 with adult abdomen protocol.
2. Display the image with a window width of 100 and window level of 0 (Fig. 10.7).
3. Place an ROI, approximately 400 mm in diameter, at the center of the image and record the HU and SD.
4. Place the same-size ROI at peripheral edges of the phantom at positions 12, 3, 6, and 9 o'clock. Record the HU and SD for each ROI.
5. Determine the difference between the mean CT number of the center ROI to the mean CT numbers for all four edge ROIs (mean CT number of center ROI − mean CT number of edge ROI).
6. Assess the image for artifacts such as rings or streaks, and record the presence and appearance of any artifacts. If artifacts are present, your medical physicist or service engineer may need to investigate and correct them.

American College of Radiology Acceptance Criteria

- All CT numbers for all five ROIs must be within ±5 HU of the center ROI mean value.
- ROIs must have correct size and location.
- Adult abdomen protocol must be used.
- Window width = 100.
- Window level = 0.
- No image artifacts should be seen.

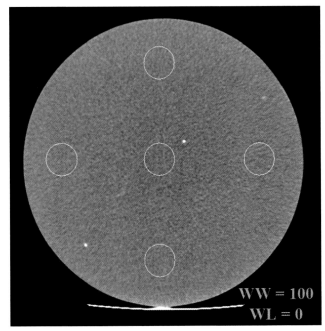

Fig. 10.7 Test image of Module 3 during uniformity testing.

Noise

Noise represents the portion of the CT image that contains no useful information. It is defined as the random variation of CT numbers about a mean value when an image of a uniform object is obtained. The contrast resolution of a CT system is primarily determined by the amount of noise in the images. Noise produces a "salt-and-pepper" appearance or grainy quality in the image. The sources of noise in a CT image include quantum (statistical) noise, electronic noise, object size, reconstruction algorithms, detector efficiency, and artifacts. Of these, the predominant source of noise is quantum noise, which is defined as the statistical variation in the number of photons detected.

Factors under the influence of the technologist that affect the amount of noise in an image are pixel size, slice thickness, reconstruction algorithm, and technique factors. Simple methods to minimize noise and help provide uniform images include tube warm-ups and daily system calibrations. Because the amount of noise contained in an image is inversely proportional to the total amount of radiation absorbed, noise can be measured by obtaining the mean and SD of the CT numbers within an ROI.

PROCEDURE: NOISE

1. Scan Module 3 with adult abdomen protocol.
2. Display the image with a window width of 100 and window level of 0.
3. Place an ROI, approximately 20 mm in diameter, at the center of the image and record the Hounsfield unit (HU) and standard deviation.

American College of Radiology Acceptance Criteria
No value given; compare with manufacturer's specifications.

Computed Tomography Number Accuracy

CT numbers represent the attenuation values of different structures within the body according to their atomic number and physical density. The CT numbers are assigned a shade of gray corresponding with the attenuation value they represent. This constitutes the gray scale or contrast scale of the displayed image. The contrast scale is determined by the CT numbers for air (−1000 HU) and water (0 HU). In CT, the scanner assigns CT numbers according to the attenuation values of X-rays passing through tissue. Water is the reference material used to determine CT numbers because it constitutes up to 90% of soft tissue mass, is easy to obtain, and is completely reproducible. Because water has a CT number value of zero, tissues with densities greater than water have positive CT numbers and those with densities less than water have negative CT numbers (Fig. 10.2C). This test is performed to determine whether the scanner is assigning CT numbers that accurately correspond to the appropriate tissue. Many radiologists use CT numbers as quantitative parameters to identify suspected pathologic conditions in the image. Calculating the CT number of known materials is necessary to measure the accuracy of the CT numbers. It is recommended that this be performed in both the axial and helical scan mode. The QC manual suggests performing these scans on alternate days to speed up the process.

PROCEDURE: COMPUTED TOMOGRAPHY NUMBER ACCURACY

1. Align Module 1 to lasers. Module 1 consists of water embedded with four cylinders of known reference materials (air, polyethylene, bone, and acrylic) (Fig. 10.8).
2. Scan with adult abdomen protocol and at all kilovolt peak (kVp) values available.
3. Place an ROI approximately 200 mm over the center of each cylinder and the water. Record all HUs.
4. Scan varying slice thicknesses and repeat step 3.

The contrast scale can vary with different X-ray energies; therefore for QC testing, each test should be repeated at the same kVp setting and for each kVp setting that can be selected. For consistent results, the same cursor size and location should be used each time the test is performed.

American College of Radiology Acceptance Criteria
- ROIs must be placed within the cylinders.
- Polyethylene mean CT number must be between −107 and −84 HU.

- Water mean CT number must be between −7 and +7 HU (±5 HU preferred).
- Acrylic mean CT number must be between +110 and +135 HU.
- Bone mean CT number must be between +850 and +970 HU.
- Air mean CT number must be between −1005 and −970 HU.
- Image data are required for all selectable kVp settings.

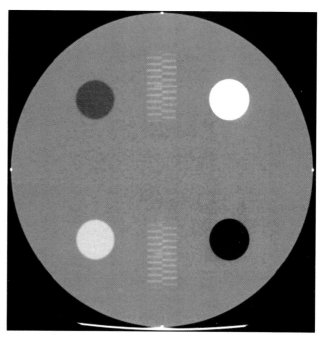

Fig. 10.8 Test image of Module 1 during CT number accuracy.

This test is performed to determine whether the scanner is assigning CT numbers that accurately correspond to the appropriate tissue. Many radiologists use CT numbers as quantitative parameters to identify suspected pathologic conditions in the image. Calculating the CT number of known materials is necessary to measure the accuracy of the CT numbers.

Slice Thickness

The slice thickness in single-slice CT is determined primarily by the collimators. The position of the collimators determines the width of the slice that falls within the view of each detector. In multidetector CT, the slice thickness is determined by the width of the active detector elements. Another factor affecting slice thickness is the focal spot size. The focal spot size can influence the penumbra, or sharpness of the edge of the X-ray beam, which can cause the edge of the slice to spread. Focal spot size in CT is determined by the technique factors or algorithm selected for the scan parameters. Slice thickness is a primary factor of image quality and spatial resolution.

Measurements of slice thickness are determined with a phantom that includes a ramp, spiral, or step wedge in the test objects. The test objects have known measurements and provide a standard to compare with the scanner. Typically, the test objects are aligned obliquely to the scan plane (Fig. 10.9).

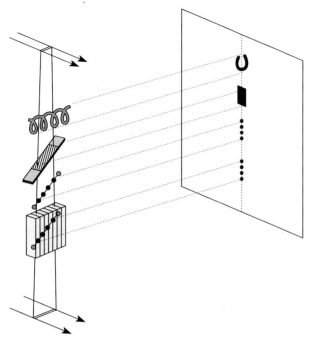

Fig. 10.9 Test objects used for determining slice thickness. (From Marshall C. *The physical basis of computed tomography.* Warren H. Green; 1982.)

If it is 5 mm or more, the slice thickness should not vary more than ±1 mm from the intended slice thickness. If it is 5 mm or less, the slice thickness should not vary more than ±0.5 mm.

Module 1 of the ACR CT Accreditation Phantom (Fig. 10.2C) is used to assess slice thickness. Embedded within Module 1 are a series of discrete wires that are positioned on a ramp inclined with respect to the axial plane such that the spacing between them equals 0.5 mm along the z-axis.

PROCEDURE: SLICE THICKNESS

1. Scan Module 1 with 3-, 5-, and 7-mm and high-resolution chest slice thicknesses.
2. Use a window width = 400 and a window level = 0 to view images.
3. Count the number of wires visualized in each of the two slice thickness ramps at each slice thickness (count the number of wires in the top and bottom ramps separately).
4. Estimate the slice thickness by counting the number of well-visualized wires at the top and bottom of each slice and divide by two. For example, if you can visualize 11 wires, 11 ÷ 2 is 5.5 mm.

American College of Radiology Acceptance Criteria
- Image data are required for high-resolution chest and 3-, 5-, and 7-mm slice thicknesses.
- The slice width must be within 1.5 mm of the prescribed width.

Linearity

Linearity refers to the relationship between CT numbers and the linear attenuation values of the scanned object with a particular kVp value. When linearity is present within an image, it is an indication that subject contrast is constant across the range of CT numbers within the image.

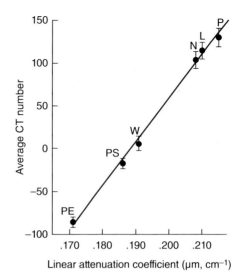

Fig. 10.10 Graph showing computed tomography (CT) linearity. *L*, Lexan; *N*, nylon; *P*, Plexiglas; *PE*, polyethylene; *PS*, polystyrene; *W*, water. (From Bushong S. *Radiologic science for technologists*, 6th ed. Mosby; 2017.)

A standard phantom containing materials with known physical and X-ray absorption properties is used for this test, such as Module 1 of the ACR Accreditation Phantom (Fig. 10.2C).

Over time, these values can vary because of changes in system components. Daily calibrations help maintain image quality by compensating for changes in detector channel variations and responses.

The plotted values should demonstrate a straight line between the average CT numbers and the linear attenuation coefficients (Fig. 10.10). Any deviation from the straight line can indicate that inaccurate CT numbers are being generated or the scanner is malfunctioning.

PROCEDURE: LINEARITY

1. Take a single scan through Module 1 of the ACR Accreditation Phantom.
2. Plot the average CT numbers as a function of the attenuation values corresponding to the materials within the phantom.

Patient Dose

Personnel should monitor the amount of radiation to which patients and staff are exposed. It is equally important for a CT technologist to realize that the patient dose can increase with changes in slice thickness, kVp, and milliampere-seconds (mAs). In addition, if it is necessary for ancillary personnel to remain within the scan room, all CT technologists should be able to direct them to the safest location within the room to avoid unnecessary radiation exposure. Figure 10.11 provides representative isodose curves for a typical CT scanner.

Specially designed ionization chambers or thermoluminescent dosimeters are used to measure the radiation dose. These specially designed radiation detectors are capable of providing measurements from which the dose can be

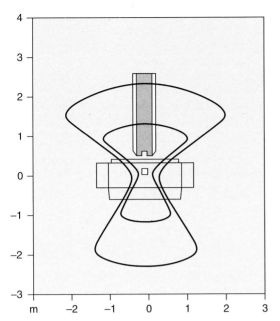

Fig. 10.11 Isodose curves for a typical computed tomography (CT) scanner. (From Wegener OH. *Whole body computed tomography.* Blackwell Scientific; 1992.)

calculated for the exposure factors used (slice thickness, mAs, and kVp).

PROCEDURE: PATIENT DOSE

1. Along with a standard phantom, position the radiation-detecting device at the location and intervals of the desired radiation measurements.
2. Initiate the appropriate scans at the selected locations and measure the resultant radiation dose. Some facilities prefer to take two scans at each location but with a change in the technique factors to simulate the difference between head and body examinations. This gives a more reliable dose estimate for a particular CT examination.

No acceptable maximum levels of radiation are specified for the permissible dose to a patient during a CT procedure. In addition, the results can vary according to patient location and distance from the X-ray source. However, most experts agree that the values should remain within ±10% of the manufacturer's specifications when a fixed technique is used.

For ACR CT accreditation purposes, a medical physicist is required to perform computed tomography dose index (CTDI) testing on every CT unit at the clinical facility. This value is measured in a cylindrical acrylic phantom placed at the scanner isocenter and obtained by using a 100-mm-long, pencil-shaped ionization chamber in one of two phantom sizes. A 16-cm phantom is used to calculate the CTDI for head examinations and a 32-cm phantom is used to calculate the CTDI for body examinations. Because multislice CT units have become the prevalent system in CT departments, a more appropriate dose descriptor of volume computed tomography dose index (CTDIvol) is now used. This value incorporates the CTDI values at both the center and periphery of the

TABLE 10.1   American College of Radiology CT Accreditation Dose Pass/Fail Criteria and Reference Levels

Examination	Pass/Fail Criteria CTDI$_{vol}$ (mGy)	Reference Levels CTDI$_{vol}$ (mGy)
Adult head	80	75
Adult abdomen	30	25
Pediatric head (1 year old)	40	35
Pediatric abdomen (40–50 lb)—16 cm phantom	20	15
Pediatric abdomen (40–50 lb)—32 cm phantom	10	7.5

CT, Computed tomography; *CTDIvol*, volume computed tomography dose index.

acrylic phantom, as well as the pitch factor and slice thickness. For a given scanner and set of scanning parameters being used (i.e., kVp, mA, tube rotation time, beam width, and CT pitch), the CTDIvol is fixed and is not affected by patient size or scan length. This means that CTDIvol does not measure how much a specific patient receives, but rather indicates the intensity of radiation that is being directed at that patient. For the CT unit to pass the phantom image quality tests, it has to be demonstrated that the scanner meets the ACR dose reference levels. The ACR has recently updated the ACR CT accreditation dose pass/fail criteria and reference levels (Table 10.1).

American College of Radiology Computed Tomography Technologist's Quality Control Testing Requirements

In addition to the medical physicist's testing, the ACR also requires that CT technologists perform QC tests on a regular basis and that the test results are properly documented. These results should be reviewed with the medical physicist and radiologist regularly. The technologists' QC tests include:

Procedure	Minimum Frequency	Approximate Time (min)
Water computed tomography number and standard deviation	Daily	5
Artifact evaluation	Daily	5 or less
Wet laser printer quality control (if film is used for primary interpretation)	Weekly	10
Visual checklist	Monthly	5
Dry laser printer quality control (if film is used for primary interpretation)	Monthly	10
Display monitor quality control	Monthly	5

Water Computed Tomography Number and Standard Deviation (Noise)

This test is performed to ensure that the relative calibration of all CT numbers to water remains within acceptable limits and that quantum noise and electronic system noise do not increase (this would cause a decrease in low-contrast detectability). Images of the water phantom provided by the scanner manufacturer or the ACR CT phantom are obtained before the first clinical scan of the day (or the equivalent for scanners used around the clock). Images of the water phantom are acquired in both the axial and helical scan modes using predetermined scan techniques.

Artifact Evaluation

The images of the water phantom or ACR CT phantom obtained in the water number and SD procedure should be reviewed daily to identify and correct artifacts in images before they become severe enough to be detected in patient images. Data are recorded on the CT Equipment Quality Control Data Form (Fig. 10.12).

PROCEDURE: WATER COMPUTED TOMOGRAPHY NUMBER AND STANDARD DEVIATION

1. Warm up the scanner's X-ray tubes according to manufacturer's recommendations.
2. Perform calibration scans (often called air-calibration scans) according to scanner manufacturer's recommendations.
3. Place the QC phantom on the holder device provided. Center the phantom at the isocenter of the scanner using the laser alignment lights of the scanner and the alignment marks on the phantom surface.
4. Set up a scan of the QC phantom using the scanner's daily QC scan parameter settings. It is strongly recommended that the QC scan protocols be preprogrammed for consistency. Usually, these scan protocols will follow the parameter settings recommended by the scanner's manufacturer. Water mean and SD values should be monitored for both axial and helical scan modes. If the scanner's manufacturer specifies only one of these modes, the medical physicist should assist the QC technologist in establishing and preprogramming a similar scan protocol for the other mode.
5. While viewing the phantom image, place an ROI at the center of the image. If a group of images was obtained on a multislice CT scanner, select an image from the central portion of the group to analyze. If the size of this ROI is not specified by the manufacturer, use an area of about 400 mm². Record the value reported for the water mean and SD on the CT Equipment Quality Control Data Form (see Fig. 10.12).
6. Repeat the previous measurement for an image that is either at the leading or trailing edge of the fan beam during the acquisition (i.e., an image at the beginning or end of the stack).
7. Repeat steps 5 and 6 for image(s) acquired in the second scan mode.
8. The water values should be 0 ± 5 HU, but must be 0 ± 7 HU. The medical physicist will establish limit criteria for noise (SD) for both axial and helical modes after consulting the manufacturer's recommendations.
9. If either the mean CT number or the noise (SD) is not within the criteria limit for three days in a row or three times within a 7-day period, corrective action should be taken by reporting the problem to service personnel.

Wet Laser Printer Quality Control

This test must be performed weekly if film is used for primary interpretation. For printers that are used infrequently (i.e., backup printers), this test should be performed before clinical use. Equipment necessary for this test is a densitometer, laser film QC chart (Fig. 10.13), and an SMPTE (Society of Motion Picture and Television Engineers) test pattern (see Chapter 8).

Visual Checklist

A visual checklist should be performed on a monthly basis (at minimum) to ensure that the CT system's patient bed transport, alignment and system indicator lights, intercom, the emergency cart, room safety lights, signage, and monitors are present, are working properly, and are mechanically and electrically stable. Results should be recorded on the visual checklist form (see Fig. 10.12). Specific items on the form include:

Gantry—All involve checks of items that are on the gantry or patient table.

- Table height indicator functioning: Display above gantry opening indicating the table height. Is it operating and appearing to track properly with table height change?
- Table position indicator functioning: Display above gantry opening indicating the table position. Is it operating and appearing to track properly with table position change?
- Angulation indicator functioning: This is the display above the gantry opening indicating the tilt of the gantry in degrees. Is it operating and appearing to track properly with gantry tilt changes?
- Laser localization lights functioning: Are the vertical laser lights indicating the patient's scan positioning, both in the scan plane and external to the scan plane, operating properly? Are the vertical laser lights indicating the patient's left/right (L-R) positioning operating properly? Are the horizontal laser lights indicating the patient's anterior/posterior (A-P) positioning (height) operating properly and are they consistent from both sides?
- Smoothness of table motion acceptable: Is the motion jerky or otherwise not as smooth as normal?
- X-ray on indicator functioning: Does the X-ray "On" indicator above the gantry opening turn on when the X-rays are on?

Control console—checks all involve checks of items that are on the console outside of the patient room.

CT EQUIPMENT QUALITY CONTROL DATA FORM

Facility Name: _____

Month: _____   Year: _____   CT Scanner: _____

Day	Warm up	Air Cals	Mode	CT$_{water}$ (HU)	Noise (SD)	Artifacts	P/F	Initials
1			Axial					
2			Helical					
3			Axial					
4			Helical					
5			Axial					
6			Helical					
7			Axial					
8			Helical					
9			Axial					
10			Helical					
11			Axial					
12			Helical					
13			Axial					
14			Helical					
15			Axial					
16			Helical					
17			Axial					
18			Helical					
19			Axial					
20			Helical					
21			Axial					
22			Helical					
23			Axial					
24			Helical					
25			Axial					
26			Helical					
27			Axial					
28			Helical					
29			Axial					
30			Helical					
31			Axial					

Action Limits: CT$_{water}$ = 0 ± 5 HU   SD: A: ____-____   H: ____-____

Comments/Corrective Action

Monthly Visual Checklist		☑
GANTRY	Table height indicator functioning...........	
	Table position indicator functioning........	
	Angulation indicator functioning.............	
	Laser localization light functioning..........	
	Acceptable smoothness of table motion.	
	X-ray on indicator functioning................	
CONTROL CONSOLE	Exposure switch functioning..................	
	Panel switches/lights/meters working.....	
	X-ray on indicator functioning................	
	Warning labels present..........................	
	Intercom system functioning..................	
OTHER	Postings present...................................	
	Service records maintained/accessible....	

Monthly Display Monitor Gray Level		☑
SMPTE PATTERN	5% patch in 0%–5% is discernible...........	
	95% patch in 95%–100% is discernible......	
	Distinct gray level steps.........................	

Window: _____   Level: _____

Monthly Large Artifact Check

If available, scan manufacturer's large phantom

Artifacts:

Date of Monthly QA: _____   Initials: _____

PASS = P or ✓   FAIL = F   NOT APPLICABLE = NA

A = Axial   H = Helical

Notes:
Warm up and Air Cals frequency are per manufacturer recommendation.
Continue Comments/Corrective action on back of sheet, if needed.

_____   _____
Qualified Medical Physicist Reviewer   Date of Review

Fig. 10.12 American College of Radiology CT Equipment Quality Control Data Form.

- Exposure switch functioning: Does the system tell you when to press the "move to scan" and the "start scan" buttons, and do these buttons operate properly?
- Display window width/level: Do the present WW/WL keys work properly and do the WW/WL control keys (up-down, left-right) work properly?

- X-ray on indicator functioning: Does the "Exposure" indicator above the keyboard light up when the X-rays are on?
- Panel switches/lights/meters working: This is a catch-all for all other items on the control console. Are any not working properly?

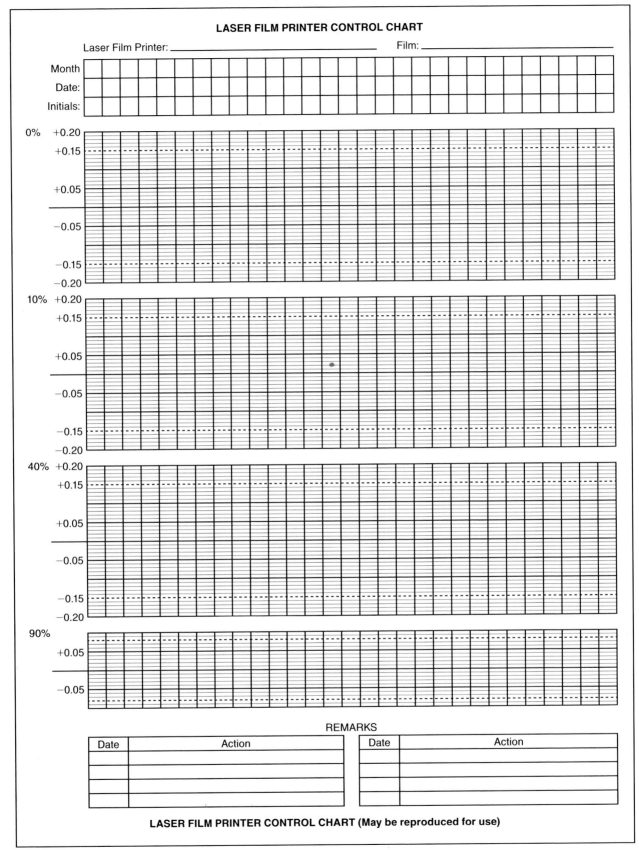

Fig. 10.13 American College of Radiology Laser Film Printer Control Chart.

- Warning labels present: Specifically the warning label about X-rays above the keypad.
- Intercom system functioning: Can voices be clearly heard by the patient and by the operator without excessive static or distortion? Do the volume controls operate properly? Does the talk switch operate properly? Check and adjust the volume if needed at this time.

Items missing from the room should be replaced immediately. Malfunctioning equipment should be reported to the CT service engineer for repair or replacement as soon as possible.

PROCEDURE: ARTIFACT EVALUATION

1. View the images obtained in the water number and SD procedure using the appropriate window width/level setting and scan for artifacts (additional images may be necessary). The artifact images should (1) be the thinnest axial images possible on the scanner and (2) span the z-axis of the detector array on the scanner.
2. Look for rings in the image, which can be darker or lighter than the water portion. Also look for streaks, lines, and the like, which should not be present in the image. Record the findings on the data form.
3. Ring artifacts typically indicate detector or data channel imbalance. Repeating the air-calibration procedure (step 2 of the water number procedure) may smooth out these imbalances. If they are not corrected after performing several air-calibration procedures, service of the scanner should be arranged.

PROCEDURE: LASER PRINTER QUALITY CONTROL

1. Display the SMPTE test pattern on the filming console. Set the display window width/level to the manufacturer-specified values for the SMPTE pattern.
2. Film the SMPTE pattern. Use a 6-on-1 format and capture the pattern in all six frames.
3. Using a film densitometer, measure the optical density of the 0, 10%, 40%, and 90% gray-level patches of the SMPTE pattern in the upper left frame of the film.
4. Plot these optical densities in the appropriate places on the laser film QC chart. Circle any points that fall outside the control limit.

SMPTE Patch	Optical Density	Control Limits
0	3.00	±0.15
10%	2.20	±0.15
40%	1.15	±0.15
90%	0.30	±0.15

5. Put the film on a viewbox and inspect it for streaks, uneven densities, and other artifacts.
6. If optical densities fall outside of control limit or if artifacts are found, corrective action should be taken.

Hard Copy Image Quality Control of Dry Laser Printers

This test must be performed monthly if film is used for primary interpretation. For printers used infrequently (i.e., backup printers), this test should be performed before clinical use. The equipment required and procedures are exactly the same as those used for the Wet Laser Printer Quality Control.

Gray Level Performance of Computed Tomography Scanner Display Monitors

This test must be performed monthly (or whenever a significant change is made to the imager's display monitors) to ensure that images on the monitors of the CT scanner display the entire range of gray shades produced by the CT scanner.

PROCEDURE: GRAY-LEVEL PERFORMANCE OF COMPUTED TOMOGRAPHY SCANNER DISPLAY MONITOR

1. Display an SMPTE Test Pattern (or American Association of Physicists in Medicine TG 18QC Test Pattern) on the imaging console. Set the display window width/level to the manufacturer-specified values for the test pattern. The monitor should be positioned so that there is no glare from room lighting.
2. Examine the pattern to confirm that the gray-level display on the imaging console is subjectively correct. The visual impression should indicate an even progression of gray levels around the ring of gray-level patches. Verify the following: (1) the small square at 5% contrast can be distinguished from the larger surrounding square at 0% contrast; (2) the small square at 95% contrast can be distinguished from the large surrounding square at 100% contrast; and (3) all the gray-level steps around the ring of gray levels are distinct from adjacent steps. This means that each of the squares around the center of the pattern should have a visibly different brightness level from each other. These squares are labeled 0%–50% on the left and from 50%–100% on the right.
3. If these conditions are not met, corrective action is needed. This may be as simple as reducing ambient light in the room. Otherwise, perform the manufacturer's recommended procedures for monitor contrast and brightness adjustment. If this still does not correct the problem, have the medical physicist or service engineer make adjustments.

COMPUTED TOMOGRAPHY DEPARTMENT COMPLIANCE STANDARDS

In addition to the CT equipment QC standards that have just been discussed in this chapter, accrediting bodies also have specific department standards that must be met, including:

1. Staff dosimetry results are to be reviewed quarterly by the radiation safety officer, medical physicist, or health physicist.
2. Equipment QC and maintenance activities are to be identified and time frames are to be established for how often they are to be performed.
3. Equipment QC and maintenance activities are to be performed and QC logs are to be completed.
4. At least annually:
   - The radiation dose (CTDI) is to be measured for adult brain, adult abdomen, pediatric brain, pediatric abdomen, or other commonly used protocols.

Medical Physicist CT Survey Report

This report summarizes the results of tests performed in accordance with the American College of Radiology CT QC Manual.

Facility Name _____ **Unit ID** _____

Address 1 _____ **Manufacturer** _____

Address 2 _____ **Model** _____

City, State, ZIP _____ **Serial Number** _____

Date of Manufacture _____

CTAP # (if applicable) _____

Survey Date _____

Medical Physicist _____ **Report Date** _____

Signature _____

Medical Physicist Tests	Pass/Fail	Technologist QC Evaluation	Pass/Fail/NA
Review of CT Protocols		Water CT Number and SD (Daily)	
Scout Prescription Accuracy		Artifact Evaluation (Daily)	
Alignment Light Accuracy		Wet Laser QC (Weekly)	
Table Travel Accuracy		Visual Checklist (Monthly)	
Radiation Beam Width		Dry Laser QC (Monthly)	
Low-Contrast Performance		Acquisition Display QC (Monthly)	
Spatial Resolution			
CT Number Accuracy			
Artifact Evaluation			
Dosimetry			
CT Number Uniformity			
Acquisition Display Calibration			

Comments

Fig. 10.14 American College of Radiology medical physicist computed tomography survey report.

- The radiation dose for each protocol is verified to be within 20% of the dose displayed.
- The measurement and dose verifications are done by a medical physicist.

5. A performance evaluation is to be performed annually by a medical physicist and includes all required tests, and that evaluation/testing results are documented (see Fig. 10.14).

6. A performance evaluation that includes all required tests and parameters is to be performed annually on each image acquisition monitor by a medical physicist.

7. A structured radiation shielding design assessment is to be conducted by a medical physicist or health physicist before imaging equipment installation.

8. A radiation protection survey is to be conducted after installation of imaging equipment or construction. The survey must be done before clinical use of the room and be conducted by a medical physicist or health physicist.

9. Documentation must be available for verification of specified qualifications for each medical physicist supporting CT services.

10. Documentation of staff annual training and ongoing education must be available. The training includes:
    - Radiation dose optimization techniques
    - Safe operation of CT equipment
11. A radiation dose index is to be documented for every CT examination. The dose index is examination specific, summarized by series or anatomic area, and retrievable.
12. Ensure that correct patient imaging site, imaging protocol, scanner parameters, and patient positioning are verified before the examination.
13. Imaging protocols are to be established or adopted based on current standards of practice and include expected radiation dose index range.
14. Imaging protocols are to be reviewed and kept current. Input is to be provided by an interpreting physician, medical physicist, and imaging technologist. These protocols are to be reviewed per established time frames.
15. Incidents where radiation dose indices exceeded expected dose index range are to be documented, reviewed, and analyzed. These incidents are to be compared with external benchmarks.

SUMMARY

An effective quality assurance program provides a method for systematic monitoring of the CT system's performance and image quality. The collected data are beneficial in identifying specific problems or malfunctions. Increasingly, it is becoming the responsibility of the CT technologist to perform and document the routine QC tests. However, more extensive quality assurance procedures should be performed periodically by the department physicist or service engineer. As with all quality management and accreditation processes, documentation of all QC testing and maintenance of all records is imperative for program success.

Refer to the Evolve website at https://evolve.elsevier.com for Student Experiment 101: Computed Tomography (CT) Quality Control.

REVIEW QUESTIONS

1. What is used as the reference material for CT number calibrations?
   a. Bone
   b. Liver
   c. Water
   d. Lung
2. Which of the following is the expected result of a CT number calibration test?
   a. 0 ± 5
   b. 1000 ± 5
   c. 0 ± 3
   d. 1000 ± 3
3. Noise in a CT scanner increases with an increase in:
   a. kVp
   b. mA
   c. Pixel size
   d. Slice thickness
4. Which term describes the ability of a CT scanner to differentiate objects with minimal differences in attenuation coefficients?
   a. Spatial resolution
   b. Contrast resolution
   c. Linearity
   d. Modulation
5. Which of the following factors can affect the accuracy of a density (HU) measurement in a CT image?
   a. System calibration
   b. Window width setting
   c. Window level setting
   d. Display field of view
6. Increasing which of the following factors can improve spatial resolution?
   a. Field of view
   b. Matrix
   c. Pixel size
   d. Slice thickness
7. Which of the following is the main limiting factor for contrast resolution?
   a. Noise
   b. Pixel depth
   c. Voxel volume
   d. Focal spot size
8. Which of the following is measured using the modulation transfer function method?
   a. Low-contrast resolution
   b. High-contrast spatial resolution
   c. Attenuation
   d. Section thickness
9. A test to evaluate the water CT number should ensure that the HU for water should be within what range of its standard value?
   a. ± 1
   b. ± 5
   c. ± 7
   d. ± 10
10. During uniformity testing with an ACR CT Phantom, the CT number measured at the center location must be within how many HU from those measured at the periphery?
    a. ± 3
    b. ± 5
    c. ± 10
    d. ± 15

11

Quality Control for Magnetic Resonance Imaging Equipment

Lorrie Kelley*

OUTLINE

OBJECTIVES

*At the completion of this chapter, the reader will be able to do
the following:*
- Describe the various types of phantoms used in magnetic
  resonance (MR) scanners
- Understand the frequency of quality control testing of
  various MR parameters
- Describe the concept of signal-to-noise ratio

- Understand the concept of center frequency
- Describe the required weekly quality control testing
  performed by the MRI technologist as required by the
  American College of Radiology
- Describe the required annual quality control testing
  performed by a medical physicist or MR imaging scientist
  as required by the American College of Radiology

KEY TERMS

Center frequency
Geometric accuracy
High-contrast resolution
Low-contrast resolution

Percent signal ghosting
Signal-to-noise ratio
Slice position accuracy
Transmit gain

Volume coil percent image
  uniformity

Quality assurance (QA) procedures for magnetic resonance imaging (MRI) equipment are designed to establish a standard of measurement for daily system performance and the documentation of any variance thereof. Although the definition of *standard* varies from scanner to scanner, the goal of quality control (QC) is the detection of any changes or potential changes in the system performance. Documentation

of daily QC measurements is considered an essential part of the MRI QC program and must be done properly. The ultimate goal is to maintain high image quality and patient safety.

MRI is a relatively new imaging modality that has seen tremendous growth and technologic advancements in recent years. The rapid proliferation of new and used magnetic resonance (MR) units, in conjunction with the older units still in place, has contributed to increasing variation in MRI quality across the country. In an effort to address those concerns and to establish a reasonable standard of image quality, the

---

*The author and publisher with to acknowledge the previous edition's contributor.

American College of Radiology (ACR) developed an MRI Accreditation Program. The MRI Accreditation Program was designed to review the qualifications of the radiologists, MR scientists/medical physicists, and technologists, as well as the clinical image quality and effectiveness of QC testing procedures of each site applying for accreditation. In November 1996, the ACR approved the MRI Accreditation Program for implementation. More information about the MRI accreditation process can be obtained by contacting the ACR (www.acr.org). In the summer of 2008, Congress passed the Medicare Improvements for Patients and Providers Act of 2008, which mandates that any nonhospital institution performing advanced diagnostic services (such as MRI) must be accredited by a Centers for Medicare & Medicaid Services (CMS)–designated accrediting organization to receive federal funding (Medicare reimbursement). As of the writing of this edition, CMS has approved four national accreditation organizations: the ACR, the Intersocietal Accreditation Commission, RadSite and The Joint Commission. This rule affects providers of MRI, computed tomography, positron emission tomography, and nuclear medicine imaging services for Medicare beneficiaries on an outpatient basis. The accreditation applies only to the suppliers of the images and not to the physician's interpretation of the image. Hospital-based MRI units are covered under hospital accreditation organizations that were covered in Chapter 1. Therefore accreditation programs are becoming mandatory for MRI departments to succeed.

PHANTOMS

Typically, the phantoms for routine QC tests are provided by the manufacturer of the MR system. A user's manual and charts for documenting standardized tests also are provided. Use of the equipment can be taught easily to the technologists during the site installation. Specific actions for obtaining and documenting QC results vary among manufacturers.

In general, QC phantoms are paramagnetic materials in an oil or water solution. Ions such as copper, aluminum, manganese, and nickel often are used. The materials used are designed to mimic biological tissues or to shorten T1 relaxation times for strong MR signals. The relaxation rates vary with each material, main magnetic field strength (B_0), and temperature. Other considerations for materials are minimal chemical shifts and thermal and chemical stability. For the sake of the scan time, when QC tests are performed, the T1 repetition time (TR) of the phantom material should be compatible with a short TR, and the T2 TR should be long enough for any echo time value that can be obtained.

QC phantoms are designed with various shapes, sizes, and geometric variables. The same type of phantom may be used for signal-to-noise ratio (SNR) and resonant frequency tests, whereas a different phantom is required for spatial resolution and linearity tests. Regardless of the type of test being performed, any QC phantom must be placed in the magnet at the isocenter, unless specified otherwise. The scanning

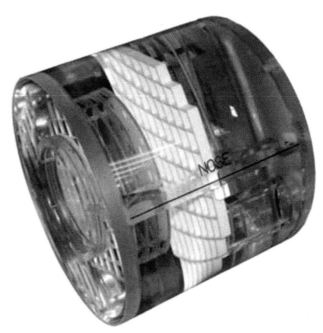

Fig. 11.1 American College of Radiology MRI Accreditation Phantom.

parameters used (e.g., TR, echo time, flip angle, slice thickness, matrix, and coil) should be documented.

The ACR MRI Accreditation Committee developed a specially designed MR phantom along with test protocols for use in establishing QA programs for clinical MRI scanners. The ACR MRI Accreditation Phantom is designed to examine several important instrument parameters within a single phantom, which means that each test can be accomplished in a reasonable amount of time. The phantom is a short, hollow cylinder constructed of acrylic plastic, and is filled with a solution of nickel chloride and sodium chloride to simulate biological tissue relaxation properties. Structures located within the phantom provide the tools necessary for quantitative assessment of seven important equipment performance parameters affecting image quality (Fig. 11.1).

QUALITY CONTROL TESTING FREQUENCY

QC tests should be performed regularly by an MR technologist and/or service engineer under the supervision of a qualified MR scientist/medical physicist. Planning and preparing for the QC tests should be part of the site installation process. The ACR states that a qualified medical physicist must have the responsibility of overseeing the equipment QC program. The medical physicist, in conjunction with the service engineer, system manufacturer specialist, and site technologist, should discuss goals and potential outcomes for regular QC tests. It can then be decided which tests should be performed at certain intervals and by which personnel. Although all of the tests are important, not all are required at the same frequency. Testing can be thought of as monitoring essential fluids in a car: the windshield washer fluid may be checked infrequently, the oil checked more regularly, and the gasoline monitored daily. The ACR requires that, at a minimum, the clinical site perform the following tests on a weekly basis: center frequency, table positioning, setup and scanning, geometric accuracy, high-contrast resolution, low-contrast resolution, artifact analysis, film QC, and visual checklist. In addition to the weekly test requirements, the ACR requires the following tests be performed annually: magnetic field homogeneity, slice position accuracy, slice thickness accuracy, radio frequency (RF) coil checks, and soft copy display devices. The decision of how frequently to perform QC testing is commonly dictated by personnel convenience and time constraints. However, performing QC tests daily will provide a site with enough quantitative data to spot negative trends much faster than if QC testing is done weekly, which might take several months to acquire enough data to spot the trends. The factors listed here are unanimously believed to be essential indicators of MR system performance. For information on MRI safety, refer to the website www.MRIsafety.com.

Although the following tests can be performed with phantoms supplied by the MR system's vendor, where appropriate, the methodology of the following QC tests will include the ACR MRI Accreditation Phantom and testing criteria. The Weekly MRI Equipment Quality Control Form to document the weekly technologist's QC tests are found in Fig. 11.2A for small phantom testing of smaller machines such as those for extremity and breast imaging or Fig. 11.2B for large phantom testing.

WEEKLY TESTS

Setup and Table Positioning Accuracy

This entails an overview of the general condition of the system's functions, including table movement, console function, prescan, data entry, and table positioning. The goal is to ensure the safe operation of the scanner during patient setup.

WEEKLY MRI EQUIPMENT QUALITY CONTROL FOR SMALL PHANTOM

MR Facility Name:　　　　　　　　　　　　　　　　　　　MR Scanner Identifier:

1	2	3	4	5	6	7	8	9	10	11	12		
	Setup & Table Position Accuracy		Center Freq (Hz)	TX Gain or Attenuation (dB)	Geometric Accuracy Measurements (Axial Slice #5 Diameter)			High-Contrast Spatial Resolution (Slice 1-Highest Resolved)		Low-Contrast Detectability (Slice # ___)	Artifact Evaluation	Tested By	Notes
Date	Accuracy OK?	Console OK?			H/F Sagittal Localizer Length (mm)	A/P (mm)	R/L (mm)	Upper Left	Lower Right	# of Spokes	Any present?		
Action limits:	± 5 mm	Yes/No			100 ± 2 mm	100 ± 2 mm	100 ± 2mm	≤ 0.8 mm	≤ 0.8 mm		Yes/No		

Reviewed by: _____　　　　Date of Review: _____

Qualified Medical Physicist/MRI Scientist

MR Weekly QC Forms_6-12-15 (2)

A

Fig. 11.2 (A) American College of Radiology (ACR) data form for Weekly MRI Equipment Quality Control for Small Phantom. (B) ACR data form for Weekly MRI Equipment Quality Control for Large Phantom. *MR*, Magnetic resonance; *TX*, transmitter.

WEEKLY MRI EQUIPMENT QUALITY CONTROL FOR LARGE PHANTOM

MRI Facility Name: MRI Scanner Identifier:

	2	3	4	5	6	7	8	9	10	11	12		
1	Setup & Table Position Accuracy		Center Freq (Hz)	TX Gain or Attenua-tion (dB)	Geometric Accuracy Measurements (Axial Slice #5 Diameter)			High-Contrast Spatial Resolution (Slice 1-Highest Resolved)		Low-Contrast Detectability (Slice # ____)	Artifact Evaluation	Tested By	Notes
Date	Accuracy OK?	Console OK?			H/F Sagittal Localizer Length (mm)	A/P (mm)	R/L (mm)	Upper Left	Lower Right	# of Spokes	Any present?		
Action limits:	± 5 mm	Yes/No			148 ± 2 mm	190 ± 2 mm	190 ± 2mm	≤ 1.0 mm	≤ 1.0 mm		Yes/No		

Reviewed by: _____   Date of Review: _____

Qualified Medical Physicist/MRI Scientist

MR Weekly QC Forms_6-12-15 (2)

B

Fig. 11.2, cont'd

Any problems noted with the scanner interface, computer bootup, table movement (including docking), or table positioning should be noted.

PROCEDURE: SETUP AND TABLE POSITION ACCURACY

1. Place the ACR phantom in the head coil, making sure that the crosshairs engraved on the phantom are moved into the center of the magnet.
2. Fine-tune the position of the phantom along all three axes with the nonmetallic bubble level enclosed with the ACR phantom.
3. Verify the accuracy of the phantom positioning by performing sagittal and, if necessary, coronal localizer scans. The center of the sagittal image of the phantom should be within ±2 mm of the central grid structure on the phantom.
4. Once the phantom is correctly aligned, leave the phantom in place for the rest of the series of scans used for QC testing. Also verify that the computer booted without problem and the scanner interface works properly.

Center (Resonance) Frequency

Center frequency is defined as the RF that matches the static magnetic field (B_0) according to the Larmor equation. It is recommended that the resonance frequency be checked before QA procedures are initiated and each time the phantom is changed. An example of the Larmor equation follows, where B_0 is the magnetic field strength and the gyromagnetic ratio for hydrogen is 42.57 MHz/T.

$$B_0 \times \text{gyromagnetic ratio} = \text{Resonance frequency}$$
$$\text{Examples}: 1.5\,T \times 42.57\,\text{MHz}/T = 63.86\,\text{MHz}$$
$$1\,T \times 42.57\,\text{MHz}/T = 42.57\,\text{MHz}$$
$$0.5\,T \times 42.57\,\text{MHz}/T = 21.29\,\text{MHz}$$
$$0.3\,T \times 42.57\,\text{MHz}/T = 12.77\,\text{MHZ}$$

The term *center frequency* is used interchangeably with *resonance frequency* and *Larmor frequency*. Conveniently, the center frequency can be obtained during the prescan mode of the ACR phantom test. Most manufacturers provide an automated way to determine the resonance frequency.

PROCEDURE: CENTER FREQUENCY

1. Use the ACR phantom.
2. Place the phantom in the center of the magnet.
3. Use the ACR T1-weighted axial series protocol and perform a prescan. Record the center frequency (usually displayed on the control console) on the required data form (Fig. 11.2) for large phantom testing.
4. If the prescribed action limit is exceeded, repeat the prescan a second time.
5. If the action limit is still exceeded, report the change to the service engineer and medical physicist.

If a notable change in the resonance frequency occurs, the service engineer should be notified. As determined by the Larmor equation (mentioned previously), a change in the center frequency indicates that there is a change in the strength of the main magnetic field, B_0. This could be a result of cryogen boil-off, the presence of external ferromagnetic materials, shim coil failure, and/or changes in the current of the main coil windings.

Checking the center frequency is important in magnets that undergo frequent ramping of the magnetic field (e.g., mobile units, resistive magnets). In a superconducting magnet, the cryogen levels should be routinely monitored. Although most systems have a cryogen alarm, monitoring is the best way to avoid an urgent situation (similar to running out of gas in a car). If the superconductor uses liquid helium and liquid nitrogen, both should be monitored. The service organization should be notified if the cryogens seem to be decreasing more than usual between replenishments.

Significant changes in the center frequency indicate changes in the SNR.

The center frequency should not deviate by more than 1.5 parts per million (ppm) between successive measurements.

Transmit Gain (Attenuation)

Transmit gain is a measure of the RF power that is required to produce a 90-degree flip of the patient's magnetic vector during imaging. During the prescan process and after establishing the center frequency, the system acquires several signals with varying levels of transmit gain to determine the appropriate RF flip angles for a given pulse sequence. Fluctuations in the transmit gain could indicate problems in the RF transmitter or the receive coils anywhere along the RF chain or circuitry. Transmitter gain or attenuation values are usually recorded in units of decibel. The decibel provides a logarithmic scale where a small change in decibel represents a large change in the transmit gain.

The transmit gain measurements should be compared with the standards set at acceptance testing. Any changes that exceed those limits should be reported.

PROCEDURE: TRANSMITTER GAIN OR ATTENUATION

1. Determine where the transmitter attenuation or gain is displayed on the scanner console.
2. Record the value displayed in column 5 on the Weekly MRI Equipment Quality Control Data Form (Fig. 11.2A–B).
3. If the change in decibels exceeds the action limits, report the problem to the qualified medical physicist or MRI scientist.

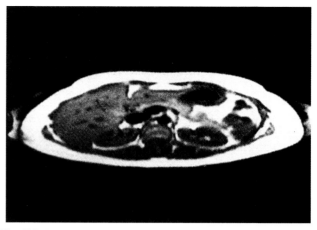

Fig. 11.3 Example of gradient amplitude falloff resulting in A-P minification of a T1-weighted axial image of the upper abdomen. (From Ros PR, Bidgood WD. *Abdominal magnetic resonance imaging.* Mosby; 1993. Courtesy GE Medical Systems, Milwaukee, Wisconsin.)

GEOMETRIC ACCURACY (THREE AXES)

Geometric accuracy, also referred to as *spatial linearity,* refers to the amount of geometric distortion in the image from displacement or improper scaling of the distance between points being displayed on the image (Fig. 11.3). This is affected primarily by the homogeneity of the main magnetic field and the linearity of the magnetic field gradients. Other factors contributing to geometric inaccuracies are low receiver bandwidth, poor eddy current compensation, and gradient miscalibration. When using the ACR MRI Accreditation Phantom, geometric accuracy measurements are considered acceptable when they are less than or equal to 2 mm of the true values when measured over a 25-cm field of view (FOV). The greatest amount of distortion is typically seen near the edges of the FOV, or increasingly distorted as you move farther from the magnet isocenter. Although these edge distortions are commonly expected, consideration should be given to procedures guided by the MR image such as surgical and treatment planning, in which distance measurements are critical. The results of this test also can be used to verify reported FOV and the accuracy of the scanner's distance-measuring tools. The most common cause of failure of this test is one or more miscalibrated gradients (which can also cause slice position errors). It is normal for gradient calibration to drift over time and to require recalibration by a service engineer.

PROCEDURE: GEOMETRIC ACCURACY

1. Seven measurements of known lengths are made from the scans acquired from the ACR phantom using the MR system's length measurement tools for on-screen display. Follow the ACR requirements for setting the window width and window level for display of the phantom images for the purposes of taking length measurements.
2. Using the sagittal localizer image, measure the end-to-end length of the phantom along a line near the center of the phantom (Fig. 11.4). Use slice 1 and measure the diameter of the phantom in the top to bottom and left to right directions (Fig. 11.5). Use slice 5 and measure the phantom in four directions: top to bottom, left to right, and both diagonals (Fig. 11.6).

3. The length measurements are compared with the known values of the distances within the ACR phantom, which are inside end-to-end length = 148 mm and inside diameter = 190 mm.
4. All measurements should be within ±2 mm of their true values.

Site engineers often perform geometric accuracy tests on systems when they perform the regularly scheduled preventive maintenance. If you find there have been changes in geometric accuracy, simply reshimming the magnet or removing lost ferromagnetic objects (e.g., paper clips, coins, bobby pins) from the magnet bore may improve the system's performance.

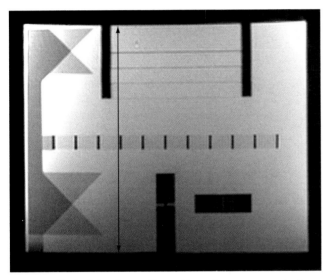

Fig. 11.4 Sagittal localizer with end-to-end measurement shown *(arrow)*. (Courtesy St. Luke's Health System.)

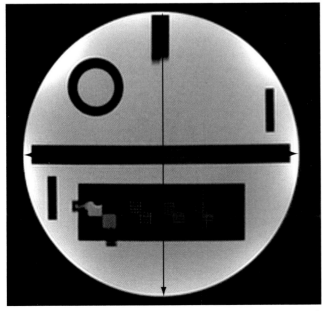

Fig. 11.5 Slice 1 from American College of Radiology T1 series with diameter measurements shown *(arrows)*. (Courtesy St. Luke's Health System.)

High-Contrast Resolution (Spatial Resolution)

High-contrast resolution (also known as spatial resolution) is the MR system's ability to resolve small objects. The phantom used for this test is unlike those previously discussed. It should consist of an array of pegs, bars, rods, or holes of known sizes. A typical spatial resolution phantom may have an array of varying element sizes. Slice 1 of the ACR MR Accreditation Phantom has inserts with arrays of holes in various diameters of 0.9, 1, and 1.1 mm.

The scanning sequence can be any multislice sequence as long as the SNR parameters are chosen to minimize noise. The testing parameters are those that affect the pixel size, slice thickness, matrix, and FOV. A two-dimensional pixel size can be determined by dividing the acquisition matrix into the FOV.

Example:

$$FOV : 200 \text{ mm } FOV_p \times 240 \text{ mm } FOVf$$

$$Matrix : 192 \text{ phase encodings} \times 256 \text{ frequency encodings}$$

$$200 \text{ mm } FOV_p \text{ divided by } 192 \text{ phase encodings} = 1.04 \text{ mm}$$

$$240 \text{ mm } FOVf \text{ divided by } 256 \text{ frequency encodings} = 0.93 \text{ mm}$$

Therefore the pixel size or in-plane resolution would be 1.04 mm by 0.93 mm.

PROCEDURE: HIGH-CONTRAST SPATIAL RESOLUTION

1. Use slice 1 acquired with the ACR phantom, using the T1 and T2 axial series test protocols (Fig. 11.7).
2. Keeping the resolution insert visible, magnify the image by a factor between 2 and 4 (Fig. 11.8).
3. Adjust the window level and width to best demonstrate the insert.
4. Identify and record the smallest hole size that can be resolved in both the right-to-left and top-to-bottom directions.
5. The ACR test protocol uses a field of view and matrix size for the axial series that should produce a resolution of 1.0 mm in both directions.

The ACR standard is a measurement of 1 mm or better in both directions.

Although resolution is traditionally known as *line pairs per millimeter*, here, it is determined by the pixel size and what the human eye can resolve on the image. Resolution is determined by the smallest array element (e.g., a bar, rod) visible that is completely separated by distance from the adjacent element. The calculated pixel size is then compared with the smallest resolvable element. Excessive filtering, poor eddy current compensation, excessive image ghosting, and geometric errors are common causes for failure of this test.

This QC test may be routinely performed by the site engineer during the preventive maintenance of the system. This test is likely to fail in conjunction with the failure of the geometric accuracy test. The gradient amplitude, the gradient duty cycle, and reconstruction filters can easily affect the spatial resolution.

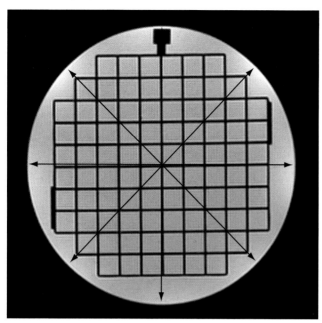

Fig. 11.6 Slice 5 from American College of Radiology T1 series with diameter measurements shown *(arrows)*. (Courtesy St. Luke's Health System.)

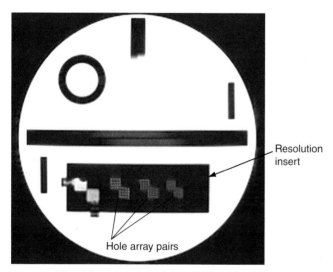

Fig. 11.7 Slice 1 from American College of Radiology T2 series demonstrating resolution insert and hole array pairs. (Courtesy St. Luke's Health System.)

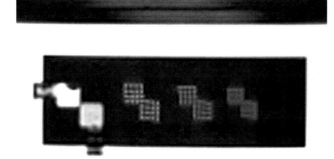

Fig. 11.8 Magnified portion of slice 1 displayed for visual assessment of high-contrast resolution. (Courtesy St. Luke's Health System.)

Low-Contrast Resolution (Detectability)

Low-contrast resolution is a measure of the MR system's ability to differentiate between adjacent tissues having minimal differences in signal intensities. Several factors can influence low-contrast resolution, including increased noise, ghosting artifacts, improper phantom positioning, RF coil malfunctions, and improper use of image filters.

Typically, low-contrast resolution is expressed in one of two ways: the smallest diameter of an object with a specific contrast that can be detected or the smallest difference in signal intensity that can be discriminated for an object of a specific diameter. A phantom that contains objects of varying size and contrast should be selected. Slices 8 through 11 of the ACR MRI Accreditation Phantom consists of three rows of low-contrast objects that radiate from the center in a circular arrangement. Each row contains 10 holes of varying diameters (from 7 to 1.5 mm). Slices acquired from four locations within the phantom provide contrast values of 1.4%, 2.5%, 3.6%, and 5.1%.

PROCEDURE: LOW-CONTRAST RESOLUTION

1. When using the ACR phantom, measurements for this test are made by counting the number of complete spokes, seen in each of the images.
2. Use slices 8–11 from the ACR phantom test series.
3. Starting with slice 11, adjust the window width and level display settings for best visibility of the objects (typically a narrow window width; Fig. 11.9).
4. Begin counting the number of complete spokes, starting with the spokes with the largest diameter disks (positioned at 12 o'clock or just slightly to the right of 12 o'clock). Count clockwise from spoke 1 until reaching a spoke where one or more of the disks is not distinguishable from the background. The number of complete spokes counted is the score for the slice. Repeat the counting procedure with slices 8–10.
5. MR systems with field strengths less than 3 T should have a total score of at least 9 spokes for each ACR series, and there should be a score of 37 spokes for MR systems with field strengths of 3 T.

Note: A spoke can be counted as complete only if all three of its disks are discernible.

According to the action limits of the ACR, an MR scanner with a field strength less than 3 T should be able to display 9 spokes of holes from the low-contrast inserts and 3-T MR systems should be able to display 37 spokes. The ACR requires that an MR scanner pass on both of the ACR T1 and T2 series or on both of the site's T1 and T2 series. The most frequent cause of failure of this test is incorrectly positioned slices. It can also occur because of the phantom being tilted.

Artifact Analysis

Various artifacts can occur during the routine QC testing procedures (Fig. 11.10). Artifacts can vary according to imaging conditions, pulse sequence parameters, choice of RF coils, and with individual patients. The presence of artifacts can be an early indication of equipment failure. The MR technologist

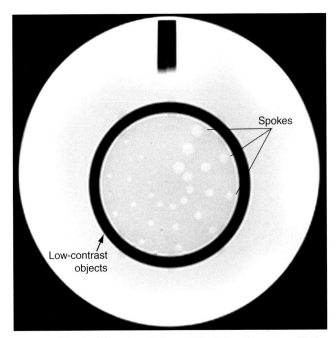

Fig. 11.9 Slice 2 of American College of Radiology T1 series with the circle of low-contrast objects displayed. (Courtesy St. Luke's Health System.)

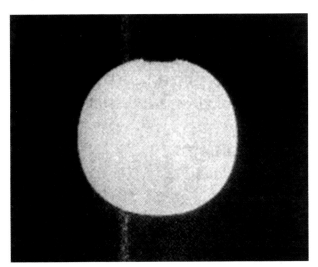

Fig. 11.10 Radio frequency interference from a steady carrier frequency source. A strong signal from the nitrogen fill–monitor circuit is detected within the pass-band of the magnetic resonance imaging receiver. It is displayed as a full vertical column perpendicular to the x coordinate that corresponds to the frequency of the spurious signal. The overall receiver performance is degraded by intermodulation distortion, which causes the background noise level to rise in comparison with the signal of the phantom. (From Ros PR, Bidgood WD. *Abdominal magnetic resonance imaging.* Mosby; 1993. Courtesy Siemens Medical Systems, Iselin, New Jersey.)

should become familiar with the common appearances of artifacts that are due to particular subsystems of the MR scanner. These include the RF system, gradient system, image and data processing, and magnetic field homogeneity.

During each QC test, the MR technologist should be evaluating each image for signs of ghosting, geometric

distortion, discrepancies in signal intensities, and any other interference with the known parameters of the image. The ACR requirement for assessment of image artifacts follows the following procedure:

PROCEDURE: ARTIFACT EVALUATION

1. Use the image slices from the ACR T1-weighted slices.
2. Adjust the display window width and window level to show the full range of pixel values for each image.
3. On each image, validate the following: the phantom appears circular and is not distorted, there are no ghost images of the phantom, there are no streaks or spots, and there are no abnormal or new elements in the image.

Hard-copy Quality Control

Some MRI departments may use dry laser film printers to print hard copies of MRI images. If so, QC testing must be performed weekly to ensure artifact-free laser films with consistent gray levels that match the image appearance on the display monitor. Any digital modality is challenged to provide hard-copy images that match the grayscale display of the system's monitor. One way to verify accurate representation of the grayscale between the monitor and hard copy is with a Society of Motion Picture and Television Engineers (SMPTE) test pattern.

PROCEDURE: FILM PRINTER QUALITY CONTROL

1. Display SMPTE test pattern on the console's monitor. Be sure to use the manufacturer-specified window width and level for display settings.
2. Verify that 0/5% and 95/100% gray-level patches are visible and note any artifacts.
3. Film the SMPTE test pattern using a 6-on-1 format.
4. Use a film densitometer to plot the optical density of the 10%, 40%, and 90% gray-level patches.
5. Plot the optical densities on a QC chart (Fig. 11.11) and circle any points that fall outside the control limits.

ACR control limits for the SMPTE test pattern:

SMPTE Test Pattern	Control Limits
0	±0.15
10%	±0.15
40%	±0.15
90%	±0.8

Visual Checklist

The visual inspection is a method to quantitatively and qualitatively verify that all equipment is available and working properly. The inspection can be scanner specific depending on the use of the equipment. Items that are typically included in a visual inspection are the patient table smoothness of motion and stability, alignment lights, high-tension cable/other cable integrity, monitors, RF door contacts, RF window-screen integrity, operator console switches/lights/meters,

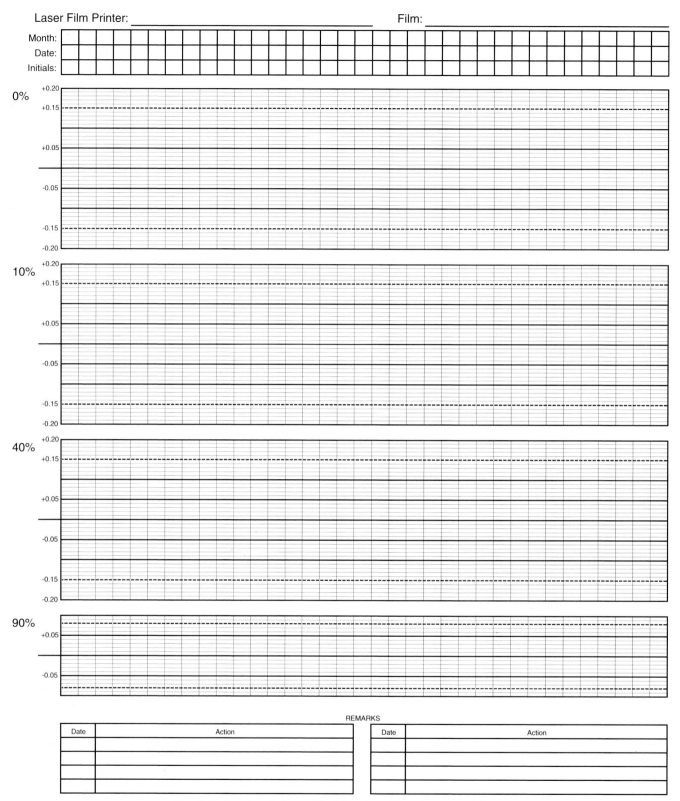

Fig. 11.11 American College of Radiology laser film printer control chart.

patient monitors, patient intercom, and room temperature and relative humidity. The visual inspection checklist should also include a section on facility safety that would include the emergency cart, safety warning signage, door indicator switch (if installed), cryogen level indicator, and oxygen monitor. Items that are missing or malfunctioning should be repaired or replaced as soon as possible. A visual inspection checklist can be provided by the equipment manufacturer or the facility's accreditation agency. Fig. 11.12 contains the ACR visual checklist form.

MRI Accreditation Program Visual Checklist

MRI Facility Name: MRI Scanner Identifier:

	Date:																																						
Patient Transport and Gantry	Table position and other displays																																							
	Alignment lights																																							
	Horizontal smoothness of motion and stability																																							
	Vertical motion smoothness and stability																																							
Filming Viewing	Laser camera																																							
	Light boxes																																							
RF Integrity and Control Room	RF door contacts																																							
	RF window-screen integrity																																							
	Operator console switches/lights/meters																																							
	Patient monitor (if present)																																							
	Patient intercom																																							
	Room temperature/room humidity																																							
Facility Safety	Emergency cart																																							
	Safety warning signage																																							
	Door indicator switch (if installed)																																							
	Cryogen level indicator																																							
Pass = ☑ Fail =F Does Not Apply = NA																																							
Technologist Initials:																																							

Reviewed by: _____   Date of Review: _____

Qualified Medical Physicist/MRI Scientist

MR Weekly QC Forms_6-12-15 (2)

Fig. 11.12 American College of Radiology MRI Facility Quality Control Visual Checklist. *MRI,* Magnetic resonance imaging; *RF,* radio frequency.

ANNUAL TESTS

As stated previously, all QC measurements are considered essential for overall system performance. Box 11.1 lists abbreviated definitions of tests that should be performed by a medical physicist or system engineer. These tests should be performed on a regular schedule and also whenever there are changes to the site scanner and environment such as hardware and software upgrades, magnet quench, or facility construction. The ACR requires that the following tests be performed on an annual basis to meet the ACR MRI Accreditation Standard. The ACR form to document the results of the annual tests is found in Fig. 11.13. The ACR requires that these tests be performed by a medical physicist or MRI scientist. The first nine annual tests are the same as the weekly QC tests performed by the MRI technologists (but are performed by a medical physicist or MRI scientist), namely:

1. Setup and Table Position Accuracy
2. Center Frequency
3. Transmitter Gain or Attenuation
4. Geometric Accuracy Measurements
5. High-Contrast Spatial Resolution
6. Low-Contrast Detectability
7. Artifact Evaluation
8. Film Printer Quality Control (if applicable)
9. Visual Checklist

The remainder of the annual MRI Equipment Evaluation Test is described in the following section.

Magnetic Field Homogeneity

The homogeneity of a system's magnetic field is an indication of the quality or uniformity of its field. Homogeneity is usually expressed in parts per million within a given spherical volume. A spherical volume is given as the diameter of a spherical volume (DSV). MRI system manufacturers provide specifications for their magnets, and values obtained from QC tests should be compared with those specified. The medical physicist can choose from a couple of methods for measuring the magnetic field homogeneity. The spectral peak method uses a uniform spherical phantom to measure the full width at half maximum of the spectral peak over the

BOX 11.1   Quality Control Tests Performed by a Medical Physicist or Magnetic Resonance Imaging Scientist

Receiver Gain (Attenuation): The receiver setting is the amount by which MR signals are amplified before digitization.

Transmitter Setting: The transmitter setting is a number expressed in decibels that influences the flip angle of each RF pulse.

Coil Q: Known as the quality factor, coil Q describes the performance of a coil used to receive MR signals.

Ghost Intensity: Ghost intensity is an expression of the intensity of background ghosts relative to the intensity of a phantom.

RF Shielding Effectiveness: The RF shielding effectiveness test verifies that the RF shield is attenuating radio waves originating from outside the scan room.

Surface Coil Performance: For the surface coil performance to be checked, a separate test is done on each surface coil to determine the SNR and image uniformity.

Slice Thickness: Slice thickness is the FWHM of a slice profile, the region from which MR signals are emitted.

Maximum Gradient Strength: The maximum gradient strength determines whether gradients are still achieving the maximum amplitude specified by the manufacturer and originally measured.

Specific Absorption Rate Monitor: The SAR monitor verifies that the imaging procedures do not cause excessive RF power to be deposited into a patient.

FWHM, Full width at half maximum; *MR*, magnetic resonance; *MRI*, magnetic resonance imaging; *RF*, radio frequency; *SAR*, specific absorption rate; *SNR*, signal-to-noise ratio.

imaging volume. The other method uses a phase difference map to calculate the magnetic field inhomogeneity. Using phase-contrast images, a medical physicist can calculate the change in phase across images acquired from a uniformity phantom as proportional to the inhomogeneity of the magnetic field. For a superconducting magnet, typical values are 2 ppm over a 30-cm to 40-cm DSV. For MR systems with spectroscopy capabilities, the suggested value is less than or equal to 0.5 ppm at 35 cm DSV.

Poor homogeneity can result in poor image quality and artifacts. Changes in homogeneity can be due to ferromagnetic objects located within the bore of the magnet and external ferromagnetic structures that may be neighboring the magnetic field. Sometimes magnetic inhomogeneities can be improved with gradient adjustments or shimming.

Slice Position Accuracy

The slice position accuracy test is performed to ensure that the landmarking location is actually centered to the magnet bore. Misalignment can simply be due to mechanical problems with the table, positioning devices, or alignment light beams. Other causes of poor performance include operator error, gradient miscalibration, magnetic field inhomogeneities, and table positioning shift.

PROCEDURE: SLICE POSITION ACCURACY

1. Use slices 1 and 11 of the ACR T1 and T2 phantom test series and magnify the images by a factor of 2–4, making sure to keep the vertical bars of the crossed wedges within the displayed image (Figs. 11.14 and 11.15).
2. Using a fairly narrow display window width, measure the difference in length between the left and right bars of the crossed wedges in each image.

Note: Because the crossed wedges have a 45-degree slope, the measured bar length difference is really twice the actual slice displacement, meaning that if the measurement of the bar length difference is 6.0 mm, the slice is displaced superiorly by 3.0 mm (Fig. 11.16).

The ACR MR Accreditation Phantom uses crossed wedges from slices 1 and 11 as a reference. On slices 1 and 11, the crossed wedges appear as a pair of dark bars at the top of the phantom. The ACR criterion is that the absolute bar length difference should be equal to or less than 5 mm. Causes of failure in this test can be an error by the scanner operator in the prescriptions of the slice locations, bad gradient calibration, or poor B_0 homogeneity.

Slice Thickness Accuracy

Slice thickness is an important image quality parameter. The accuracy of slice thickness is especially important for stereotactic and interventional procedures. The thickness of each slice is determined by both the transmit RF bandwidth and the amplitude of the slice select gradient. Factors that influence slice thickness include gradient calibration and the RF pulse profile. Inaccuracies in slice thickness can cause interslice interference (cross talk) in multislice acquisitions and can alter the validity of SNR measurements in all pulse sequences. When the ACR MRI Accreditation Phantom is used to perform this test, the lengths of two signal ramps located within the slice thickness insert in slice 1 are measured. To meet the ACR criteria, the measured slice thickness should be 5.0 mm ±0.7 mm. Causes of failure of this test include radio frequency amplifier nonlinearity, bad gradient calibration, or poor gradient switching performance.

PROCEDURE: SLICE THICKNESS ACCURACY

1. Use slice 1 of the ACR T1 and T2 phantom test series and magnify the images by a factor of 2–4, making sure to keep the slice thickness insert visible within the displayed image (Fig. 11.17).
2. Display the images with a narrow window level and window width to provide optimal visualization of the signal ramps.
3. Place a rectangular region of interest (ROI) at the middle of each signal ramp and note the mean signal values for both ROIs, then average the two values together.
4. Lower the window level of the display to half of the average of the ramp signal calculated in step 3.
5. Measure the length of the top and bottom ramps and record their lengths (Fig. 11.18).

Note: The following formula is used to calculate slice thickness:

$$\text{slice thickness} = 0.2 \times (\text{top} \times \text{bottom}) / (\text{top} + \text{bottom})$$

MRI Equipment Performance Evaluation Data Form

Site: _____ Date: _____

MRAP Number: _____ Serial Number: _____

Equipment:

    MRI System Manufacturer: _____ Model: _____

    Film Processor Manufacturer: _____ Model: _____

    PACS Manufacturer: _____ Model: _____

    ACR MRAP Phantom Number used: _____

1. Magnetic Field Homogeneity

    Method Used (check one):   Spectral Peak _____ Phase Difference _____

                              Other (describe) _____

    Measured Homogeneity: Diameter of Sperical   Homogeneity

                                     Volume (cm)   (ppm)

                                     _____   _____

                                   _____   _____

                                   _____   _____

2. Slice Position Accuracy

From Slice Positions #1 and #11 of the ACR Phantom:

Wedge (mm)

        [▢] = −   [▢] = +

Slice Location #1   _____

Slice Location #11   _____

3. Slice Thickness Accuracy

From Slice Position #1 of the ACR Phantom:

Slice Thickness   Top: _____   Calculated slice

(fwhm in mm)   Bottom: _____   Thickness (mm): _____

4. RF Coil Performance Evaluation

A. Volume RF Coil—

RF coil description: _____ Date: _____

Phantom description: _____

Pulse sequence: Type: _____ TR: _____ TE: _____ flip angle: _____degrees

FOV: _____ cm² Matrix: _____ BW: _____kHz; NSA: _____

               Slice thickness: _____mm; spacing: _____mm

               TX attenuation (or gain): _____

Data Collected: _____

Mean Signal	Maximum Signal	Minimum Signal	Background Signal	Noise Standard Deviation	Ghost Signal

Calculated Values: Max − Min = _____; Max + Min = _____

Signal-to-Noise Ratio	Percent Image Uniformity	Percent Signal Ghosting

B. Volume RF Coil—

RF coil description: _____ Date: _____

Phantom description: _____

Pulse sequence: Type: _____ TR: _____ TE: _____FOV: _____cm²

Orientation: Matrix: _____ BW: _____ kHz; NSA: _____

               Slice thickness: _____ mm; spacing: _____mm

               Flip angle: _____ degrees   TX attenuation (or gain): _____

Fig. 11.13 MRI Equipment Performance Evaluation Data Form.

Continued

Maximum Signal	Noise Standard Deviation	Maximum Signal-to-Noise Ratio

Image uniformity distribution OK? _____

Image ghosting OK? _____

HARD COPY IMAGE: WINDOW WIDTH: _____   Window level: _____

5. Inter-slice RF Evaluation

Phantom description: _____

Pulse sequence: Type: _____ TR: _____ TE: _____FOV: _____cm^2

Matrix: _____ BW: _____ kHz; NSA: _____

Number of slices: _____ Flip angle: _____degrees

Series Number	Slice Gap mm	Signal-to-Noise Ratio
1		
2		
3		
4		

Measured SNR — 100%, 90%, 80%, 70%

Inter-slice Gap (percent of slice thickness): 0 25% 50% 75% 100%

6. Soft Copy Displays

Luminance Meter Make/Model: _____   Cal expires: _____

Monitor Description: _____

Luminance measured: Cd m^{-2} Ft. lamberts   (Circle correct units)

Monitor Description	Center of Image Display	Top Left Corner	Top Right Corner	Bottom Right Corner	Bottom Left Corner
Console					

Luminance Uniformity:

Average of values obtained in four corners of screen: _____Cd m^{-2}.

Percent difference: _____%

$$\text{\% difference} = 200^* (L_{max} - L_{min}) / (L_{max} + L_{min})$$

7. Evaluation of Site's Technologist QC Program

1. Set up and positioning accuracy: (weekly)

2. Center frequency: (weekly)

3. Transmitter attenuation or gain: (weekly)

4. Geometric accuracy measurements: (weekly)

5. Spatial resolution measurements: (weekly)

6. Low-contrast detectability: (weekly)

7. Film quality control: (weekly)

8. Visual checklist: (weekly)

SPECIFIC COMMENTS:

_____

_____

_____

_____

Fig. 11.13, cont'd

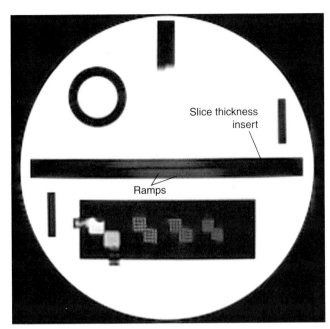

Fig. 11.14 Slice 1 from American College of Radiology T2 series, demonstrating the slice thickness insert and signal ramps. (Courtesy St. Luke's Health System.)

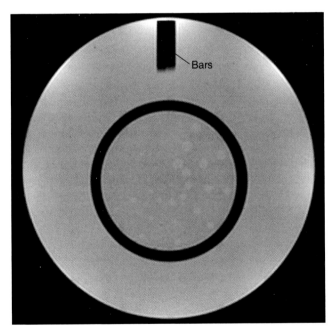

Fig. 11.15 Slice 2 of American College of Radiology T1 series, with a pair of dark vertical bars from the 45-degree crossed wedges indicated. (Courtesy St. Luke's Health System.)

Radio Frequency Coil Checks

The performance of the RF coils used to generate MR images is critical to the overall performance of the MR system as a whole. Currently, the ACR requires three different measurements for volume coils and one measurement for surface coils. The QC tests required for volume coils provide measurements of SNR, volume coil percent image uniformity (PIU), and **percent signal ghosting** (PSG). The QC test used for surface coils measures only the maximum SNR.

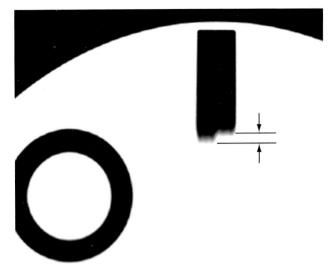

Fig. 11.16 Magnified portion of slice 1, showing measurement for slice position error. The *arrows* indicate the difference in bar length. (Courtesy St. Luke's Health System.)

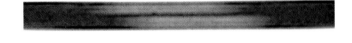

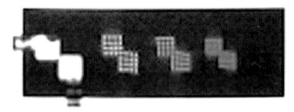

Fig. 11.17 Magnified portion of slice 1, showing placement for rectangular regions of interest to measure average signal in the ramps. (Courtesy St. Luke's Health System.)

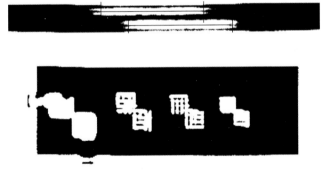

Fig. 11.18 Magnified portion of slice 1, showing measurements for the slice thickness signal ramps. (Courtesy St. Luke's Health System.)

Signal-to-Noise Ratio

The ratio of signal intensity in the image to the noise level is the **signal-to-noise ratio**. Although some describe it in complicated mathematical calculations, others simplify it as a measure of the graininess of the image. One simple method to determine SNR is to calculate the signal, which is the mean intensity within a uniform phantom

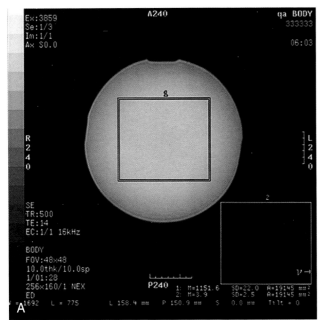

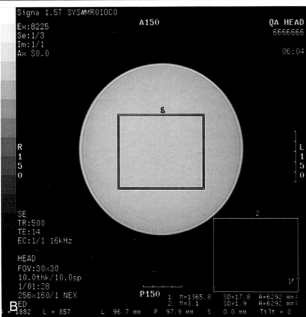

Fig. 11.19 (A) A signal-to-noise ratio (SNR) test performed with the body coil phantom. (B) An SNR test performed with the head coil phantom. Note that the head coil yields a higher SNR.

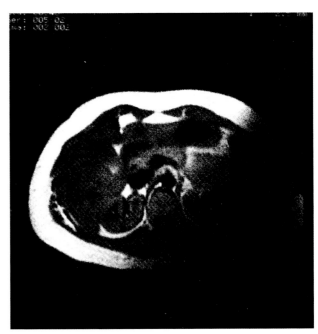

Fig. 11.20 Nonuniformity of image intensity produced by radio frequency field inhomogeneity. Note the region of hypointensity in the left flank. The cause in this case is improper setting of active shim coil current; an unwanted focal gradient is produced in the main magnetic field. (From Ros PR, Bidgood WD. *Abdominal magnetic resonance imaging.* Mosby; 1993. Courtesy GE Medical Systems, Milwaukee, Wisconsin.)

BOX 11.2 Volume Coil Percent Image Uniformity Calculation

For a simple calculation of the volume coil PIU, a multislice acquisition (approximately three) is made with a large slice gap and an FOV slightly larger than the phantom. Once the chosen image is displayed, the ROI should be approximately 75% of the center phantom area. Determine the maximum and minimum intensities within the ROI, using the display window. The following equation then can be used:

$$PIU = \frac{(1 - I_{max} - I_{min})}{(I_{max} + I_{min})} \times 100$$

where PIU = percent image uniformity and I = intensity. Although ideal uniformity is 100%, large FOVs yield less uniformity. In general, uniformity should be higher than 80%.

FOV, Field of view; *PIU*, percent image uniformity; *ROI*, region of interest.

ROI divided by the noise (Fig. 11.19), which is the standard deviation within an ROI in the background. Most MR systems have a means to calculate the SNR automatically. When performing tests to measure SNR, one must be aware that incorrect placement of ROIs can result in apparent artifacts that will impede SNR calculations. Several factors can influence SNR: resonance frequency, RF shielding, scanning parameters, field strength, RF coil performance, and general system calibration.

Volume coil percent image uniformity. Volume coil percent image uniformity is a parameter that describes the spatial sensitivity of RF coils. An image intensity uniformity test measures the image intensity over a large uniform area of a homogeneous phantom lying in the sensitive region of a volume RF coil. Nonuniformity of the radio frequency field can result in an image artifact (Fig. 11.20). See Box 11.2 for calculation of PIU value. For ACR accreditation, slice 7 of the ACR Accreditation Phantom is used. Common causes of failure of this test include improper centering of the coil, image ghosting, or failure of components in the coil.

PROCEDURE: VOLUME COIL PERCENT IMAGE UNIFORMITY

1. Place the phantom in the center of the magnet and perform a typical multislice acquisition from a commonly used clinical protocol with a slice thickness of 10 mm in the axial plane.
2. Select an image and place an ROI over the center of the image. The ROI should cover at least 10% of the area of the phantom or 100 pixels, whichever is greater. The mean pixel value from the ROI represents the signal.
3. Place the same ROI over the background and record the standard deviation, which represents the noise inherent in the system.
4. The formula for calculating the SNR is 1.41 × (mean ÷ standard deviation).

Percent signal ghosting. Artifacts that appear as a faint copy of the imaged object or as multiple replications of the object smeared along the phase encode direction are called phase-encode ghosts. Ghost artifacts are created as a result of signal instability between pulse cycle repetitions. The PSG test assesses the level of ghosting in the images. During testing, ghosting can be caused by motion or vibration of the phantom during testing as well as hardware problems.

The following procedure uses the ACR MRI Accreditation Phantom to measure the SNR, percent image uniformity, and PSG of volume coils:

PROCEDURE: PERCENT SIGNAL GHOSTING

1. Use slice 7 (see Fig. 11.21) of the ACR phantom test series.
2. Create an ROI that encompasses approximately 80% of the phantom and place over the center of the phantom. Record the mean signal on the data form.
3. Adjust the window width and window level so that the region of greatest signal intensity is depicted.
4. Create an ROI (measurement ROI) that is approximately 0.15% of the area of the FOV. For a 128 × 256 matrix, the ROI would be about 50 pixels; for a 256 × 256 matrix, the ROI would be approximately 100 pixels. Center this ROI over the position of the greatest signal intensity within the "mean signal ROI" from step 2. Record the mean signal as the maximum signal on the data form.
5. Move the measurement ROI to the position of the lowest signal intensity within the "mean signal ROI" from step 2. Record the mean signal from this ROI measurement as the minimum signal on the data form.
6. Move the measurement ROI outside the phantom along the frequency encode direction. Record the mean value of all pixel intensities within this measurement ROI as the noise ROI on the data form.
7. Determine the noise standard deviation as the root mean square value of all the pixel intensities in the "noise ROI." Record the value on the data form.
8. Place four elliptical ROIs outside the phantom along the four edges of the field of view. The elliptical ROIs should have a length-to-width ratio of 4:1 and a total area of about 10 cm. Record the mean value for each ROI and label them according to position: left, right, top, and bottom.

9. The SNR is calculated by dividing the mean signal by the standard deviation.
10. The PIU is calculated using the following formula:

$$PIU = 100 \times \left[1 - \frac{(\text{maximum signal} - \text{minimum signal})}{(\text{maximum signal} + \text{minimum signal})} \right]$$

11. The PSG is calculated using the following formula, which gives the value for ghosting as a fraction of the primary signal:

$$\text{ghost ratio} = \left[(\text{top} + \text{bottom}) - \frac{(\text{left} + \text{right})}{[2 \times (\text{mean signal})]} \right]$$

The ACR criteria for SNR, PIU, and PSG are:
SNR: no significant change from baseline
PIU ≥87.5% for MR systems with field strengths less than 3 T and ≥82.0% for 3 T MR systems ghosting ratio: ≤0.025.

Soft Copy (Monitor) Quality Control

Soft-copy display has replaced film images as the industry standard for diagnosis. As a primary diagnostic tool, soft-copy devices should be tested at acceptance testing and at regular intervals thereafter for maximum and minimum luminance, luminance uniformity, resolution, and spatial accuracy using the procedures discussed in Chapter 8. The ACR's suggested performance criteria for soft-copy display devices are as follows:

1. Maximum luminance should exceed 90 Cd m^{-2}, and minimum luminance should be less than 1.2 Cd m^{-2}.
2. Luminance uniformity should be within 30% of the maximum brightness measured in the center of the screen.

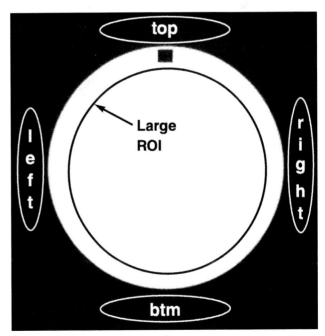

Fig. 11.21 Image of slice 7 illustrating size and placement of the large, 200 cm^2 region of interest *(ROI)* for image intensity uniformity measurements. *btm*, Bottom.

3. Spatial resolution: the monitor should display a resolution bar pattern of 100% contrast when the spatial frequency of the bar phantom is equal to half the monitor line frequency in vertical and horizontal directions.
4. Spatial accuracy: lines displayed on the monitor should be straight to within +5 mm.

MAGNETIC RESONANCE SAFETY PROGRAM ASSESSMENT

The medical physicist or MRI scientist must also assess the MR safety program on a yearly basis. This program must confirm that the site's written MRI safety policy addresses the following in a satisfactory manner:
- Designated MR medical director
- Site access restrictions (MR zones)
- Documented MR safety education/training for all personnel
- Patient and non-MR personnel screening
- Pediatric patients
- Magnetic quench
- Cryogen safety
- Acoustic noise
- Pregnant patients and staff
- Contrast agent safety
- Sedations
- Thermal burns
- Emergency code procedures
- Device and object screening
- Designation of MR safe/MR conditional status
- Reporting of MR safety incidents or adverse incidents
- Patient communication
- Infection control and medical waste
- Written policies present and readily available to facility staff
- Written policies reviewed and updated on a regular basis
- Facility has appropriate MR safety warning signage and methods of controlled access

Documentation for the MRI Safety Program Assessment can be documented using the checklist shown in Fig. 11.22.

OPTIONAL TESTS

Signal-to-Noise Ratio Consistency

The repeatability of an RF coil's performance can be tested during the annual testing of the RF coil's performance. This is done by conducting SNR tests on a specific coil several times, separated by a few hours. Variations of more than a few percentage points can reflect intermittent system or noise problems.

Magnetic Fringe Field

Periodically checking the magnet's fringe field is a good idea to ensure that all spaces over 5 G have appropriate warning signs. Many instances of a magnet's fringe field exceeding the posted 5 G line have occurred. This violates the Food and Drug Administration requirements and could present a potential source of liability.

For ACR Accreditation, the medical physicist or MRI scientist must submit an MRI Equipment Evaluation Summary Form to document the results of the annual QC inspection (Fig. 11.23).

MAGNETIC RESONANCE IMAGING DEPARTMENT COMPLIANCE STANDARDS

In addition to the MRI equipment QC standards that have just been discussed in this chapter, accrediting bodies also have specific department standards that must be met, including:
1. Processes must be in place to address the following MRI safety risks (staff can describe the processes for):
   - Patients with claustrophobia, anxiety, and emotional distress
   - Urgent/emergent patient care needs
   - Patients with medical implants, devices, and embedded metallic objects
   - Preventing entry of ferromagnetic objects into MRI area (only MRI-safe equipment, e.g., fire extinguishers)
   - Protecting patients from acoustic noise
2. Ensure that access to the MRI area is restricted:
   - All staff and patients are screened before entering the MRI area.
   - There are controls in place to prevent unauthorized access to the MRI area.
   - Warning signage is posted at the entrance to the MRI scanner.
   - Signage is posted indicating that the magnet is always on (as applicable).
3. Equipment QC and maintenance activities are to be identified and time frames are established for how often they are to be performed.
4. Equipment QC and maintenance activities are to be performed and QC logs are completed. Preventive maintenance shall be scheduled, performed, and documented by a qualified service engineer on a regular basis. Service performed to correct system deficiencies shall also be documented and service records maintained by the MR site.
5. A performance evaluation is to be conducted annually by a medical physicist or MRI scientist, and all required tests and evaluation/testing results are to be documented.
6. A performance evaluation that includes all requires tests and parameters is to be conducted on each image acquisition monitor annually by a medical physicist or MRI scientist.
7. Documentation of staff annual training and ongoing education on all topics must be available.
8. Data are to be collected on:
   - Any MRI-related patient thermal injuries
   - Incidents where anyone has unintentionally entered the MRI scanner room
   - Injuries resulting from the presence of ferromagnetic objects in the MRI scanner room

MRI Safety Program Assessment Checklist

Site:_____

The site's written MRI safety policy addresses the following: **Yes/No/NA**

1. Designated MR medical director
2. Site access restrictions (MR zones)
3. Documented MR Safety education/training for all personnel
4. Patient and non-MR personnel screening
5. Pediatric patients
6. Magnet quench
7. Cryogen safety
8. Acoustic noise
9. Pregnant patients and staff
10. Contrast agent safety
11. Sedations
12. Thermal burns
13. Emergency code procedures
14. Device and object screening
15. Designation of MR safe/MR conditional status
16. Reporting of MR safety incidents or adverse incidents
17. Patient communication
18. Infection control and medical waste

ACR criteria for compliance: **Yes/No/NA**

1. Written policies are present and readily available to facility staff.
2. Written policies are reviewed and updated on a regular basis.
3. Facility has appropriate MR safety warning signage and methods of controlled access.

Overall Pass/Fail [   ]

Comments

[   ]

Reviewed by: _____   _____

Qualified Medical Physicist/MR Scientist   Date

Fig. 11.22 American College of Radiology Safety Program Assessment Checklist. *ACR,* American College of Radiology; *MR,* magnetic resonance; *MRI,* magnetic resonance imaging; *NA,* not applicable.

MRI Equipment Evaluation Summary

Site: _____

System MRAP#: _____

MRI System Manufacturer: _____   Model: _____

Medical Physicist/MRI Scientist: _____

Signature: _____

Report Date: _____

Survey Date: _____

Equipment Evaluation Tests	Pass/Fail/NA
1. Setup and Table Position Accuracy	
2. Center Frequency	
3. Transmitter Gain or Attenuation	
4. *Geometric Accuracy Measurements**	
5. *High-Contrast Spatial Resolution**	
6. *Low-Contrast Detectability**	
7. Artifact Evaluation	
8. Film Printer Quality Control (if applicable)	
9. Visual Checklist	
10. Magnetic Field Homogeneity	
Method of Testing	
11. *Slice-Position Accuracy**	
12. *Slice-Thickness Accuracy**	
13. Radiofrequency Coil Checks	
Were all clinically used coils evaluated? (Yes/No)	
a. SNR	
b. Volume Coil Percent Image Uniformity (PIU)	
c. Percent Signal Ghosting (PSG)	
14. Soft Copy (Monitor) Quality Control	
15. MR Safety Program Assessment	

* tests that can be performed by scanning the ACR MRI Phantom

Evaluation of Site's Technologist QC Program	Pass/ Fail
1. Setup and Table Position Accuracy *(weekly)*	
2. Center Frequency *(weekly)*	
3. Transmitter Gain or Attenuation *(weekly)*	
4. Geometric Accuracy Measurements *(weekly)*	
5. High-Contrast Spatial Resolution *(weekly)*	
6. Low-Contrast Detectability *(weekly)*	
7. Artifact Evaluation *(weekly)*	
8. Film Printer Quality Control (if applicable) *(weekly)*	
9. Visual Checklist *(weekly)*	

Medical Physicist's or MRI Scientist's Recommendations for Quality Improvement

Fig. 11.23 American College of Radiology MRI Equipment Evaluation Summary Form.

SUMMARY

QC procedures for MRI are becoming more prevalent because of the introduction of the MR Site Accreditation program by the ACR in the spring of 1997. The ACR has a dedicated QC component to the application for the accreditation process. A specific phantom must be used, and information about the entire process can be obtained by contacting the ACR (www.acr.org). As with all quality management and accreditation processes, documentation of all QC testing and maintenance of all records is imperative for program success. Many imaging facilities where QC was not routinely performed now have to be educated on the various testing methods and quality factors. Although some facilities do only what is necessary to get by, others with dedicated QA departments likely have a comprehensive program for each imaging modality. In MRI, this can include assessment of the placement of a warning sign, fire alarms and extinguishers, magnet quench

procedures, computer room air conditioners, the patient/technologist intercom, the resetting of halon systems, the start-up and shutdown of MR systems, and even jam clearing in the camera and processor.

Training and competency assessment of new and existing MR personnel help maintain the overall quality of the facility. With a limited operating budget, MR technologists often are required to do a considerable amount of error troubleshooting before calling for service. Ironically, productivity issues may drive QA programs, whereas QA should be thought of as enhancing productivity. A summary of the weekly and annual QC tests for MR systems is found in Box 11.3.

Refer to the Evolve website at https://evolve.elsevier.com for Student Experiments 11.1: Magnetic Resonance Scanners, and 11.2: MRI Visual Inspection.

BOX 11.3 Summary of Quality Control Testing for Magnetic Resonance Imaging Systems

Technologist's Weekly QC Tests Required by ACR
- Setup and Table Position Accuracy
- Center Frequency
- Transmitter Gain or Attenuation
- Geometric Accuracy
- High-Contrast Spatial Resolution
- Low-Contrast Detectability
- Artifact Evaluation
- Film Printer Quality Control (if applicable)
- Visual Checklist

Physicist's/MR Scientist's Annual QC Tests Required by ACR
- Magnetic Field Homogeneity
- Slice Position Accuracy
- Slice Thickness Accuracy
- Radio Frequency Coil Checks
- Soft Copy (Monitor) Quality Control
- MR Safety Program Assessment
- Evaluation of Technologist Weekly QC

ACR, American College of Radiology; *MR*, magnetic resonance; *MRI*, magnetic resonance imaging; *QC*, quality control.

REVIEW QUESTIONS

1. Phantoms for MRI QC tests are made with which material?
   a. Aluminum
   b. Copper
   c. Manganese
   d. All of the above
2. Daily QC tests should be performed by which employee?
   a. Medical physicist
   b. MR technologist
   c. Service engineer
   d. System specialist
3. When the SNR test is performed, changing the imaging parameters does not affect the resulting SNR.
   a. False
   b. True
4. Which equation is used to calculate the system's resonance frequency?
   a. Bloch
   b. Fourier
   c. Larmor
   d. Plank

5. Between which of the following should image uniformity values range?
   a. 20% and 40%
   b. 40% and 60%
   c. 60% and 80%
   d. 80% and 100%
6. The phantom used for the spatial linearity test can be the same as the phantom for the resonance frequency test.
   a. False
   b. True
7. Which of the following terms identifies the QC test performed to ensure that the landmarking location is at the isocenter?
   a. Slice position
   b. Slice thickness
   c. Slice uniformity
   d. Spatial localization
8. An acquisition with a 20-cm FOV and a 1282 matrix yields a pixel of what size?
   a. 0.78 mm^2
   b. 1.56 mm^2
   c. 1.92 mm^2
   d. 2.56 mm^2

9. What term is used to describe the quality factor of the coil used to receive signals?
   a. Coil Q
   b. Receiver setting
   c. Resonance frequency
   d. SNR

10. Which of the following personnel are considered key to a good QC MR program?
    a. Medical physicist
    b. MR technologist
    c. MR scientist
    d. All of the above

12

Ultrasound Equipment Quality Assurance

James A. Zagzebski, James M. Kofler*

OUTLINE

OBJECTIVES

At the completion of this chapter, the reader will be able to do the following:

- Discuss the importance of quality assurance for ultrasound equipment
- Describe the various phantoms used in ultrasound quality assurance

- Identify the basic quality control tests for ultrasound
- Explain the importance of documentation of quality assurance testing
- Describe the basic quality control testing for Doppler color flow equipment

KEY TERMS

Axial resolution
Axial or vertical distance measurement
Depth of penetration (DOP)
Elevational resolution

Lateral or horizontal distance
    measurement
Lateral resolution
Phantom

Scan image uniformity
Sensitivity
Slice thickness
String test

In an imaging facility, quality assurance (QA) is a process carried out to ensure that equipment is operating consistently at its expected level of performance. During routine scanning, each sonographer is vigilant for equipment changes that can lead to suboptimal imaging and might require service. Thus in some ways, ultrasound equipment QA is carried out every day, even when it is not identified as a process itself.

QA steps to be discussed here go beyond judgments of scanner performance that are made during routine ultrasound imaging. They involve prospective actions to identify problem situations, even before obvious equipment malfunctions occur. QA testing provides confidence that image data

*The author and publisher wish to acknowledge the previous edition's contributor.

such as distance measurements and area estimations are accurate and that the image is of the best possible quality from the imaging instrument.

COMPONENTS OF AN ULTRASOUND QA PROGRAM

QA and Preventive Maintenance

Various approaches are used by ultrasound facilities when setting up a QA program for their scanners. Sometimes these programs include both preventive maintenance procedures performed by trained equipment service personnel and in-house testing of scanners with phantoms and test objects. Some facilities rely on only one of these measures. For preventive maintenance, emphasis is usually given to invasive electronic testing of system components such as voltage measurements at test points inside the scanner. Sometimes preventive maintenance also involves an assessment of the imaging capability by scanning a phantom.

In-house scanner QA programs usually involve imaging phantoms or test objects and assessing the results. In-house tests may be performed by sonographers, physicians, medical physicists, clinical engineers, or equipment maintenance personnel. Detailed recommendations from professional organizations and experts in ultrasound on establishing an in-house QA program are available elsewhere (ACR Ultrasound Accreditation Program, 2017; Goodsitt et al, 1998; Zagzebski, 2000). Both the American College of Radiology (both ultrasound and breast ultrasound) and the American Institute of Ultrasound in Medicine offer accreditation programs for ultrasound imaging departments.

Tissue-Mimicking Phantoms

In-house scanner QA tests most often are performed with tissue-mimicking phantoms. In medical ultrasound, a phantom is a device that mimics soft tissues in its ultrasound transmission characteristics. Phantoms represent "constant patients," and images can be taken at different times for close comparison. Image penetration capabilities, for example, are readily evaluated for changes over time when images of a phantom are available for comparison. Phantoms also have targets in known positions, and so images can be compared closely with the region that is scanned. Examples include simulated cysts, echogenic structures, and thin "line targets."

Tissue Properties Represented in Phantoms

Tissue characteristics mimicked in commercially available phantoms are the speed of sound (speed of sound in phantom material is the same as that of human soft tissue, 1540 m/s); ultrasonic attenuation; and, to some degree, echogenicity (i.e., the ultrasonic scattering level). Phantoms cannot exactly replicate the acoustic properties of soft tissue. This is partially because of the complexity and variability of tissues. Instead, phantom manufacturers construct these objects to have acoustic properties that represent the average properties of many different tissues. Sometimes the term *tissue equivalent* is used when phantoms are described; however, this term should not be interpreted literally, because most phantom materials are not acoustically equivalent to any specific tissue.

Typical QA Phantom Design

An example of a general-purpose ultrasound QA phantom is shown in Fig. 12.1. Such phantoms are examined with scanner settings that are similar to those used when patients are being scanned. The phantom images have grayscale characteristics that are analogous to characteristics of organs, although the actual structures are not anatomically represented.

Fig. 12.1B, shows the internal structure of this phantom. The tissue-mimicking material within the phantom consists of a water-based gelatin in which microscopic particles are mixed uniformly throughout the volume (Burlew et al, 1980; Madsen et al, 1978). The speed of sound in this material is about 1540 m/s, the same speed assumed in the calibration of ultrasound instruments. The ultrasonic attenuation coefficient versus frequency is one of two values: either 0.5 or 0.7 dB/cm per megahertz (Box 12.1). Some users prefer the lower-attenuating material because they find it easier to image objects in the phantom. However, standards groups recommend the higher attenuation because it challenges machines more thoroughly (Zagzebski, 2000).

Attenuation in the gel-graphite material in the phantom is proportional to the ultrasound frequency and mimics the behavior in tissues (Lu et al, 1999; Madsen et al, 1978; Maklad et al, 1984). Other types of materials have been used in phantoms, but only water-based gels laced with powder have both speed of sound and attenuation with tissue-like properties (Madsen et al, 1978; Zagzebski, 2000).

Small scatterers are distributed throughout the tissue-mimicking material; therefore the phantoms appear echogenic when scanned with ultrasound imaging equipment (see Fig. 12.1C). Many phantoms have simulated "cysts," which are low-attenuating, nonechogenic cylinders. These should appear echo-free on B-mode images and should exhibit distal echo enhancement. Some tissue phantoms provide additional image contrast by having simulated masses or test objects of varying echogenicity. Such objects are evident in Fig. 12.1C.

Most QA phantoms also contain discrete reflectors such as nylon-line targets to be used mainly for evaluating the distance measurement accuracy of a scanner. Tests of the accuracy of distance measurements rely on the manufacturer of the phantom to have filled the device with a material with a sound propagation speed of 1540 m/s or at least close enough to this speed that no appreciable errors are introduced in calibrations. These phantoms also rely on the manufacturer placing the target or reflector positions accurately. With the correct speed of sound (1540 m/s) and precisely known distances between point-like reflectors, it is easy to check the accuracy of distance measurements with calipers, as described later.

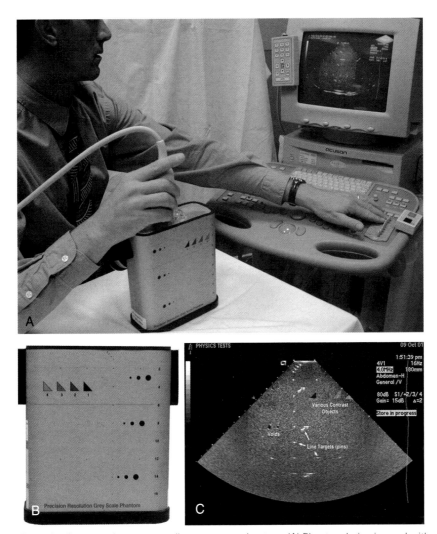

Fig. 12.1 Example of a general-purpose quality assurance phantom. (A) Phantom being imaged with an ultrasound scanner. (B) Close-up of phantom, with diagram of interior contents. (C) B-mode image of the phantom.

BOX 12.1   Tissue Attenuation Coefficients

Attenuation coefficients are normally specified in decibels per centimeter. To include the dependence of attenuation on frequency, phantom manufacturers divide the attenuation coefficient by the frequency at which the measurement is done. This yields units of decibels per centimeter per megahertz. Strictly speaking, this approach should be used only when attenuation is directly proportional to the frequency, as we often assume for tissues. The value of 0.7 dB/cm/MHz is representative of the attenuation coefficient in difficult-to-penetrate fatty liver. The depth that structures can be visualized within tissue-mimicking material having this amount of attenuation more closely correlates with clinical penetration.

From Lu ZF, Lee FT, Zagzebski JA. Ultrasonic backscatter and attenuation in diffuse liver disease. *Ultrasound Med Biol* 1999;25:1047.

Phantoms often contain a column of reflectors, each separated by 1 or 2 cm, for vertical measurement accuracy tests. One or more horizontal rows of reflectors are used for assessing horizontal measurement accuracy. Additional sets of reflectors may be found for assessing the axial resolution and the lateral resolution of scanners.

Cautions About Phantom Desiccation

When a phantom made of water-based gels is used, loss of water (desiccation) may become a problem as the phantom ages. If this occurs, the speed of sound in the phantom may have changed. A scanning surface that has become concave is an indication of severe desiccation. Occasionally, water losses become so problematic that air entering the phantom window leads to the inability to image the phantom effectively. Users should follow the instructions given by the phantom manufacturer to avoid significant desiccation. For example, some manufacturers recommend storage in a humid, airtight container, and this practice should be adhered to if so stated.

Desiccation is not a problem with rubber-based phantom materials (Fig. 12.2) produced by some manufacturers. Storing these phantoms with the tissue-mimicking material directly exposed to the environment can be an advantage compared with water-based gels. The main disadvantages of rubber materials are that their speed of sound is lower than 1540 m/s (≈1450 m/s in some rubber-based phantoms) and that their attenuation is not proportional to the ultrasound frequency (Zagzebski, 2000). Therefore they may not be as effective as water-based gel phantoms when imaging over a large frequency range.

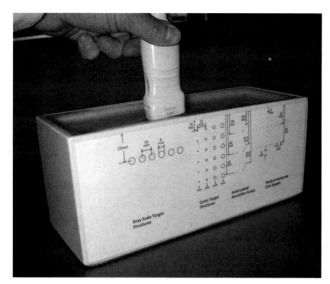

Fig. 12.2 A phantom with rubber-based, tissue-mimicking small parts. Although the acoustic properties are not as precise as the water-based phantoms, less care is required during manufacturing and with on-site storage to minimize changes over time.

BASIC QUALITY CONTROL TESTS

A recommended set of instrument quality control tests includes checks for the consistency of instrument sensitivity; evaluation of image uniformity; assessment of grayscale photography or image workstation brightness levels; and, where necessary, checks of both vertical and horizontal distance measurement accuracy (ACR Ultrasound Accreditation Program, 2017; Goodsitt et al, 1998; Zagzebski, 2000). This group of tests can be performed by a sonographer in 10–15 min, which includes the time for recording the results on a worksheet or in a notebook.

Visual Inspection

The visual inspection is used to evaluate the physical condition of the scanner's mechanical components, along with a few quick scan tests. This should be performed monthly or according to the user manual provided by the manufacturer. A checklist for documentation of the visual inspection is found in Fig. 12.3. Some of the items to check during the visual inspection are described as follows.

Transducers: Cables, housings, and transmitting surfaces should be checked for fraying, cracks, separations, delamination, and discolorations. Any bent or loose prongs on the plug should be fixed. Transducers should be intact, with no cracks or delaminations. Also verify that the transducers are cleaned after each use.

Power cord: The cable and plug should be checked for any fraying, cracks, discoloration, and damage.

Control panel: Check for dirty or broken switches and knobs as well as any burnt-out indicator lights. Also verify that the keyboard is clean and free of debris.

Video monitor: The video display monitor should be clean and free of scratches. The brightness and contrast controls should be set at proper levels.

Wheels and wheel locks: All wheels should be checked to ensure that they rotate freely and that the unit is easy to maneuver. The wheels also should be seated and fastened securely, and wheel locks should be checked to ensure that they lock securely.

Dust filters: Dust filters should be inspected and free of lint and clumps of dirt. Otherwise, overheating of the internal electronic components can occur and shorten the life span of the unit.

Scanner housing: The unit should be inspected for dents or other cosmetic damage, which could indicate events that might have caused damage to the internal components. Also, verify that all accessories (DVR, cameras, etc.) are fastened securely to the ultrasound unit.

Transducer Choice

Results of some test procedures depend on which transducer/frequency combination is used with the instrument. On systems in which several transducers are available, tests should be done with two transducers (ACR Ultrasound Accreditation Program, 2017). Choose the most common transducer used in most examinations; additionally, it is preferable to test another transducer that has a different frequency range and a different scan format. For example, with a general-purpose scanner, a low-frequency (2–5 MHz) curvilinear or phased array and an intermediate-frequency (5–8 MHz) or even a high-frequency linear array are appropriate. This transducer combination should be used for all subsequent test procedures. All necessary transducer assembly identification information should be checked, including the frequency, size, and serial number so that future tests will be conducted with the same probe. If several identical scanners are available, the same transducer/scanner pairs should be used for all subsequent testing.

System Sensitivity

The sensitivity of an instrument refers to the weakest echo signal level that can be detected and displayed clearly enough to be discernible on an image. Most scanners have controls that vary the receiver amplification (gain) and the transmit level (e.g., output or power). These are used to adjust the sensitivity during clinical examinations. The *maximum sensitivity* of the instrument occurs when these controls are at maximum practical settings. Often, the maximum sensitivity is limited by electrical noise that appears on the display when the receiver gain is at maximum levels. The noise may be generated externally, for example, by electronic communication networks or by computer terminals. More commonly, the noise arises from within the instrument itself, such as in the first preamplification stage of the receiver amplifier.

Concerns during QA tests are usually centered on whether notable variations in sensitivity have occurred since the last QA test. Such variations might result from a variety of causes, such as damaged transducers, damaged transducer cables, or electronic drift in the pulser-receiver components of the scanner. Questions related to the sensitivity of a

SYSTEM INSPECTION – ULTRASOUND
DEPARTMENT OF DIAGNOSTIC IMAGING

ULTRASOUND SYSTEM: _____

SYSTEM ID: _____

CHECKED BY: _____

PASS = ✓
FAIL = F (explain in remarks)
DOES NOT APPLY = NA

		Month																			
		Day																			
CONTROL PANEL	Knobs, trackball, buttons, etc.																				
	Lights																				
MAIN UNIT	Scratches, dents, etc.																				
	Wheels (function and park)																				
	Cables not tangled																				
	Power cord not damaged																				
	Air filters																				
	Excessive noise, heat, etc.																				
TRANSDUCERS	Cables																				
	Cracks, scratches, etc.																				
	Lens delamination																				
	Connections																				
	Other																				
MISC	Hard copy imager																				
	Display monitor																				

Date	Remarks

Fig. 12.3 Ultrasound system visual checklist.

scanner sometimes occur during clinical imaging; a quick scan of the QA phantom and comparison with results of the most recent QA test help determine whether there is cause for concern.

A commonly used technique for detecting variations in maximum sensitivity is the measure of the maximum depth of penetration (DOP) for signals from scattered echoes in the tissue-mimicking phantom (ACR Ultrasound Accreditation Program, 2017; American Institute of Ultrasound in Medicine, 1990; Carson and Goodsitt, 1995; Goodsitt et al, 1998; Zagzebski, 2000). The DOP can be defined as the greatest depth at which echo signals can be distinguished from the noise. The technique includes the following:

1. Adjust the output power transmit levels and receiver sensitivity controls so that echo signals are obtained from as deep as possible into the phantom. The depth of field must be larger than DOP (if possible). Place a focal zone as close as possible to the DOP. Now the output power control is positioned for maximum output, and the receiver gain is adjusted for the highest values without excessive noise on the display. (Experience helps in establishing these control settings; they should be recorded in the quality control worksheet, which is described later.)

2. Scan the phantom and estimate the maximum depth of visualization of texture echo signals (Fig. 12.4).

3. File a digital or hard-copy image of the phantom.

In the examples in Fig. 12.4, the maximum depth of penetration is 16.8 cm at 4 MHz. With a 2-MHz mode, the maximum depth of penetration is at least as deep as the length of the phantom, and so it cannot be measured with this

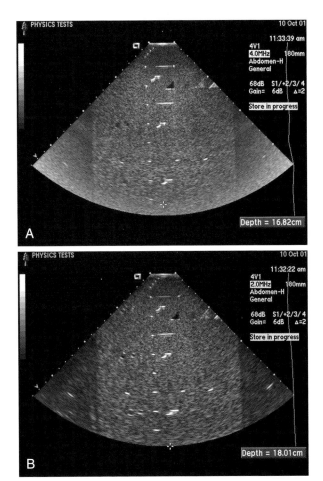

Fig. 12.4 Images obtained for the maximum depth of the visualization quality assurance test with a multifrequency array transducer. The phantom has an attenuation coefficient of 0.7 dB/cm/MHz. (A) At 4 MHz, the maximum depth of visualization is 16.8 cm. (B) At 2 MHz, the maximum depth of visualization cannot be determined with this phantom because visualization remains excellent all the way to the bottom of the phantom.

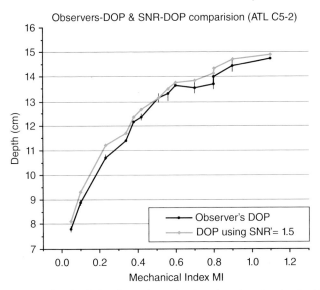

Fig. 12.5 Graph of signal-to-noise ratio plotted against the depth of penetration.

likely associated with the scanner and not the transducer assemblies. Medical physicists may also use a quantitative measurement of signal-to-noise ratio to evaluation system sensitivity (described in International Electrotechnical Commission (IEC) 61391-2) (Fig. 12.5).

Photography and Grayscale Hard Copy

Perhaps the most frequent source of ultrasound instrument variability over time is related to image photography. Too often, drift in the imaging instrument, in the hard-copy cameras, or in film processing reduces image quality to the point that significant amounts of detail related to echo signal amplitude variations are lost on hard-copy B-mode images. However, if image-viewing monitors and recording devices are set up properly and if sufficient attention is given to photography during routine quality control, these problems can be reduced. The advent of laser printers with automatic (or semiautomatic) calibration has greatly reduced much of the variability of producing a hard-copy image. However, even laser printers have problems.

Monitor Setup and Recording Devices

Most instruments provide both an image display monitor, which is viewed during scan buildup, and an image recording device. As a general rule, the display monitor should be set up properly first, and then adjustments should be made, if necessary, to the laser printers or other hard-copy recording devices to produce an acceptable grayscale on hard-copy images. The establishment of proper settings is expected only during the installation of a scanner, major upgrades, or detection of image problems. Changes made to the display settings are not automatically reflected in the printed image. Changing the display settings requires adjustment of the hardcopy device to properly match the printed image to the displayed image; therefore image display settings should not be shifted routinely. Many facilities go so far as to remove the control

phantom. The lower frequency results in a lower attenuation and therefore greater maximum depth of penetration.

For the test results to be interpreted, a comparison is made with maximum visualization results from a previous test, perhaps 6 months earlier. Results should agree within 0.6 cm. Normal trial-to-trial variations in scanning and interpretation prohibit closer calls than this. However, with digital or hard-copy images and records of maximum depth of visualization tests, ascertaining whether a scanner/transducer combination has drifted significantly over time in echo detection capabilities should be possible.

In addition to this measurement being made with the standard transducer, occasionally performing the test with different transducers is useful. For example, the test can be performed with all of the transducers that are available for each instrument when quality control tests are first established and semiannually thereafter. This method helps pinpoint the source of any decrease in the maximum sensitivity. If the maximum depth of visualization decreases on all of the transducers tested on a specific scanner, the problem is most

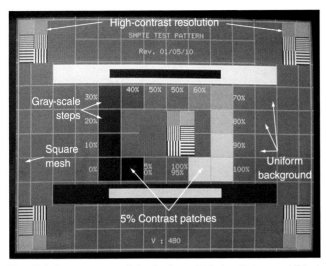

Fig. 12.6 A test pattern of the Society of Motion Picture and Television Engineers (SMPTE). The pattern contains a grayscale range in increments of 10% video level. There are also 5% contrast patches at the 0% *(black)* and 100% *(white)* levels, a mesh pattern to check for spatial distortions, and several resolution patterns.

knobs on image monitors once the contrast and brightness are adjusted to an acceptable level; thus the temptation to change settings casually is removed.

An effective method for setting up both viewing and hard copy devices is discussed in Chapter 8.

It is recommended that adjustments be done with an image that contains a clinically representative sampling of gray shades.

1. First, attend to the display monitor viewed during scanning. With the contrast settings of the monitor initially set at minimum settings, adjust the brightness to a level that just allows television raster lines to be discernible.
2. After the adjustment, increase the monitor contrast until just before the text on the display begins to become distorted (the text, which is typically displayed at a maximum brightness, begins to smear to the left and right if the contrast is too high). Use a clinical image to verify that the settings are adequate. After the viewing monitor is properly adjusted, make provisions to prevent casual changes in settings by department personnel.
3. Adjust the image recording device to obtain the same gray shades that appear on the display monitor. This adjustment may require several repetitions, varying the contrast and the overall brightness, until satisfactory results are obtained. Many manufacturers provide grayscale test patterns such as the one by the Society of Motion Picture and Television Engineers (SMPTE) (Fig. 12.6) that can be displayed on the scanner. These patterns are useful for matching the hard-copy image to the display image. If such a pattern is unavailable, a small grayscale bar is usually presented on the real-time image.

Routine QA of Image Recording

Routine checks should be performed on the quality of grayscale photography or other hard-copy recording media.

Detailed analysis performed in some installations includes film sensitometry and film-emulsion batch crossovers. These processes are well established and documented in Chapter 4 and are not explained in detail. The procedure for the evaluation of dry laser printers is covered in Chapter 8. Images of a tissue-mimicking phantom, along with the graybar pattern that appears on the edge of most image displays, can be used for routinely assessing photography settings. In photography and processing, all brightness variations in the viewing monitor image should be successfully recorded on the hard copy image.

A quick check of grayscale recording can be done as follows:

1. On an image of a tissue-mimicking phantom (or of a patient), check to see whether weak echo signal dots appearing on the viewing monitor are successfully recorded on film.
2. Determine whether the entire gray-bar is visible and whether all gray levels are distinguishable. For example, for a scanner with a gray bar including 15 levels of gray, along with the background, the hard copy image should portray distinctions among all of the different levels. Continuous gray bars are more of a visual challenge when display bars are compared with printed gray levels. In this case focus attention on the light and dark ends of the patterns and compare the differences in the extent of white and black areas on the bars. The suggested action level is any optical density that is greater than or equal to 0.2 optical density units from the baseline.
3. The entire length of the gray-bar pattern displayed on the viewing monitor should be visible on the final image (see Fig. 12.4B). For multiple images on a single sheet of film or paper, all images should have the same background brightness and should display the gray-bar pattern in the same manner. These images can be verified from clinical images taken on the same day the QA tests are taken, or from the QA films themselves.
4. Some laser printers offer features for setting other characteristics of the printed image such as border width and background density. These settings should be decided, usually by trial and error, by all of those involved in reading the images. Once a conclusion has been reached, the settings should be installed in all printing devices used for ultrasound and documented for future reference.

Many imaging facilities now use digital images archived on computer systems and image workstations, rather than film recording. Workstation displays require periodic evaluation to ensure optimum performance. The displays should be cleaned periodically and before any QA testing. Ideally, a lint-free cloth should be used for wiping the surface of the display. Cleaning solution should be applied to the cloth and not sprayed directly on the display. Some displays, especially flat-panel displays, may require specific cleaning products because of antiglare or other special coatings on the screen surface, so check the manufacturer's cleaning instructions before applying any chemical product to the display. Storing a cloth and cleaner solution next to the workstation display is a convenient practice to promote a dust-free, clean display screen.

The SMPTE pattern (see Fig. 12.6) is useful for the routine QA of displays. The large squares on the SMPTE pattern are used to note any distortions caused by the display; they should appear as an array of perfect squares over the entire screen. Degradation of monitor resolution can be noted by viewing the high-contrast resolution patterns and the text on the SMPTE pattern. These should appear well defined, not blurry or smeared. The 95% density patch within the 100% video *(white)* and the 5% density patch within the 0% video *(black)* square should be visible. The gray background of the SMPTE pattern should be uniformly gray across the entire display.

The following characteristics should be noted when performing display QA (Groth et al, 2001):

- *Monitor cleanliness.* The display screen should be free of dust or other markings (e.g., pen markings, fingerprints).
- *Spatial distortion.* The display should be serviced if the squares on the SMPTE pattern are distorted at the corners or if their aspect ratios (width/height) are not correct (e.g., a square shape that appears to be rectangular). Some displays provide controls that allow the user to correct minor spatial distortions.
- *Monitor resolution (edge definition).* Any high-contrast boundary such as white text on a dark background should be well defined.
- *Grayscale uniformity.* The intensity on the display should be consistent over the entire screen. This requires a test pattern that contains a constant gray level over the entire screen or at least at all four sides and in the center. Moving a small uniform image from one side of the screen to the other is typically an ineffective alternative to a single large image.
- *Low-contrast visibility.* The 5% difference in video level (on black and on white) of the SMPTE pattern should be noticeable on the display. Room lighting should be minimal when viewing low-contrast objects. Alternatively, the entire gray-bar pattern seen on the scanner monitor should be visualized on the workstation monitor.
- *Display artifacts.* The display should not contain streaks, lines, or dark/light patches. If a test pattern of uniform brightness is unavailable, the brightest pattern available

should be used. In this case the observer must look through the test objects at the background of the image. A few nonfunctioning (dropped) pixels, which appear as small black dots, may be tolerable. However, a group of dropped pixels or several dropped pixels scattered over the screen warrants replacement of the display. Also look for the presence of stuck (white) pixels.

Scan Image Uniformity

Ultrasound phantoms typically contain a background material that is distributed throughout the phantom. However, with most phantoms, it is impossible to acquire a view that does not contain any test objects. In these cases, scan image uniformity can be assessed by focusing attention solely on the background material of the phantom. Ideally, when a region within a phantom is scanned and the machine's gain settings are adjusted properly, the resultant image has a uniform brightness throughout (Fig. 12.7A). Nonuniformities caused by the ultrasound imager can occur because of the following situations:

- Bad elements in a linear or curved array or loose connections in beam former board plug-ins can lead to vertically oriented nonuniformities (Fig. 12.7B). (Boards can be loosened if the scanner is wheeled over bumps or if it is transported by a van to other hospitals or clinics.)
- Inadequate side-to-side image compensation in the machine can lead to variations in brightness from one side of the image to another.
- Inadequate blending of pixel data between transmit and receive focal zones can lead to horizontal or curved streaks parallel to the transducer surface. QA testing is an ideal time to assess whether such faults are noticeable. An image is taken of a uniform region in the QA phantom, and the image is inspected for these problems.

A uniformity image is useful in the detection of subtle artifacts that may not be readily evident on the clinical images. Care should be taken to inspect the image thoroughly for any vertical or radially oriented streaks, any dark or light patches, or any grayscale gradients in the axial or lateral directions. Occasionally a swirling pattern with the background texture

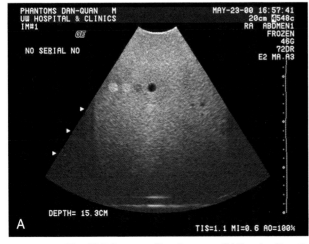
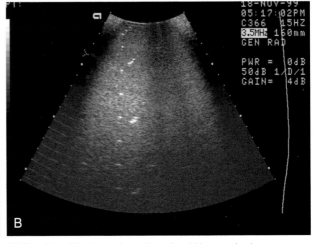

Fig. 12.7 Image uniformity tests. (A) Good uniformity. (B) Results with a transducer that should be repaired or replaced. Note the vertical streaks that are evidence of element dropout for this linear array transducer.

may be noticed. However, this pattern is typically a result of the phantom manufacturing process, which can be verified by comparison with uniformity images from other transducers. The suggested action level would be nonuniformity greater than or equal to 4dB or any consistent measurable change from the baseline.

Distance Measurement Accuracy

Instruments used for measuring structure dimensions, organ sizes, and areas can be tested periodically for accuracy of distance indicators. However, many individuals think that routine distance measurement accuracy checks are not useful because digital measurement systems on scanners exhibit satisfactory stability over time (ACR Ultrasound Accreditation Program, 2017; Goodsitt et al, 1998).

Distance indicators usually include 1-cm-deep markers on M-mode and B-mode scanning displays and electronic calipers on B-mode scanning systems. Calipers on workstations that are part of computer archiving systems also should be checked for accuracy. The principal distance measurement tests are separated into two parts: one part is for measurements along the sound beam axis, which is referred to as the *axial or vertical distance measurement* test, or the *axial distance measurement test,* and the other part is for measurements taken perpendicular to the sound beam axis, which is called the *lateral or horizontal distance measurement* test.

Axial or Vertical Distance Measurements

Vertical distance measurement accuracy also is called *depth calibration accuracy* in some texts.
1. To evaluate a scanner's vertical distance measurement accuracy, scan the phantom, ensuring that the vertical column of reflectors in the phantom is clearly imaged (Fig. 12.8).
2. Position the digital calipers to measure the distance between any two reflectors in this column.
3. Correct caliper placement is from the top of the echo from the first reflector to the top of the echo from the second reflector or from any position on the first reflector to the corresponding position on the second reflector.
4. When testing general-purpose scanners, choose reflectors positioned at least 8–10 cm apart for this test. Most laboratories also measure a smaller spacing such as 4 cm. For small-parts scanners and probes, use a distance of 1 or 2 cm. In general, the largest separation allowed by the transducer/frequency combination and the target placement in the phantom is appropriate for the distance accuracy test.
5. Determine that the measured distance agrees with the actual distance given by the phantom manufacturer to within 1 mm or 1.5%, whichever is greater. If a larger discrepancy occurs, consult with the ultrasound scanner manufacturer for possible corrective measures.

Lateral or Horizontal Distance Measurements

Horizontal measurement accuracy should be checked in a manner similar to vertical distance measurement. Measurements obtained in this direction (Fig. 12.9) are frequently less accurate because of beam width effects and scanner inaccuracies.

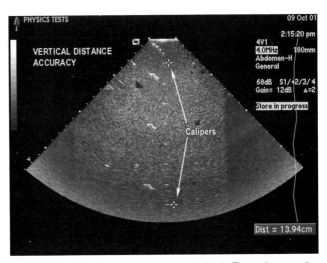

Fig. 12.8 Vertical distance measurement check. The caliper reading (13.94 cm) is compared with the actual separation (14 cm) between pins positioned along a vertical column in the phantom. Shorter distances should be used when high-frequency transducers are evaluated.

Nevertheless results should agree with the phantom manufacturer's distances to within 3 mm or 3%, whichever is greater. Correct caliper placement for this test is from the center of one reflector to the center of the second reflector. For the example in Fig. 12.9, measurement results are within 1 mm of the actual distance between the reflectors examined. This is well within the expected level of accuracy.

Other Important Instrument QA Tasks

During routine performance testing, it is a good idea to perform other equipment-related chores that require occasional attention. These include cleaning air filters on instruments that require this service (most do), checking for loose and frayed electrical cables, looking for loose handles or control arms on the scanner, checking the wheels and wheel locks, and performing recommended preventive maintenance of photography equipment, which may include dusting or cleaning of photographic monitors and maintenance chores on cameras.

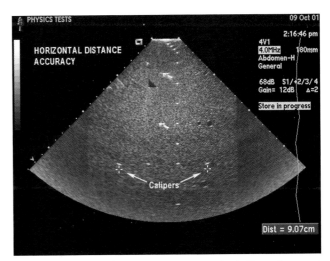

Fig. 12.9 Horizontal distance measurement check. The caliper reading (90.7 mm) is for a measurement taken horizontally on the image and compared with the actual pin separation (90 mm).

BOX 12.2   Sample Ultrasound Quality Control Results

Machine: Acuson 128

Transducer assembly: I.D.: V4

Date: 9/09/97

Instrument settings:

Room: E3 315

Serial no: 555–1212

Phantom: RMI 403 GS

Power 0 dB

Dynamic range: 50 dB

Pre 0/Persis 3/Post 0

Gain: 12 dB

Transmit focus: 16 cm

Image magnification: 18 cm

1. Depth measurement accuracy

Electronic calipers

Measured distance ....98.8 mm

Actual distance ....100 mm

Error ....1.2 mm

2. Horizontal measurement accuracy

Electronic calipers

Measured distance .... 30.5 mm

Actual distance .... 30 mm

Error .... 0.5 mm

3. Depth of penetration (4 MHz)

Measured distance ....152 mm

Baseline distance .... 150 mm

Variation from baseline .... 2 mm

4. Image uniformity

Significant Nonuniformity   Excellent Uniformity

1   2   3   4   5

5. Photography

Gray bars

Number of gray bars visible 13

Number of gray bars visible on baseline 15

Variation 2

Low-level echoes

All echoes displayed on viewing monitor also seen on film:

Yes X__ No___.

Contrast and brightness

Level of agreement between contrast and brightness on viewing monitor and film:

Poor   Excellent

1   2   3   4   5

6. Filters

Clean _____   Dusty X____

DOCUMENTATION

An important aspect of a QA program is keeping track of the test results. Most laboratories want to adopt a standardized worksheet on which to write the test results. The worksheet helps the user carry out the tests in a consistent manner by having enough information to assist recall of transducers, phantoms, and machine settings. It also includes blank spaces for recording the results. An example is shown in Box 12.2. Fig. 12.10 contains the American College of Radiology (ACR) Ultrasound/Breast Ultrasound Equipment Annual

Ultrasound/Breast Ultrasound Equipment Annual Survey Summary

Facility Name:		
UAP/BUAP #:	Unit #:	Report Date:
Serial Number:		Survey Date:
System Manufacturer:		Model:
Medical Physicist or designee (Print name):		
Medical Physicist or designee (Signature):		

Equipment Evaluation Tests

Required	Pass/Fail *	Comments
1. Physical and Mechanical Inspection		
2. Image Uniformity and Artifact Survey		
3. System Sensitivity		
4. Scanner Electronic Image Display Performance		

Were all clinically used transducers tested? ⌊ YES   ⌊ NO

Optional		
1. Primary Interpretation Display Performance		
2. Contrast Resolution		
3. Spatial Resolution		
4. Geometric Accuracy		

Overall comments:

*If any Fail result is indicated above, documentation of corrective action is required.

Revised 10/27/2020

Fig. 12.10 American College of Radiology Ultrasound/Breast Ultrasound Equipment Annual Survey Summary.

Survey Summary, to be completed by the medical physicist. Fig. 12.11 contains the ACR Evaluation of Site's Routine QC Program, to be completed by the technologist. Box 12.3 contains a summary of the ACR Annual System Performance Evaluation Requirements.

SPATIAL RESOLUTION TESTS

Some ultrasound departments include spatial resolution in their QA testing. Measurements of spatial resolution generally require more exacting techniques to achieve results that allow intercomparisons of scanners; therefore many centers

| Facility UAP #: | | Facility BUAP #: | | Survey Date: | |

Evaluation of Site's Routine QC Program

Test	Minimum Frequency	Pass/ Fail	Comments
1. Physical and Mechanical Inspection	semiannually		
2. Image Uniformity and Artifact Survey	semiannually		
3. Geometric Accuracy (mechanically scanned transducers only)	semiannually		
4. Scanner Electronic Image Display Performance	semiannually		
5. Primary Interpretation Display Performance*,**	semiannually		

* If located at the facility where ultrasound is performed
** Semiannually, or as judged appropriate based on the specific display technology, or prior QC testing data

Specific Comments:

Fig. 12.11 Evaluation of Site's Routine Quality Control Program.

BOX 12.3 American College of Radiology Annual System Performance Evaluation Requirements

Annual Quality Control Test

Physical and Mechanical Inspection

Image Uniformity and Artifact Survey

Geometric Accuracy (Optional)

System Sensitivity

Ultrasound Scanner Electronic Image Display Performance

Primary Interpretation Display Performance (Optional)
Only required if located at the facility where ultrasound is performed.

Contrast Resolution (Optional)

Spatial Resolution (Optional)

Evaluation of QC Program (if applicable)

QC, Quality control.

do not do such performance tests routinely but may do so only during equipment acceptance tests (Carson and Goodsitt, 1995). Common methods for determining spatial resolution to measure axial resolution, lateral resolution, and elevational resolution (for 3D and 4D scanners) are discussed in this section (Fig. 12.12).

Axial Resolution

Axial resolution is a measure of how close two reflectors can be to one another along the axis of an ultrasound beam and still be resolved as separate reflectors. Axial resolution also is related to the crispness of the image of a reflector arranged perpendicularly to the ultrasound beam.

Axial resolution can be estimated by measuring the thickness of the image of a line target in the QA phantom. Alternatively, some phantoms contain sets of reflectors for axial resolution testing. Fig. 12.13 shows both approaches. The axial separations between successive targets in this phantom are 2, 1, 0.5, and 0.25 mm. The targets are offset horizontally to minimize the effects of shallow targets shadowing the deeper ones. The pair most closely spaced yet clearly distinguishable in the axial direction indicates the axial resolution. This implies that to be considered resolved, the axial extent of one-pin depiction does not overlap with that of the next one below, even though the two pins may be distinguishable because of their lateral separation. Often, as in this phantom, the target pair separations are not finely spaced enough to allow a good measure of axial resolution; that is, the 0.25-mm pair in this example

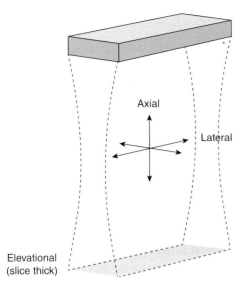

Fig. 12.12 Axial, lateral, and elevational dimensions of ultrasound beam.

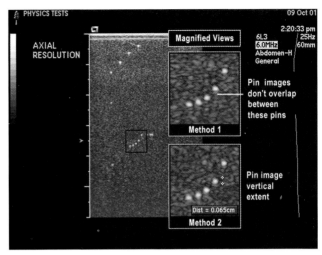

Fig. 12.13 Axial resolution measurement. The thickness of the pin target is 0.65 mm. In the axial resolution target set (vertical separation 2, 1, 0.5, and 0.25 mm), the 1-mm pair is separated a sufficient distance vertically so that there is no vertical overlap of the images of these two targets, whereas the 0.5-mm pair overlaps if the two targets are on a vertical line. The axial resolution is just over 0.5 mm, in agreement with the estimate made from the thickness of the single target image.

is not clearly resolved, whereas the 1-mm pair certainly is, and the 0.5 mm is almost resolved. The vertical thickness of a single target (0.6 mm in this case) is sometimes used (Burlew et al, 1980) to obtain more detailed indication of the axial resolution (*Method 2* in Fig. 12.13). The suggested action level is 1 mm or less for central frequencies (f_c) >4 MHz 2 mm or less for f_c <4 MHz or measurable change from baseline.

Lateral Resolution

Lateral resolution is a measure of how close two reflectors can be to one another, be perpendicular to the beam axis, and still be distinguished as separate reflectors on an image. One approach that is used for lateral resolution tests is to measure the width on the display of a point-like target such as a line target inside a phantom. For example, Fig. 12.14 shows such a measurement. The cursors indicate that the displayed width is 0.7 mm for this case. The displayed response width is related to the lateral resolution at the depth of the target. Through the imaging of targets at different depths, it is easy to see that the lateral resolution usually varies with depth for most transducers. Additionally, the lateral resolution measurement is sensitive to any focal zone placement. The suggested action level is 2.5 × focal length/(frequency in MHz × aperture in mm) or change >1 mm from baseline value.

Elevational Resolution

Three-dimensional probes can image an entire volume of tissue, so elevational resolution (slice thickness) should also be evaluated. Resolution in the elevational dimension can be measured directly with an inclined plane phantom (Fig. 12.15). It can be measured indirectly by assessing overall resolution (all three dimensions) of low echogenic targets of different sizes at different depths.

Cautions About Resolution Tests With Discrete Targets

The lateral and axial dimensions of the displayed image of a point-like target depend on the power and gain settings on

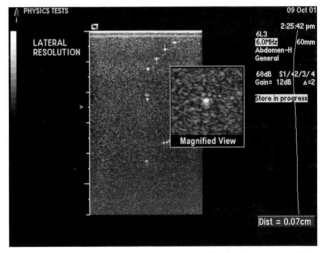

Fig. 12.14 Lateral resolution measurement. The horizontal size of the pin target is 0.7 mm.

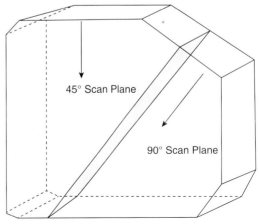

Fig. 12.15 Inclined plane ultrasound phantom.

the machine. Such dependency is one of the difficulties of adopting such tests in routine testing. Quantitative results for axial and lateral resolution have been obtained by measuring the dimensions of point-like targets when they are imaged at specified sensitivity levels above the threshold for their display (American Institute of Ultrasound in Medicine, 1990; Carson and Goodsitt, 1995). The procedure is as follows:

1. Obtain an image with the sensitivity of the scanner set so that the target is barely visible on the display.
2. Next, obtain a second image, with the scanner sensitivity increased 20 dB above the setting for display threshold.
3. Set the calipers to measure the lateral resolution at this scanner setting. Additional information is available elsewhere (Goodsitt et al, 1998; Zagzebski, 2000).

OTHER TEST OBJECTS AND PHANTOMS

Most general-purpose phantoms contain additional objects for the evaluation of image performance. Although these tests are not considered essential to a routine QA program, they may be useful for testing or optimizing specific imaging configurations. These tests are subjective; therefore the comparison of results with those acquired previously is essential.

Anechoic Voids

Many phantom designs include cylindrical anechoic voids (Fig. 12.16). These voids appear as dark, circular objects on an ultrasound image and can yield a wide range of information about the performance of a scanner. The void depictions can be inspected for spatial distortions; the voids should not be elliptical. The edges of the voids should be relatively sharp, and the interior of the voids should be echo-free. If voids of different sizes are available, the smallest visualized void can be noted.

Objects of Various Echogenicity

Many phantoms also include a set of objects with different inherent contrasts (Fig. 12.17). These objects can be visually assessed as a means of comparing one scan configuration with another or the performance of a specific scan configuration over time. For example, these objects may be useful to demonstrate the effect of changing the log compression. However, there must be caution when the impressions obtained by the set of various contrast objects are extrapolated into the clinical environment, because the entire clinical range of inherent object contrasts may not be completely represented by the test objects. As with the anechoic voids, the perimeter of the objects can be inspected for edge definition.

Spherical Object Phantom

Another phantom becoming increasingly popular for spatial resolution tests is one that has simulated focal lesions embedded within echogenic tissue-mimicking material (American Institute of Ultrasound in Medicine, 1990; Madsen et al, 1991). Different simulated lesion sizes and different object

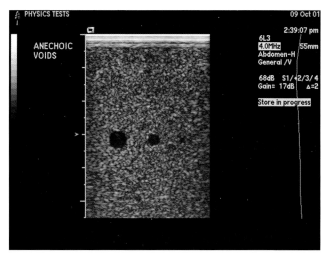

Fig. 12.16 B-mode image of a phantom containing three anechoic cylinders of different sizes (6-mm, 4-mm, and 2-mm diameter) acquired with a 4-MHz linear transducer. Some echoes are evident within the voids, and the edges are well defined. The smallest void is easily detectable.

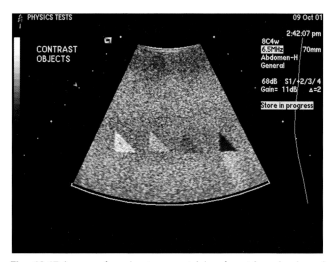

Fig. 12.17 Image of a phantom containing four triangular-shaped objects of different contrast values acquired with a 6.5-MHz curvilinear transducer. The higher-contrast objects (the outer two) are clearly visualized. The second object from the right is barely visible. The corners of the two inner objects are poorly defined.

contrast levels (e.g., relative echogenicity) have been tried (Madsen et al, 1991). An example is shown in Fig. 12.18, in which the phantom imaged contained 4-mm-diameter, low-echo masses. The centers of the masses are coplanar and distributed in a well-defined matrix.

A test of the ultrasound imaging system is used to determine the imaging zone for detection of masses of a given size and object contrast (Madsen et al, 1991). The 5-MHz phased array used for Fig. 12.18 can successfully detect the masses over a 5-cm to 12-cm depth range. The slice thickness (Goodsitt et al, 1998) is too large for this transducer to pick up these structures at more shallow depths.

A particularly useful aspect of spherical mass phantoms is that they present realistic imaging tasks that readily demonstrate resolution capabilities in terms of resolution.

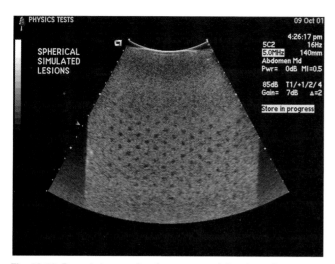

Fig. 12.18 B-mode image of a phantom containing 4-mm low-scattering spheres that mimic cysts. The spheres are centered in a regular array within a plane, and the scanning plane is carefully aligned to coincide with the plane containing the spheres. They can be visualized from depths of 5.0–12.0 cm with this transducer.

For three-dimensional spherical targets, the resolution is a combined effective resolution composed of axial, lateral, and slice thicknesses. If two-dimensional cylindrical objects are used as phantoms, only two dimensions, usually axial and lateral, are involved in their visualization. Because slice thickness is usually the worst measure of spatial resolution with array transducers, cylindrical objects can be misleading in terms of translating minimum sizes resolved into resolution of actual focal masses. The spherical lesion phantom is superior in this regard.

DOPPLER TESTING

Limited evaluations of Doppler and color flow equipment also can be made in the clinic. A number of devices, including string test objects, flow velocity test objects, and flow phantoms, are available to clinical users for carrying out tests of Doppler equipment (Hoskins et al, 1994; Performance criteria and measurements for Doppler ultrasound devices, 1993; Zagzebski, 1995).

String Test Objects

String test objects consist of a thin string wound around a pulley and motor-drive mechanism. The string is echogenic, so it produces echoes that are detected by an ultrasound instrument. The drive moves the string at precise velocities, either continuously or after a programmed waveform. This provides a way to evaluate the velocity measurement accuracy of Doppler devices. String test objects also may be used to evaluate the lateral and axial resolution in Doppler mode and can be used to determine the accuracy of gate registration on duplex Doppler systems (Hoskins et al, 1994).

The advantage of the string test object is that it provides a small target moving at a precisely known velocity. The disadvantages are that the echogenic characteristics of the string are not the same as those of blood and that actual blood flow,

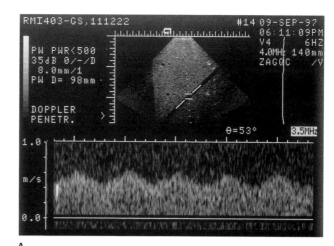

A

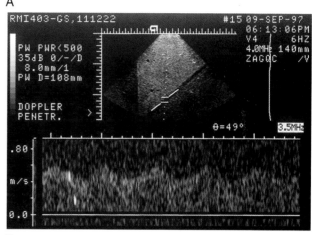

B

Fig. 12.19 B-mode and spectral Doppler display of a flow phantom for evaluating Doppler penetration. (A) A strong Doppler signal and a good signal-to-noise ratio is obtained when the sample volume is at a depth of 9.8 cm. (B) The Doppler signal is just detectable above the electronic noise when the sample volume is at a depth of 10.8 cm. The maximum depth of detection of the Doppler signal in this case is 10.8 cm.

with its characteristic distribution of velocities across the vessel, is not mimicked.

Doppler Flow Phantoms

Doppler flow phantoms (Figs. 12.19 and 12.20) consist of one or more hollow tubes coursing through a block of tissue-mimicking material. A blood-mimicking fluid is pumped through the tube(s) to simulate blood flowing through vessels in the body. Usually the blood-mimicking fluid is a solution of water and glycerol that has small plastic particles suspended in it. The blood-mimicking material should provide the same echogenicity as whole human blood at the ultrasound frequencies of the machine; reasonable representative blood-mimicking materials are now available for use in these phantoms. If the tissue-mimicking material in the body of the phantom has a representative amount of beam attenuation, the depth-dependent echogenicity of the fluid within the phantom is representative of signal levels from actual vessels in vivo.

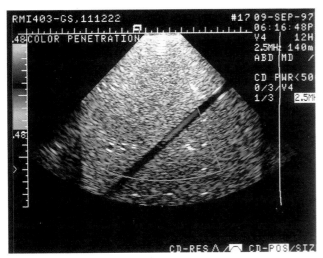

Fig. 12.20 An example of a color flow image of a Doppler flow phantom used to determine the maximum penetration in color.

Doppler flow phantoms are used for the following types of tests of Doppler and flow-imaging equipment (Hoskins et al, 1994; Zagzebski, 1995):

- *Maximum detection depth.* The maximum depth at which flow waveforms can be detected in the phantom has been used to assess whether the Doppler sensitivity has varied from one QA test to another.[1] This is shown in Fig. 12.20. Penetration in this case is 10.8 cm.
- *Alignment.* The phantom can be used to evaluate whether the pulsed Doppler sample volume is aligned with the volume indicated on the B-mode image.
- *Volume flow accuracy.* Some Doppler flow phantoms have precise volume flow-measuring equipment. A flow phantom can thus be used in assessments of the accuracy of flow-measuring algorithms on Doppler devices.
- *Velocity accuracy.* If the velocity of the fluid within the phantoms can be determined accurately, then this can be used to evaluate velocity displays on Doppler and color flow machines.
- *Color flow penetration* (see Fig. 12.20). System sensitivity settings are at their maximum levels without excessive electronic noise. The maximum depth at which color data can be recorded in the flow phantom is noted. Any changes over time such as greater than 1 cm indicate a change in the sensitivity of the instrument.
- *Color display and grayscale image congruency* (image congruency test). This test checks whether the color flow image and B-mode image are aligned so that they agree spatially. Color images of vessels should be completely contained within the B-mode image of the vessel. Sometimes

---

[1]This measurement may be useful for consistency checks, which are an essential part of quality assurance, in attempting to verify that equipment is operating at least as well as when it was delivered or last upgraded. As an absolute measure of Doppler sensitivity, it is controversial because many factors are involved in the concept of Doppler sensitivity (Performance criteria and measurements for Doppler ultrasound devices, 1993).

bleeding out occurs, and this can be corrected by equipment service personnel.

ELECTRONIC PROBE TESTS

Nonfunctioning elements in ultrasound transducer arrays frequently cause nonuniformity on B-mode images. We previously saw that nonfunctioning elements in a transducer array often result in dark shadow-type regions emanating from the transducer as seen on a B-mode image.

Quantitative tools for assessing transducer integrity now are becoming available. One of these is a mode on a scanning machine for testing transducers. Although not available generally, such modes would greatly facilitate routine QA in the clinic and would allow operators to do tests quickly and routinely. Beta versions of the transducer test mode separately address each element in the transducer and channel in the machine. The test mode excites the element with the system pulser and measures the resultant ring-down signal. Criteria are then applied to the signal to judge whether the element is operating normally or is faulty. In this way, a profile of the array functionality can be obtained. Although such modes are not yet available on scanners, manufacturers are encouraged to provide this information to enable more convenient assessment of transducer integrity than can be done at present.

An alternative, more sensitive means to evaluate transducer function is to use an electronic probe tester. Special-purpose transducer testers, such as the Aperio by Sonora (Longmont, Colorado; Fig. 12.21), are available. Analogous to the probe testing mode just described, the function of the probe tester is to evaluate each element in an array transducer, testing its transmission and echo detection capability and its acoustic and electrical properties.

The transducer to be tested is immersed in water and oriented to transmit waves toward a specular interface (Fig. 12.21). Users select a planar interface for testing linear arrays (Fig. 12.21B) and phased arrays, whereas a concave-shaped interface is selected for testing curvilinear arrays. Transducer data provided by the probe tester manufacturer guide placement of the transducer, and a screen that displays the echo amplitude and exact distance between selected elements and the reflector aids users to achieve the correct transducer orientation. When alignment is satisfactory, users switch the software into test mode. In this mode, each element is isolated, a short electrical pulse is applied to it, and the resultant echo from the interface is detected and analyzed. Information including the amplitude of the signal produced by the element, the frequency content of this echo, and the electrical capacitance is provided.

Graphs that depict the amplitude of the signal from each array element (Fig. 12.22) are used to evaluate the condition of the transducer. The top record in this figure shows that this transducer has eight elements that are compromised in some way, as seen by the relative amplitudes of their signals. The electrical capacitance test in the lower figure helps engineers pinpoint whether the problem is likely caused by electrical malfunctions or by mechanical

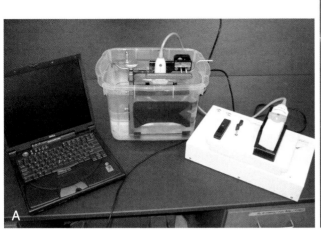 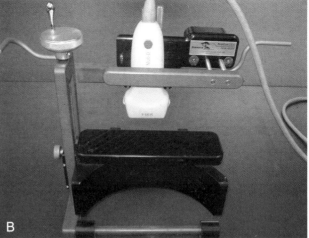

Fig. 12.21 (A) Arrangement for testing transducers using an electronic probe tester. The transducer is connected to the tester through its port. The tester may have various special ports to adapt to different manufacturer's transducer connectors. The face of the probe is immersed in water and directed toward a smooth reflector. A computer controls the tester and produces printouts of test reports. (B) Typical arrangement for testing a linear array transducer. Positioners on the holder enable users to orient the transducer so that beams are perpendicular to the smooth reflecting surface. The mount is immersed in a water bath so that the path from the transducer to the reflector is water.

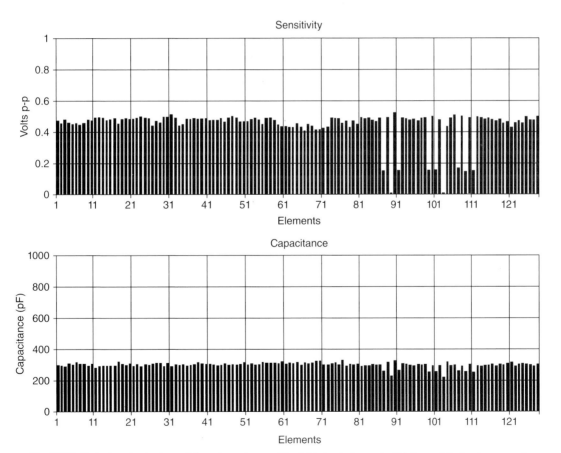

Fig. 12.22 Typical probe test result for a transducer with eight dead elements. "Volts p–p" in the top record indicates the relative amplitude of the echo signal detected by each element from the specular reflector. For eight of the elements, the signal clearly is much weaker than for the other elements. The lower record displays the electrical capacitance of each element and its electric lead.

problems, such as delaminations of the matching layers that exist between the transducer and the medium. This transducer was operating poorly enough to warrant replacement following the test.

Advantages of the probe tester include the following:

1. This is a more sensitive test than the use of images of uniform phantoms for establishing whether a transducer is functioning well or not.
2. Users can readily establish objective pass-fail criteria for a transducer. For example, the test manufacturer suggests that if there are three or more nonfunctioning elements in a typical 128-element transducer, the probe should be replaced.
3. Often, the data provided by the electronic probe tester enable users to determine the cause of any dead elements and consider whether repair is possible. An auxiliary test of the electrical capacitance of transducer elements helps pinpoint whether a dead or weak element is a result of a disconnect in the electrical path between the probe cover and the transducer housing, or whether the flaw is caused by delaminations between the element and the lens material or matching layers.

Disadvantages of the system include the following:

1. The system is costly. Besides the basic test unit and target fixture, individual transducer adapters are needed for different manufacturers' transducers.
2. Not all transducers are testable. The pin connection of transducer connectors are not standardized in the probe industry, requiring extensive testing by the electronic probe tester manufacturer to provide "probe definition files" that apply to each transducer.
3. New transducers such as multidimensional and two-dimensional arrays are less likely to have probe definition files available because of the complicated nature in which these transducers must operate.

Despite these shortcomings, many large imaging centers where dozens of transducers are available and must be evaluated in a QA testing environment find electronic probe testers essential to their routine ultrasound quality management program. For ACR Ultrasound accreditation, Box 12.3 lists the required and optional quality control testing requirements.

Refer to the Evolve website at https://evolve.elsevier.com for Student Experiment 12.1: Ultrasound System Visual Inspection.

REVIEW QUESTIONS

1. Which term best describes routine tests done to determine that an ultrasound scanner is operating at its expected level of performance?
   a. Equipment acceptance tests
   b. General equipment maintenance
   c. Quality assurance
   d. Instrument upgrades

2. Which one of the following statements is true about QA tests of ultrasound scanners?
   a. They require the expertise of a hospital engineer or physicist.
   b. QA for each scanner takes approximately 2 hours per week.
   c. Good record keeping is an essential component.
   d. Quantitative results generally are not necessary.

3. In-house QA programs usually involve all but which of the following?
   a. Tests with phantoms
   b. Inspection and cleaning of air filters
   c. Records and worksheets with test results
   d. Voltage measurements at specified points

4. Material making up the body of a typical QA phantom is "tissue-like" in terms of its _____ properties.
   a. Attenuation and perfusion
   b. Sound speed and attenuation
   c. Sound speed and reflector location
   d. Echogenicity and reflector location

5. To be used for tests of geometric accuracy, the _____ and _____ in a phantom must be precisely specified.
   a. Echogenicity; reflector location
   b. Sound speed; reflector location
   c. Attenuation; reflector location
   d. Echogenicity; attenuation

6. What is the percentage error in the caliper readout if the actual distance between two reflectors in a phantom is 4 cm but the digital caliper readout indicates it is 3.8 cm?
   a. Less than 1%
   b. 1.5%
   c. 5%
   d. 10%

7. Which of the following tests does not need to be performed routinely as part of a QA program?
   a. Uniformity
   b. Distance accuracy
   c. Axial resolution
   d. Maximum depth of visualization

8. What is a string phantom useful for measuring?
   a. The maximum depth of Doppler signal detection
   b. Velocity accuracy on a spectral Doppler display
   c. Axial resolution in B-mode
   d. Vertical distance measurement accuracy

9. What are Doppler flow phantoms useful for determining?
   a. The maximum depth of Doppler signal detection
   b. The vertical distance measurement accuracy
   c. The acoustic output during color flow imaging
   d. The horizontal distance measurement accuracy

10. For echo signals to be produced that are of a similar magnitude as blood in the body, what two factors in a Doppler phantom must be comparable to human tissues?
    a. Phantom material attenuation and mimicking material blood echogenicity
    b. Phantom material density and mimicking material blood attenuation
    c. Mimicking material blood viscosity and attenuation
    d. Mimicking material blood velocity and acceleration

REFERENCES AND BIBLIOGRAPHY

ACR Ultrasound Accreditation Program. *ACR Ultrasound Accreditation Program 2017*. American College of Radiology; 2017.

American Institute of Ultrasound in Medicine. *AIUM Standard Methods for Measuring Performance of Ultrasound Pulse-Echo Equipment*. American Institute of Ultrasound in Medicine; 1990.

Burlew M, et al. A new ultrasound tissue-equivalent material with a high melting point and extended speed of sound range. *Radiology*. 1980;134:517.

Carson P, Goodsitt MM. Acceptance testing of pulse-echo ultrasound equipment. In: Goldman L, Fowlkes B, eds. *Medical CT and Ultrasound: Current Technology and Applications*. Advanced Medical Publishers; 1995.

Goodsitt M, et al. Real-time B-mode ultrasound quality control test procedures. Report of AAPM Ultrasound Task Group No. 1. *Med Phys*. 1998;25:1385–1406.

Gray J. Test pattern for video display and hard copy cameras. *Radiology*. 1985;154:519.

Groth D, et al. Cathode ray tube quality control and acceptance program: initial results for clinical PACS displays. *Radiographics*. 2001;21:719.

Hoskins PR, Sheriff SB, Evans JA. *Testing of Doppler Ultrasound Equipment*. The Institute of Physical Sciences in Medicine; 1994.

Lu ZF, Lee FT, Zagzebski JA. Ultrasonic backscatter and attenuation in diffuse liver disease. *Ultrasound Med Biol*. 1999;25:1047.

Madsen L, et al. Tissue mimicking material for ultrasound phantoms. *Med Phys*. 1978;5:391.

Madsen L, et al. Ultrasound lesion detectability phantoms. *Med Phys*. 1991;18:1771.

Maklad N, Ophir J, Balara V. Attenuation of ultrasound in normal and diffuse liver disease in vivo. *Ultrason Imaging*. 1984;6:117.

Moore GW, et al. The need for evidence-based quality assurance in the modern ultrasound clinical laboratory. *Ultrasound*. 2005;13:158–162.

Performance Criteria and Measurements for Doppler Ultrasound Devices: Technical Discussion. 2nd edition. 2007; American Institute of Ultrasound in Medicine.

Routine Quality Assurance for Diagnostic Ultrasound Equipment 2008. American Institute of Ultrasound in Medicine; 2008.

Thijssen JM, et al. Objective performance testing and quality assurance of medical ultrasound equipment. *Ultrasound Med Biol*. 2007;33:460–471.

Zagzebski J. Acceptance tests for Doppler ultrasound equipment. In: Goldman L, Fowlkes B, eds. *Medical CT and Ultrasound: Current Technology and Applications*. Advanced Medical Publishers; 1995.

Zagzebski J. US quality assurance with phantoms. In: Goldman L, Fowlkes B, eds. *Categorical Course in Diagnostic Radiology Physics: CT and US Cross-Sectional Imaging*. Radiological Society of North America; 2000.

13

Quality Assurance in Nuclear Medicine

*Joanne M. Metler**

OBJECTIVES

At the completion of this chapter, the reader should be able to do the following:

- Describe the principles of radiation detection and measurement
- Describe the scintillation crystal
- Describe the basic principles of the gamma camera
- Describe the scintillation camera performance characteristics of image linearity, image uniformity, intrinsic spatial resolution, detection efficiency, and counting rate problems
- Describe the design and performance characteristics of commonly used collimators
- Describe planar camera quality control testing methods of calibration, gamma energy spectrum, window determination, daily floods (intrinsic and extrinsic), weekly resolution (intrinsic and extrinsic), counting efficiency and sensitivity, and multiwindow spatial registration

- Describe gamma camera single-photon emission computed tomography (SPECT) systems
- Describe SPECT quality control (i.e., flood uniformity, center of rotation, attenuation correction, and pixel size)
- Describe positron emission tomography and its quality control
- Describe nuclear medicine nonimaging equipment and related quality control procedures (i.e., gas-filled detectors such as dose calibrators, survey meters, Geiger–Müller meters, and scintillation detectors such as the multichannel analyzer and thyroid probe)
- Describe quality control procedures in a radiopharmacy and radionuclide generator quality control evaluation of contaminant such as molybdenum, aluminum, and hydrolyzed reduced technetium

---

*The author and publisher wish to acknowledge the previous edition's contributor.

KEY TERMS

American College of Radiology

Bioassay

Center of rotation

Chemical impurity

Chi-square test

Chromatography

Collimator

Count rate

Counts per minute

Disintegrations per minute

Dose calibrator

Energy resolution

Field uniformity

Gas-filled detector

Geiger–Müller (GM) meters

Hydrolyzed reduced technetium

Molybdenum-99

Multichannel analyzer

Nuclear Regulatory Commission

Occupational Safety and Health Administration

Optically stimulated luminescent dosimeter

Photomultiplier tubes

Photon

Photopeak

Pixel size

Positron emission tomography

Pulse height analyzer

Radionuclide impurity

Scintillation crystal

Scintillation detectors

Scintillation gamma camera

Sensitivity

Single-photon emission computed tomography

Spatial linearity

Spatial resolution

Spectrum

Standardized uptake value (SUV)

Technetium-99m

Technetium-99m pertechnetate

The Joint Commission

Thermoluminescent dosimeter

Uniformity correction flood

Nuclear medicine technology is a scientific and clinical discipline involving the diagnostic, therapeutic, and investigative use of radionuclides. The nuclear medicine professional performs a variety of responsibilities in a typical day, including formulating, dispensing, and administering radiopharmaceuticals; performing in vivo and in vitro laboratory procedures; acquiring, processing, and analyzing patient studies on a computer; performing all daily equipment testing; preparing the patient for the studies; operating the imaging and nonimaging equipment; and maintaining a radiation safety program. Because of the variety of responsibilities in the nuclear medicine department, The Joint Commission (TJC) has recognized the necessity for an established quality assurance (QA) program in nuclear medicine. TJC states, "There shall be quality control policies and procedures governing nuclear medicine activities that assure diagnostic and therapeutic reliability and safety of the patients and personnel" (Accreditation Manual for Hospitals, 1993). The American College of Radiology (ACR) also offers accreditation of nuclear medicine departments and mandates that certain QA procedures be performed. This chapter discusses the many QA procedures routinely performed in nuclear medicine. In the summer of 2008, Congress passed the Medicare Improvements for Patients and Providers Act of 2008, which mandates that any nonhospital institution performing advanced diagnostic services (such as nuclear medicine) must be accredited by a Centers for Medicare & Medicaid Services–designated accrediting organization to receive federal funding (Medicare reimbursement). As of the writing of this edition, Centers for Medicare & Medicaid Services has approved three national accreditation organizations: ACR, the Intersocietal Accreditation Commission, and TJC. This rule affects providers of magnetic resonance imaging (MRI), computed tomography (CT), positron emission tomography (PET), and nuclear medicine imaging services for Medicare beneficiaries on an outpatient basis. The accreditation applies only to the suppliers of the images and

not to the physician's interpretation of the image. Therefore, accreditation programs are mandatory for nuclear medicine departments to succeed.

THE SCINTILLATION GAMMA CAMERA

The scintillation gamma camera was first developed by Hal Anger in 1958 and has undergone many changes in design and electrical sophistication since its inception. However, the basic components of the gamma camera remain the same (Fig. 13.1) (Anger, 1958). The camera consists of a circular or rectangular detector mounted on a gantry, which allows flexible manipulation around a patient, and electronic processing

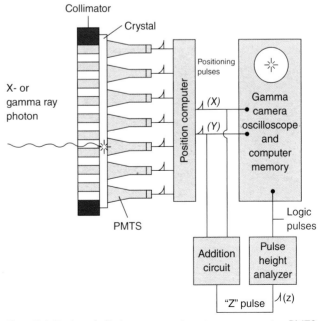

Fig. 13.1 Basic scintillation camera detector components. *PMTS,* Photomultiplier tubes. (From Thrall JH, Ziessman HA. *Nuclear Medicine: The Requisites.* St Louis: Mosby; 1995.)

and display components. In addition, the camera system is interfaced to a computer to control study acquisition, analysis, and display. The detector head contains a thallium-activated sodium iodide [NaI(T1)] crystal, photomultiplier tubes (PMTs), preamplifiers, a position energy circuit, a pulse height analyzer (PHA), and a display mechanism.

Because radiation is a random process, gamma rays are not easy to control. The energy of the ionizing gamma radiation is too high to be deflected like visible light. However, the gamma photon can be directed through holes in a collimator while it blocks tangential or scattered photons. For a resolving image to be obtained, the collimator must be placed on the face of the detector head; this placement allows the desirable gamma photons to pass through to the NaI(T1) crystal. A collimator is a lead-filtering device that consists of holes through which a gamma photon can pass. These holes are separated by lead septa (Fig. 13.2). The photons that are not absorbed or scattered by the lead septa pass straight through to the NaI(T1) crystal and subsequently create an image of the isotope distribution from the patient. With high-energy photons, thicker lead septa are required to prevent scatter from degrading the image.

Collimators are available from several manufacturers. The collimator chosen for a patient study depends on the isotope energy and resolution required for the specific diagnostic procedure. Collimators commonly used in nuclear medicine include low-energy, medium-energy, and high-energy parallel hole; high-resolution parallel hole; high-sensitivity parallel hole; general all-purpose parallel hole; pinhole; and converging and diverging collimators (Early and Sodee, 1995). Because collimators are made specifically to operate within a gamma photon's energy range, a nuclear medicine

department must have collimators suitable for several types of applications. The most common type used for diagnostic studies is the parallel-hole collimator. The parallel-hole collimator is preferred because it directs photons from a patient onto the scintillation crystal without varying the image. Once the photon passes through the collimator, it reaches the NaI(T1) scintillation crystal and is converted to light. The number of light photons produced is directly proportional to the energy of the gamma photon. Typically, 30 photons are produced per kiloelectron volt (keV) of energy (Murray and Ell, 1994). The NaI(T1) crystals vary in diameter, shape, and thickness. Changing the parameters of the crystal affects sensitivity or resolution (i.e., if sensitivity is increased by the use of a thicker crystal, then the resolution is compromised and vice versa). The NaI(T1) crystal is hygroscopic and extremely sensitive to sudden temperature changes. The environment of the gamma camera must remain stable, and precautions must be taken to prevent moisture from entering the NaI(T1) crystal and sudden temperature shifts (Early and Sodee, 1995). In addition, an accidental impact may cause the crystal to crack.

The scintillation, or light, photon interacts with the PMT. The light generated in the NaI(T1) crystal is then converted to electrical signals. The electrons produced are amplified and accelerated a million-fold in the PMT system. After conversion to an electrical pulse, a position circuit produces x and y position signals, which are directly related to the location of the photon interaction on the NaI(T1) crystal. Because of the high potential of ionizing radiation interacting with matter, not all of the gamma photons detected by the NaI(T1) crystal are the original primary gamma photons of interest. The interactions with matter from the patient and through the

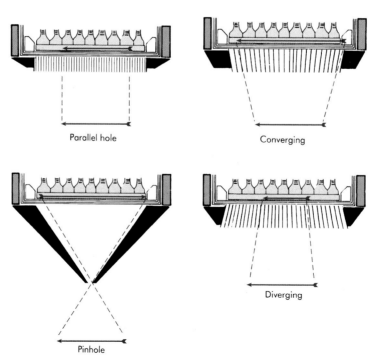

Fig. 13.2 Four common types of collimators used on gamma cameras. (From Bernier DB, Christian PE, Langan JM, et al. *Nuclear Medicine: Technology and Techniques*. 4th ed. St Louis: Mosby; 1997.)

camera system can cause scatter radiation. Too much scatter radiation can cause degradation in the resolution of the final image. It is therefore possible to electronically exclude undesirable photons by only accepting the gamma ray photons above a certain energy.

The discrimination and selection of the gamma photon are performed with a pulse height analyzer (PHA). The PHA can be preset to accept only specific energy signals from the detector. The gamma photon energy required is specified by creating an energy "window" in the PHA. The energy window designates lower and upper limits of the gamma photon energy of interest. The model and age of equipment determine how a window is set; three different methods can be used. A threshold window may be set with a window reading above it; the reading is usually expressed in a percentage of total kiloelectron volts of the gamma energy in question. A midline energy may be set at the energy of the gamma ray or at the maximum count position of the voltage or gain adjustment. The percent window is then applied above and below this midpoint or peak. Finally, some instruments allow setting window thresholds at any position, including overlapping energies and multiple discrete windows for multiple isotope studies. Multiple windows also may be set up for those radionuclides that emit more than one gamma ray (e.g., thallium-201, indium-111, gallium-67). The signal is then sent to a display controller to produce a numeric display and an image. The display can occur simultaneously on a cathode-ray tube, a scalar, a film, and a computer screen. Many camera systems can display an analog or a digital image, or both. An analog camera allows the image to be displayed directly onto film in a cassette with or without the use of a computer. The analog camera also may be interfaced to a computer that simultaneously collects the image in the computer and displays it digitally. Finally, a digital camera digitizes the output of each PMT to create a digital image.

Various gamma camera configurations are available. The gamma camera detector may have a small or large field of imaging capability. The detector also may be circular or rectangular. In addition, the gamma camera system may hold one, two, or three detectors. These configurations are better known as single-head, dual-head, or triple-head cameras. In addition, some gamma cameras are fixed, whereas others are mobile. The scintillation gamma camera system is a complex mechanism accompanied by a variety of components that are crucial to producing a reliable and factual clinical image. The quality of the nuclear medicine image is determined by a variety of parameters. These parameters must be perpetually evaluated to guarantee that the image the physician is interpreting is accurate and truly diagnostic of the patient's pathologic condition.

According to the National Electrical Manufacturers Association (NEMA), 12 acceptance test standards are performed at the factory on all gamma cameras (Murphy, 1987; National Electrical Manufacturers Association, 1980, 1986). Box 13.1 lists the tests that are performed. The quality control measures taken at the factory ensure the good working condition of the new system. However, once the gamma cameras are in

---

BOX 13.1 NEMA Acceptance Tests for Scintillation Cameras (SPECT)

Intrinsic Spatial Resolution
Intrinsic Energy Resolution
Intrinsic Field Uniformity
Intrinsic Count Rate Performance
Intrinsic Spatial Linearity
Multiple Spatial Registration
Sensitivity
Angular Variation of Spatial Position
Angular Variation of Flood Field Uniformity and Sensitivity
Reconstructed System Spatial Resolution
Spatial Resolution with and without Scatter
System Count Rate Performance with Scatter

NEMA, National Electrical Manufacturers Association; *SPECT*, single-photon emission computerized tomography.
From National Electrical Manufacturers Association (1986).

TABLE 13.1 Gamma Camera Quality Control

Quality Control Procedure	Frequency
Peaking	Daily and before each new radionuclide used
Counting rate limits	Daily
Field uniformity	Daily after repair
Spatial resolution	Weekly after repair
Spatial linearity	Weekly after repair
Sensitivity	Quarterly

---

the nuclear medicine department, it is impractical and sometimes impossible for all of the NEMA standard acceptance tests to be performed (Sorenson and Phelps, 1987). However, the quality control procedures listed in Table 13.1 are required by TJC (Accreditation Manual for Hospitals, 1993) and regulatory agencies and are to be performed routinely (Rao et al, 1986). The quality control procedures performed on all imaging equipment ensure that the patient's diagnostic study is safe and accurate.

QUALITY CONTROL PROCEDURES FOR IMAGING EQUIPMENT

Energy Resolution and Photopeaking

Before any quality control or patient procedure, the correct energy setting for the radionuclide being used must be selected and the primary gamma ray energy, or photopeak, centered around an energy window. The quality control is performed daily, either manually or automatically, depending on the manufacturer's specifications. The PHA is centered about the photopeak(s) of the radionuclide of interest, usually with a 5%–10% window. This is generally referred to as "peaking" the camera. It is accomplished by adjusting the baseline window setting of the PHA around the specific energy of the gamma ray. For example, technetium-99m (^{99m}Tc) is used daily in a nuclear medicine department. The primary gamma ray of

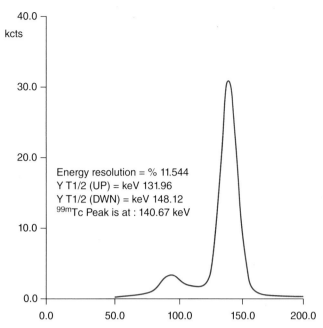

Fig. 13.3 Energy spectrum of the radionuclide technetium-99m (99mTc). *kcts*, Kilocounts; *keV*, kiloelectron volt.

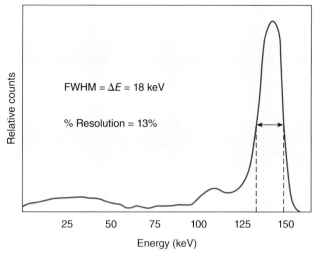

Fig. 13.4 Energy spectrum of technetium-99m (99mTc). The full width at half maximum (*FWHM*) is 18 kiloelectron volts (*keV*). The energy resolution is 13%. Δ*E*, Change in energy. (From Thrall JH, Ziessman HA. *Nuclear Medicine: The Requisites.* St Louis: Mosby; 1995.)

99mTc has an energy of 140 keV. The window generally used for imaging is 20% around 140 keV; therefore resetting a 20% window "tells" the PHA to accept only gamma photons with energies from 126–154 keV and to center the photopeak at 140 keV. The camera must be peaked before any radionuclide is used.

Because radioactive decay is random, each step in converting the radiation to an electrical current is subject to random error. The **spectrum** (curve) of the radionuclide of interest is not a straight line representing complete absorption of the gamma ray but a Gaussian distribution resulting from random error, Compton scattering, or material attenuation (Fig. 13.3). The light photons emitted by the NaI(T1) crystal are given off in all directions with random probability. The **energy resolution** can then be expressed as the spread, or width, of the spectrum divided by the center photopeak. The spread of the spectrum or the full width at half maximum (FWHM) measurement is the energy range of the widest width of the spectrum, which is halfway down from the photopeak (Fig. 13.4). The energy resolution is calculated as follows:

$$\text{Percent energy resolution} = \frac{\text{FWHM at half maximum}}{\text{Photopeak center}} \times 100$$

The narrower the curve, the better the energy resolution of the detector. A good energy resolution is between 8% and 12%, which enables the camera system to better discern gamma rays with close energies. A reliable energy resolution is significant because it represents the system's ability to accurately depict two separate events in space, time, or energy. The ability of a system to detect separate radiation events becomes clinically relevant, especially when used for in vitro or in vivo counting, which potentially leads to a patient's clinical diagnosis. Performing a test of energy resolution also verifies that

scatter rejection is sufficient to provide optimal contrast in clinical studies.

Counting Rate Limits

The sensitivity (counting ability) of a gamma camera generally decreases with increased amounts of activity. If the activity is too high, the detector is "paralyzed" and cannot count. The system's inability to count is referred to as *dead time*. Dead time describes the duration the detector requires to process the ionizing events as they occur in the NaI(T1) crystal. The manufacturer's specification of the **count rate** limit per second states that the observed count rate through a 20% window should not exceed 20% of the counts lost as a result of dead time (Greer et al, 1985). The electronic circuitry of most contemporary gamma cameras reaches counting limits of 120,000–150,000 counts per second before experiencing a 20% loss because of dead time (Henkin et al, 1996). Before any quality control procedure is performed, the count rate of the radioactive point or flood source must be determined to ensure that the counts per second do not exceed the manufacturer's specifications. Once the count rate is determined to be within the counting rate limits for that gamma camera, only then can the quality control testing continue. The procedures to determine count rate are simple: The radioactive source is placed at the appropriate location necessary for quality control, and the time/count scalar continuously displays the counts per second. Count rates that exceed the gamma camera's design limits can result in degradation of the images and loss of counts (Henkin et al, 1996). If the counts-per-second rate is too high and it is necessary to decrease the count rate, the radioactive source is repositioned at an increased distance, or the amount of radioactivity in the source is decreased.

Field Uniformity

Field uniformity refers to the gamma camera's ability to detect a uniform source of radiation and respond exactly the same at

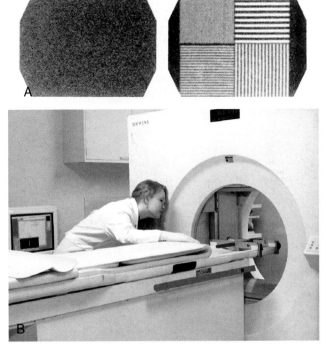

Fig. 13.5 (A) Field uniformity flood and resolution pattern. (B) Nuclear medicine technologist preparing to obtain a field flood uniformity on a dual-head camera system. (Courtesy Northwest Community Hospital, Arlington Heights, Illinois.)

any location within the imaging field. The uniform response of the gamma camera results in an image with an even distribution of radioactivity (Fig. 13.5). The uniformity of the gamma camera depends on the uniform response of the NaI(T1) crystal and the PMTs. The response of each PMT must match that of all the other PMTs. In addition, the counting window must be centered around the photopeak. Mispositioning the photopeak may alter the field

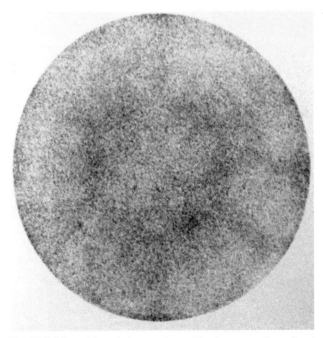

Fig. 13.6 Mispositioned photopeak resulting in a nonuniform flood.

uniformity (Fig. 13.6). Nonuniformity also may arise because of, for example, the use of the incorrect photopeak for a specific radionuclide, a malfunctioning PMT, a cracked NaI(T1) crystal, or total system malfunction (Fig. 13.7). Because the uniformity of the camera determines the accuracy of a patient's image and, ultimately, the diagnosis, it is imperative that the field uniformity or flood be performed daily. This quality control procedure must be performed before any patient studies.

The measurement of the daily field uniformity can be performed intrinsically or extrinsically. Intrinsic uniformity is the measurement of the uniformity of the gamma camera detector with no collimator in place. The procedure is generally performed with a point source of radioactivity placed at a distance equivalent to four to five diameters of the detector's field of imaging (Scintillation Camera Acceptance Testing and Performance Evaluation, 1980). Caution should be taken that the counts-per-second rate does not exceed that particular system's limits. The intrinsic uniformity determines the integrity of the NaI(T1) crystal and its electronic components. The phenomenon known as *edge packing* can show up as a bright rim of activity around the perimeter of the flood. To prevent edge packing, most manufacturers provide a lead-shielded ring that masks the effect when attached to the edge of the camera head. These tests also monitor a scintillation unit for electronic problems and crystal deterioration (hydration).

Extrinsic uniformity testing is also the measurement of the camera's field uniformity; however, it is performed with the collimator (which is used for imaging) in place. A uniform flood source of radioactivity is placed directly on the collimated camera (Fig. 13.8). The two commonly used extrinsic radioactive sources are (1) an acrylic plastic (Plexiglas) container filled with water and generally 1–10 mCi of ^{99m}Tc and (2) a solid-sealed 10 mCi cobalt-57 sheet (Steves, 1992). The ^{99m}Tc liquid-filled acrylic plastic (Plexiglas) source does have some disadvantages. It must be manually filled with technetium and thoroughly mixed to secure even distribution of the radionuclide. The procedure increases the risk of radioactive contamination to the technologist and equipment; thus the technologist's risk of radiation exposure is increased. The extrinsic uniformity, in addition to evaluating the NaI(T1) crystal and electrical components, allows visualization of a defect or damage to the collimator. Annual inspection of collimators with extrinsic field uniformity testing is recommended and should become a routine part of any QA program. A defect in a collimator will visualize in an image as photopenic areas (Fig. 13.9).

A flood field image of 1–3 million is generally acquired whether the intrinsic or extrinsic method is used. However, it is recommended that the quality control for each gamma camera should be carefully evaluated according to the manufacturer's specifications and the department's needs. The quality control test used should remain consistent. The consistency allows visual inspection of any nonuniformity of the camera system to be easily monitored. The uniformity flood must be performed daily on every piece of imaging equipment. Visual inspection of the flood and comparison with that of the previous day reveals any subtle changes in uniformity that are

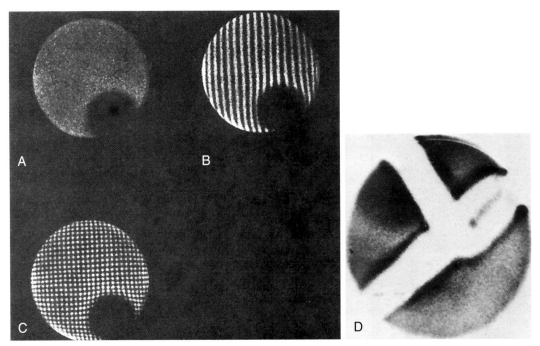

Fig. 13.7 (A) Example of a nonfunctioning photomultiplier tube seen in the flood field; (B) the orthogonal hole resolution pattern; and (C) the parallel-line equal space phantom. (D) Examples of nonuniform flood fields caused by a cracked crystal. (A): From Rollo FD: *Nuclear Medicine Physics, Instrumentation, and Agents*, St Louis, 1997, Mosby. (B): From Early PJ, Sodee BD. *Principles and Practices of Nuclear Medicine*. 2nd ed. St Louis: Mosby; 1995.)

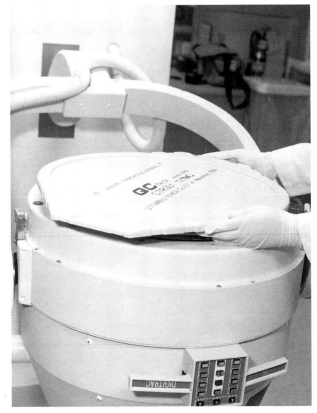

Fig. 13.8 Extrinsic flood uniformity with a cobalt-57 (^{57}Co) sheet source.

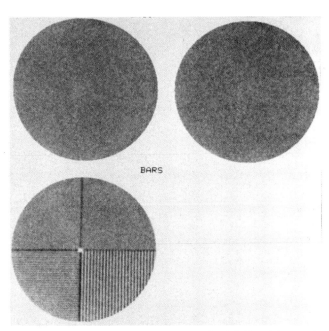

Fig. 13.9 Note the photopenic area in the flood field and the resolution bar pattern. These are due to collimator damage.

not always apparent by looking at one image. Any areas of nonuniformity of the detector must be noted and repaired before clinical use. In addition to the performance of daily floods, the TJC QA program recommends that every piece of equipment also has a preventive maintenance program performed biannually (Accreditation Manual for Hospitals, 1993).

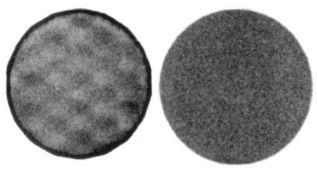

Fig. 13.10 An uncorrected and a microprocessor-corrected uniformity flood.

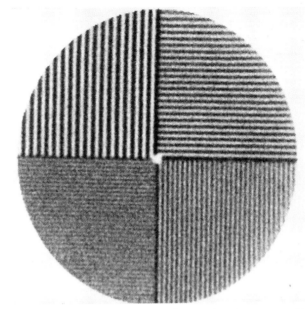

Fig. 13.11 Spatial resolution with a four-quadrant bar pattern. Four images are obtained 90 degrees apart.

Gamma cameras of the late 1970s until the present have been developed to correct some of the nonuniformities seen in older images. A microprocessor built into the gamma camera generates a correction factor for each pixel of the matrix according to the variation in counts of different pixels (Saha, 1993). Fig. 13.10 demonstrates the difference between an uncorrected and corrected uniformity flood. Subsequently, when patient images are generated, the correction factors are applied to each pixel; thus nonuniformity is reduced (Saha, 1993).

Spatial Resolution and Spatial Linearity

Spatial resolution is the gamma camera's ability to reproduce small details of a radioactive distribution (Greer et al, 1985). The smaller the details that a camera can reproduce, the better the spatial resolution is for that system. The spatial resolution quality control procedure is required to be performed a minimum of once a week on every imaging system. The quality control determines the camera's ability to detect and image fine differences of a radioactive distribution that exist in closely spaced areas. In essence, the gamma camera detects the small abnormalities of different radioactive concentrations that may subsequently be seen on patient images. For the exact spatial resolution of a gamma camera system to be determined, one of the following resolution test pattern transmission sources must be used: four-quadrant bar phantom with varying size bars, parallel-line equal space (PLES) bar pattern with constant bar and spacing sizes, or an orthogonal hole phantom with varying sizes of holes (Bernier et al, 1997; Eisner, 1985).

The manufacturer of every gamma camera system determines the intrinsic spatial resolution specific for the gamma camera. This is important when choosing the type and size of a transmission resolution pattern. For example, if the manufacturer specifications say that gamma camera 1 has an intrinsic spatial resolution of 3 mm, then the four-quadrant bar phantom used must have bars between 2 and 5 mm. The resolution pattern is placed on the collimator or camera for an intrinsic resolution quality control test and on the collimator for an extrinsic resolution quality control test. The resolution pattern is placed in the center of the field of view (FOV) in such a way that the center of the pattern is directly over the center of the detector. A ^{99m}Tc or cobalt-57 (^{57}Co) sheet source is then placed on the resolution pattern so that the radioactivity is transmitted through the resolution pattern. It is recommended that when the four-quadrant bar pattern is used, four images should be obtained at 90 degrees between positions (Bernier et al, 1997; Henkin et al, 1996). This allows verification of the spatial resolution in the x and y positions and allows the bars barely resolved to be evaluated in each quadrant of the FOV (Fig. 13.11). The ACR Phantom criteria for spatial resolution for planar-only images using the four-quadrant bar phantom are in Table 13.2.

TABLE 13.2 ACR Phantom Criteria for Spatial Resolution for Planar-Only Images Using the Four-Quadrant Bar Phantom

Tc^{99m} or Co^{57}:

Intrinsic spatial resolution images:

Satisfactory:	2.5- to 2.9-mm bars are resolved in one quadrant of a four-quadrant pattern and they have low contrast
Marginal:	3.0- to 3.4-mm bars resolved in one quadrant of a four-quadrant pattern

System spatial resolution images:

Satisfactory:	3.0- to 3.4-mm bars are resolved in one quadrant of a four-quadrant pattern
Marginal:	3.5- to 3.9-mm bars resolved in one quadrant of a four-quadrant pattern

Tl^{201}, Ga^{67}, or In^{111}:

Intrinsic spatial resolution images:

Satisfactory:	3.0- to 3.4-mm bars are resolved in one quadrant of a four-quadrant pattern and they have low contrast
Marginal:	3.5- to 3.9-mm bars resolved in one quadrant of a four-quadrant pattern

System spatial resolution images:

Satisfactory:	3.5- to 3.9-mm bars are resolved in one quadrant of a four-quadrant pattern

ACR, American College of Radiology.

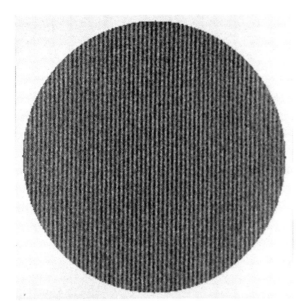

Fig. 13.12 Parallel-line equal space bar resolution pattern.

The PLES bar resolution pattern is sometimes preferable to the four-quadrant pattern. A PLES pattern is preferable for testing spatial resolution because it is specifically designed to minimize the number of images that are actually required to evaluate resolution (Henkin et al, 1996). Only two images are required to evaluate the camera spatial resolution because the size of the bars and the spacing between the bars are constant (Fig. 13.12). The orthogonal hole phantom is a hexagonal lead sheet containing holes of equal diameter at right angles to each other. Only one image is required to determine the resolution and uniformity over the entire FOV of the camera detector.

Regardless of which resolution test pattern is used routinely for a gamma camera system, it is important to inspect each image visually to detect any fluctuation in resolution. This inspection is made by the comparison of the weekly resolution image with the previous ones. A change in the resolution can be caused by several factors. If there is a change in resolution, the photopeak, window, source, source distance, gamma photon, energy, and type of collimator used should all be verified. Any malfunction or misposition of these factors can detrimentally affect the spatial resolution. If all of the factors are properly functioning and are in proper position, the crystal must then be evaluated for damage or degradation.

The **spatial linearity** of a gamma camera system is its ability to produce a linear image with straight lines corresponding to the same straight lines of the bar pattern. Most modern gamma camera systems have circuits that correct for nonlinearity. Linearity is generally assessed and can be seen by visual inspection of any of the spatial resolution test pattern images. This is done by carefully inspecting the linearity of the bars or holes in both the x and y positions and comparing the results with the acceptance test results and the results from previous weeks. Any nonlinearity can cause extreme image artifacts, especially in reconstructed

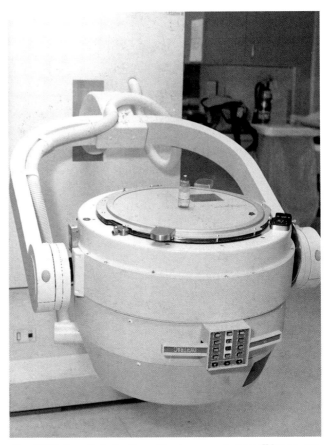

Fig. 13.13 Sensitivity testing with a known cobalt-57 (^{57}Co) source.

tomographic images. A nonlinear image indicates that the gamma camera should be serviced and reevaluated before further clinical use. The service and reevaluation ensure the accuracy of the diagnostic images, both planar and tomographic.

Sensitivity

Sensitivity is another quality control procedure performed to determine the gamma camera detector's ability to detect the ionizing events that occur in the NaI(T1) crystal. The events recorded as **counts per minute** (cpm) are calculated and expressed as counts per minute per microcurie (µCi) of activity present. The sensitivity quality control is performed biannually. It is performed by placing a sealed point source such as ^{57}Co at different locations (center and at least four peripheral locations) on the camera head and by counting for a set time (Fig. 13.13; Eisner, 1985; National Electrical Manufacturers Association, 1980). The sensitivity is equal to the net counts per time divided by the actual activity of the sealed source:

$$\text{Sensitivity} = \frac{\text{Net counts/time}}{\text{Activity of the scaled source in µCi (on that day)}}$$

The sensitivity is compared with the previous documented sensitivity tests and the manufacturer's specifications to

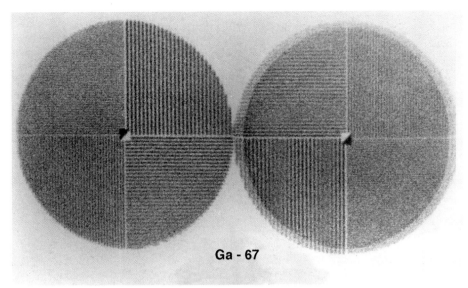

Ga - 67

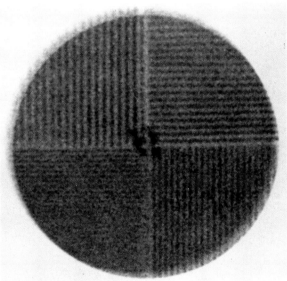

Fig. 13.14 Multiwindow spatial resolution testing. Ga-67, Gallium 67. (From Henkin RE, et al. *Nuclear Medicine.* Vol. 1. St Louis: Mosby; 1996.)

ensure that there is no change in the ability of the gamma camera to detect ionizing events.

Multiple-Window Spatial Registration

Gamma cameras are equipped with multiple PHA windows to use with photons of different energies. The multiplicity capability must be evaluated for spatial registration. The position of the x and y signals must be the same for each energy window. If a study is performed with a radionuclide that has multiple gamma photons of different energies, the photons must be received by their perspective windows and positioned on the cathode-ray tube in the same locations. If they are received in different locations, the resolution of that image is compromised. NEMA recommends that a gallium-67 (^{67}Ga) source be used with a bar pattern phantom and sequential images acquired with the three imaging gamma peaks of ^{67}Ga (93, 184, and 296 keV). The individual images are then acquired with each peak individually, and the final images are made with

combinations of two peaks. The images are then evaluated for best time and best resolution. In addition, the three floods are superimposed on each other to evaluate the match (Fig. 13.14; Early and Sodee, 1995).

QUALITY ASSURANCE OF SINGLE-PHOTON EMISSION COMPUTED TOMOGRAPHY CAMERAS

Tomographic techniques have been developed in nuclear medicine for both single-photon emission computed tomography (SPECT) and PET (Eisner, 1985; English, 1995; Esser et al, 1983). The research and development of various tomographic systems have given way to the rotating gamma camera. The rotating system, with the aid of a computer and reconstruction software, has the ability to perform true transaxial tomography. Rotational SPECT, CT, and PET all share

TABLE 13.3 **SPECT Gamma Camera Quality Control***	
Quality Control Procedure	**Frequency**
Uniformity correction flood	Weekly
COR	Weekly for every collimator used for tomography
Pixel size	Monthly
Cine to detect patient motion	After each patient acquisition

COR, Center of rotation; *SPECT*, single-photon emitting computerized tomography.
*Quality control procedure in addition to routine gamma camera quality control procedures.

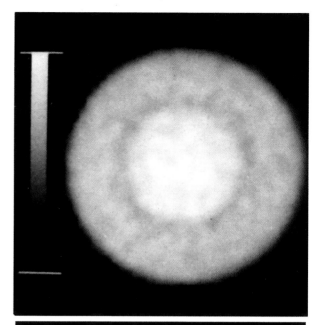

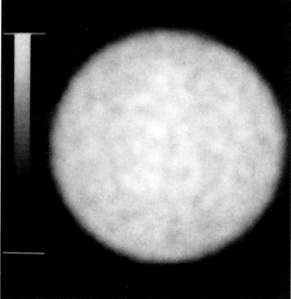

Fig. 13.15 *(Top)* Ring artifact. *(Bottom)* Normal image without the artifact. (Reproduced with permission from the Society of Nuclear Medicine from Greer K. Quality control in SPECT. *J Nucl Med Technol.* 1985;13:76.)

the characteristic that using only data that arise in the particular image plane in the reconstruction of the tomographic image allows higher image contrast (Bernier et al, 1997). SPECT systems are commercially available with single, dual, triple, and quadruple heads. The multiple-head SPECT systems are becoming the preferred model because more information with increased resolution can be obtained in a given period.

The camera head(s) are attached to a mechanical gantry that allows them to rotate 360 degrees in a circular or elliptical orbit about the patient. The gantry unit is designed to enable the camera head to come as close to the patient as possible to ensure the best resolution at the face of the detector head. Some cameras also are designed to follow the patient's body contour in a noncircular orbit (whole-body scanner capability). SPECT systems also require a computer to control the gantry, acquire the data, and reconstruct the tomographic images. The QA of a SPECT system requires stricter controls. SPECT QA procedures are not as tolerant as those for planar imaging. For example, a ±5% field uniformity is acceptable for planar imaging; however, variations in uniformity for SPECT cannot exceed ±1% (Henkin et al, 1996; National Electrical Manufacturers Association, 1980). In addition, the camera coordinates must be properly aligned with the axis of rotation of the gantry and the computer image matrix. The SPECT system must adhere to the required quality control procedures of the scintillation gamma camera as recently discussed (i.e., energy calibration, field uniformity, spatial resolution and linearity, sensitivity, and multiple window registration). However, additional procedures must be performed to ensure maximum SPECT camera performance (Graham et al, 1996; Greer et al, 1985). Table 13.3 lists the required and recommended quality control procedures of a SPECT system (Graham et al, 1996).

Uniformity Correction Flood

Field uniformity corrections are much more critical in SPECT imaging than in other forms of imaging. Small changes in extrinsic uniformity may alter the reconstructed images. Acquiring the 1–3 million counts needed in a planar system is just not adequate for the SPECT. Acquiring fewer than 30 million counts for a uniformity correction flood may result in a ring artifact (Fig. 13.15). The 30-million-count figure used for uniformity correction is acquired so that there are about 10,000 counts per pixel in a 64 × 64 matrix. The system's manufacturer requires that a camera with a collimator in place must have uniformity with variations of less than 1%. In addition, some internal software programs are used to verify a 1% standard deviation (SD). Acquiring 10,000 counts per pixel is necessary to obtain the recommended percent relative SD of 1%.

$$\text{Percent SD} = \frac{100}{\sqrt{10,000}} = 1$$

A uniform ^{99m}Tc or ^{57}Co source is placed on the collimator. The uniformity correction flood of 30–60 million counts with a 64 × 64 matrix is acquired weekly for each collimator used. The image is stored in the computer and later used to correct raw data used in reconstruction of the tomographic images.

Center of Rotation

No misalignment must exist between the physical or mechanical center of rotation (COR) of the SPECT system and the COR in the reconstruction computer matrix. The pixel matrix that forms the projection images of the SPECT acquisition is a function of the computer, not the camera. The alignment of the computer matrix may not be perfectly aligned with the camera head or gantry, or both. The basic mechanical parts of the SPECT system, such as the gears and bearings, as well as patient diversity, prevent a consistent symmetry. In addition, daily use and wear and tear on the system could cause rotational discrepancies (English, 1995; Greer et al, 1985). The COR is important to all SPECT systems, from single-head to quadruple-head systems. However, multiple-head systems also require software to guarantee synchronization between the heads.

The COR is properly calibrated if a point source placed in the center of the detector head orbit projects to the center of the 64 × 64 computer matrix, or pixel 32. The COR discrepancies of most SPECT systems are less than 2 mm from the center of the matrix, but the goal is to be no more than 1 mm from pixel 32 (English, 1995; Greer et al, 1985). A point source of ^{57}Co or ^{99m}Tc is used to calculate the COR and the pixel size. A SPECT study is performed on the point source, and the images are reconstructed. A misaligned COR shows the point source to appear larger, blurred, or containing a ring artifact. A COR shift of 3 mm or more can affect the quality of the reconstructed images. The COR quality control must be performed weekly on all SPECT systems. Many SPECT systems now use computer processing to construct a linear representation to ensure stability. If there is a deviation or a misalignment, the computer generates a straight line with areas appearing outside the line.

Pixel Size

Pixel size of the matrix must be calibrated properly because pixels take on the three-dimensional characteristic of depth in SPECT. Any variation in the pixel size changes depth or distance and subsequently alters attenuation correction factors used in the tomographic reconstructed images. The sizes of the pixels should be monitored monthly for any fluctuations. The pixel size can be adjusted by setting analog-to-digital converters and should be checked in both the x and y directions (Thrall and Ziessman, 1995). The pixel width should be the same in both directions. Any difference in the pixel dimensions causes problems in reformatting of the image data. In addition, a shift in the analog-to-digital converter also can move the COR matrix.

Single-Photon Emission Computed Tomography Quality Control During and After Patient Procedures

SPECT quality control of the camera and computer systems is important to ensure accurate and optimal image quality for the patient. However, in addition to the quality control of the mechanics of the SPECT system, QA must be practiced during a patient study. It is important to remove any materials from the patient's body that might attenuate the radioisotope being imaged or interfere with image acquisition and reconstruction. This is especially crucial when imaging myocardial perfusion. Examples of external attenuators on a patient are metal coins left in a shirt pocket, a necklace with a hanging metal, an electrocardiogram lead left on, or a prosthesis. Breast tissue also may attenuate data and should be noted. Many software programs are able to correct such attenuation. The patient also must be closely monitored for motion. Any vertical or horizontal motion can create artifacts in the reconstruction. In addition, the camera head must be level when the acquisition begins and remain level throughout the study. Once the study acquisition is completed, patient motion can be detected on the computer. The computer programs used today allow inspection for patient motion by summed projection, sinograms, or cine displays. In a summed projection, patient motion appears as a change in the height of the organ imaged. A sinogram is a plot of each projection. If the patient does not move during the acquisition, the plot appears as a bright line. A break in the line indicates patient motion from left to right. A cine display, a raw motion picture of the acquired projections, is a simple way to detect patient motion. If the motion is significant, the study is invalid and must be repeated (Fig. 13.16). The ACR Phantom Criteria for their accreditation program is listed in Table 13.4. The ACR Nuclear Medicine (NM) Equipment Evaluation Summary for both standard NM scanners and SPECT systems is found in Fig. 13.17.

POSITRON EMISSION TOMOGRAPHY

PET is a fast-growing imaging modality of nuclear medicine that produces tomographic images of the distribution of positron-emitting radiopharmaceuticals. The excitement surrounding PET technology is that the images depict both physiologic and biochemical processes of the human body. According to the study of nuclear physics, positrons are emitted from proton-rich nuclei that only travel a short distance before encountering an electron; this encounter results in annihilation of both particles. On annihilation, two gamma rays of 511 keV are produced and travel 180 degrees apart in opposite directions. A great quantity of energy is required for positron emission to occur. The radionuclides that emit positrons must be artificially produced in a linear or cyclotron accelerator. Examples of the more common radioisotopes used for PET are carbon-11, oxygen-15, nitrogen-13, and fluorine-18. In addition, generator-produced positron-emitting radioisotopes rubidium-82, copper-62, germanium-68, and

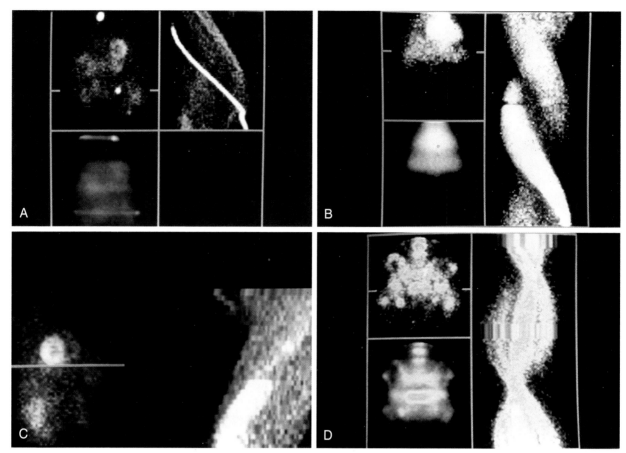

Fig. 13.16 Problems identified with the patient motion quality control displays. (A) Single-photon emission computerized tomography catches patient's bed during rotation. (B) Patient sits up during acquisition. (C) Patient's bed translates axial during acquisition. (D) Gantry stops before completion of study. (From Henkin RE, et al. *Nuclear Medicine.* Vol. 1. St Louis: Mosby; 1996.)

TABLE 13.4 ACR SPECT Phantom Criteria

ACR Phantom Spatial Resolution Tc99m using the ACR-approved SPECT Phantom	
(At least 75% of the rods in a segment must be visualized to qualify a set as "seen.")	
General purpose parallel hole collimators:	
Satisfactory:	9.5-mm rods resolved with high contrast
Marginal:	9.5-mm rods resolved with low contrast
High-resolution parallel hole collimators:	
Satisfactory:	7.9-mm rods resolved with high contrast
Marginal:	7.9-mm rods resolved with low contrast
ACR Phantom Spatial Resolution Tl^{201}, Ga^{67}, or In^{111} using the ACR-approved SPECT Phantom	
(At least 50% of the rods in a segment must be visualized to qualify a set as "seen.")	
General purpose parallel hole collimators (Tl^{201}) or Medium energy general purpose parallel hole collimators (Ga^{67} or In^{111})	
Satisfactory:	11.1-mm rods visible
Marginal:	12.7-mm rods visible
High-resolution parallel hole collimators (Tl^{201})	
Satisfactory:	9.5-mm rods visible
Marginal:	11.1-mm rods visible

TABLE 13.4   ACR SPECT Phantom Criteria—cont'd

Nuclear Medicine SPECT Phantom:

(Deluxe Phantom. If a phantom receives 2 scores of Marginal, this equals a FAIL)

Uniformity (GP and HR), Tc99m SPECT:

Satisfactory [3]:	Artifacts are seen in only a few slices of the complete set but are not thought to be clinically significant.
Marginal [2]:	Significant artifacts visualized in one or more slices, but they probably would not affect the interpretation of clinical studies.
Fail [1]:	Strong artifacts visualized in one or more slices of such magnitude that they probably will affect the interpretation of clinical studies; and the instrument should not be used for clinical studies.

Spatial Resolution (GP and HR):

Satisfactory:	11.1-mm rods resolved with low contrast
Marginal:	12.7-mm rods resolved with high contrast

Contrast (GP and HR):

Satisfactory:	19.1-mm and larger spheres resolved with high contrast
Marginal:	25.4-mm and larger spheres resolved with low contrast

ACR, American College of Radiology; *GP*, pho gamma; *HR*, high resolution; *SPECT*, single-photon emitting computerized tomography.

gallium-68 also are used. The chemical characteristics of the radioisotopes used for PET enable the synthesis of molecules that are used in tissue metabolism. The metabolic radiopharmaceuticals currently being studied and researched entail diagnostic applications in tumor biology, neurology, psychiatry, and cardiology.

The PET camera is a system that has many crystal detectors, which are placed in a circular configuration about the patient. The most common detector materials now in use are lutetium oxyorthosilicate and gadolinium oxyorthosilicate. The system hardware configuration looks similar to the CT; however, the operation has no similarity. A positron-emitting radiopharmaceutical is administered to the patient. The crystal detectors are paired off 180 degrees apart to count simultaneously, and the 511-keV photons are detected (Esser et al, 1983). The PET system then establishes where the event occurred simultaneously and acquires the data (Esser et al, 1983). The computer software then manipulates the data and reconstructs tomographic slices of the original images.

The PET system is a complicated detection device that can have literally thousands of crystals. Specific quality control testing varies according to scanner manufacturer, but some common requirements include the following:

- Adjustments of PMT gain—should be performed daily
- Crystal and energy map—a crystal map converts the analog position of a detected event to a specific crystal within the detector block (daily)
- Coincidence timing calibration—adjusts for timing delays so that events from each block are time stamped equivalently (daily)
- Detector drift check—based on change in sonogram (visual or numeric comparison) or drifts of baseline or peaks (daily)
- Blank scan—used with the transmission data in the computation of attenuation correction factors to monitor system stability. These are acquired daily using transmission rod sources.
- Normalization—compensates for the variation in efficiency in each line of response in the sonogram and for axial sensitivity variation in some scanners (monthly or as required)
- Calibration—used to convert the reconstructed image pixel values into activity concentration (monthly or as required)
- Phantom image evaluation—allows for evaluation of tomographic uniformity, region of interest, spatial resolution, noise, and the standardized uptake value (SUV), which is a measure of fluoro-d-glucose uptake, contrast, and scatter/attenuation. It is determined by the following equation:

$$SUV = \frac{r}{\alpha'/\omega}$$

where r is the radioactivity concentration (in kilobecquerels (kBq) per milliliter) measured by the PET scanner within a region of interest, α' is the decay-corrected amount of injected radiolabeled fluoro-D-glucose measured in kBq, and ω is the weight of the patient (70 kg is used during phantom testing). The following figure contains the ACR SUV Analysis Worksheet.

NM Equipment Evaluation Summary

System: _____   Report Date: _____
Address: _____
System NMAP# - Unit #: _____   Survey Date: _____
System Manufacturer: _____   Model: _____
Medical Physicist: _____
Physicist Signiture: _____

Equipment Evaluation Tests

Pass/Fail/NA

#	Test	
1	Intrinsic uniformity	
2	System Uniformity with all commonly used collimators	
3	Intrinsic or System Spatial Resolution	
4	System Sensitivity (count rate/unit activity)	
5	Relative Sensitivity	
6	Energy Resolution	
7	Count Rate Parameters	
8	Monitor Evaluation	
9	System Interlocks	
10	Overall System Performance for SPECT Systems	
	a. Uniformity	
	b. Resolution	
	c. Contrast	

Evaluation of Site's QC Program

Pass/ Fail

#	Test	Date	
1.	Daily Uniformity Check		
2.	Daily CT check (SPECT/CT systems)		
3	Weekly Bar Phantom		
4	Semi-annual (quarterly preferred) SPECT ACR phantom		
5	Uniformity Calibration (monthly or as specified by manufacturer)		
6	Center-of-Rotation/Head Alignment (SPECT Systems)		
7	Dose Calibrator Tests		
	a. Accuracy		
	b. Linearity		
	c. Constancy		

Medical Physicist's Recommendations for Quality Improvement and Comments on Testing Procedures

[blank box]

Fig. 13.17 ACR Nuclear Medicine (NM) Equipment Evaluation Summary for gamma and SPECT cameras. *ACR*, American College of Radiology; *CT*, computed tomography; *NA*, not applicable; *NM*, nuclear medicine; *NMAP*, nuclear medicine accreditation program; *SPECT*, single photon emission computed tomography; *QC*, quality control.

The PASS/FAIL CRITERIA for SUV values are:
Mean background: 0.85–1.15
25 mm cylinder: >1.8 to <2.8
16/25 ratio: >0.7
The ACR-approved PET phantom is a cylinder with an internal diameter of 20.4 cm. The faceplate has walled cylinders (8, 12, 16, and 25-mm in diameter); two additional 25-mm cylinders, one for air and one for "cold" water; and a Teflon cylinder.

The quality control tests required at installation and thereafter and described and outlined in depth by Karp and colleagues (1991) and NEMA (National Electrical Manufacturers Association, 2001) are radial resolution, tangential resolution, axial resolution, sensitivity, linearity, uniformity, attenuation accuracy, scatter determination, and dead time corrections (National Electrical Manufacturers Association, 2001). The ACR PET Phantom criteria for their accreditation program are in Table 13.5.

SUV Analysis Worksheet

Patient Dose: _____   PET(/CT) Model: _____

For SUV calculations, enter the following into the site's computer: Use the patient dose previously selected from the phantom dose chart on page 10. DO NOT use the value of dose B. Use 70 kg (154 pounds) as the patient's weight. Use the ROI data obtained for the minimum (min.), maximum (max.) and mean SUV values to complete tables 1 & 2 below.

A) Contrast – Table 1

	Hot Vial 8 mm	Hot Vial 12 mm	Hot Vial 16 mm	Hot Vial 25 mm
max. SUV				

B) Scatter/Attenuation – Table 2

	Background	Bone	Air	Water
mean SUV				
min. SUV	■■■			

C) Ratio Calculations (using data from Tables 1 & 2 above):

max. vial SUV to mean background SUV e.g., Contrast = 8mm SUV / bkgd SUV	8mm/bkgd	12mm/bkgd	16mm/bkgd	25mm/bkgd

max. vial SUV to max. 25 mm vial e.g., Contrast = max16 mm SUV / max 25 mm SUV	8mm/25mm	12mm/25mm	16mm/25mm

min. air or water to min. bone e.g., ratio = min air SUV / min bone SUV	air/bone	water/bone

ACR SUV Analysis Worksheet.

TABLE 13.5   ACR PET Phantom Criteria
PET Phantom:
(If a phantom receives 2 scores of Marginal, this equals a FAIL)

Contrast:
Satisfactory: 12-mm vial is resolved with low contrast; larger vials resolved with high contrast
Marginal: 16-mm vial is resolved with acceptable contrast; larger vials resolved with high contrast

Spatial Resolution:
Satisfactory: 9.5-mm rods are resolved with low contrast; larger rods are resolved with high contrast
Marginal: 11.1-mm rods are resolved with low contrast; larger rods are resolved with high contrast

Uniformity:
Satisfactory: Artifacts are seen in only a few slices of the complete set but are not thought to be clinically significant
Marginal: Strong artifacts are seen in a small number of slices

A phantom acquisition with two or more marginal scores for any category will be failed. *ACR*, American College of Radiology; *PET*, positron emission tomography.

POSITRON EMISSION TOMOGRAPHY/COMPUTED TOMOGRAPHY SYSTEMS

Systems combining PET scanning capability and CT scanning into the same machinery are rapidly becoming commonplace in diagnostic imaging departments. With these systems, quality control testing of the PET scanning circuitry and the CT circuitry must be performed separately using procedures discussed here and in Chapter 10. Additional quality control testing such as spatial coregistration between CT and PET image data also must be performed. Figure 13.18 contains the ACR PET Equipment Evaluation Summary for PET and PET/CT systems.

QUALITY CONTROL OF NONIMAGING EQUIPMENT

In addition to the variety of imaging systems used in nuclear medicine, nonimaging equipment is essential for the function and safety of all nuclear medicine departments. Nonimaging devices are used daily in radiation protection, in vitro studies, and all radiopharmacy procedures. A radiation protection QA program is essential and required by TJC (Accreditation Manual for Hospitals) and the Nuclear Regulatory Commission (NRC; USNRC Title 10, 2013). A radiation protection program ensures that the workplace, employees, and patients are safe and not needlessly exposed to any ionizing radiation. A QA program is also crucial in the radiopharmacy of any nuclear medicine department. Radionuclides must be produced, and radiopharmaceuticals prepared and subsequently dispensed and administered to the correct patients. In addition, the procedure of Standard Precautions, enacted into law and enforced by the Occupational Safety and Health Administration (OSHA) (Strasinger and Di Lorenzo, 1996), must be an integral component of any nuclear medicine QA program to secure a safe environment for both the patient and the healthcare worker. This is especially important to all individuals who may come in contact with needles and blood products.

PET Equipment Evaluation Summary

System: Report Date:
Address: Survey Date:
System PETAP# - Unit #:
PET System Manufacturer: Model:
Medical Physicist:
Signature:

Equipment Evaluation Tests

* Optional ** Not required for PET/MR systems

	Pass/Fail/NA
Spatial Resolution	
Count Rate Performance (count rate versus activity), including count loss	
Sensitivity	
Image Uniformity	
Image Quality Phantom	
Accuracy of CT# **	
Accuracy of standard uptake value (SUV) measurement	
Image Co-registration	
Monitor Evaluation	
Safety Evaluation	
Mechanical	
Electrical	

Evaluation of Site's QC Program

		Pass/Fail
Daily PET Detector Check		
Daily CT Check		
Semi-annual (quarterly preferred) PET ACR Phantom		
Dose Calibrator Tests	Date	
a. a. Accuracy		
b. b. Linearity		
c. c. Constancy		

Medical Physicist's Recommendations for Quality Improvement and Comments on Testing

PET Equipment Evaluation Summary and QC Review Form 2/24/21   022421

Fig. 13.18 ACR PET Equipment Evaluation Summary for PET and PET/CT systems. *ACR*, American College of Radiology; *CT*, computed tomography; *MR*, magnetic resonance; *NA*, not applicable; *PET*, positron-emission tomography; *PETAP*, positron emission tomography accreditation program.

For the guarantee of safe and accurate diagnostic and therapeutic studies, it is imperative to have quality control procedures in place from the moment a radionuclide is produced or received until the patient study is completed.

Gas-Filled Detectors

Many radiation detection devices not only detect radiation but also quantitate the amount of ionizing radiation present. The gas-filled detector is one type of radiation detection device. The gas-filled detector is a mechanism that consists of a chamber filled with a gas, an anode, a cathode, an external voltage source, and a display meter. The operation of gas-filled detectors is based on the principle that the ionization-induced electrical currents are produced within the gas chambers of these detectors. As radiation passes through the gas chamber, ions are produced, and the positive ions migrate to the cathode, whereas the electrons migrate to the anode. The amount of ion pairs collected is a function of the voltage applied and is directly proportional to the energy and quantity of gamma rays entering the chamber. The detector then responds to the presence of radiation by discovering the ionization-induced electrical currents and displaying the current to read in radiation units. Ionization chambers and Geiger–Müller (GM) meters are the most common gas-filled detectors used in nuclear medicine. *The NRC Regulation Title 10 Code of Federal Regulations Part 35.63* (USNRC Title 10, 2013) (10 CFR 35.63) requires that nuclear medicine departments must assay all radionuclides administered to patients in a dose calibrator, a specialized ionization chamber.

Ion-Detecting Radiation Detectors

Three types of ion-detecting radiation detectors are commonly used in nuclear medicine. The ionization survey meter, which includes the "cutie-pie"[†] type, measures radiation exposure rates (roentgens [R] per hour); the dose calibrator measures the quantity of the radiation dosage in microcuries to curies (Ci); and the GM survey meter and room monitor measure qualitative exposure rates. The NRC requires that nuclear medicine departments possess all three types of radiation detectors (Henkin et al, 1996).

The ionization survey meter is generally battery operated and portable. The ionization survey meter is commonly used in the nuclear medicine department to secure radiation safety of the personnel and the work environment. The NRC states in Section 35 of the CFR (USNRC Title 10, 2013) that any licensee using radioactive materials or radiopharmaceuticals is required to possess a portable radiation survey meter (Henkin et al, 1996). In addition, the NRC regulations state that a daily area survey must be performed in any area where radioactive materials are used and stored. Unrestricted areas must not exceed 2 mrem in any 1 hour (USNRC Regulatory Guide, 1977). The NRC requires that the survey meter be capable of detection of dose rate from 0.1–100 mR/h (Henkin et al, 1996; USNRC Regulatory Guide, 1977).

The radiation monitoring equipment must function accurately and properly to ensure that all monitoring and daily survey radiation exposure readings are true values and conform to the NRC regulations. The NRC requires that all survey meters undergo an annual calibration and a daily reference check before use. The survey meter must be calibrated; otherwise, the values it produces when exposed to radiation have no meaning. The survey meter must be calibrated against a point source that is traceable to a standard certified within 5% accuracy by the US National Institute of Standards and Technology (NIST; Thrall and Ziessman, 1995). The survey meter is adjusted if necessary to read the calculated value of the standard (i.e., cesium-137). The survey meter should be calibrated on three to five scales (0.1, 10, 100). The procedure and requirements of the NRC can be found in 10 CFR 35.61 (USNRC Title 10, 2013).

The reference check is a simple procedure. It requires that the instrument measure a standard, long-lived, radioactive source at the same geometry. The readings obtained in the reference check must be within 20% of the exposure rate checked at calibration, which must always be posted on the side of the instrument (USNRC Title 10, 2013). The reference check of the survey meter ensures that the instrument is maintaining calibration. In addition, because the survey meter is battery operated, it is good practice to perform a battery check on the instrument before each use.

Geiger–Müller Meters

The GM meter is a survey meter used mainly as a survey instrument and an area monitor. One of its uses is as a room monitor. The audible mechanism allows a quick and inexpensive way to determine the presence of ionizing radiation and is a reminder to work quickly. The intensity of the sound increases with the intensity of the ionizing radiation field. However, the GM meter is not capable of accurately measuring and quantitating radiation exposure caused by diverse energy photons commonly found in a nuclear medicine department. The GM meter cannot accurately measure radiation exposure or dose rate, although it is calibrated in milliroentgens per hour or counts per minute. It can only indicate the presence of ionizing radiation. The NRC requires that all GM meters undergo the same quality control as the ionization survey meters. The GM meter must be calibrated annually, and the reference and battery checked before use (USNRC Title 10, 2013).

Dose Calibrator

A dose calibrator is an ionization chamber that is used to verify radioactivity measurements of all radionuclides, radiochemicals, and radiopharmaceutical doses subsequent to their administration to the patient. Confusion of the terminology used in the radiopharmacy can be avoided by knowing the following definitions of the "radio" terms:

- *Radionuclide:* any radioactive atom
- *Radiochemical:* a radionuclide that has combined with a nonradioactive chemical molecule
- *Radiopharmaceutical:* a radionuclide combined with a biologically active molecule

---

[†]The "cutie-pie" is considered more accurate and linear over all ranges compared with the GM tubes.

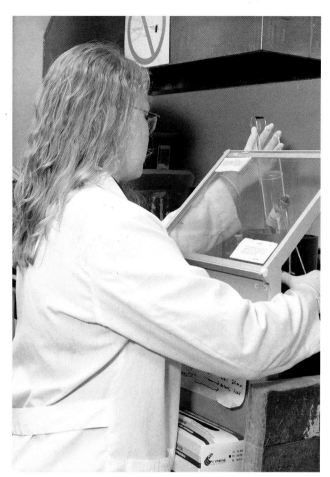

Fig. 13.19 Nuclear medicine technologist performing the quality control tests on a dose calibrator.

Radioactive material may require the addition of stabilizers, reagents, or buffering agents. In addition, a radiopharmaceutical requires approval by the Food and Drug Administration before clinical use (Thrall and Ziessman, 1995). The four NRC-required quality control tests performed on a dose calibrator are accuracy, constancy, geometry, and linearity.

The accuracy test evaluates the ability of the radionuclide dose calibrator to measure the activity of standard sources such as ^{57}Co, cesium-55, and barium-133 accurately. These reference sources must be traceable to the NIST. The accuracy test, performed annually, compares the actual activity of the standard sources with the observed readings of the dose calibrator. If the dose calibrator readings vary from the reference sources by more than 10%, then the instrument must be recalibrated, repaired, or replaced (Fig. 13.19).[‡]

The constancy test assesses and verifies the precision of the dose calibrator. A long-lived sealed reference source such as ^{57}Co, ^{137}Cs, or radium-226 is assayed daily on all commonly used radionuclide settings, and the readings are compared with the standard reference source. *The dose calibrator readings must not vary from the reference source activity by more than 10%.*

[‡]The 10% variance refers to the NRC regulations. The accepted variance is 5% in most agreement states. Please check with your individual state's regulations for the correct value.

There may be significant variation in measured values versus actual radioactivity present as a result of a variation of sample volume. For example, 10 mCi (370 megabecquerels [MBq]) contained in the volume of a 1-mL syringe or a 20-mL syringe or vial might vary significantly. If the geometric variations cause the actual measurements to vary by more than 10% from the true value, correction factors are calculated and used for that specific volume. The geometric variation test is required on installation of the dose calibrator and after any repair.

Radionuclide dose calibrators should display the actual radioactivity of a sample. A linearity test determines the accuracy of the dose calibrator's response to measure a wide range of activities. The dose calibrator should be able to measure a full range of activities from microcuries to millicuries. *Two methods are readily used and accepted by the NRC.* The first linearity test requires assaying a decaying source of ^{99m}Tc sequentially over 3–5 days. The readings are compared with the actual decay of ^{99m}Tc at the same time intervals. The second method involves the use of precalibrated lead sleeves that are placed sequentially over the same source. The advantage of using the lead sleeves is that the procedure takes only about 5 min and results in a much lower level of radiation exposure to the technologist. The linearity test is performed at installation, at 3-month intervals, and after any repair. *The observed values in either method must be within 10% of the actual calculated activities.*[‡]

Nonimaging Scintillation Detectors

Along with the scintillation gamma camera systems mentioned previously, there are also nonimaging systems found in nuclear medicine that use the NaI(T1) crystal and detect radiation with the same basic principle of scintillation. The scintillation detectors used in nuclear medicine have many functions. The single-channel or multichannel analyzers (well counters) are scintillation detectors that are used to count blood and urine samples obtained from in vitro procedures such as red cell mass and plasma volume determinations and Schilling tests. In addition to in vitro patient studies, well counters are used to count the quality control chromatography strips required to evaluate radionuclides and radiopharmaceuticals (Zimmer, 1991). The advantage of the multichannel over the single-channel analyzer is that samples with multiple radioisotopes presenting low to high energy can be analyzed simultaneously. In addition, because the spectrum display is directly proportional to the radionuclide energy, it is possible to determine the unknown radiation that might be present in some contamination. It is also possible to see at a glance the whole spectrum and proper peaking over the energy of interest. This is important when performing NRC-required, daily, area-wipe surveys to locate, identify, and quantitate any contamination. The quality control procedures required for a scintillation detector are listed in Table 13.6.

Calibration is performed to determine and preset the correct operating voltage that is necessary for the detector to place the gamma energy peak in the center of the spectrum

TABLE 13.6   Scintillation Detector Quality Control

Quality Control Procedure	Frequency
Energy calibration	Daily
Peaking	Daily and before each new radionuclide used
Background	Daily and before each new radionuclide used
Constancy	Daily
Instrument calibration	Annually after repair
Energy resolution	Annually after repair
Efficiency	Annually after repair
Chi-square test (reproducibility)	Quarterly; weekly recommended

window. This results in achieving the highest and most accurate count rate. In general, a long-lived radionuclide such as ^{137}Cs, with a gamma photon energy of 662 keV, is used. The voltage is adjusted so that the pulse height of 662 keV is at the center of the spectrum and the window is spaced equally above and below 662 keV.

Because the scintillation detectors count a variety of radionuclides (e.g., ^{99m}Tc, iodine-123, iodine-125, iodine-131, ^{57}Co), the detector must be photopeaked before each new radionuclide is counted. Once this is accomplished, the detector's high voltage is adjusted properly for that specific radionuclide. When environmental samples are counted for contamination, windows are set wide to capture the gamma rays of all radionuclides that may be potentially released as contaminants. Matching the photopeaks on the spectrum to specific energies allows identification of the radionuclide in the sample.

A background measurement with no radionuclide present is taken to ensure that no contaminating radioactivity will affect the true counts. The background is taken for the same period that the sample is counted. The background counts must be subtracted from each sample's gross counts to obtain the true, or net, counts (i.e., net counts = gross counts − background counts). A new background count must be taken for each radionuclide and for each separate procedure to obtain accurate clinical data.

A constancy test is performed daily to verify the stability of the detector. A long-lived source such as ^{137}Cs is counted, and the counts per minute per microcurie are determined and compared with the counts per minute per microcurie at the time of calibration. A change of more than 10% indicates that repair is necessary (Graham et al, 1996).

An annual calibration is performed to regulate the gain and high-voltage settings in such a way that dial settings of the channels read directly to the energy kiloelectron volt of the radionuclide. A ^{137}Cs source is used in the detector, and the energy peak is set on 662 keV with a 5% window. The voltage and gain are adjusted until the center, or photopeak, is exactly centered on 662 keV.

The energy resolution can be thought of as the ability of the scintillation detector to accurately discern two different energies as separate. Energy resolution quality control is discussed in the section on quality control of imaging equipment. To review, the energy resolution can then be expressed as the spread or width of the spectrum divided by the center photopeak. The spread of the spectrum or the FWHM is the energy range of the widest width of the spectrum, which is halfway down from the photopeak. The energy resolution is calculated as follows:

$$\text{Percent energy resolution} = \frac{\text{FWHM at half maximum}}{\text{Photopeak center}} \times 100$$

The energy resolution of most scintillation systems that use ^{137}Cs is between 8% and 12% (Bernier et al, 1997).

The efficiency of a counting detector is measuring the sensitivity of the detector. It is expressed as the observed count rate divided by the disintegration rate of a radioactive sample (Sorenson and Phelps, 1987).

$$\text{Percent efficiency} = \frac{\text{Counts per minute}}{\text{Disintegrations per minute}}$$

This concept is important because counts per minute must be converted into disintegrations per minute (dpm) for the technologist to know whether regulatory requirements are being met for keeping environmental contamination within specific contamination limits for both fixed and removable contamination. For the same sample activity and geometry, every instrument registers a different count per minute on the basis of several detector design factors; therefore an efficiency factor must be determined for each instrument used to count in counts per minute and convert to disintegrations per minute.

Radioactive decay of an atom is a random process, and so when a radioactive source is said to undergo a number of disintegrations per second, the value represents only the average. Because the number of disintegrations per unit time varies, it can be expected that the counts obtained also vary. The variation to be expected when counting the same sample is due to random error. A statistical test called the chi-square test is used to evaluate the reliability of the detector. The results of the chi-square test indicate whether the error that exists in counting is due to randomness. If the error is due to some other problem such as a technical or mechanical error, the detector must be serviced before clinical use. The chi-square quality control test is easy to perform. A radioactive sample is counted 10 times for 1 min each time. The sample must be placed at a distance from the detector that results in a minimum of 10,000 counts. The 10,000 counts are necessary to obtain good statistical data within 1% SD. The data are then used to determine the chi-square value:

$$\text{Chi} - \text{square} = \frac{\text{Sum}\,(x_i - \text{mean})^2}{\text{Mean}}$$

where x_i = individual count rates.

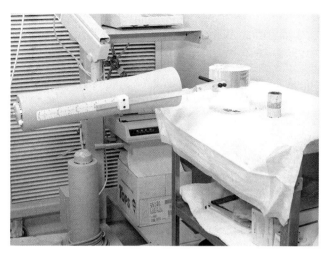

Fig. 13.20 Thyroid probe quality control with a neck phantom.

The result is then located on the table of chi-square values to determine the probability that the discrepancy between the observed and expected frequency is due to random error. Most scintillation detectors are computer driven and maintain the statistical programs that automatically calculate the chi-square values.

Another NaI(T1) scintillation detector used in nuclear medicine is the thyroid uptake probe. The thyroid probe is used clinically to determine the function of the patient's thyroid. A percent uptake of an ingested radioisotope of iodine is calculated. The thyroid uptake probe is a multichannel analyzer with a flat-face crystal and PMT encased in an open-field collimator that faces the patient's thyroid during the procedure. The collimator is generally 20–30 cm long, which is the length required to obtain the proper counting geometry of the patient's thyroid. All of the quality control procedures required for a scintillation detector are performed on the thyroid probe. However, because distance and geometry are crucial in measuring a patient's iodine uptake, a thyroid phantom is used in all daily quality control procedures (Fig. 13.20). The thyroid phantom has been designed to mimic the location of a thyroid in a patient. The phantom ensures that the quality control procedures are accurate and can be related to the patient study.

QUALITY ASSURANCE IN THE RADIOPHARMACY

Sealed Radioactive Source

The sealed sources used in the previously mentioned calibrations and for calibration of other nonimaging and imaging equipment must be tested for any leakage of radioactive material. The NRC requires that all photon-emitting sealed sources containing 100 μCi or more be tested for leakage biannually (USNRC Regulatory Guide, 1977). Any sealed sources with more than 0.005 μCi of removable activity per test must immediately be removed, properly stored, and reported to the NRC (USNRC Title 10, 2013). In addition, the NRC requires that all sealed sources be inventoried and surveyed quarterly for radiation exposure.

Molybdenum-99/Technetium-99 Radionuclide Generator

The radionuclide generator system, a long-lived parent yielding to a shorter-lived daughter, allows the production of useful radionuclides for clinical use. The combination of half-lives of the radionuclides in the generator system makes the shipping of radionuclides from a commercial pharmacy to a hospital more cost-effective; deliveries are required once a week rather than daily. Most of the radiopharmaceuticals prepared by the nuclear medicine technologist are labeled with ^{99m}Tc. The most commonly used generator system in hospitals and clinics is the **molybdenum-99/technetium-99m** (^{99}Mo/^{99m}Tc) system. The ^{99}Mo/^{99m}Tc generator is an alumina ion-exchange column onto which ^{99}Mo, the parent, has a high affinity. Subsequently, ^{99m}Tc has a lower affinity to the column; therefore the separation of ^{99m}Tc from the parent, ^{99}Mo, is simple. When saline solution is pulled through the alumina column by means of an evacuated collection vial, the daughter, ^{99m}Tc, is removed, or eluted, from the column. The technetium eluted is in the radiochemical form ^{99m}TcO$_4^-$ **(technetium-99m pertechnetate)**, and the ^{99m}Tc is in the valence state of +7. Quality control procedures are essential on the technetium eluent each time the generator is eluted, to ensure that the eluent does not contain any contaminants or impurities including **radionuclide impurity** of ^{99}Mo, molybdate, **chemical impurity** of Al^{+3}, alumina, or radiochemical impurity of **hydrolyzed reduced technetium** (HR-Tc).

A common contaminant found in the generator eluent is the parent, ^{99}Mo. The appearance of ^{99}Mo in the eluent is called *moly breakthrough.* If any ^{99}Mo is injected into a patient, the liver absorbs the ^{99}Mo and receives unnecessary radiation.

Testing for moly breakthrough is simple to perform. A lead container, which absorbs the ^{99m}Tc 140-keV energy but allows the passage of the higher-energy 740 and 780 keV ^{99}Mo photons, is used. The generator eluent vial is placed in the moly lead shield and assayed in the dose calibrator. The amount of ^{99}Mo contamination is calculated by dividing the total amount of ^{99}Mo assayed by the total amount of ^{99m}Tc. *The NRC allowable limit is 0.15 μCi of ^{99}Mo activity per 1 mCi of ^{99m}Tc activity at the time of injection of the administered dose (*USNRC Title 10, 2013). *This is critical because the concentration of ^{99}Mo/^{99m}Tc may creep up and exceed limits several hours after elution.*

The chemical impurity that can be present in the generator eluent is alumina, Al^{+3}, which comes from the ion-exchange column. The US Pharmacopoeia (USP) has established that the Al^{+3} concentration limits not exceed 10 μg of Al^{+3} per milliliter eluent. Aurin tricarboxylic acid is used for colorimetric spot testing (Thrall and Ziessman, 1995). The color reaction for a standard alumina sample is compared with the generator eluate. The comparison is qualitative and made by visual inspection. Excessive levels of aluminum can interfere with normal distribution of some radiopharmaceuticals.

In addition, the radiochemical impurity that may exist in the eluent solution is HR-Tc. Technetium that is eluted is expected to have a valence state of +7, which is the desired chemical form for most kit preparations. If the ^{99m}Tc is present in other forms, then the distribution of the final radiopharmaceutical product in a patient is altered. Unbound, or free, ^{99m}TcO$_4^-$ accumulates in the stomach, thyroid gland, and salivary gland. ^{99m}Tc-colloidal uptake occurs in the reticuloendothelial system, especially the liver. The USP standard for the generator eluent is that 95% or more of the technetium activity be in the *+7 valence state* (Klingensmith et al, 1995).

Radiopharmaceuticals

Because radiopharmaceuticals are intended for diagnostic and therapeutic patient procedures, quality control procedures are crucial in ensuring the safety and effectiveness of these preparations (Zimmer, 1991). When a nuclear medicine department uses unit doses provided by a commercial nuclear pharmacy, the preparations undergo extensive quality control procedures by the manufacturer or the commercial nuclear pharmacy. However, many radiopharmaceutical preparations are prepared with lyophilized radiopharmaceutical preparation kits and short-lived radionuclides such as ^{99m}Tc. As a result, the absolute responsibility for the QA of the radiopharmaceuticals lies with the radiopharmacist or the nuclear medicine technologist preparing the kits.

Whether the radiopharmaceuticals are prepared by commercial manufacturers or at the hospital nuclear pharmacy, they must be subjected to physiochemical and biological testing, including physical state examination and osmolality, pH, chemical, radionuclidic and radiochemical purity, sterility, and pyrogenicity testing (Zimmer, 1991).

Sterility represents the absence of metabolic products such as endotoxins in the final product. Sterility testing uses USP standard media such as thioglycollate and soybean casein digest media to determine the presence of bacteria and fungi in the radiopharmaceutical solution (Thrall and Ziessman, 1995). Because many radiopharmaceuticals are prepared just before patient administration, the sterility test must be performed retrospectively. Pyrogens or microorganism metabolites that may exist in the radiopharmaceutical solution can cause a fever if injected into a patient. The pyrogen test uses the USP limulus amebocyte lysate test to detect the presence of pyrogens.

The radiochemical and radionuclidic purity of a radiopharmaceutical may be assessed by many different methods, including paper chromatography, thin layer chromatography, high-performance liquid chromatography, and gel electrophoresis (Robbins, 1984; Zimmer, 1991; Zimmer and Pavel, 1977; Zimmer and Spies, 1991). Because of the characteristics of short-lived radionuclides used in the preparation of radiopharmaceuticals, time is critical. Miniaturized chromatography procedures are used to evaluate the radiochemical purity of radiopharmaceuticals because they are rapid and easy to use (Webber et al, 1983; Zimmer and Pavel, 1977). The miniaturized chromatography system developed by Zimmer (Zimmer and Spies, 1991) uses a support medium such as thin-layer chromatography and a developing solvent to routinely evaluate radiopharmaceutical

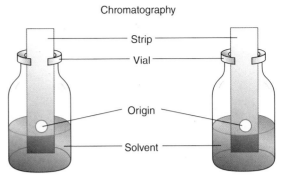

Chromatography

Fig. 13.21 Eluting chromatography strips.

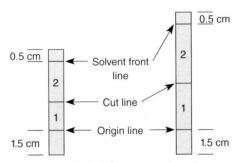

Fig. 13.22 Typical chromatography strips.

preparations subsequent to patient administration (Taukulis et al, 1979).

The chromatography procedures involve spotting the radiopharmaceutical being tested on the origin line of the respective paper strips and eluting the strips in the designated solvent system (Fig. 13.21). After solvent migration to the solvent front line, the strips are removed, cut at the cut line, and counted for activity with appropriate counting systems such as the dose calibrator or the well counter (Fig. 13.22). The labeling efficiency or the fraction of total radioactivity incorporated into the radiolabeled material is calculated by subtracting the sum of the fraction of the impurities of free technetium and HR-Tc from 100%.

Percent labeling efficiency = 100 − (Sum of all impurities).

The percent labeling efficacy for most radiopharmaceuticals should be more than 98% (The Joint Commission, 2013).

Radiation Protection of Nuclear Medicine Personnel

Through mutual cooperation, several regulatory agencies control the radiation exposure of radiation workers in the United States. The Department of Transportation, the Environmental Protection Agency, OSHA, individual state nuclear safety agencies, and the US Nuclear Regulatory Commission Council on Radiation Protection and Measurements determined and provided the radiation dose exposure recommendations used for establishing the regulations and statutes of the NRC (Bernier et al, 1997). Table 13.7 lists the current acceptable radiation dose limits for occupational radiation workers (USNRC Title 10, 2013).

TABLE 13.7 Nuclear Regulatory Commission Dose Equivalent Limits per Year

Anatomic Category	Dose Equivalent Limit/Year
Whole body, head, trunk, blood-forming organs, gonads, and lens of the eyes	50 rem (500 mSv)
Hands, forearms, feet, and ankles	5 rem (50 mSv)
Skin of whole body	30 rem (300 mSv)
Fetus of radiation worker	0.5 rem (5 mSv)*

mSv, Millisievert; *rem*, roentgen equivalent man.
*Dose equivalent for entire gestation period.

To ensure that the occupational radiation worker maintains an exposure far below the federal limits, the radiology communities adhere to the philosophy that the radiation dose exposure be "as low as reasonably achievable," or ALARA (Bernier et al, 1997). The NRC states that the ALARA concept should maintain radiation doses to personnel working in radiation areas of a medical institution to less than 10% of the federal limits of occupational exposure (Bernier et al, 1997).

Personnel Monitoring

All radiation workers in the medical institution who may run the risk of exposure to ionizing radiation during routine duties must be provided with and wear a film badge dosimeter, thermoluminescent dosimeter (TLD), or optically stimulated luminescent dosimeter personnel monitoring device. The detector must be worn on the body part likely to receive the highest radiation exposure. It is recommended that the detector be worn between the shoulders and the waist. Nuclear medicine technologists or others who handle radionuclides or radiopharmaceuticals also must wear a ring or wrist radiation monitor (usually a TLD) so that radiation exposure of fingers and extremities can be estimated. A female technologist who has a declared pregnancy should be issued a second monitoring device to be worn at the waist area to determine any fetal dose. The average period that a radiation worker routinely wears the personnel monitoring device is recommended not to exceed 1 month for film badge dosimeters and optically stimulated luminescent dosimeters and 3 months for TLDs. In addition, it is the responsibility of the radiation safety officer to review at least quarterly the results of personnel radiation monitoring and investigate and document any radiation dose exposure exceeding action level II (30% of the federal limit; Regulatory Guide 8.7, 1992).

In addition to personnel monitoring, any individual handling certain amounts of radioiodine (10 CFR 35.315(a)(8)) must have a bioassay performed. The bioassay is performed to determine whether any iodine activity in the thyroid is due to ingestion or inhalation. The assay is performed with the thyroid uptake probe. The bioassay must be performed between 6 and 72 hours after handling for any individual dispensing, preparing, or administering a therapeutic dose of sodium iodide-131. Individuals who handle less than 30 mCi of iodine are required to undergo a bioassay each calendar quarter if it is volatile. The NRC recommends that corrective action be taken if the ^{131}I thyroid activity of the radiation worker exceeds 40 nCi.

Area Monitors

In addition to monitoring radiation exposure with personal dosimeters, individuals working in areas with radioactive materials also must monitor themselves before meals and before going home. The individuals can use a portable survey instrument such as a survey meter to determine any contamination to the body or clothing. In addition, each radiation work area must be surveyed daily to ensure that only background levels of radiation are present. If an area exceeds background radiation, it must be decontaminated. Because the survey meter is the best instrument to detect radiation but not quantitate or identify radionuclide contaminant, a daily wipe test also is required in any radiation areas. The wipe test is a survey designed to detect any removable radiation contamination by wiping the area to be evaluated with a cotton swab or some other absorbent paper such as filter paper. The wipe sample is analyzed in a scintillation detector such as a well counter or multichannel analyzer to determine the extent of the radionuclidic contamination. Although the NRC only requires a detector sensitive enough to detect any contamination of 2000 dpm, it recommends that if the wipe sample results are more than or equal to 200 dpm/100 cm², *the specific area must be decontaminated and checked again* (USNRC Regulatory Guide, 1977).

The NRC mandates that areas where radioactive gaseous materials are used such as the nuclear pharmacy, as well as rooms where xenon-133 lung ventilation studies are performed, have negative airflow pressure with respect to surrounding areas (USNRC Title 10, 2013). With this pressure, airborne activity that might be generated within the room can be removed through the exhaust system. The negative airflow pressure does not permit xenon-133 to passively diffuse into any surrounding areas. The exhaust must be a dedicated system and provide enough ventilation to dilute and remove radioactive concentrations that may be released into the room (USNRC Regulatory Guide, 1977). The exhaust also must release at a distance away from the public such as the roof top and meet Environmental Protection Agency regulations for effluents released. Quality control procedures must be performed to demonstrate that the air flow at the perimeters of these rooms is toward the room (Regulatory Guide 8.25, 1992). The air flow must be checked a minimum of every 6 months to demonstrate proper and unchanged ventilation.

Radioactivity Signposting

Specific signs are required by the NRC (Bernier et al, 1997; Early and Sodee, 1995; USNRC Regulatory Guide, 1977). They must be posted near the entrance to any room where

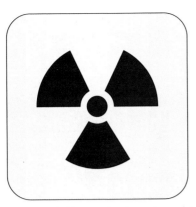

Fig. 13.23 The three-bladed international warning symbol for ionizing radiation.

TABLE 13.8	Radiation Signs
Type of Sign	**Radiation Exposure Potential**
Caution, radioactive materials	Areas in which radioactive material is stored or used in amounts not exceeding 5 mrem in 1 h
Caution, radiation area	Areas in which an exposure could result in excess of 100 mrem in any 1 h
Caution, high-radiation area	Areas in which an exposure could be >5 mrem in 1 h or >100 mrem in 5 consecutive days
Caution, airborne-radioactivity area	Areas in which the airborne radioactivity level may exceed the restricted limit or may exceed 25% of the restricted area limit when averaged over 1 week

mrem, Millirem.

radioactive material may be used or stored. This is done to inform anyone entering the area of the potential hazard of radiation exposure. Each sign must bear the three-bladed international warning symbol for ionizing radiation (Fig. 13.23). The three-bladed symbol can be either magenta, purple, or black on a yellow background. Four different signs are used depending on the amount of potential exposure, as listed in Table 13.8.

Package Shipment, Receipt, and Opening

NRC Regulation Part 20 recommends that all radioactive materials be monitored on receipt or within 3 hours if received during normal working hours or within 18 hours if received after normal working hours (USNRC Title 10, 2013). A good QA program recommends that any radioactive package be handled with disposable gloves, visually inspected, verified for contents, and checked for breakage or leaks. The radiation safety officer is to be notified of any irregularities. The package must then be monitored with a survey meter at the surface of the package and at 3 ft from the package. In addition, a wipe survey of the exterior surface is performed to determine any removable contamination present. *Any value in excess of 0.01 μCi/100 cm²* of surface area tested is a reportable level and must be

decontaminated. In addition, exposure levels exceeding 200 mR/h on the surface or 100 mR/h at 3 ft from the package require notification of the radiation safety officer (USNRC Title 10, 2013). *These must be documented daily on receiving forms.*

Infection and Radiation Exposure Control

Protective shielding in a variety of forms must be used when working with radioactive material. Several protective measures must be followed to minimize radiation contamination and exposure. Some examples of shielding protection materials are lead bricks, disposable gloves, leaded glass, shielded bench tops, syringe shields, vial lead containers, lead container "pigs" to transport the dose, lead-shielded containers to transport radioactive materials outside of the nuclear medicine department, and shielded waste receptacles. Use of the gloves and shielding are considered mandatory for the nuclear medicine worker. The department/institution must have a plan in place in case of a spill of radiopharmaceuticals, and training of nonnuclear medicine personnel must be provided and documented.

In addition, OSHA requires that all personnel who work with needles and blood products minimize their chance of exposure to the human immunodeficiency virus and the hepatitis virus by practicing Standard Precautions. When working with patient procedures that include needles and patient blood products, personnel are now required to wear disposable gloves. The standard precaution guidelines assert the prevention of recapping of needles at all costs. The used syringe must be placed in an approved infectious control needle and syringe receptacle or sharps container (Fig. 13.24). Because nuclear medicine deals with radioactive needles and syringes, the sharps container also must be properly shielded, be decayed, and been stored a minimum of 10 half-lives before disposal to the biohazard department.

Radiopharmaceutical Administration

After preparation and quality control testing, the radiopharmaceutical is ready to be dispensed and administered to

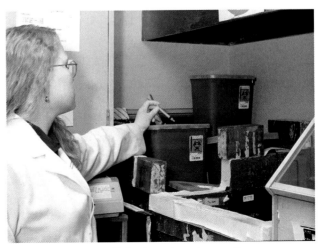

Fig. 13.24 Following universal precautions.

a patient. QA does not stop here. The individual who is dispensing and injecting the radiopharmaceutical should again verify the requisition, the identity of the radiopharmaceutical, the activity, and the patient. The following information must be visually inspected and verified on each request before the nuclear medicine procedure is initiated:

- Patient's name
- Hospital identification number and room number
- Requesting physician's name
- Patient history, condition, and preliminary diagnosis
- Examination agreement with the physician's orders and possible diagnosis of the patient
- Correct radiopharmaceutical for the examination
- Contraindications that can interfere with the radiopharmaceutical biodistribution
- Patient's physical limitations
- Allergies or potential drug interactions
- Potential nuclear medicine radiopharmaceutical interference with other diagnostic or therapeutic procedures
- Patient concerns

After the information has been checked and it is determined that the examination is correct, the person who is administering the radiopharmaceutical must continue to practice good QA. The radiopharmaceutical, the activity, and the volume to be administered must be verified. Before administration, the patient's name and hospital identification number must be verified on the patient's wristband. Finally, if an outpatient is being treated, they must be identified through name, birth date, and Social Security number. If misadministration occurs, the radiation safety officer must be notified immediately. The radiation safety officer determines what NRC classification of misadministration has occurred and immediately takes appropriate action (USNRC Title 10, 2013), including notification of ordering physician, medical director, patient, and NRC or agreement state. An investigation must be conducted to determine all factors contributing to the misadministration and a plan made for corrective action, including training to prevent future occurrences.

NUCLEAR MEDICINE DEPARTMENT COMPLIANCE STANDARDS

In addition to the nuclear medicine equipment quality control standards that have just been discussed in this chapter, accrediting bodies also have specific department standards that must be met, including:

1. Staff dosimetry results are to be reviewed quarterly by the radiation safety officer, medical physicist or health physicist.
2. Equipment quality control and maintenance activities are to be identified and time frames are established for how often they are to be done.
3. Equipment quality control and maintenance activities are to be performed and quality control logs must be completed.
4. A performance evaluation is to be performed annually by a medical physicist and includes all required tests, and that evaluation/testing results are documented.
5. A performance evaluation that includes all required tests and parameters is to be performed on each image acquisition monitor annually by a medical physicist.
6. A structured radiation shielding design assessment is to be conducted by a medical physicist or health physicist before imaging equipment installation.
7. A radiation protection survey is to be conducted after installation of imaging equipment or construction. The survey must be done before clinical use of the room and is conducted by a medical physicist or health physicist.
8. Correct patient, image site, and patient positioning are to be verified before the examination.

REVIEW QUESTIONS

1. The scintillation detector is based on the principle that certain crystals _____ after deposition of energy by some ionizing radiation.
   a. Vibrate
   b. Refract
   c. Emit light
   d. Trap
2. The crystal that is used in most planar and SPECT gamma cameras is the _____ crystal.
   a. Cesium iodide (CsI(T1))
   b. Cesium fluoride (CsF)
   c. Lithium iodide LiI(Eu)
   d. NaI(T1)
3. _____ testing involves performing a quality control performance evaluation of the camera system without the collimator.
   a. Extrinsic
   b. Intrinsic
   c. Phantom
   d. Dead time
4. What are the two most important quality control procedures that must be performed on a scintillation gamma camera?
   a. Intensity; persistence
   b. Counting efficiency; sensitivity
   c. Flood field uniformity; spatial resolution
   d. Linearity; geometry

5. A dose calibrator is an example of an ionization chamber. The following quality control procedures are mandated by the NRC except for which of the following?
   a. Geometry
   b. Chi-square
   c. Linearity
   d. Accuracy
   e. Constancy

6. Which of the following values is the allowable (NRC) limit of molybdenum in the generator eluent of ^{99m}Tc pertechnetate?
   a. 0.0015 µCi/mCi
   b. 0.015 µCi/mCi
   c. 0.15 µCi/mCi
   d. 1.5 µCi/mCi
   e. 1.5 mCi/µCi

7. _____ is the gamma camera's ability to see detail in any image.
   a. Spatial linearity
   b. Spatial resolution
   c. Relative position
   d. Energy resolution

8. In addition to the routine QA procedures required for planar gamma cameras, the SPECT systems require evaluation of its tomographic performances as well as reconstruction algorithms. Uncorrected center-of-rotation errors greater than 1/2 pixel can produce significant loss of spatial resolution. The quality control procedure COR aligns the COR projected onto the computer matrix with the center of the _____ used for reconstruction.
   a. Camera
   b. Patient
   c. Computer matrix
   d. Camera gantry

9. Evaluating the equipment used in a SPECT system is important, as is evaluating each patient study for artifacts or errors. The sinogram of a selected tomographic slice is a summed image of all the projection data. It is useful in detecting _____, which can degrade the quality of the SPECT study.
   a. Patient motion
   b. Dead time
   c. Correct acquisition time
   d. Incorrect radionuclide energy

10. Impurities found in radiopharmaceutical preparations are placed in all of the following categories except which of the following?
    a. Chemical impurities
    b. Nuclidic impurities
    c. Radionuclide impurities
    d. Radiochemical impurities

REFERENCES AND BIBLIOGRAPHY

Accreditation Manual for Hospitals. Vol. 1. Oakbrook Terrace, IL: Joint Commission on Accreditation of Healthcare Organizations Standards; 1993.

Anger HO. Scintillation camera. 1958;29:27.

Bernier DB, Christian PE, Langan JM, et al. *Nuclear Medicine: Technology and Techniques.* 4th ed. Mosby; 1997.

Christian P, Waterman-Rich K. *Nuclear Medicine and PET/CT.* 7th ed. Mosby; 2013.

Early PJ, Sodee BD. *Principles and Practices of Nuclear Medicine.* 2nd ed. Mosby; 1995.

Eisner R. Principles of instrumentation in SPECT. *J Nucl Med Technol.* 1985;13:23.

English RJ. *SPECT Single-Photon Emission Computerized Tomography: A Primer.* 3rd ed. The Society of Nuclear Medicine; 1995.

Esser PD, Sorenson JA, Westerman BR. *Emission Computed Tomography.* The Society of Nuclear Medicine; 1983.

Graham SL, Kirchner PT, Siegel BA. *Nuclear Medicine: Self Study Program II: Instrumentation.* The Society of Nuclear Medicine; 1996.

Greer K, Jaszczak R, Harris C, et al. Quality control in SPECT. *J Nucl Med Technol.* 1985;13:76.

Henkin RE, et al. *Nuclear Medicine.* Vol. 1. Mosby; 1996.

Karp JS, et al. Performance standards in positron emission tomography. *J Nucl Med.* 1991;2:2342.

Klingensmith III WC, Eshima D, Goddard J. *Nuclear Medicine Procedure Manual: 1995–1996.* Wick; 1995.

Murphy PH. Acceptance testing and quality control of gamma cameras including SPECT. *J Nucl Med.* 1987;28:1221.

Murray IPC, Ell PJ. *Nuclear Medicine in Clinical Diagnosis and Treatment.* Vol. 1. Churchill Livingstone; 1994.

National Electrical Manufacturers Association. *NEMA Standards for Performance Measurements of Scintillation Cameras*; 1986.

National Electrical Manufacturers Association. *NEMA Standards for Performance Measurement of Positron Emission Tomographs.* Publication 2-2001; 2001.

National Electrical Manufacturers Association. *Performance Measurements Of Scintillation Camera*; 1980.

Rao DV, Early PJ, Chu RY, et al. *Radiation Control and Quality Assurance Surveys: Nuclear Medicine—a Suggested Protocol.* American College of Medical Physicists; 1986.

Regulatory Guide 8.25. *Air Sampling in the Workplace.* US Nuclear Regulatory Commission; 1992.

Regulatory Guide 8.7. *Instructions for Recording and Reporting Occupational Radiation Exposure Data.* US Nuclear Regulatory Commission; 1992.

Robbins PJ. *Chromatography of Technetium-99M Radiopharmaceuticals: A Practical Guide.* The Society of Nuclear Medicine; 1984.

Saha GP. *Physics and Radiobiology of Nuclear Medicine.* Springer-Verlag; 1993.

Scintillation camera acceptance testing and performance evaluation. American Association of Physicists in Medicine; 1980.

Sorenson JA, Phelps ME. *Physics in Nuclear Medicine.* 2nd ed. WB Saunders; 1987.

Steves AM. *Review of Nuclear Medicine Technology.* The Society of Nuclear Medicine; 1992.

Strasinger SK, Di Lorenzo MA. *Phlebotomy Workbook for the Multiskilled Healthcare Professional.* FA Davis; 1996.

Taukulis RA, et al. Technical parameters associated with miniaturized chromatography systems. *J Nucl Med Technol.* 1979;7:19.

The Joint Commission. *Accreditation Manual.* The Joint Commission; 2013.

Thrall JH, Ziessman HA. *Nuclear Medicine: The Requisites.* Mosby; 1995.

USNRC Regulatory Guide. 8.18. *Information Relevant to Insuring That Occupational Radiation Exposures at Medical Institutions Will be as Low as Reasonably Achievable.* US Nuclear Regulatory Commission; 1977.

USNRC Title 10. Code of Federal Regulations, Part 20: standards for protection against radiation. *Fed Reg.* 2013;56(89):23390.

USNRC Title 10. *Code of Federal Regulations, Part 35: Human Uses of Byproduct Material.* US Nuclear Regulatory Commission.

Webber DI, Zimmer AM, Spies SM. Common errors associated with miniaturized chromatography. 1983;11:66.

Zimmer AM. *Miniaturized Chromatography Procedures for Radiopharmaceuticals.* Northwestern University Medical Center; 1991.

Zimmer AM, Pavel DG. Rapid miniaturized chromatographic quality control procedures for Tc-99m radiopharmaceuticals. *J Nucl Med.* 1977;18:1230.

Zimmer AM, Spies SM. Quality control procedure for newer radiopharmaceuticals. *J Nucl Med Technol.* 1991;19:210.

Agencies, Organizations, and Committees in Quality Assurance

Agency for Healthcare Research and Quality 540 Gaither Road, Rockville, MD 20850 https://www.ahrq.gov

American Association of Physicists in Medicine One Physics Ellipse, College Park, MD 20740 https://www.aapm.org

American College of Medical Physics 11250 Roger Bacon Drive, Suite 8, Reston, VA 20190-5202

American College of Nuclear Medicine PO Box 175, Landisville, PA 17538-0175 https://www.acnucmed.org

American College of Radiology 1891 Preston White Drive, Reston, VA 20191-4397 https://www.acr.org

American Institute of Ultrasound in Medicine 14750 Sweitzer Lane, Suite 100, Laurel, MD 20707-5906 https://www.aium.org

American Society of Radiologic Technologists 15000 Central Avenue SE, Albuquerque, NM 87123-3917 https://www.asrt.org

Centers for Medicare and Medicaid Services 7500 Security Blvd, Baltimore, MD 21244 https://www.cms.gov

Conference of Radiation Control Program Directors 205 Capital Avenue, Frankfort, KY 40601 https://www.crcpd.org

DNV-GL 400 Techne Center Drive, Milford, OH 45150 http://dnvgl.com

FDA/CDRH 5600 Fishers Lane, Rockville, MD 20857 https://www.FDA.gov

FDA/CDRH/Mammography 1350 Piccard Drive, Rockville, MD 20850 https://www.FDA.gov/cdrh/mammography

Fluke Biomedical 6920 Seaway Blvd, Everett, WA 98203 https://www.flukebiomedical.com

Sun Nuclear 3275 Suntree Blvd, Melbourne, FL 32940 www.sunnuclear.com

Healthcare Information and Management Systems Society (HIMSS) 230 East Ohio Street, Suite 500, Chicago, IL 60611-3270 https://www.himss.org

Integrating Healthcare Enterprise (IHE) 820 Jorie Blvd, Oak Brook, IL 60523 https://www.ihe.net

Intersocietal Accreditation Commission (IAC) 6021 University Blvd, Suite 500, Ellicott City, MD 21043 https://www.intersocietal.org

National Council on Radiation Protection and Measurements 7910 Woodmont Avenue, Suite 800, Bethesda, MD 20814-3095 https://www.ncrp.com

National Electrical Manufacturers Association 1300 N. 17th Street, Suite 1752, Rosslyn, VA 22209 https://www.nema.org

Radiological Society of North America, Inc. 820 Jorie Blvd, Oak Brook, IL 60523-2251 https://www.rsna.org

Society for Computer Applications in Radiology 10105 Cottesmore Court, Great Falls, VA 22066 https://www.scarnet.org

The Joint Commission 1 Renaissance Blvd, Oakbrook Terrace, IL 60181 https://www.jointcommission.org

United States Department of Health and Human Services 200 Independence Ave SW, Washington, DC 20201 https://www.hhs.gov

BIBLIOGRAPHY

Adams H, Arora S. *Total Quality in RadioRogy*. GR/St Lucie Press, 1994.

Adler A, Carlton R. *Principles of Radiographic Imaging*. 6th ed. Cengage, 2020.

Al-Assaf A, Schmele J. *The Textbook of Total Quality in Healthcare*. GR/St Lucie Press, 1993.

American Association of Physicists in Medicine. *Basic Quality Assurance in Diagnostic Radiology, 1977*. The Association.

American Association of Physicists in Medicine. *Quality Control in Diagnostic Radiology, 1994*. The Association.

American Association of Physicists in Medicine. *Assessment of Display Performance for Medical Imaging Systems, 2005*. The Association.

American Association of Physicists in Medicine. *An Exposure Indicator for Digital Radiography, 2009*. The Association.

American Association of Physicists in Medicine. *Report No. 272 – Comprehensive Acceptance Testing and Evaluation of Fluoroscopy Imaging Systems, 2022*. The Association.

American College of Radiology Committee on Quality Assurance in Mammography. *Mammography Quality Control Manual: Digital Mammography. 2nd Edition.* May 2020. American College of Radiology.

American College of Radiology. *ACR-AAPM-SIIM Practice Guideline for Digital Radiography, 2022*. American College of Radiology.

American College of Radiology. *ACR Computed Tomography Quality Control Manual, 2017*. American College of Radiology.

American College of Radiology. *MRI Quality Control Manual, 2015*. American College of Radiology.

Anderson R. Darkroom disease: a matter of debate. *ASTR Scanner*. 1996;28(10):1.

Ball J, Price T. *Chesneys' Radiologic Imaging*. 6th ed. Wiley, 1995.

Balter S. Fundamental properties of digital imaging. *Radiographics*. 1993;13:129.

Bonnick S, Lewis L. *Bone Densitometry for Technologists*. Humana Press, 2006.

Bushberg J. *The Essential Physics of Medical Imaging*. 4th ed. Walters Kluwer/Lippincott Williams & Wilkins, 2020.

Bushong S. *Radiologic Science for Technologists: Physics, Biology, and Protection*. 12th ed. Mosby, 2021.

Carlton R, Adler A. *Principles of Radiologic Imaging*. 6th ed. Delmar, 2020.

Carroll Q. *Fuchs' Principles of Radiologic Exposure*. 7th ed. Charles C Thomas, 2003.

Carroll Q. *Radiography in the Digital Age*. 3rd ed. Charles C Thomas, 2018.

Carter C, Veale B. *Digital Radiography and PACS*. 4th ed. Elsevier, 2023.

Curry T. *Christensen's Physics of Diagnostic Radiology*. 4th ed. Lea & Febiger, 1990.

Deming WE. *Out of the Crisis*. MIT Press, 2018.

Forster E. *Equipment for Diagnostic Radiography*. MPT Press, 1985.

Gaucher E, Coggey R. *Total Quality in Health Care*. Jossey-Bass, 1993.

Graham N. *Quality in Health Care*. Aspen, 1995.

Gray J. *Quality Control in Diagnostic Imaging*. University Park Press, 1983.

Haus A, Jaskulski S. *The Basics of Film Processing in Medical Imaging*. Medical Physics Publishing, 1997.

Hendee WR, Ritenour ER. *Medical Imaging Physics*. 5th ed. Wiley-Liss, 2019.

Hendrick RE. *Digital Mammography Quality Control Manual*. 2nd ed. American College of Radiology, 2020.

Huda W, Slone R. *Review of Radiologic Physics*. 2nd ed. Lippincott Williams & Wilkins, 2003.

Joint Commission on Accreditation of Healthcare Organizations. *Forms, Charts & Other Tools for Performance Improvement*. The Joint Commission, 1995.

Judson K, Harrison C. *Law & Ethics for the Health Professions*. 9th ed. McGraw-Hill, 2021.

Lederer W. *Regulatory Chemicals of Health and Environmental Concerns*. Van Nostrand Reinhold, 1985.

Lorh KN. Outcomes measurement: concept and questions. *Inquiry*. 1988;25:37.

Mammography Quality Standards. 21 CFR part 900. *Fed Reg*. 1994;21:471.

McKinney W. *Radiographic Processing & Quality Control*. JP Lippincott, 1988.

McLemore J. *Quality Assurance in Diagnostic Radiology*. Mosby, 1981.

Meisenheimer C. *Improving Quality*. 2nd ed. Aspen, 1997.

National Council on Radiation Protection. The Council, Rep No 99, 1988.

National Council on Radiation Protection. The Council, Rep No 105, 1990.

National Council on Radiation Protection. The Council, Rep No 116, 1993.

Obergfell A. *Law & Ethics in Diagnostic Imaging and Therapeutic Radiology*. WB Saunders, 1995.

Parelli R. *Principles of Fluoroscopic Image Intensification and Television Systems*. Delray Beach, FL: GR/St Lucie Press, 1996.

Samei E. *Assessment of Display Performance for Medical Imaging Systems*. Task Group 18, Version 10: *Draft Report of the American Association of Physicists in Medicine (AAPM)*; 2004.

Shepard C. *Radiographic Image Production and Manipulation*. New York: McGraw-Hill, 2002.

Shleien B, Slaback L, Birky B. *Handbook of Health Physics and Radiological Health*. 3rd ed. Baltimore: Williams & Wilkins, 2017.

Siegel E, Kolodner R. *Filmless Radiology (Formerly Computers in Health Care)*. New York: Springer, 1999.

Sollecito W, Johnson J. *McLaughlin and Kaluzny's Continuous Quality Improvement in Health Care*. 5th ed. Burlington, MA: Jones & Bartlett, 2018.

Thompson M. *Principles of Imaging Science and Protection*. Philadelphia: WB Saunders, 1994.

Tortorici M. *Medical Radiographic Imaging*. WB Saunders, 1992.

Vyborny C, Schmidt R. Mammography as a radiographic examination: an overview. *Radiographics*. 1989;9:723.

Wentz G. *Mammography for Radiologic Technologists*. New York: McGraw-Hill, 1996.

Wolbarst A. *Physics of Radiology*. Norwalk, CT: Appleton & Lange, 2005.

Zandlerk A. *Managing Outcomes Through Collaborative Care*. Chicago: American Hospital Publishing, 2013.

Acceptance testing Quality control testing performed on new equipment on delivery and installation.

Accreditation A method used to assess organizations and determine if they meet minimum established standards.

Accuracy The extent to which a measurement is close to the true value.

Achievable dose an optimization goal, based on survey data, and typically defined as the median value (50th percentile) of the dose distribution of standard techniques and technologies in widespread use

Action The activity portion of a process that will achieve the desired outcome.

Action or control limit A part of a control chart that allows you to identify common and special cause variation

Active matrix array (AMA) A large-area (the size of conventional film/screen image receptors) integrated circuit that consists of millions of identical semiconductor elements deposited on a glass base that acts as the flat-panel image receptor.

Actual focal spot The actual area of the x-ray tube target from which x-rays are emitted.

Adverse event A harmful or unintended incident that may occur during any diagnostic procedure.

Aggregate data indicator Quantifies a process or outcome related to many cases.

Agitation Stirring, swirling, or shaking of processing solutions.

Air Kerma An acronym for kinetic energy released in matter, and it measures the amount of kinetic energy released from particles of matter (such as electrons created during Compton and photoelectric interactions) from exposure to x-rays into air molecules.

Air Kerma Rate (AKR) The amount of air kerma measured per unit time.

Algorithm A step-by-step procedure or mathematical process for solving a problem or accomplishing a specific task.

American College of Radiology Founded in 1923, the American College of Radiology® is an organization representing more than 41,000 diagnostic and interventional radiologists, radiation oncologists, nuclear medicine physicians and medical physicists.

American Recovery and Reinvestment Act The American Recovery and Reinvestment Act of 2009 (ARRA) was fiscal stimulus legislation passed by the U.S. Congress to alleviate the Great Recession of 2008.

Amorphous Without form.

Analog-to-digital convertor (ADC) Device for converting an analog electronic signal into a digital electronic signal for processing by a computer.

Annotations the process of labeling medical imaging data

Application program interface (API) A system that specifies how certain software components in a picture archiving and communication system (PACS) should interact with other software components.

Appropriateness of care Whether the type of care is necessary.

Archival film Film images made before 1974 and containing 20% more silver than film made afterward.

Archival quality How well an image can be stored over time.

Archive test Test performed on PACS servers to ensure that they can both send and retrieve images.

Artifact The appearance in a diagnostic image of anything that is not a part of the patient's anatomy.

Artificial intelligence A field which combines computer science and robust datasets, to enable problem-solving.

As low as reasonably achievable (ALARA) Philosophy of keeping radiation exposure to a minimum.

Aspect ratio The ratio of the width of the image displayed on a computer or video monitor to the height of the display.

Assess A system for evaluating performance, as in the delivery of services or the quality of products provided to consumers, customers, or patients.

Automatic brightness control (ABC) Also called *automatic brightness stabilization* (ABS), is an electronic method of regulating fluoroscopic image brightness level for variations of patient thickness and attenuation.

Automatic brightness stabilization Electronic method of regulating fluoroscopic image brightness. Also known as *automatic brightness control.*

Automatic exposure control (AEC) Electronic system that terminates the x-ray exposure once an adequate amount of radiation has been emitted.

Automatic exposure rate control (AERC) A system used in fluoroscopy to maintains the radiation dose per frame at a predetermined level.

Automatic gain control Electronic method of regulating image brightness.

Avoirdupois ounce Unit of weight in the English system more commonly known as the *standard ounce.*

Axial or Vertical distance resolution Minimum reflector spacing along the axis of an ultrasound beam that results in separate, distinguishable echoes on the display.

Background radiation Radiation exposures from naturally occurring radioactivity and extraterrestrial cosmic radiation.

Bandwidth The range of frequencies that can be satisfactorily transmitted or processed by a system.

Base + fog Inherent optical densities in film resulting from the tint added to the base of the film and silver grains not exposed to radiation.

Benchmarking Involves comparing one organization's performance with that of another.

Beryllium window A portion of the mammographic x-ray tube where the useful beam exits.

Bioassay The laboratory determination of the concentration of a drug or other substance in a specimen.

Bit Binary digit; the smallest unit of computer memory that holds one of two values, one or zero.

Brainstorming A group process used to develop a large collection of ideas without regard to their merit or validity.

Brightness gain The degree of image-brightness increase obtained with an image intensifier.

Bromide drag Decrease in optical density caused by halides being deposited on trailing areas of the film during automatic processing.

Capture element The top portion of an active matrix array image receptor that will absorb the x-rays that exit the patient (much like the photostimulable phosphor [PSP] in computed radiography [CR] systems).

Cause-and-effect diagram A causal analysis tool. Also known as a *fishbone chart* or *Ishikawa diagram.*

Center frequency A relatively fine adjustment in MRI systems that tells the scanner at *exactly* what frequency the protons of interest are resonating in the magnet's isocenter.

Center of rotation (COR) The fulcrum, or pivot point, of tomographic equipment motion.

Central tendency The central position of a sample frequency.

Channeling A potential problem in certain metallic replacement silver recovery units whereby the fixer forms a straight channel that reduces efficiency.

Charge-coupled device (CCD) A two-dimensional electronic array for converting light patterns into electronic signals.

Chatter Artifact that appears as bands of increased optical density that occur perpendicular to film direction because of inconsistent motion of the transport system; usually the result of slippage of the drive gears or drive chain.

Chemical activity How well the processing solutions perform their desired function.

Chemical impurity The presence of a chemical or other substance that normally should not be present.

Chi-square A statistic test for an association between observed data and expected data represented by frequencies.

Chromatography Any one of several processes for separating and analyzing various gaseous or dissolved chemical materials.

Cinefluorography The recording of a fluoroscopic image onto motion picture film.

Collection element The bottom portion of the active matrix array image receptor that will collect the charge and send it through an analog-to-digital convertor and onto the computer for processing. This can be made up of a photodiode, thin-film transistor (TFT) of CCD chip, depending on the system.

Collimator (1) A device that regulates the area of x-ray beam exposure. (2) A device for improving image resolution in nuclear medicine procedures.

Comparator A portion of an automatic exposure control system that compares the amount of radiation detected with a preset value.

Complementary metallic oxide semiconductor (CMOS) An integrated circuit design on a printed circuit board (PCB) that uses semiconductor technology, often found in video cameras.

Compression Applying pressure to a body area to reduce part thickness.

Compression ratio The ratio of the size of the original file to the compressed image file.

Computed radiography (CR) A process of creating a digitized radiographic image using a photostimulable phosphor.

Computed tomography volume dose index (CTDI$_{vol}$) A measure of patient dose in multislice CT scans that incorporates CTDI values measured at both the center of the acrylic phantom as well as the slice thickness.

Concurrent data Data collected during the time of care.

Consolidated Appropriations Act of 2016 Provides FY2016 appropriations; extends expiring tax provisions; and affects policies in areas including oil exports, intelligence, cybersecurity, health care, financial services, visa waivers, and conservation.

Consumer An individual who chooses to comment or complain in reference to an examination including the patient or representative of the patient (e.g., family member or referring physician).

Continuity of care The degree to which the care is coordinated among practitioners or organizations, or both.

Continuous variables Variables that have an infinite range of mathematic values.

Contrast-detail curve Used to identify a limit to visual perceptual performance in the context of detectability of space-occupying lesions in homogeneous background.

Contrast indicator Value obtained during sensitometric testing, which indicates film contrast.

Contrast resolution The ability of an imaging system to distinguish structures with similar transmission as separate entities.

Contrast scale The change in linear attenuation coefficient per computed tomographic number relative to water.

Contrast-to-noise ratio (CNR) The ratio between the image contrast to the amount of image noise (both quantum mottle and/or electronic); can be used to describe image quality.

Contrast ratio the ratio of the maximum white level (L_{max}) to the minimum black level (L_{min}), OR L_{max}/L_{min}, of an image display monitor.

Control chart A modification of the trend chart in which statistically determined upper and lower control limits are placed.

Control console Part of a diagnostic imaging system whereby technical and imaging parameters are selected and operated.

Cosine Law States that when a monitor is viewed straight on, the luminous intensity is at its maximum.

Cost of quality A methodology that allows an organization to determine the extent to which its resources are used for activities that prevent poor quality, that appraise the quality of the organization's products or services, and that result from internal and external failures.

Coulomb per kilogram International System of Units' radiation intensity equivalent to 3876 R.

Count rate Measurement of the activity of a radioactive substance.

Counts per minute A measure of the decay rate of ionizing emissions by radioactive substances.

Coupling element The portion of the active matrix array image receptor that will transfer the x-ray–generated electronic signal to a collection element. It can be made up of fiber optics, lens coupling, or amorphous selenium depending on the system.

Critical path Documents the basic treatment or action sequence in an effort to eliminate unnecessary variation.

Customer A person, department, or organization that needs or wants the desired outcome.

Daily Testing Quality control tests that are performed on a daily basis.

Dashboards A condition-specific, actionable web-based application for quality reporting and population management that is integrated into the Electronic Health Record (EHR).

Darkroom Area protected from white light where films are processed.

Data or Data set The information or measurements that were acquired by evaluating the particular sample.

Database An organized collection of data stored and accessed electronically through the use of a database management system.

Daylight system A system for loading and unloading film from image receptors outside of a darkroom.

Densitometer Electronic device for measuring the optical density of a film.

Deficit Reduction Act Federal legislation enacted in 2005 to help reduce Medicare and Medicaid spending.

Dependent variable Variables that are studied under the supposition or demand that they depend, by some law or rule

Depth of visualization Depth into a patient or phantom at which signals from scattered echoes can create an image.

Design Systematic planning and implementation of and function or process.

Det Norske Veritas Norway-based agency approved by the Centers for Medicare and Medicaid Reimbursement in 2008 to accredit healthcare organizations.

Detective quantum efficiency (DQE) One of the fundamental physical variables related to image quality in radiography and refers to the efficiency of a detector in converting incident x-ray energy into an image signal.

Detector Also known as the *sensor*, is a radiation detector that monitors the radiation exposure at or near the patient and produces a corresponding electric current that is proportional to the quantity of x-rays detected.

Detector element (DEL) The small, individual components of a digital x-ray detector.

Developer A processing solution responsible for conversion of the latent image to a manifest image in film.

Deviation Index (DI) This measures how far the actual EI value deviates from the projection-specific Target Exposure Index

Diagnostic reference levels (DRLs) An investigational level used to identify unusually high radiation doses for common diagnostic medical x-ray imaging procedures.

Dichotomous variables Variables that have only two values or choices.

DICOM broker Changes the format between the HL7 information in the EHR and the DICOM information in PACS.

DICOM grayscale standard display function (GSDF) Specifies a standardized display function that would convert digital pixel values to luminance values for consistent display of grayscale images on different devices and monitors, and that these values, which are displayed, are perceived as being equal by human viewers.

Digital breast tomosynthesis (DBT) (also known as 3D mammography) Process that requires multiple images from many angles to generate tomographic slices that can eliminate overlapping structures.

Digital fluoroscopy Computerized enhancement of fluoroscopic images.

Digital Imaging and Communications in Medicine (DICOM) A system of computer software standards that allows different digital imaging programs to understand one another.

Digital radiography (DR) A method of obtaining a digitized radiographic image using an active matrix array.

Digital subtraction angiography An electronic method of enhancing visibility of vascular structures involving digital fluoroscopy.

Direct-to-digital radiographic (DDR) systems Method of creating digital radiographic images, also known as *flat-panel* or *flat-plate imaging*; involves the installation of a flat-panel image receptor in the Bucky of a radiographic table or upright Bucky, which sends an electronic signal directly to a digital image processor.

Discrimination The ability of a radiation detector to separate signals from different types or energies of radiation.

Disintegrations per minute (DPM) A measure of the rate of ionizing emissions by radioactive substances.

Dose area product (DAP) Measurement that incorporates the total dosage of radiation along with the area of field that is being used.

Dose calibrator A component in nuclear medicine equipment for determining the amount of radionuclide.

Dose creep Increase in patient dose in CR and DR (as compared to film/screen) caused by overexposure of the image receptor to avoid quantum mottle.

Dropped pixels Artifact occurring in digital imaging whereby certain pixels data does not appear in the final image.

Dual-energy x-ray absorptiometry (DEXA) X-rays with two separate energies used to obtain bone density data.

Dwell time The amount of time that the fixer solution is in contact with the active portion of the silver recovery device.

Edge enhancement The enhancement of structure margins (edges) using digital processing techniques.

Edge spread function A graphic indication of image resolution.

Effective focal spot The area of the x-ray tube target that emits x-rays when viewed from the perspective of the image receptor.

Effectiveness of care The level of benefit when services are rendered under ordinary circumstances by average practitioners for typical patients.

Efficacy of care The level of benefit expected when healthcare services are applied under ideal conditions.

Efficiency of care The highest quality of care delivered in the shortest amount of time with the least amount of expense and a positive outcome.

Electron beam computed tomography (EBCT) A fifth-generation CT scanner design used in cardiac imaging.

Electrolysis A process in which an electric charge causes a chemical change in a solution or molten substance.

Elevational resolution Sometimes referred to as slice thickness, it is the extent to which an ultrasound system is able to resolve objects within an axis perpendicular to the plane formed by the axial and lateral dimensions

Emission spectrum Graphic demonstration of the component energies of emitted electromagnetic radiation.

Energy resolution The amount of variation in pulse size or spreading of the spectrum produced by a detector.

Enterprise data warehouse (EDW) A database, or collection of databases, that centralizes a business's information from multiple sources and applications, and makes it available for analytics and use across the organization

Error A deviation from the desired outcome or product.

Expectation The criteria that customers use to evaluate the value of products, services and experiences.

Exposure Index (EI) An index of exposure to the image receptor in a relevant region.

Extended processing A method of film processing that extends the normal developer time to increase image contrast.

F-center Empty lattice sites in photostimulable phosphors where crystal electrons are trapped following exposure to x-ray energy.

Field uniformity Refers to the even distribution of magnetic field strength in the region of interest.

File transfer protocol (FTP) A method for transferring files across a computer network.

Fill factor The percentage of pixel area that is sensitive to the image signal (contains the x-ray detector). The fill factor for most current systems is approximately 80% because some of the pixel area must be devoted to electronic conductors and the thin-film transistor (TFT).

Fixer Processing solution responsible for removal of undeveloped silver halide and hardening of the film emulsion.

Flat fielding A software correction used in digital imaging to equalize the response of each pixel to make the image more uniform.

Flat panel sensor (detector) An alternate name for the active matrix array of radiation detectors used in DR and fluoroscopic systems in place of tube-type image intensifiers.

Flood replenishment A timed method of replenishing processing solutions with an automatic processor.

Flowchart A pictorial representation of the individual steps required in a process.

Flow meter A device for measuring the volume of liquid flowing through it.

Fluorescence The type of luminescence that is desired for use in intensifying screens because it occurs when certain crystals emit light within 10^{-8} s after being exposed to radiation.

Flux gain The gain in image brightness occurring with an image intensifier during fluoroscopy resulting from the high voltage across the tube.

Failure mode and effects analysis (FMEA) A procedure for analysis of potential failure within a system, classifying the severity or determining the failure's effect upon the system, and help determine remedial actions to overcome these failures.

Focal spot blooming An increase in stated focal spot size, usually as a result of an increase in milliampere.

Focus group Group dynamic tool for problem identification and analysis.

FOCUS-PDCA A quality management method developed by the Hospital Corporation of America.

Foot-candle Measurement of illuminance lumens per square foot = foot-candles.

Frame rate Also known as refresh rate, it refers to how many times each second that a display monitor rewrites or updates the image on the display. This can be measured in either frames/second or hertz.

Frequency The number of repetitions of any phenomenon within a fixed period.

Full-width half maximum (FWHM) A measure of resolution equal to the width of an image of a line source at points where the intensity is reduced to half the maximum.

Fusion imaging A combination of two images such as positron emission tomography (PET) and CT.

Gamma camera A device used for image acquisition in many nuclear medicine procedures.

Gantry Portion of equipment that holds radiation detectors and/or a radiation source used to diagnose or treat a patient's illness.

Gas-filled detector A category of radiation detector consisting of a gas-filled chamber.

Gaussian distribution A mathematical distribution that is symmetric about the mean value of the measurement set with the spread of the measurements, also known as a normal distribution.

Geiger-Müller (GM) meter A survey meter used mainly for radiation protection purposes as a survey instrument and an area monitor.

Geiger-Müller tube A type of gas-filled radiation detector.

Geometric accuracy The closeness of a measurement to its true value or the accurate representation of anatomical structures in diagnostic imaging.

Gray (Gy) SI unit of absorbed dose and air kerma.

Grayscale processing Conversion of patient data into gray shades that represent anatomical structures.

Grayscale Standard Display Function (GSDF) The mathematically defined mapping of patient data into to Luminance values according to DICOM standards.

Green film Film that has not been processed.

Grid latitude The margin of error in centering the central ray of the x-ray beam to the center of the grid.

Grid uniformity Quality control test to ensure that grid strips are uniformly distriuted throughout the grid.

Half-value layer The amount of filtering material that reduces the intensity of radiation to one half of its previous value.

Health Information Technology for Economic and Clinical Health Act (HITECH) Part of the American Recovery and Reinvestment Act that amended HIPAA's enforcement regulations by adding several categories of violations and established ranges of penalty amounts for each category of violation.

High-contrast resolution The ability to resolve small, thin black-and-white areas.

High-contrast spatial resolution The minimum distance between two objects that allows them to be seen as separate and distinct.

High-frequency generator A type of x-ray generator that dramatically increases the frequency of alternating current sent to the x-ray tube.

Health Insurance Portability and Account-ability Act (HIPAA)   Enacted in 1996 (also known as the Kennedy–Kassebaum Act or Public Law 104191) to simplify healthcare standards and save money for healthcare businesses by encouraging electronic transactions.

Histogram   A data display tool in the form of a bar graph that plots the most frequent occurrence of a quantity in the center.

Histogram error   Improper optical density resulting from selection of an incorrect preprocessing histogram in a cathode-ray system (such as using an adult histogram when radiographing a pediatric chest).

Homogenous phantom   A device used in quality control testing that is uniform in thickness and density.

Horizontal distance measurement   A quality control test for ultrasound equipment requiring measurements taken perpendicular to the sound beam axis.

Humidity   A measurement of the relative level of moisture in the air.

Hydrolyzed reduced technetium   A type of technetium-99m used in radionuclide imaging.

Hydrometer   A device for measuring specific gravity.

Hyporetention   A residue of fixer components remaining on a film after processing.

Illuminance   The brightness of light projected on a given surface, measured in lux or foot-candles.

Image compression   A reduction of the space required to store or time required to transfer a digital image.

Image enhancement   The use of a computer to improve or enhance an image.

Image intensifier   An electronic device that brightens a fluoroscopic image.

Image inversion   Allows converting of a negative image (standard radiographic image) into a positive image (meaning a reverse of the negative image where white areas on the negative image are black on the positive image and vice versa).

Image lag   An image persisting on a cathode-ray tube even after termination of radiation.

Image management and communication system (IMACS)   A computerized system for storing patient images and medical records.

Image orthicon   A type of video camera tube used in fluoroscopic systems.

Image restoration   A process in digital imaging whereby the final image is displayed.

Image uniformity   A uniform brightness level throughout the image when visualizing a homogenous phantom.

Improve   Corrective action taken to fix or correct a process.

Incident   Any occurrence that is not consistent with the routine care of a patient or the normal course of events at a particular facility.

Incident light   The emitted light from its source before striking the film.

Indicator   A valid and reliable quantitative process or outcome measure related to one or more dimensions of performance.

Input   Information or knowledge necessary to achieve the desired outcome.

Intensification factor   A measurement of intensifying screen speed.

Interpolation   A display monitor function that allows it to show an image created of one matrix size to display as another size.

Ion chamber   A type of gas-filled radiation detector.

K-edge   The binding energy of K-shell electrons.

Kerma   An acronym for kinetic energy released in matter, it measures the amount of kinetic energy that is released into particles of matter (such as electrons created during Compton and photoelectric interactions) from exposure to x-rays.

Kerma area product (KAP)   An average of the air kerma (in Gy) multiplied by the corresponding x-ray beam cross-sectional area (in cm^2)

Key input variable   A key process input variable (KPIV) is a process input that provides a significant impact on the output variation of a process or a system

Key output variable   A key process output variable (KPOV) is the factor that results as output from a process

Key performance indicator   Metrics that measure the progress of a specific project toward the defined goals

Kilowatt rating   A rating of power output for x-ray generators.

Latensification   The increase in sensitivity of a film after it has been exposed to light or ionizing radiation (such as in a cassette during a radiographic examination) so that it can be as much as two to eight times more sensitive to subsequent exposure as an unexposed film (depending on the type of emulsion).

Latent image   An invisible image present after exposure but before processing.

Lateral resolution   A measure of how close two reflectors can be to one another perpendicular to the beam axis and still be distinguished as separate.

Law of reciprocity   Law stating that the amount of x-ray intensity should remain constant at a specific milliampere-second value despite the milliampere and time combination.

Lean process improvement   A systematic approach to identifying and eliminating waste, where waste is defined as any nonvalued tasks.

Level of expectation   A preestablished level of performance applied to a specific indicator.

Line focus principle   A principle stating that the effective focal spot always appears smaller than the actual focal spot because of the anode angle.

Line spread function   A graphic indication of image resolution.

Linear tomography   A type of conventional tomography whereby the x-ray source and image receptor undergo reciprocal motion in a straight line.

Linearity   Sequential increases in milliampere-seconds should produce the same sequential increase in exposure rate.

Liquid crystal display (LCD)   Flat-panel display form for viewing monitors.

Locational effect   A variation in film quality caused by the sensitometric test film being inserted in different portions of the feed tray.

Look-up table (LUT)   A table used to assign (transform) digital data into image brightness values.

Loss potential   Any activity that costs a facility either money or its reputation.

Low-contrast resolution   Performance variable measuring the ability to image structures of similar density.

Luminance   The amount of luminous intensity emitted by a source of light.

Luminescence   The emission of light resulting from x-rays exiting the patient, which energize the phosphor crystals. It can occur by one of two different processes, fluorescence or phosphorescence.

Lux   The unit of illuminance, or luminous flux per unit area, in the International System of Units (SI).

Machine learning   A branch of artificial intelligence (AI) and computer science which focuses on the use of data and algorithms to imitate the way that humans learn, gradually improving its accuracy.

Magnification   Electronic digital zoom with software manipulation that can reduce the need to take additional magnification views, as with film/screen mammography.

Mammography Quality Standards Act (MQSA)   Federal legislation mandating quality standards for all mammographic procedures.

Mammography Quality Standards Reauthorization Act (MQSRA)   1998 law that made the MQSA standards permanent.

Manifest image   The final visible image.

Matrix size   The number of pixels allocated to each linear dimension in a digital image.

Mean   The average set of observations.

Mean computed tomography number   Average pixel value calculated by dividing the total computed tomography value by the total number of pixels in a sample.

Meaningful use rules   A term used to define minimum U.S. government standards for electronic health records (EHR), outlining how clinical patient data should be exchanged between healthcare providers, between providers and insurers and between providers and patients.

Measure   Quality measures are standards for measuring the performance and improvement of population health or of health plans, providers of services, and other clinicians in the delivery of health care services.

Median   A point on a scale of measurement above which are exactly one half of the values and below which are the other half of the values.

Medicare Access and Children's Health Insurance Program Reauthorization Act of 2015 (MACRA) A bipartisan legislation signed into law on April 16, 2015 that changes the way that Medicare rewards clinicians for value over time..

Medicare Improvements for Patients and Providers Act (MIPPA) 2008 law that mandates that any non-hospital institution performing advanced diagnostic procedures must be accredited in order to receive federal funding.

Metallic replacement A method of silver recovery from used fixer solution.

Metrics Measures of quantitative assessment commonly used for assessing, comparing, and tracking performance

Minification gain An increase in brightness with image intensifier tubes as a result of the difference in size between the input and output phosphors.

Mobile x-ray generator A smaller-size x-ray generator mounted on wheels that can be transported to various locations.

Mode The one value that occurs with the most frequency.

Modulation transfer function (MTF) A graphic or numeric indication of image resolution.

Molybdenum-99 The parent element of technetium-99m.

Monthly Tests Quality control testing that is performed on a monthly basis.

Multichannel analyzer A specialized scintillation detector that can select specific energy levels for detection.

Multifield image intensifier A specialized image intensifier that allows for magnified fluoroscopic images.

Negative predictive value Negative predictive value is the proportion of the cases giving negative test results who are already healthy

Nit A unit to measure luminance, equivalent to candela per square meter.

Noise Random signals or disturbances that interfere with proper image formation or demonstration.

Nuclear Regulatory Commission (NRC) Federal agency that enforces radiation safety guidelines.

Nyquist frequency The highest spatial frequency resolved by an imaging system, measured in line pairs per millimeter (lp/mm).

Objective plane The region remaining relatively sharp in detail during tomographic procedures.

Occupational Safety and Health Administration (OSHA) Federal agency that oversees the workplace environment.

Optical disk A large-capacity digital data storage device used to store digital images.

Optically stimulated luminescent dosimeter A personal monitoring device that uses aluminum oxide crystals that will absorb ionizing radiation. When exposed to light from a laser, the crystal will emit light

in proportion to the original amount of ionizing radiation that struck the crystal. This light can then be measured and an exact dose measurement can be obtained.

Orthicon A type of television camera tube.

Orthochromatic A type of film that is sensitive mainly to light in the green portion of the visible light spectrum.

Output A specific product or result which you expect to be produced by a process.

Oxidation/reduction reaction A chemical change in which electrons are removed (oxidation) from an atom, ion, or molecule, accompanied by a simultaneous transfer of electrons to another atom, ion, or molecule (reduction). Also known as *redux*.

Panchromatic A type of film that is sensitive to all wavelengths of the visible light spectrum.

Pareto chart A causal analysis tool that is a variation of a histogram.

Patient Protection and Affordable Care Act A law that provides numerous rights and protections that make health coverage more fair and easy to understand, along with subsidies (through "premium tax credits" and "cost-sharing reductions") to make it more affordable.

Percent signal ghosting A type of structured noise appearing as repeated versions of the main object (or parts thereof) in an MR image.

Phantom A quality control test tool used to simulate human tissue or body parts or demonstrate certain image characteristics.

Phosphorescence Delayed emission of light—often called *afterglow* or *lag*—not desired for use in intensifying screens that occurs when certain crystals emit light sometime after 10−8 s after exposure to radiation.

Photodetector An electronic device used for detecting photons of light, x-rays, or gamma rays.

Photoemission The emission of electrons from a material after exposure to light or other ionizing radiation.

Photofluorospot A method of recording static images during fluoroscopy.

Photometry The study and measurement of light.

Photomultiplier tube (PMT) A device used in many radiation detection applications that converts low levels of light into electronic pulses.

Photon The smallest quantity of electromagnetic energy.

Photopeak The peak amplitude on an oscilloscope display.

Photostimulated luminescence Emission of light from crystals that have been exposed to ionizing radiation (such as x-rays) following exposure from laser light; it is used in CR systems to obtain the image.

Photostimulable phosphor A barium fluorohalide material used to capture radiographic images in computed radiography (CR) systems.

Picture archiving and communication system (PACS) A computerized system that stores patient images to allow access from remote locations.

Pincushion distortion A type of distortion in image-intensified images caused by the projection of a curved image onto a flat surface.

Pixel Abbreviation for picture elements. Small cells of information that make up the digital image on a computer monitor screen.

Pixel size The size of the picture element found in the matrix of a computer-generated image; the smaller the pixel size, the greater the spatial resolution.

Plumbicon A type of television camera tube.

Pluridirectional tomography A specialized type of tomographic unit that allows for multiple-direction motion of the x-ray source and image receptor.

Point spread function A graphic demonstration of image resolution.

Population Any group measured for some variable characteristic from which samples may be taken for statistical purposes.

Portable x-ray generator A type of x-ray generator that is small enough to be carried from place to place by one person.

Positive predictive value Positive predictive value is the proportion of cases giving positive test results who are already patients

Positron emission tomography (PET) An imaging technique whereby a positron-emitting radionuclide is administered to a patient, and the result is the release of photons by an annihilation reaction.

Postprocessing A manipulation of the image data in the memory of the computer, before the image is displayed on a monitor.

Poisson distribution A discrete probability distribution that expresses the probability of a given number of events occurring in a fixed interval of time or space

Precipitation A process whereby silver particles are made to settle out of a used fixer solution.

Precision how close data measurements are to each other

Prejudice Also known as bias, it is a systematic or nonrandom difference between the true value of a property and individual measurements of that property.

Prevalence The proportion of a population who have a specific characteristic in a given time period.

Problem A situation, person, or thing that needs attention and needs to be dealt with or solved

Process An ordered series of steps that help achieve a desired outcome.

Protecting Access to Medicare Act of 2014 Prevented a scheduled payment reduction for physicians and other practitioners who treat Medicare patients from taking effect on April 1, 2014.

Performance management A forward-looking process that is used to set goals and regularly check progress toward achieving those goals.

Performance measurement   A process by which a healthcare organization monitors important aspects of its programs, systems, and processes.

Psychrometer   An instrument used to measure relative humidity.

Pulse height analyzer (PHA)   A device that accepts or rejects electronic pulses according to their amplitude or energy.

Qualitative data   Data that approximates and characterizes. Qualitative data can be observed and recorded. This data type is non-numerical.

Quality assessment   the data collection and analysis through which the degree of conformity to predetermined standards and criteria are exemplified.

Quality assurance   An all-encompassing management program used to ensure excellence.

Quality control   The part of the quality assurance program that deals with techniques used in monitoring and maintenance of technical systems.

Quality improvement team   A group of individuals who are responsible for implementing the solutions that were derived by a focus group.

Quality of Care   The data collection and analysis through which the degree of conformity to predetermined standards and criteria are exemplified.

Quantitive data   The value of data in the form of counts or numbers where each data set has a unique numerical value.

Quantum mottle   Image noise caused by statistical fluctuations in the number of photons creating the image.

Radiation Exposure Monitoring (REM) Integration Profile   Specifies how details of radiation exposure resulting from imaging procedures are exchanged among the imaging systems, local dose information management systems, and cross-institutional systems such as dose registries.

Radionuclide impurity   The presence of other substance(s) in the radiopharmaceutical for nuclear medicine procedures.

RAID   Redundant array of inexpensive disks, a computer storage medium with rapid image access time and fault tolerance.

Range   The difference between the highest and lowest values, and is a measure of the dispersion of the data distribution.

Receiver operator characteristic (ROC)   A curve that plots the true-positive fraction versus the false-positive fraction and is used to evaluate imaging performance.

Reciprocity   The amount of x-ray intensity should remain constant at a specific milliampere-second value despite the milliampere and time combination.

Recirculating electrolytic   A type of electrolytic silver recovery device that recirculates fixer back into the processor after silver reclamation.

Rectification   The process of converting an alternating current (AC) into a direct current (DC).

Refresh rate   This refers to how many times each second that a video or computer monitor rewrites or updates the image on the display (also known as the frame rate or vertical scan frequency) of the monitor.

Region of interest (ROI)   A specified region of the image selected for display or analysis.

Reject or Repeat analysis   A systematic process of cataloging rejected images and determining the nature of the rejects.

Regulation   Standards written into local, state, or federal law that are employed in controlling, directing, or managing an activity, organization, or system.

Relative conversion factor   Measures the amount of light produced by the output phosphor per unit of x-radiation incident on the input phosphor.

Relative speed   A relative number indicating the speed of an intensifying screen imaging system.

Reliability   The accuracy, dependability, or validity of the data that has been collected.

Repeat analysis   A data collection of repeat images to determine the cause of the repeats so that they may be prevented in the future.

Reproducibility   The same technique setting should always create the same exposure rate at any time.

Resonance frequency   (1) The frequency for which the response of a transducer to an ultrasound beam is a maximum. (2) In magnetic resonance imaging, the frequency at which a nucleus absorbs radio energy when placed in a magnetic field.

Reticulation marks   Network of fine grooves on film-based x-ray images caused by uneven solution temperatures.

Risk   The likelihood and severity of hazardous events.

Risk management   The ability to identify potential risks to patients, employees, and visitors to the healthcare institution and institute processes that minimize these risks.

Root cause analysis (RCA)   A system to identify the root causes of faults or problems within the process.

Roentgen   The special unit of radiation exposure or intensity.

S distortion   An artifact that can occur in image intensifier tubes consisting of a warping of the image along an S-shaped axis.

Safelight   A light source that does not fog film.

Safe Medical Devices Act (SMDA)   Legislation of 1991 that requires a medical facility to report to the Food and Drug Administration any medical devices that have caused a serious injury or death of a patient (e.g., malfunctioning bed, nonworking defibrillator, nonworking pacemaker, malfunctioning radiation therapy unit) or employee. It also authorizes civil penalties to be imposed on healthcare workers or facilities that do not report defects and failures in medical devices.

Safety   The freedom from the occurrence or risk of injury, danger, or loss

Sample   The number of items that are actually measured from a population.

Saturation   Occurs when a CR image plate receives more than a 500% overexposure to x-rays. This results in the image appearing black despite all postprocessing attempts to brighten the image.

Scan image uniformity   The uniformity in brightness of an image created with a homogenous phantom.

Scatter plot   A graph that demonstrates a possible correlation between two variables.

Scheduled workflow integration profile   This profile establishes the continuity and integrity of basic departmental imaging data.

Scintillation crystal   A sodium iodide crystal used in scintillation detectors.

Scintillation detector   A radiation detector consisting of a sodium iodide crystal coupled to a photomultiplier tube.

Scintillation gamma camera   The most commonly used imaging device in nuclear medicine.

Scrap exposed film   Exposed and processed film that is not of diagnostic use and is disposed of for silver recovery.

Screen speed   The amount of light that is emitted from an intensifying screen for a given amount of x-ray exposure.

Semiannual tests   Quality control tests that are performed every six months.

Sensitivity   Indicates the likelihood of obtaining a positive diagnosis in a patient with the disease.

Sensitometer   An electrical device that exposes the film to a premeasured light source for quality control purposes.

Sensitometry   The study of the relationship between the amount of radiation exposing a film and the optical density that is produced.

Sensor   The radiation detector assembly in an automatic exposure control system.

Sentinel event indicator   An individual event or phenomenon that is significant enough to trigger further review each time it occurs.

Serious adverse event   An adverse event that may significantly compromise clinical outcomes or an adverse event for which a facility fails to take appropriate corrective action in a timely manner.

Serious complaint   A report of a serious adverse event.

Signal-to-noise ratio (SNR)   Used to describe the relative contributions to a detected signal of the true signal and random superimposed signals or noise.

Single-phase   A type of x-ray generator with a single source of alternating current.

Single-photon emission computerized tomography (SPECT)   A nuclear medicine procedure that creates cross-sectional images.

Six sigma   A management strategy that seeks to identify and remove the causes of errors in business processes.

Slice position accuracy   The relative position of the image section and the patient.

Slice thickness The thickness of the image section.

Solarization A decrease in optical density with an increase in exposure. Also known as *image reversal*.

Solid-state detector A radiation detector with silicon or germanium crystals.

Spatial linearity The ability of a gamma camera system to produce a linear image with straight lines corresponding to the same straight lines of the bar pattern or the amount of geometric distortion in the image as affected by the homogeneity of the main magnetic field and the linearity of the magnetic field gradients.

Spatial resolution The ability of an imaging process to distinguish small, adjacent, high-contrast structures in the object.

Special procedures laboratory Fluoroscopic room where diagnostic and interventional procedures are performed.

Specificity Indicates the likelihood of a patient obtaining a negative diagnosis when no disease is present.

Spectral matching The matching of film sensitivity with the color of light emitted by the intensifying screen.

Spectrum A display of electromagnetic energy on the basis of wavelength and frequency.

Specular reflection A type of reflection coming from the surface of an electronic display that produces a mirror image of the light source creating it.

Speed indicator The step closest to one above the base + fog on a sensitometric test film.

Standard Something established as a measure or model to which other similar things should conform

Standard deviation The amount of variance in a sample.

Standardized uptake value (SUV) A measure of the rate and/or total amount of FDG accumulation in tumors during PET scanning.

Static electricity Electrical charges created by friction, which can cause artifacts on unprocessed film.

Steradian The unit of solid angle in the International System of Units (SI)

String test A quality control test for Doppler ultrasound equipment.

Sulfurization A buildup of sulfur on the electrodes in an electrolytic silver recovery unit as a result of incorrect amperage setting.

Supplier One who provides goods or services.

SWOT analysis Analysis tool that allows assessment of strengths, weaknesses, opportunities and threats.

Synergism The action of two agents working together is greater than the sum of the action of the agents working independently.

System A group of related processes.

Transmit gain The amount of amplification used in sending a signal (MRI or ultrasound) into the patient.

Target composition Refers to the elemental composition of the x-ray tube anode.

Target Exposure Index (EI$_t$) The target reference exposure that is obtained when the image receptor is properly exposed, and will differ for each body part and projection.

Technetium-99m The isotope of technetium whose primary gamma ray has an energy of 140 kiloelectron volts.

Technetium pertechnetate A radionuclide used in nuclear medicine procedures that consists of technetium-99m.

Temperature A measure of the average kinetic energy in atoms and molecules of matter.

Terminal electrolytic An electrolytic silver recovery device in which the used fixer is removed for disposal.

The Joint Commission (TJC) A private agency (formerly known as JCAHO) responsible for accreditation of healthcare systems.

Thin-film transistor (TFT) Switches for each pixel of an array connected to circuitry that allows all switches in a row of the array to be operated simultaneously.

Thread test Evaluates how the PACS passes data from module to module to ensure that they link up appropriately.

Three-phase An alternating-current power source made up of three single-phase currents that are staggered by 120°.

Threshold A preestablished level of performance applied to a specific indicator.

Time of day variability A possible variable in sensitometric testing in which test films are processed at different times during the day, varying in optical density.

Tissue equalization Image processing that compensates for varying breast tissue densities so that the entire breast (from the chest wall to the skin line) can be visualized in a single image.

Thermoluminescent dosimeter (TLD) A type of radiation detector with crystals such as lithium fluoride that release light when heated that is proportional to the amount of incident radiation.

Tomography A radiographic process whereby specific slices of the body are imaged.

Tomosynthesis An image option available with some DR systems that requires multiple images from many angles to generate tomographic slices that can eliminate overlapping structures. Playback of the sequence of slices is via a cine loop, similar to that used in CT imaging.

Transmitted light The amount of viewbox light that is transmitted through a film image.

Trending To show a general tendency.

Trend chart A graph that pictorially demonstrates whether key indicators are moving up or down over a given period. Also called a *run chart*.

Troy ounce A unit of weight used for precious metals such as silver; 14.58 troy ounces = 16 standard ounces.

Ultraviolet radiation A type of electromagnetic radiation in between visible light and x-rays.

Uniformity correction flood A quality control procedure for nuclear medicine equipment.

Validity Establishes the existence and strength of the co-variation between the cause and effect variables

Variance A numeric representation of the dispersion of data around the mean in a given sample.

Variation A change or slight difference in a level, amount, or quantity

Veiling glare Glare caused by light being reflected from the window of the output phosphor in an image intensifier. Also known as *flare*.

Ventilation The process by which air is changed into and out of a specific area.

Vertical distance measurement A quality control test variable for ultrasound equipment measuring along the sound beam axis. Also known as *depth calibration accuracy*.

Vidicon A type of television camera tube.

Viewbox illuminator An electronic device for viewing transparency images such as radiographs.

Vignetting A decrease in brightness toward the periphery of a fluoroscopic image when using an image intensifier tube.

Visibility of detail How well anatomic structures are visible in diagnostic imaging.

Voltage ripple The variation from the peak voltage through the x-ray tube in an x-ray generator.

Volume coil percent image uniformity A method of MR image uniformity analysis

Volume replenishment A type of system in an automatic processor that replenishes a volume of solution for each film introduced.

Weekly testing Quality control testing performed on a weekly basis.

Window level A value in digital imaging that selects the level of the displayed band of values within the complete range.

Window leveling A manipulation of the dynamic range, allowing for the selection of more or less shades of gray to enhance image contrast.

Window width A value in digital imaging that selects the width of the band of values in the digital signal that can be represented as gray tones in the image.

Workflow Encompasses a few actions which include ordering, scheduling, imaging acquisition, storage and viewing activities associated with radiology exams.

Workstation Functionality Test Test on PACS to ensure each function is available.

INDEX

Note: Page number followed by *f*, *t* and *b* indicates figure, table and box respectively.